AF615378

Reflections on Pharmacy
by the Remington Medalists
1919–2003

■

SECOND EDITION OF
THE REMINGTON LECTURES (1994)

■

George Griffenhagen, Senior Editor
Grover C. Bowles, Jr., Co-Editor
Richard P. Penna, Co-Editor
Dennis B. Worthen, Co-Editor

2004
American Pharmacists Association
2215 Constitution Avenue, N.W.
Washington, D.C.

Published by the American Pharmacists Association, 2215 Constitution Avenue, N.W., Washington, D.C., 20037-2985.

Book Design by Mac Designs, Oak Hill, Virginia
Printed by United Book Press

Publication supported by a grant from Aventis Pharmaceuticals

Printed in the United States of America
ISBN #1-58212-070-6

Library of Congress Cataloging-in-Publication Data
Reflections on pharmacy by the Remington medalists 1919-2003; the Remington lectures (1994)/George Griffenhagen, senior editor ... [et al.].--2nd ed.
p.cm.
Includes index.
ISBN 1-58212-070-6
1. Pharmacy--United states--History. 2. Pharmacy--Awards--United States. I. Griffenhagen, George B.

RS67.U6R44 2004
615'.1'0973--dc22

2003063899

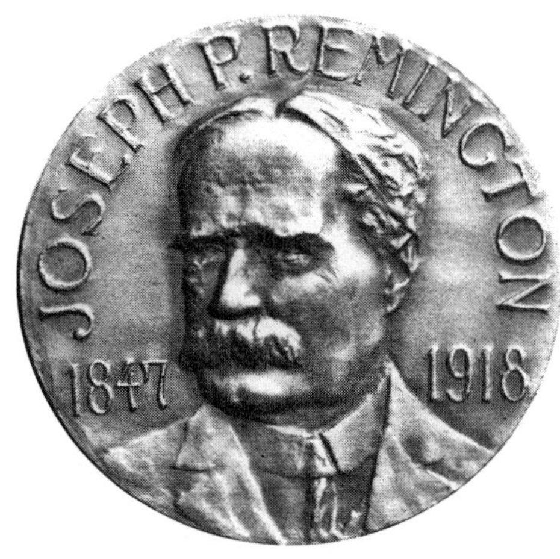

Joseph Price Remington
(1847-1918)

Joseph Price Remington was born into a Philadelphia Quaker family on March 26, 1847. His father, Isaac Remington, was a well-known physician. His mother, Lydia Hart, was a descendant of Townsend Speakman, an 18th century Philadelphia apothecary. Joseph exhibited an early interest in science, even to the point of equipping "a chemical laboratory in which most of the apparatus was of his own devising and construction." His family planned that he would enter college and take an academic degree, but this hope had to be abandoned when his father died in 1862.

One of Joseph's older sisters married Henry M. Troth, whose father was a founder of the Philadelphia College of Pharmacy. Troth guided Remington to the pharmacy of Charles Ellis, Son & Company to serve his apprenticeship during the years 1863-1866. This fortunate arrangement placed the young Remington under the tutelage of one of the most influential pharmacists in Philadelphia. Remington's experience with Ellis was very broad since the store manufactured medicines on a broad scale as well as serving its retail clientele. Ellis encouraged Remington to attend lectures at the Philadelphia College of Pharmacy during his apprenticeship. Lectures were held in the evenings; the course normally took two years to complete. Remington graduated with a Ph.G. in 1866.

In 1867 Remington joined Edward Robinson Squibb in the latter's Brooklyn-based pharmaceutical and chemical manufacturing company. Remington's first task was to sweep the basement. However, he was soon learning how to make ether and assay cinchona bark. Squibb also had Remington help in experiments on carbolic acid. Joseph W. England identified Squibb as "probably the most painstaking and conscientious manufacturing pharmacist of the country." Squibb detested dishonesty. He believed in sharing the results of his research and disdained secrecy, refusing to patent any of his discoveries. Remington lived with the Squibb family and remained with the firm for three years. Later Remington spoke of this period as one of the most decisively influential of his life.

Remington returned to Philadelphia when his mother died. Once there he continued to pursue his interest in pharmaceutical manufacturing and took a position in 1870 with Powers and Weightman, one of the first American manufacturers of quinine. While employed there, he also accepted an appointment as an assistant to Edward Parrish, the professor of pharmacy at the Philadelphia College of Pharmacy. After Parrish died in 1872, William Procter, Jr., returned to the position of professor of pharmacy and retained the young Remington as his assistant. In 1872 Remington bought a drug store in Philadelphia, which he retained for 13 years. This experience deepened his understanding of the profession, in particular, the need to organize pharmacists and provide them information on an ongoing basis.

In 1874 Remington married Elizabeth Baily Collins, another Philadelphian raised in the Quaker tradition. The couple had five children: Arthur Hart, Joseph Percy, William Procter, Anna Collins, and Elizabeth Baily.

When Procter died in 1874, Remington was elected to the position of professor of pharmacy, a position he would hold until his death 44 years later. Remington was an early and strong advocate of laboratory instruction for pharmacy students. In 1877 he helped establish a pharmaceutical laboratory at the College, which he furnished, in part, with his own funds. In 1893 he succeeded John M. Maisch as the dean of the College.

Remington was remembered as a master teacher and a friend to students by the thousands who graduated from the College during his decades of service. However, his greatest accolade might well have been the recognition that he was the teacher of teachers for, as one eulogist wrote, "most of the successful teachers of pharmacy in America to-day have been pupils of his at some time in their careers." Many among the alumni, including Charles La Wall, E. Fullerton Cook, Ivor Griffith, Henry V. Arny, and Eugene Eberle, went on to distinguished careers in pharmacy education; all are Reminton medalists.

Remington embodied the role of professor in its broadest sense. In addition to the daily routine of teaching at the Philadelphia College of Pharmacy, he was an influential writer and editor. In 1879, after the death of George B. Wood, one of the founders of the *United States Dispensatory*, Remington was invited to become an associate editor, a post he retained for the rest of his life. The first edition of Remington's *Practice of Pharmacy* was published in 1885. In the textbook, Remington combined his practical experience with an understanding of the needs of both students and practitioners.

Joseph Price Remington was an untiring leader in professional organizations. He joined the American Pharmaceutical Association in 1867 and served in many Association offices during his 50 years of membership. Among his most noteworthy accomplishments was the creation of the APhA Council (now the Board of Trustees). At the 1879 APhA meeting, Remington noted that a great deal of time was expended dealing with necessary but trivial matters. He suggested establishing a Council that would work with the permanent secretary to transact the business of the Association between the annual meetings. In 1887 Remington suggested the plan to organize the association membership into three sections - one for scientific papers, one for education and legislation, and the last for commercial interests. APhA frequently appointed him as its representative to the American Medical Association. This working relationship led to the creation of a Section on Materia Medica and Pharmacy (later renamed the Section of Pharmacology and Therapeutics) within AMA. Remington served as president of APhA in 1892-1893.

Another of Remington's great professional legacies was his work and leadership on the *United States Pharmacopeia (USP)*. His first connection with the *USP* was in 1877, when he was appointed by the College to serve on the Auxiliary Committee of Revision. The excellence of his work led to his leadership role in the 1880 and 1890 *USP* revisions. In 1900 Remington was elected vice-chairman of the Committee of Revision. When committee chair Charles Rice died in 1901, Remington was elected to that post, which he retained until his own death.

Speaking of his old professor when he received the Remington Medal in 1931, E. Fullerton Cook noted that "the master passion of his life was his pride in pharmacy and his confidence in its future. He gave to its development all of his own great powers and cooperated with every sane movement of his day which promised the advancement of the art and science he loved."

Joseph Price Remington left an indelible mark on his beloved profession of pharmacy. His impact as an educator went beyond the classroom, and his voice continues to be heard by generations of pharmacists, for whom his publications are an integral part of professional formation and practice. "His power to organize other men and get them to work together in harmony" is remembered in the highest award in professional pharmacy -- the Remington Medal.

This biography is based on the "Heroes of Pharmacy" essay on Joseph Price Remington by Dennis B. Worthen published in the *Journal of the American Pharmaceutical Association* (2002; 42: 664-666) and is used with permission. See also numerous recollections of Remington medalists in this volume.

Acknowledgements & Recognition

The American Pharmacists Association gratefully recognizes the support provided by Aventis Pharmaceuticals for the publication of *Reflections on Pharmacy by the Remington Medalists 1919-2003,* the second edition of *The Remington Lectures* published in 1994.

APhA also pays tribute to John Uri Lloyd, the 1920 Remington Medalist, who founded Lloyd Brothers, which eventually became Aventis Pharmaceuticals.

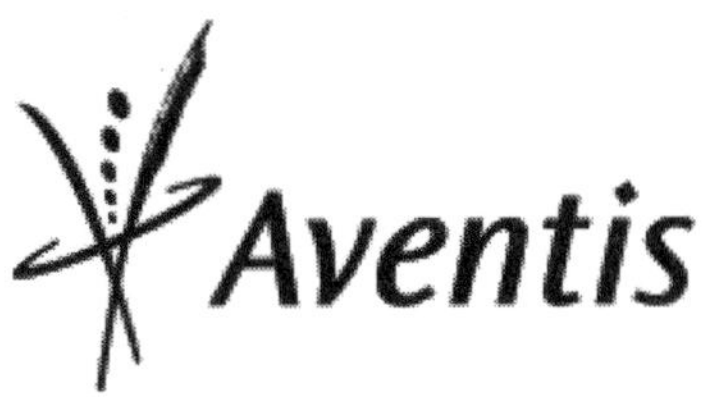

Table of Contents

Remington Medalists

Alphabetical Listing

INTRODUCTION

"While not all Remington addresses were masterpieces, many represent the considered thinking of some of pharmacy's best minds at the time and even today make interesting reading."

This is how Grover Bowles introduced the concept of using the Remington lectures to record the evolution of American pharmacy. Shortly thereafter, William Blockstein and David Krigstein jointly proposed publishing all Remington addresses in a single volume. When Blockstein and Krigstein learned that APhA was considering such a project in 1985, they offered assistance that would result in what they called a "finely produced, scholarly prepared, and appropriately edited volume - the Remington Lectures that all in pharmacy could receive with pride and satisfaction." But the project lay dormant until 1990 when newly elected APhA executive vice president, John A. Gans, solicited support from a number of pharmaceutical manufacturers who had one or more employees or executives that had been named a Remington medalist. Funds were subsequently pledged, and George Griffenhagen was assigned as senior editor, with William Blockstein and David Krigstein as co-editors. The first edition of *The Remington Lectures* was published in 1994 with a sub-title of *A Century in American Pharmacy.*

Almost immediately after publication of the first edition, it was decided that a second edition would follow in about ten years incorporating the lectures of the Remington medalists from 1994 to 2003; updating the biographical sketches contained in the first edition; and including a new Subject Index. Since the two co-editors of the first edition had died, senior editor George Griffenhagen has been joined by three co-editors: Grover C. Bowles, Richard P. Penna, and Dennis B. Worthen.

This second volume is dedicated to the previous co-editors: William Leonard Blockstein (1925-1995) and David Jacob Krigstein (1924-2003). The title of this second volume has also been revised to make it clear that they are not lectures by Joseph P. Remington. Hence the new title is *Reflections on Pharmacy by the Remington Medalists 1919-2003.*

No attempt was made in the first edition to provide extended biographical data for Joseph Price Remington, the man whom Kremers and Urdang's *History of Pharmacy* calls "one of the most versatile and influential American pharmacists of his time." However we have included in this second edition a modification of the Remington article in the "Heroes of Pharmacy" series by Dennis B. Worthen that was published in the *Journal of the American Pharmaceutical Association*, volume 42, pp. 664-666, 2002. In addition, it should be noted that many of the early Remington lectures provide first hand accounts of the medalist's relationship with Remington. Especially noteworthy are the anecdotes told by the 1931 Remington Medalist, E. Fullerton Cook, who served for many years as Remington's assistant.

Origin and Evolution

Brooklyn, New York, pharmacist, pharmaceutical educator, and long-time APhA treasurer, Hugo H. Schaefer, recommended at the March 11, 1918, meeting of the APhA New York Branch, the creation of:

> "A gold medallion suitably named [to] be awarded annually to the man or woman who has done most for American Pharmacy during the proceeding year, or whose efforts during a number of years have culminated to a point during the preceding year where

the results of these efforts would be considered as being the most important and advantageous for American Pharmacy."

Schaefer further suggested that "the medal be awarded by a standing committee of all past presidents of the American Pharmaceutical Association," and "the New York Branch devote one meeting annually to the presentation of this medal." This proposal was adopted, and a committee was appointed to further study the proposal. On April 8, 1918, the APhA New York Branch approved the recommendation that "the committee be empowered to obtain the moral support and consent of the Parent Organization, and take steps towards raising a $1,000.00 fund."

When the request was submitted to the APhA Council [now Board of Trustees}, it included the first reference to the fact that the New York Branch had decided to call the award the "Joseph P. Remington Medal in honor of Joseph Price Remington who had died on January 2, 1918." The submission further noted that "a fund of $1,000.00 would be raised commencing with a $200.00 contribution from the New York Branch, and the remainder would be made up by voluntary contributions from the members and firms in New York City and vicinity... to be invested in Liberty Bonds held in trust by the APhA Treasurer."

The APhA Council discussion included comments on the actual presentation, which it assumed "would probably be held during the winter months in New York [City], bringing many representative members of APhA from various parts of the country and would, in a way, establish a kind of mid-winter [APhA] meeting." The motion was subsequently approved by the APhA Council on June 4, 1918.

Hugo Schaefer then presented a detailed procedure for the selection of the Remington Honor Medalist at the September 1918 meeting of the APhA New York Branch which included the following provisions:

"Each living former president of the APhA shall be requested by the Secretary [of the Committee] to present before February 1st of each year the names of not more than three personages whom he deems worthy of the distinction.

"The Secretary shall promptly submit these names to the Committee for a vote by mail. The three names receiving the highest number of votes shall then be considered as candidates or nominees for the award.

"The Secretary shall then send a ballot containing the names of the nominees so chosen to each member of the Committee, and the ballots must be returned within fifteen days. The person receiving a majority of the votes shall be declared the recipient of the award."

Not everyone was happy with this procedure, and several alternatives were proposed. One proposal would have the presidents of APhA, AACP, and NABP each designate two persons to a nominating committee who shall select three candidates to be submitted for final selection to all APhA past presidents. Another proposal would have "the three junior APhA past presidents receive suggestions and then select and submit three nominees to all APhA past presidents for the final selection." But Henry M. Whelpley pointed out that either plan could result in "the ex-presidents of APhA having to elect for the Honor Medal one of three, no matter how large a proportion of the ex-presidents should favor one not on the list of three candidates."

Thus it was decided that all APhA past presidents would both nominate as well as select the Remington Medalist from all candidates nominated." Funding also remained a problem, as reported by Hugo Schaefer at the January 13, 1919, meeting of the New York Branch, but APhA Treasurer Henry M. Whelpley reported on August 15, 1919, that the Joseph Remington Fund now exceeded the goal of $1,000.00.

Even though it was proposed that the first Remington Medal would be awarded at a special April 1919 meeting of the APhA New York Branch, the first award was presented to James Hartley Beal on August 26, 1919, at the first general session of the 67th APhA annual meeting held in New York City. The second Remington Medal was presented to John Uri Lloyd at a special meeting of the APhA New York Branch convened on April 19, 1920, at the Hotel Pennsylvania in New York City. It was reported that "nearly one hundred guests assembled in one of the beautiful and spacious banquet rooms of the hotel; there were present representatives of all national pharmaceutical associations and several state associations, and a number of pharmacy schools and universities."

The selection process ran into its first problem in 1921 when there was a tie between George Beringer and Henry Arny with one remaining APhA past president refusing to cast the tie-breaking vote. It was suggested that two medals be awarded, but the final decision was not to make any award in 1921. Arny was subsequently selected for the 1922 award, and Beringer received the 1924 award.

In most instances, the presentation ceremonies took place at a dinner, and from 1920 to 1972 they were held mainly in New York City, usually at the Hotel Pennsylvania or the Roosevelt Hotel. The 1924 Remington Dinner was held at the Robert Trent Hotel in Newark, New Jersey, for George Beringer, but was hosted exclusively by the APhA New York Branch. The 1932 dinner for Eugene Eberle was held at the Hotel Emerson in Baltimore, Maryland, hosted by both the New York and Baltimore APhA Branches, while the 1935 dinner for Samuel Hilton was held at the Mayflower Hotel in Washington, D.C., in cooperation with the District of Columbia Pharmaceutical Association.

In addition to the first Remington Honor Medal, which was presented at the 1919 APhA annual meeting in New York City, the 1930 and the 1934 Remington Medals were presented at APhA annual meetings. The 1930 Remington Medalist (Edward Kremers) received his medal at the Hotel Emerson in Baltimore, Maryland, during the APhA annual meeting banquet, while the 1934 Remington Medalist (Henry Wellcome) received his medal at the Shoreham Hotel in Washington, D.C., during the 82nd APhA annual meeting. Two presentations were made posthumously without dinners (1948 at the University of Maryland in Baltimore to Andrew DuMez, and 1950 at Columbia University in New York City to Edwin Newcomb). Both medalists died after they were selected but before a Remington Dinner could be held.

Attendance at Remington Dinners in New York City varied from year to year with more than 550 attending the 1943 function honoring Robert P. Fischelis, and with an all-time record attendance of "more than 900" attending the 1951 dinner honoring Hugo H. Schaefer - a most fitting tribute to the man who conceived this award. After 1951, attendance started to drop to an average of 200 persons, and it was decided to regularly hold the Remington Dinner as a separate function at each APhA annual meeting commencing in 1974. At this point the "1973 Medalist" received his award at the 1974 Remington Dinner, continuing through the 1979 Remington Dinner which honored the "1978 Medalist."

In 1977, Arthur G. Zupko, then chairman of the Remington Medal Committee, announced "a new procedure to select candidates for the Remington Medal" which "will insure a broader input from all facets of the profession." Accordingly, all pharmacists were invited to submit nominees. A committee was established by the APhA New York Chapter to screen the larger number of nominations, and only three nominees were submitted to all living APhA past presidents for final selection. But several APhA past presidents expressed dissatisfaction with this screening process, claiming that "the past presidents no longer select the recipient of their choice, and the prestige of the Remington Medal will be best preserved by returning to the original procedure when the award was established." [We are reminded of similar concerns expressed in 1919 when the original nomination and selection process was established.]

APhA Assumes Responsibility

On May 31, 1979, the APhA Board of Canvassers certified the vote by which APhA active members revised the APhA Bylaws terminating authorization for APhA Branches [which were then called Chapters]. The APhA Board of Trustees voted on June 1, 1979, to retain the Remington Honor Medal "as an APhA Award in light of the termination of the APhA New York Chapter." The APhA Trustees further authorized "a five-member committee to review the entire selection procedure, as well as the arrangements surrounding the award ceremony, and to offer appropriate recommendations to the Board for the future operation of this activity."

The committee, consisting of Andrew Bartilucci, Robert C. Johnson, David Krigstein, Irving Rubin, and John J. Sciarra, recommended to the APhA Board of Trustees on October 9, 1979:

> "1. The Remington Honor Medal should be continued in a manner which retains the high prestige [in] which it has been [held] since its inception in 1918.
>
> "2. The APhA Board of Trustees chairman should annually appoint a Remington Honor Medal Selection Committee of seven persons including a chairman to solicit and screen the nominations for this Award. The Selection Committee should include substantial representation from those who were actively involved in this activity when the Remington Honor Medal was sponsored by the former New York APhA Chapter. Nominations should be encouraged from anyone, except that no self-nominations should be accepted. The Committee will select and submit no fewer than three candidates, and no more than six candidates, to the APhA Board of Trustees which should develop its own procedure for making the final selection.
>
> "3. The presentation of the Remington Honor Medal should be made at the APhA Annual Meeting opening general session with the participation of a representative of the former New York APhA Chapter. The Remington medalist should be given up to ten minutes to present a response. A printed program should be developed and printed for distribution which includes a brief history of the Medal, a list of all previous recipients, and a current biographical sketch and portrait photograph of the medalist to be honored. APhA should sponsor a reception in honor of the medalist to be held prior to or following the presentation, and should include family members and close personal friends of the recipient, past Remington medalists, APhA past presidents, the APhA Board of Trustees, and members of the Selection Committee."

The APhA Board of Trustees accepted these recommendations at their October 15-16, 1979, meeting, but then at their January 21-22, 1980, meeting, the Board decided that only three nominations are to be submitted to APhA past presidents for the final selection. The selection process preceded without complications for the 1980 recipient (Joseph Williams), but none of the three 1981 nominees received a majority of votes cast leaving the Board to declare that there would be no 1981 Remington Medalist [a situation which had been previously encountered in 1921, 1927, 1939, 1946, 1954, 1961, 1966, 1968, and 1973].

Despite the fact that new written criteria were developed in July 1981 for the selection of the Remington medalist - "the names of the two nominees receiving the highest number of votes shall be resubmitted to APhA past presidents on a second ballot" - a deadlock resulted in 1982. Then on July 8-9, 1982, the APhA Board of Trustees modified the charge to the Screening Committee to select two nominees for submission to the APhA past presidents, and agreed that "if a tie vote were to result, the two candidates would be resubmitted to the APhA past presidents for a re-vote in hopes that the tie could be broken."

Since 1983, the Remington Honor Medal has been awarded annually, but several past Remington medalists raised concern over the changes in presentation. One past Remington medalist wrote: "It grieves me that we no longer have the awards dinner followed by the address of the recipient. Presentation of the medal at the APhA opening exercises is impressive, but there is so little time for the recipient to respond." In 1986, a Remington Honor Medal Luncheon was instituted at the APhA annual meeting, which provided the Remington medalist an opportunity to make additional remarks following the presentation at the APhA annual meeting opening session. In 1991, the Remington Honor Medal Dinner was re-established, and once again Remington medalists were provided a forum for expanding their remarks following brief five-minute remarks at the APhA annual meeting opening session.

In 1991, the APhA Board of Trustees expanded the Screening Committee to 13 members by inviting all national organizations represented in the APhA House of Delegates to recommend one committee member. The 1992-1993 APhA Honors Advisory Committee recommended at their November 14, 1992, meeting that "final selection of two candidates by the Screening Committee should be conducted by telephonic conference call rather than by mail ballot."

In 1997 a two step screening process was introduced: Preliminary screening by mail ballot selecting "a total of one more than half of the number of nominations received. The final screening was made by telephone conference selecting the top two candidates. If the top two candidates cannot be determined, a second vote of the screening committee would be conducted. If no two candidates are selected, the Chairman of the screening committee shall vote to break the tie which shall be final. The APhA past presidents still make final selection; in the event of a tie, a second ballot is sent to the past presidents. If there is still a tie, the current APhA president will break tie.

A new problem surfaced in 2002 when Varro Tyler died after being selected by the Screening Committee as one of two candidates, but before these two candidates were submitted to APhA past presidents for the final selection of the Remington medalist. This led to a clarification of the rules that the Remington medal could not be presented posthumously. In addition, one or more past recipients of the Remington medal were added to the Screening Committee to provide some background on the history of the Remington medal.

Finally another layer for the screening process was established at the June 15-17, 2003, meeting of the APhA Board of Trustees. A new Remington Honor Medal Review Committee (consisting of eight members of the Nominations Committee that was previously called the Screening Committee) selects those candidates that "best meet the criteria established for the Remington Honor Medal" with the "number of candidates selected to be one more than one-half of the number of nominations received." The recommendation of the Review Committee is then forwarded to the Remington Honor Medal Nominations Committee to select the top two candidates by a telephone conference call. Should there be a tie after two votes, the chairman of the Nominations Committee votes to break the tie. The top two candidates are then forwarded to all APhA past presidents who will select the recipient of the award. In the event of a tie after two votes, the current APhA president votes to break the tie.

Sources of Remington Lectures

The process of locating the original texts for all Remington lectures commenced in 1991. It was soon discovered that not all of the Remington lectures were published in the *Journal of the American Pharmaceutical Association* or in *American Pharmacy*. However, further research revealed that additional lectures were published in other pharmacy journals. Of the remaining unpublished lectures, original manuscripts or tape recordings were located for most of the Remington lectures. For the remainder of the Remington medalists, alternate manuscripts were selected. For example, when we were unable to locate the Remington lecture of Henry Rusby, we selected a lecture which he made to the American Conference of Pharmaceutical Faculties presented three months prior to his Remington lecture representing "the explorations of the medalist, if not the actual content of the Remington lecture." Only in one instance we were unable to locate a suitable alternate lecture for Takeru Higuchi, and so we selected an editorial from the *Journal of Pharmaceutical Sciences* which was devoted in its entirety to scientific papers authored by some of Higuchi's more than 200 students and research associates, and published at the time of Higuchi receiving the Remington Honor Medal.

In one instance, what appeared to be an original Remington lecture was located at the Wisconsin State Historical Society, along with extensive background correspondence. Edward Kremers was notified that he had been selected as the 1930 Remington medalist, but Kremers refused to accept it, expressing the belief that "Professor [E. Fullerton] Cook has withdrawn his name in my favor. I cannot accept this sacrifice on his part." Even after being assured by various APhA past presidents and members of the Screening Committee that this was not the case, Kremers wrote, "I cannot alter my decision." Hugo Schaefer then sent an April 24, 1930, Western Union telegram to Kremers reading: "Decision of Committee is irrevocable. Your name will enter [the] records as 1930 medalist. Medal now being engraved and press notices have been sent out." Kremers responded by telegram: "Kindly cancel formal presentation," to which APhA president H. A. B. Dunning and APhA secretary Evander F. Kelly jointly dispatched an April 28 telegram: "Deeply regret request to cancel presentation. Arrangements made and announced for presentation at banquet Tuesday May 6th. Very embarrassing and difficult to change arrangements now. We urge your consent for simple presentation." Kremers subsequently attended the Baltimore meeting and received the 1930 Remington medal at the APhA annual meeting banquet. But upon closer examination of the "acceptance remarks" which had been uncovered in Wisconsin, it was discovered that they were described by Kremers with the following handwritten note: "Thoughts penned previous to the award at Baltimore...That I did not make use of the manuscript has already become apparent." A story appearing in the *New York Times* for May 6, 1930, indicates that Kremers, "winner of the Remington medal, deplored commercialization of the drug store in an address to the Teachers Conference on Pharmaceutical Economics." The alternate lecture included in this volume was presented at the University of Maryland School of Pharmacy four days after the Remington medal presentation, and it captures Kremers' views of the reform in American pharmaceutical education.

Great care has been exercised in retaining the original terminology of all lectures contained herein - even though we would have liked to professionalize such terms as "drugstore" and "druggist," which were commonly used until after World War II. Since every Remington lecture did not have a title, we have assigned a title to those lectures without a title so as to maintain consistency and to provide the user of this volume with some idea of the content of each lecture. It should be obvious that some of the lectures appearing in this volume are expanded versions of the actual Remington address, even though in the 1920s and 1930s, a Remington lecture took over an hour for delivery.

Profile of Remington Medalists

Who are these Remington Medalists? All but five of the 75 Remington medalists from 1919 to 2003 were born in the U.S.A.; the foreign-born medalists were Ko Kuei Chen from China, Peter Paul Lamy from

Germany, Ivor Griffith from Great Britain, and both J. Leon Lascoff and Joseph Rosin from Russia. Twelve medalists were born in Pennsylvania; six were born in Wisconsin; five each in New York and Ohio; four each in Indiana, Michigan, and New Jersey; three each in California, Delaware, Minnesota, and the District of Columbia; two each in Iowa and Massachusetts; and one each in Connecticut, Maryland, Missouri, North Carolina, North Dakota, Oregon, Virginia, Washington, and West Virginia.

Fifteen medalists obtained their first pharmacy degree from the Philadelphia College of Pharmacy and Science, while four obtained their first degree from the University of Wisconsin. Three obtained their first pharmacy degree from the University of California and the Chicago College of Pharmacy / University of Illinois. Two each obtained their first pharmacy degree from George Washington University, Massachusetts College of Pharmacy, Purdue University, Scio (Ohio) College of Pharmacy, the University of Maryland, the University of Michigan, the University of Nebraska, the University of Pittsburgh, and Wayne State University. The remainder were graduates of 24 other universities.

Twenty-eight of the Remington medalists served as APhA president, ten as APhA honorary president, five as APhA chief executive officer, and four as APhA professional staff members. Twenty-four served as president or secretary of their state pharmaceutical association, and another 19 served as dean of a college of pharmacy. Fourteen served as president or executive director of the American Association of Colleges of Pharmacy, while six served as either president or secretary of the National Association of Boards of Pharmacy. Three served as either president or chief executive officer of the American Society of Health System Pharmacists, and three served as president of the American College of Apothecaries. Three women Remington medalists are Gloria Niemeyer Francke in 1987, Linda Mae Strand in 1997, and Mary Louise Andersen in 2003.

It is hazardous to quantify Remington medalists by their principal area of practice or specialty because most of them were very active in more than one field. However, it is clear that at least 40 percent of the principal affiliation of Remington medalists is as pharmaceutical educators. In an attempt to identify the principal affiliation of the remaining Remington medalists, we find that 18 percent are mainly considered as practicing pharmacists; 16 percent climaxed their career as national pharmaceutical association executives; 13 percent are generally recognized as pharmaceutical industry executives; eight percent spent most of their career as a governmental official; and five percent are best known as pharmacy journal editors.

History of pharmacy was routinely covered in most early Remington addresses. Of special note is the presentation by Eugene Eberle in 1932 who described individuals who used their experience in pharmacy to gain fame in a variety of fields such as Egyptologist James Henry Breasted; Norwegian poet Henrik Ibsen; Danish physicist Hans Christian Oersted; and American author William Sidney Porter ("O Henry"). Later, a detailed description of a typical American pharmacy was presented by Roy Bird Cook in 1955.

Various aspects of the history of the American Pharmacists Association and its sub-divisions are included in the majority of the Remington addresses, while a history of related U.S. pharmacy organizations are selectivly covered by various Remington medalists. Among them are the American Association of Colleges of Pharmacy (Patrick Costello in 1952 and Richard Penna in 2002); the American Council on Pharmaceutical Education (Melvin Green in 1976 and Daniel Nona in 2000); the American Foundation for Pharmaceutical Education (Ernest Little in 1949 and W. Paul Briggs in 1957); the National Association of Boards of Pharmacy (Henry C. Christiansen in 1938 and Patrick Costello in 1952); and the United States Pharmacopeia (E. Fullerton Cook in 1931 and William Heller in 1984).

Two Remngton medalists devoted their

addresses to a prediction of the future; Glenn Sonnedecker in 1972 speculated what pharmacy might be like in 2072, while Jerome Halperin in 2001 prophesied the status of pharmacy in the the year 2101.

One aspect that is to be found in the vast majority of Remington addresses is the liberal use of quotations from such notables as Francis Bacon, Miguel Cervantes, Winston Churchill, Charles Dickens, Arthur Conan Doyle, T. S. Eliot, Ralph Waldo Emerson, Henry Ford, Benjamin Franklin, Robert Frost, Oliver Wendell Holmes, Hubert Humphrey, Thomas Jefferson, John F. and Robert Kennedy, Abraham Lincoln, Martin Luther King, Henry Wadsworth Longfellow, Wolfgang Mozart, Ronald Reagan, Franklin D. and Theodore Roosevelt, William Shakespeare, Adlai Stevensen, George Washington, and Oscar Wilde. Eli Lilly in 1958 went so far as to state, "The shades of Demosthenes, Cicero, Edmund Burke, and Daniel Webster have been singularly unresponsive to my desperate appeals for words, phrases, and ideas," and then he went on to offer several quotes from Oliver Wendell Holmes. The subject index at the end of this volume will aid in further identifying affiliations, activities, and contents of the addresses of the Remington medalists.

In closing, we wish to acknowledge the assistance in tracking down original manuscripts of Remington lectures contained in this volume, or in obtaining biographical data and/or portrait photographs of Remington medalists. They include the American Institute of the History of Pharmacy in Madison, Wisconsin; the American Pharmaceutical Association Foundation Archives in Washington, D.C.; George Washington University Library in Washington, D.C.; Mrs. Melvin Green of Cedar Rapids, Iowa; Willam H. Grosz of Bismark, North Dakota; Anita Martin of Eli Lilly & Company; Jeffrey L. Sturchio of Merck and Company; the Wisconsin State Historical Society; and virtually all of the living Remington medalists.

Special thanks are also due to John A. Gans, Karen Tracy, and the APhA staff for their efforts in raising the funds to support this venture, and Jim McGinnis for designing the format and seeing this volume through publication. And finally, we again express our appreciation to Aventis Pharmaceuticals for their financial support which made it possible to publish this volume. We hope you will find it as absorbing as we found our task of putting it all together.

George Griffenhagen, senior editor
Grover C. Bowles, co-editor
Richard P. Penna, co-editor
Dennis B. Worthen, co-editor
January 2004

1919 Remington Medalist

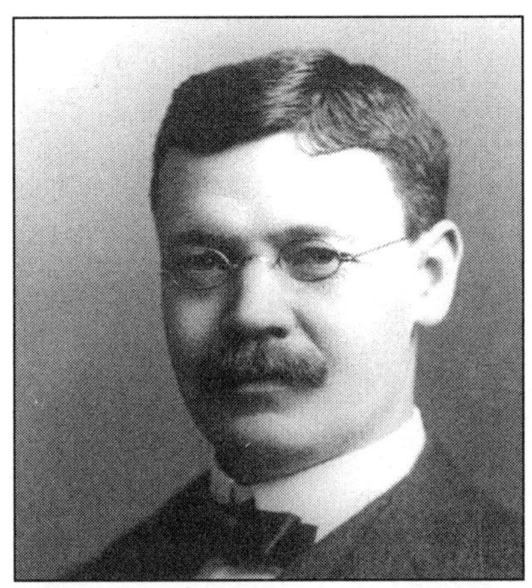

JAMES HARTLEY BEAL

(1861-1945)

James Hartley Beal was born in New Philadelphia, Ohio, received a Ph.G. degree in pharmacy in 1884 from Scio College, and obtained an LL.B. degree in 1886 from the Cincinnati School of Law. He accepted a teaching post at Scio College where he established a College of Pharmacy, serving as dean from 1887 to 1907 when the college merged with the University of Pittsburgh College of Pharmacy. He continued at the University of Pittsburgh as professor of pharmacy until 1911 when he accepted a position as director of pharmacy research at the University of Illinois 1914-1917. During this period, he served as president of the Ohio State Pharmaceutical Association 1898-1899, as a member of the Ohio State Legislature 1901-1903, as editor *of Midland Druggist and Pharmaceutical Review* 1908, as national councilor to the U.S. Chamber of Commerce 1917-1918, and as pharmaceutical expert to the War Industries Board during World War I. Beal developed the American Pharmaceutical Association's model state pharmacy act which was subsequently adopted by many states, and he variously served as chairman of the APhA Section on Education and Legislation 1897-1898, APhA second vice president 1898-1899, chairman of the APhA Council 1902-1908, APhA president 1904-1905, APhA general secretary 1911-1914, and founding editor of the *Journal of the American Pharmaceutical Association* 1912-1914. He also served variously as chairman of the USP board of trustees 1900-1930, as president of the American Association of Colleges of Pharmacy 1907-1908, and as president of the National Drug Trade Conference 1918-1919. He authored numerous textbooks including the five volume *Principles of Theory and Practice of Pharmacy* (1910).

Measuring Professional Ideals

James Hartley Beal

The first Remington Honor Medal Lecture was presented August 26, 1919, at the Hotel Pennsylvania in New York City during the First General Session of the 67th American Pharmaceutical Association annual meeting. Beal's Remington address was published in the *Journal of the American Pharmaceutical Association,* volume 8, pages 704-707, September 1919.

When I compare my own few and feeble efforts in behalf of pharmacy with the substantial achievements of so many faithful and deserving members of this Association I cannot help but wonder, as perhaps some of you have wondered, why I should have been selected to receive the first Remington medal.

However we may view the action of the committee in this particular instance, no one will question the wisdom or the laudable enterprise of the New York Branch of the American Pharmaceutical Association in establishing the means of commemorating the eminent services of one who for so many years filled so large a place in American pharmacy, both in name and in fact, as did Professor Joseph Price Remington.

When I became a member of the Association many years ago, Professor Remington was one of the first to extend the hand of professional fellowship, and from the day of that first acquaintance until the last his sympathetic advice and encouragement were unfailing. This was typical of his behavior to many other young and timid members who will always gratefully remember his approachableness, his efforts to make them feel at home at the annual meetings and to interest and encourage them in association work.

To you who knew him so well little could be said that would add to your knowledge of his personal characteristics. You still have a keen recollection of his vigorous personality, of his constant zeal in advancing the interests of this Association, of his readiness in debate, of his wisdom in counsel, and of his uniform courtesy and unfailing good humor.

Professor Remington's professional experience bridged the space between two distinct periods of pharmaceutical development. When he began his apprenticeship the apothecary, as he was then commonly called, was the principal manufacturer as well as the purveyor of medical supplies. The mineral acids and salts and most of the medicinal chemicals were purchased ready-made, but the galenicals which then ruled in the world of medicine were almost uniformly manufactured in the same establishment that dispensed them. He lived to see the period when the apothecary ceased to be the principal producer of medicinal compounds and became mainly the purveyor of preparations manufactured by others, and when the medicinal agents in most common use assumed a character that required for their successful production the resources of establishments maintained by large aggregations of capital and employing large numbers of specially trained workers.

To those who knew him intimately it was evident that although Professor Remington did not welcome the passing of the manufacturing functions of the apothecary to the large laboratory, he at length came to realize that such a change was inevitable, that it was but a natural step in the process of social evolution, and that the logical action of the apothecary was not to resist that which he could neither prevent nor change, but to readjust himself to the new conditions.

To some people optimism consists in refusing to see unwelcome facts, or in denying their existence when they are forced upon their attention. Professor Remington's optimism was of a different sort. He frankly recognized the changes that had come to pharmacy, but he had an abiding faith in its future, and in the opening of new fields of usefulness that would always require the best efforts of the best trained minds.

The historical development of a human vocation in many respects resembles the development of a river bed. Within certain rather narrow limits the stream determines its own channel; it may dig away the bank at one place and deposit a bar or build up to a point at another, but its volume of flow, its principal characters and general direction will be determined by the nature of the water-shed, by the general topography, and by other natural factors which no action of the current can control or modify. In a similar manner the members of a trade or profession are limited largely to the control of the collateral and incidental features of its development. By conscious thought and cooperation certain minor phases can be emphasized, restrained or reformed, but the general trend of its evolution will be determined by the fundamental features of the society and civilization which it serves, and by other factors beyond direction and control regardless of whether the direction of such evolution be in accordance with the ideals of its teachers and philosophers or opposed to them.

It is a common characteristic of men to cling to their early ideals for the progress of the particular calling with which they have been associated, and to feel that it will lose in power and dignity if the direction of its development chances to be along different lines than those previously marked out for it, overlooking the historical fact that the evolution of an art or a science according to preconceived ideals has been the exception rather than the rule; and also forgetting that each successive stage of development in every human vocation has brought with it opportunities for the best efforts of the best trained men and the basis for the formulation of new ideals as much worth while, or perhaps even more worth while, than the ideals that have been discarded.

After all, what is the proper measure by which to determine the correctness of professional ideals? Is not the true standard that of service, and service alone? Is not the truest and the most worth while development of an art that which brings the greatest good and the greatest service to the greatest number?

If the old method of local and individual production furnished more efficient medicinal agents than the new, then we are justified in regretting the change in the methods of production and distribution; but if the transfer of productive functions from the individual apothecary to the manufacturing laboratory has resulted in increasing the efficiency of medicinal agents, or has enlarged the extent of our control over disease, then we have no alternative but to acquiesce in the transfer, and to readjust our ideas and ideals to make them fit the new conditions.

It is not true that pharmacy has failed to progress in accordance with the spirit of the age. The improvement in the quality of its products and in the methods of their production has been as great as the improvement in any other line of productive manufacture. It is only the external form, not the substance of pharmacy, that has altered.

We must get away from the pessimistic idea that pharmacy is not pharmacy unless it is carried on in small establishments where two or three individual workers produce and dispense medicaments to a limited clientele in a small locality. The workers in the large laboratories who contribute to the improvement of therapeutic agents or who are engaged in their production on a large scale are as truly entitled to be called pharmacists as if each of the individual workers expended his entire activities behind the dispensing desk or in the back room laboratory of a small retail store.

Examined without prejudice the frequently deplored commercialization of pharmacy can be interpreted as the beginning of the separation of its merchandising features from its purely professional features. It is a part of the natural process of evolution; a first step toward a more complete specialization of functions. Its tendency is towards the same end as that sought by those who advocate legislation to create two classes of pharmacies, one class to be purely commercial, the other purely professional. We can retard the rate of this beginning cleavage between commercial and professional functions by demanding that every pharmacy shall particularly concern itself with the production and standardization of medicinal agents and the compounding of physicians' prescriptions, or we can materially advance its progress by frankly acknowledging the right of commercial pharmacy to a separate and independent existence.

The total amount of real pharmaceutical service required by the public and the medical profession is insignificant as compared with the number of existing drug stores, whereas its division among a smaller number of establishments would give a substantial portion to each and would encourage the cultivation of such work as a specialty.

It may be too early to ask for legislation dividing pharmacies into different classes according to the character of the patronage they seek, but it ought not to be too early to encourage the progress of such a separation through voluntary action on the part of their proprietors.

He must indeed be pessimistic who cannot see in present conditions the promise of a prosperous future for pharmacy. If all other signs were lacking, the fact that for years the demand for the graduates of our colleges and university schools of pharmacy has been far greater than the supply, and that the call for still better trained men is every increasing, should be evidence enough to convince the unbiased mind that pharmacy is not decadent.

Though it is true that hitherto the majority of the better trained graduates have been absorbed by the large laboratories, this is because the demand there has been most insistent. When this demand has been more nearly satisfied, we may reasonably expect to see an increasing number of establishments where the compounding of prescriptions, the making of laboratory examinations required by the physician, and the other so-called professional features of pharmacy, will be cultivated as specialties.

By some Professor Remington would probably have been denominated an opportunist, owing to the fact that at times he seemed to endorse policies which, externally at least, appeared to be inconsistent with each other. Those who were more intimately associated with him came at length to realize that he was a man of remarkable tenacity of purpose; that however much he might seem to yield in matters of detail the central thought and idea of his purpose was never lost sight of. Like a skillful commander he knew that campaigns are rarely completely carried out as planned, and that the details of their execution must be varied to meet the changing exigencies of the situation to make the central purpose of the general plan come true.

In other words, he was more intent upon final results than upon the forms or formulas by which they were obtained, and his tenacity was for things of substance rather than for mere names or for theoretical consistency. If he could meet a prejudice or lessen opposition to his general purpose by the sacrifice of some nonessential detail, or by a change of name to suit some stickler for form and method, he never hesitated to yield the point and to come to an accommodation. Not infrequently those who contested an important matter with him, later had reason to realize that although they had gained liberal concessions in the way of empty forms and minor details, Professor Remington had gained practically every substantial point involved in the contest.

It was this diplomatic disposition to yield in non-essentials in order to accomplish matters of larger consequence that enabled him to act so successfully as moderator between antagonistic views and personalities, where without such diplomatic mediation only confusion and disagreement could have resulted.

Professor Remington's position in pharmacy was not fortuitous nor was it thrust upon him by circumstance. Men do not achieve such a position of leadership as he so long enjoyed, nor continuously fill so many important and conspicuous positions, without the possession of unusual qualities of mind and character.

Even those who were occasionally forced by circumstances into positions of antagonism that sometimes verged upon bitterness will be most ready to admit his large and liberal qualities of mind and heart. In all the essential qualities of manhood he was sound and vigorous, clean alike in thought and habit, and with a personality and character that justly entitle him to rank as one of the very foremost men of the profession which he so long adorned.

Doubtless, like all men of action, he was at times responsible for decisions or policies that his own reason would not have endorsed at a later date, but even those most frequently at variance with him will concede that, weighed in any balance, his worth as a man and the value of his services to the American Pharmaceutical Association and to American pharmacy will far exceed the sum of any human frailties or errors of judgment that a critical examination of his life and character might bring to light.

No words at my command can adequately express my appreciation of the honor of having been selected as the first Remington medalist. I can only assure you that I am very deeply sensible of the distinction which you have conferred. ■

1920 Remington Medalist

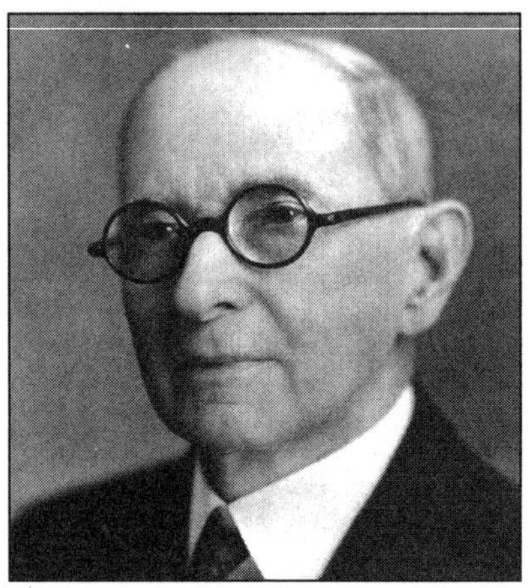

JOHN URI LLOYD
(1849-1936)

John Uri Lloyd was born in West Bloomfield, New York, but moved to Kentucky in 1853 where he obtained his education in private schools. He served as professor of pharmacy at the Cincinnati College of Pharmacy 1883-1887, president of the Eclectic Medical Institute 1896-1904, and associate editor of both the *Pharmaceutical Review* and the *Eclectic Medical Journal.* He joined the firm of William S. Merrell Company of Cincinnati, which was using indigenous plants as the basis for its pharmaceutical products, and in 1885 Lloyd organized Lloyd Brothers, which soon assumed a leading position in the field of plant preparations. He received the American Pharmaceutical Association Ebert Prize on three occasions for his research on alkaloidal assays and collodial chemistry, and he served as APhA president 1877-1878.

Among the many books that Lloyd authored are *Chemistry of Medicine* (1881), *Drugs and Medicines of North America* (1884), *Elixirs: Their History and Preparation* (1892), and *Origin and History of All the Pharmacopeial Vegetable Drugs* (1911). He was also noted for his investigation of dialect, superstition, and folklore of northern Kentucky, authoring numerous popular novels including *Stringtown on the Pike* (1900), *Warwick of the Knobs (1901), Red Head* (1903), and *Scroggins* (1904). The Lloyd Library, which he founded, remains as a lasting memorial to one of America's most versatile pharmacists.

KEEP THE HOME FIRES BURNING

John Uri Lloyd

The 1920 Remington Honor Medal Lecture was presented April 19, 1920, at the Hotel Pennsylvania in New York City. Lloyd's Remington address was published in the *Journal of the American Pharmaceutical Association,* volume 9, pages 484-487, May 1920.

When comes an opportunity to respond to the congratulations of friends concerning a something accomplished or an honor gained, comes also the privilege of crediting absent friends who have been helpful in consummating the happy event. Comes even a questioning of one's right to accept the honor without acknowledgment of the services and contributions of those silent copartners. Regardless of conventionalities, may not one who holds views such as these, injustice to himself, claim the privilege of frankly and openly dividing with absent friends the honors of the evening, sharing with them the tributes that may justly be considered their part? Especially does this apply when the recipient, past the allotted age of man, beholds not only an exceptional circle of friends present, but in mental vision, an even greater host of comrades, allies one and all, gone from human sight. May he not then speak reverently the names of a few memory cherished friends to whom this occasion would have been a joy, and but for whom the medal now bestowed could not have been extended?

As in life appears the face of this speaker's first preceptor, W.J.M. Gordon, of Cincinnati, whose methodical instruction and exacting rules, extremely severe and inflexibly enforced, guided the speaker in the beginning of his career, in the winter of 1863. Fortunate was it for that immature country bred lad that in the beginning of his career, no deviation from duty was permitted. Fortunate was it, too, that with far-sighted interest while the boy was yet an apprentice, Mr. Gordon, fifty years ago this year, filled out and signed the blank that gave to him the privilege of membership in the American Pharmaceutical Association. A hard taskmaster was Mr. Gordon; long were the hours of service, the "evenings off," one each week, Sundays for the boy, one each month. But, as the speaker looks back over the decades passed, he appreciates that had a different course then been adopted, this evening's occasion might not have been for him.

Appears now to mind's sight George Eger, the talented German apothecary who, next, in 1865, took charge of that apprentice. No pains spared he to instruct the rather tardy but yet hopeful youth. He, too, held that lad to the strictest professional accountability. Even more inflexible were his rules and processes than had been those of Mr. Gordon. Surely, those who meet here to-night will agree that but for the foundation laid during those four years' persistent instruction, this honor medal could never, to a homeless, friendless country-bred boy of sixty years ago, have been this evening awarded.

"Honor to whom honor is due." Would that all here could see, as does this speaker, the faces of these two men, talented members both of our Society, before most of those present were born! Would that both could tonight join in receiving the honors due to them by reason of their services to that apprentice!

A half century of time brings many friends, its mellowing touch makes comrades of one arid all. Come now to sight a great group of worthy men; but not as a group came they to the boy. One by one they passed into and out of his life, as one by one they severally sought the mystic domain where sleep the silent majority. Very pleasant is it in peaceful meditation to call their faces from out the mind's recesses, very helpful is it to feel that even though freed from life's activities they yet live and are of service.

Turn to the volumes of the Proceedings of our Society. Read the names recorded during the half century just passed. Not that of a cumberer of the ground, nor yet of a nonentity, he ventures to hope, has been the speaker's part in those fleeting years. Sunshine there has been, and clouds a-plenty. Blessed, is it not, that under the touch of time the brightness of other days grows still brighter in memory, while the softening influence of the fleeting years gives past-time gloom no present setting?

Turn as you may the pages of those fifty volumes of Transactions. The name of every man recorded brings only the thought of comrade, to him who this year of golden jubilee is made doubly blessed by this evening's events. Would that not alone his two preceptors, but one and all whose names are recorded in these volumes could be with us this night, for all, by what they have accomplished in the passing along, have earned the right to share in the honors this offered him who was the apprentice lad over half a century ago.

Where pharmacist and teacher alike for so many decades have in our Society taken a just part, it is impossible to make a selection of names. But as faces rise successively to view, may we not reverently venture to call out a few names, all well known even to the youngest present? Procter and Parrish came very early; famous teachers were they. Squibb and Chapman, Maisch, Ebert, Markoe, Judge, Prescott, Hoffman and Rice. Enough, enough. Need more be added? But for these men and a host of other co-laborers, this speaker could never have been privileged to hold in his hand this, your great gift.

Nor should we neglect to state that happily in those days, the members of the medical profession were close to the apothecary, who was just beginning to designate himself under the term pharmacist, as a contraction of the long established name pharmaceutist. Discussions concerning prescriptions, problems concerning drugs new and rare, natures of pharmaceutical preparations, were constant subjects of discursive argument. In this way, the apprentice of fifty years ago came in touch with the very cream of Cincinnati's professional men. King, Scudder, Pulte, Bartholow, Stevens and others akin in idealistic effort, were honored teachers. They, too, need be thankfully credited. But for them, many a phase of the apothecary's duty, in those days a prescription necessity, would never have been this speaker's opportunity. Their voices, long silent in the past, left messages that flow onward, let us hope ever onward.

Reflect over it all. If the credit-to whom credit is due be abstracted from this speaker's resources, behold, how little remains.

But one name cherished with us all, has been as yet unspoken. Very close were we two, from times far back. Decade after decade, each year we met. Pleasures and disappointments came to each in the passing along. Like ideals possessed us, though our fields of activity were far separated.

Let us again turn thought back half a century. Rises now before us the face of the then young man, now in view, little more than a lad, earnest, hopeful, inspiring to a degree. Pass next with a bound the intervening years to the one just closed. Came to that friend, as comes to everyone, the shutting of the door that time slowly but irresistibly moves to its final setting.

Listen! It seems as though it were but yesterday. In the home of this speaker, side by side, sat two old men who talked of times gone by, of men now unseen by others and events in which each had taken a part, both in life's bright beginning and in the memory of the blessed sunny passing along. The mellowness of age had come at last to both. The dock on the mantel ticked yet to both, but soon must tick for one only. Comprehending fully that they might that day part forever, they reluctantly bade each other adieu, and soon thereafter the one who left that home was ushered across the great divide into the company of friends whose faces are now but memory pictures.

Need that name be spoken? Is it not engraved in the heart of every comrade present as indelibly as it is on the cherished honor medal held before you? Let us utter it reverently, in tones that all can hear, but softly, Joseph P. Remington.

Close now this chapter, this eulogy of and credit offering to our absent friends. A word to you, who in the name of Remington make this gift, may not be amiss. This you feel tonight, each and every one. Comes to you the satisfaction of knowing that to your generous act no touch of selfishness clings, that the honor you extend in the name of Remington is given because of what Remington accomplished in his chosen field, what he did, not for himself, but for others.

An inspiration is this tribute you are offering, in behalf of ideals of the past, and service to the present. Seemingly dose together, as you look back, will lie the dates of your early meetings, yearly events, but one is scarcely passed till comes another. "Keep the home fires burning." Beautiful thought! Like the faith of the Oriental devotee who, in the far East, keeps alive the spark of fire that within the sacred sanctuary has never darkened, will be your part as recurs this beautiful ceremony year by year, that honors you in the eyes of all our friends.

And may not the recipient of the tribute this evening extended, now add a word in his own behalf, without breaking the conventions of occasions such as this? He comes this day to awaken mental greetings with friends of old, but not afar off, and to link them with friends new, close about. To weave into this story of the past the names of those who taught us how to live arid sacrifice, who, joining the past with the present, gave him the right to stand as their representative. In their name, as well as his own and his own loved ones, he wishes to thank you-his friends-for the privilege offered in this eventful occasion.

And lastly, most gratefully does he accept the honors this day bestowed, honors that can come to but one person each year.

May it not be asked? Could a more touching testimonial be devised to gladden the heart of him who, an apprentice in pharmacy still, this the evening of his seventyfirst birthday, receives this medal and celebrates also his golden anniversary of membership in this, our beloved Society? ■

1922 Remington Medalist

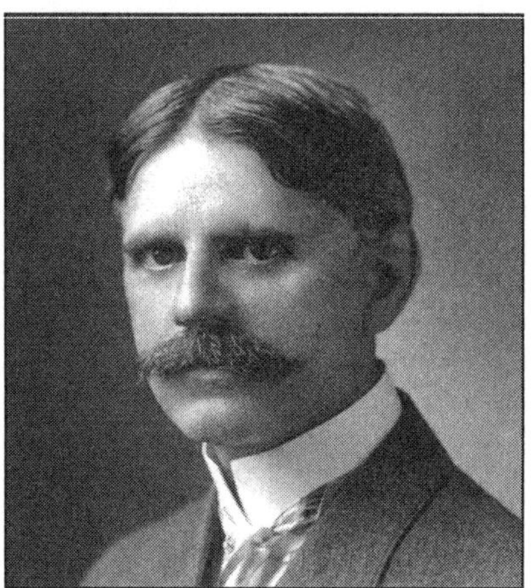

Henry Vincome Arny
(1868-1943)

Henry Vincome Arny was born in Philadelphia, Pennsylvania, but moved to New Orleans when three years old. At the age of 16, he apprenticed in the pharmacy of his brother-in-law, F.C. Godbold, and graduated with a Ph.G. degree from the Philadelphia College of Pharmacy in 1889. He continued his studies at the University of Berlin 1893-1894, and at the University of Goettingen, Germany, where he obtained a Ph.D. degree in 1896. He returned to New Orleans for one year to practice pharmacy and to serve as secretary of the Louisiana Pharmaceutical Association. He joined the faculty of Western Reserve University College of Pharmacy in Cleveland, Ohio, serving as dean 1905-1911, and then became dean of the Columbia University College of Pharmacy, serving until his retirement in 1936. During this period he served as editor of *Druggists Circular* 1914-1915, and as founding member of the American Metric Association executive committee 1916-1920.

Arny served the American Pharmaceutical Association as secretary of the APhA Scientific Section 1898-1899, as president of the New York APhA Branch 1912, as editor of the APhA *Year Book* 1916-1922, and as APhA president 1923-1924. He also served as president of the American Association of Colleges of Pharmacy 1915-1916, as a member of the committee of revision for both USP and the *National Formulary,* and as author of *Principles of Pharmacy* (1909, 4th edition 1936).

THE PLACE OF PHARMACY IN THE WORLD

Henry Vincome Arny

Presented May 15, 1922, at the Hotel Pennsylvania, New York City. Arny's Remington address was published in the *Journal of the American Pharmaceutical Association,* volume 11, pages 441-446, June 1922.

To reverently paraphrase a great saying: Before Science was Pharmacy is. I love to dream over the historic wealth of pharmacy; to think of our pharma- ceutical progenitors amid the mists of the past. First there were priests of the Egyptian templeswho prepared the medicaments; the writersof Eber's Papyrus. Then there were those inthe Bible whom I wish to continue to consider as apothecaries even though the Revised Version calls them "perfumers." The one Solomon had in mind when he wrote of the fly in the ointment; the one who had the great, though unconscious, glory of preparing theprecious ointment that the Magdalen poured upon the feet of her Lord and Master; the one whose name we know, Hananiah, the apothecary whose son helped Nehemiah to rebuild the walls of Jerusalem. Then I like to think of the pharmaceutical helpers of Dioscorides and Galen; of the seplasiarii of ancient Rome; of the medieval apothecaries of Nuremberg, whom Valerius Cordus had in mind when he prepared his *Pharmacoporum Omnium.* Then to the colonial apothecaries of our own land; to the druggists of the young Republic of 1822 and thence along through the nineteenth century, to that honored line of pharmacists, Procter, Parrish,Bedford, Rice, Maisch, Oldberg, Diehi down to my beloved teacher, that great man, Joseph Price Remington, whose kindly countenance adorns the medal just bestowed upon me, the face that I imagine greets his pupil with a smile of friendly recognition.

What lessons we can learn from these worthies of the past; these disciples of Service, these humble searchers after the Truth. For let us frankly admit that the pharmacist of the eighteenth century and earlier was an unassuming helper rather than a brilliant master. In ancient Egypt he was the assistant priest; in ancient Greece he was the doctor's pupil; in medieval Europe he was the lay brother; in Tudor England he was, to quote the quaint saying of William Bulleyn, "the physician's cook," and in Colonial America he was the small shopkeeper. But whenever and wherever he lived, he was a Man, a person whose passion was Service, whose motto was "Accuracy," whose virtue was Trustworthiness. Verily these cardinal principles represent a heritage more precious than a mere place in the Almanach de Gotha.

Moreover let us remember that up to the nineteenth century the only exalted personages were the nobles, the clergy, and the warriors. In those days, the surgeon was also the barber; the author lived only as he basked in the smiles of his noble patron; the chemist was either a soap boiler or a practitioner of black art, the banker was usually a Hebrew money lender. It is therefore not surprising that the pharmacist was little esteemed at court until Parmentier made the influence of pharmacy felt in the palace of the Fifteenth Louis of France. But any calling that has produced a Scheele, a Serturner, a Pelletier, a

Caventou, a Schiotterback, a Trimble, a Power and a Lloyd need not bow its head in the presence of the modern sciences; a calling that has developed the vast concerns headed by a Dieterich, a Wellcome, a Squibb, a Dohme, a Warner and a Seabury need not be considered insignificant when compared to other manufacturing enterprises; a calling that has been inspired by a Procter, a Prescott, a Markoe, a Searby, a Caspari and a Rusby need not be held in ill esteem in educational circles even though we have some pharmaceutical Jeremiahs who seem to think the contrary. When we come to the backbone of pharmacy, the great body of retail druggists such as Metcalf and Sheppard of Boston, Adamson and McIntyre of New York, Marshall and Blair of Philadelphia, Duhamel and Hynson of Baltimore, Ebert of Chicago, Alexander of St. Louis, Finlay of New Orleans, Jones of Louisville, Painter of San Francisco and New York and Holzhauer of Newark to say nothing of those who are still with us we will all agree that there is no class of retail merchants, who are of such vital importance to the community.

To quote inexactly from Professor Beal, the retail druggist is more than a merchant, he is a professional man in the fact that he is the only retail business man who receives family confidences that must remain as inviolate as information imparted to the physician. And then there is no retail business in which such strong emphasis must be laid upon service as in Pharmacy. I might point out that the main difference between the management of a chain of corporation stores and the business of an individual pharmacist is that the former is financed with the primary object of making money for the corporation with service as a mere selling point; while with the right sort of an individual pharmacist service to his patrons comes first with the financial rewards as the necessary complement to his primal consideration. This last statement is not as fantastic as it sounds. Of course, all of us work in order to make a living; to acquire a competence. But the gulf that divides the worthy from the unworthy is this very question of service. Is one's aim to freely give of one's time with reward sure to follow; or is it to take all one can get and give as little as possible in return? Time will not permit me to cite examples of unusual service rendered by retail pharmacists but this has been the theme of a paper I published some years since (*Druggists Circular* 1914).

I hope I have made a case for Pharmacy as an historic calling whose record of 4000 years of service is available to all of those who will only read it. But how do we pharmacists of 1922 pass along the truth as concerns pharmacy? How well are we holding aloft the torch of pharmaceutical progress, with its flame brightly burning; ready to pass along to the generations that follow us? Sometimes I fear that in accordance with efficiency and progressiveness characteristic of pharmacy we have exchanged the torch of the poet for the Bunsen burner: an instrument of greater calories but of less luminosity. It seems to me that instead of letting our "light so shine," we are too unobtrusive in furnishing our calories to those whom we are benefiting; in short, that we are too modest in letting our achievements be known.

In this virile twentieth century the keynote is publicity. Unobtrusiveness is but a foolish way of letting another calling get the credit of our achievements. While we sit humbly back and modestly deprecate our achievements, our more energetic mother, Medicine, and our younger sister, Chemistry, have caught the spirit of the age and are letting the lay world know what they are doing; are doing work that we pharmacists should be doing; and if the truth be told are appropriating to themselves some of the achievements of us pharmacists.

Is this statement extreme? Let me give some illustrations of what I mean. Scheele, Serturner, Pelletier, Caventou and other pharmacists of the past whose names are linked with their great discoveries in phytochemistry are usually classed in non-pharmaceutical literature as chemists.

In the same way those great pharmaceutical research workers of today, John Uri Lloyd and Frederick B. Power, are proudly claimed by our chemical brethren.

In a cabled news item that appeared in the American newspapers of a year or so ago the eminent Professor Bourquelot, head of the l'Ecole Superieur de Pharmacie of Paris, was cited as biologist.

Our own Dean Rusby is claimed by medicine on one hand, and on the other hand the expedition which he has recently conducted through South America with such brilliant success is considered as a botanical achievement by our friends of that calling. Amusing and yet irritating it is, that the early newspaper accounts of the undertaking dubbed the well-known pharmaceutical manufacturers of Philadelphia who financed the undertaking "a chemical firm."

In the list of research grants, research fellows and research medals published by the National Research Council, those relating to pharmacy are classified among the medical subjects, and the same thing is true as to the catalogues of certain publishers where books of pharmacy are listed in the sub-head "pharmacology."

During the war by special invitation a certain college of pharmacy sent one of its faculty down to Washington as a civilian expert on the subject of protective ointments against mustard gas. The gentleman worked on the problem during the four or five months and perfected the ointment that was adopted by our army. In the newspapers of a later date, the research was described as an achievement of the Chemical Warfare Service.

Lastly, while our newspapers employ as juicy morsels the occasional misdoings of the retail druggist, they are usually silent as to their virtues. Others get the credit for the narcotic legislation that druggists have placed upon the statute books to their own inconvenience but for the welfare of the public. Few realize the honest straightforward way that a vast majority of pharmacists have assumed the grave responsibilities that have come to them under the Eighteenth Amendment.

Those who have patiently listened to me thus far may be asking themselves "What has all this to do with the Remington Honor Medal?" It has this much to do with the subject, if I may be allowed to abruptly turn to personalities.

To me has been awarded the third Remington Honor Medal-a badge of distinguished pharmaceutical service. Far be it from my thoughts to question the wisdom of eminent jury of award, the past-presidents of the American Pharmaceutical Association, but in taking inventory of my own modest achievements it is not as easy to see why the great honor fell upon me in 1922, as it was to understand why the first medal was awarded in 1919 to James Hartley Beal and why the second medal was awarded in 1920 to John Uri Lloyd. The medal of 1919 went to Dr. Beal as the pharmacist in legislation; for no man during the last thirty years has done more to formulate the legislative status of American pharmacy than has our friend from Scio, Ohio, and Urbana, Illinois. The second medal went to Professor Lloyd as we still love to call him as the pharmacist in research; for it is no disparagement to other distinguished pharmaceutical research workers to say that Lloyd, pharmaceutical manufacturer, author and scientist, is the brightest jewel in the research crown of American pharmacy. But the third medal and its recipient? This is another matter. Some of my friends have referred to my versatility, but versatility is not enough to bring this supreme honor. Some have been good enough to refer to my capacity for performing work, but service, not mere work, is the standard set for the award of the Remington Honor Medal. May I therefore be pardoned for taking this unique opportunity in my life to dare to venture the hope that the Remington Honor Medal Committee chose me in this Year of Grace 1922, because of my humble efforts toward solving the problem that I have chosen as the topic of my address, The Proper Place of Pharmacy in the World?

I hope I have proven my contention that pharmacy is more than an ancient calling; that it is more than a humble service. I hope I have shown sufficiently clearly that as a science, as a field of service, as a profession the followers of pharmacy have proven their worth.

But that is only half of the battle. We know these facts to be true, but have we impressed them sufficiently upon the world around us; have we, in truth, absorbed these facts ourselves? I find too often that our pharmaceutical manufacturers turn to chemists untrained in pharmacy for a solution of their problems. I find at times our pharmaceutical educators sneering at their own colleagues in pharmacy and lauding the achievements of those working in other fields of scientific and educational endeavor; I find some of our younger pharmacists so ignorant of the possibilities of pharmacy that they are frankly desirous of embarking in other lines of scientific or professional endeavor.

All of these conditions so detrimental to pharmaceutical progress are due to a lack of proper illumination. I have asserted that in our modesty, we pharmacists have not properly set forth our right to recognition as a science, as an art and as a profession.

I have endeavored during my twenty-five years of teaching to impress upon my students the fact that pharmacy is something more than the mere making of a living. I have tried during the last ten or fifteen years in my various APhA activities to emphasize that pharmacy has a distinct place in the world of science as well as in the world of service and that it was the duty of every true pharmacist to maintain pharmacy's proper place in the world. I have on sundry occasions pointed out how these things can be done and at this time I will summarize what I regard as the proper means; many of them, by the way, being the methods used satisfactorily by the followers of our mother, Medicine, and our sister, Chemistry.

1. We Pharmacists Must Stick Together. There are too many of us flirting with medicine and with chemistry rather than devoting our best efforts to our own calling.

2. We Should Give Our Financial Aid to Projects for the Betterment of Pharmacy.- Those of us who have means should bestow it upon our pharmacy colleges and upon our pharmaceutical research undertakings.

3. We Should Develop Better Facilities for Acquainting the Public with the Achievements of Pharmacy.— It was my good fortune to organize a national committee on pharmaceutical publicity and during the past year it has been doing excellent work under the leadership of its accomplished chairman, Dean Robert P. Fischelis of Newark. I might, however, point out that Dr. Fischelis has had at his disposal less than $1200 per annum whereas the annual publicity appropriation of another American scientific society averages about $12,000. Such meritorious work as our publicity efforts should receive better support.

4. We Should Do More Research Work Ourselves or Should Give More Encouragement to the Research Work of Others.— In other addresses I have discussed the subject of pharmaceutical research at length and I hope to have satisfactorily demonstrated the fact that even as a selfish proposition, pharmaceutical research should be encouraged by all who make their living out of pharmacy. It is now my task to organize a national committee on pharmaceutical research and while the organization will not be effected until the time of the Cleveland meeting of APhA. I can now say that it is my earnest hope that at that time the several agencies interested in pharmaceutical research may come to a common agreement that will be of marked benefit to the whole of pharmacy. In the meanwhile there is much left for individual pharmacists to do in this direction. The only American endowment for pharmaceutical research now extant is the $16,500 of the APhA Research Fund, the net profits from sale of the *National Formulary.* This fund, which should be augmented by outside contributions, provides at present $360 per annum for research grants and has been and still is of distinct service to those performing research. But we should go further. Every teacher in a college of pharmacy should be expected to perform some research work. In every college of pharmacy, provision should be made for the maintenance of at least one research fellow.

5. We Should GiveBetterSupport to the Scientific and Professional Work of the American Pharmaceutical Association.—Practically all of us here present are members of that great organization-the American Pharmaceutical Association. Few of us appreciate the fact that it is among the oldest of America's national professional organizations. Thus, while the venerable Franklin Institute dates from 1824, the American Medical Association and also the American Association for the Advancement of Science from 1848, our own organization will celebrate its seventieth anniversary at its Cleveland meeting next August, while the American Chemical Society will have its semi-centennial in 1924.

We should do more than be merely members of APhA. We should give to it, our time, or means; yea even our prayers. How many here present know practically the last words of that great pharmacist, Albert E. Ebert, were words of affection for the APhA. Each of us should consider himself (or herself, since women have ever been as welcome in APhA as men) a committee of one to bring new members into APhA. Each of us should aid our great journal in securing more advertising patronage. Each of us should feel a personal responsibility in aiding the project of our APhA Headquarters, of erecting a building that will tell the world of the dynamic power of Pharmacy.

And then there is the APhA *Year Book.* Of course I cannot close this address without a reference to my early pharmaceutical love "the Handy Black Volume." Since I was a young man in a southern drug store, I have drawn much of my inspiration from the old APhA *Proceedings* and their successors, the *Year Books.* When the call came to me to canyon the great task of editing this magnificent work, a task to which my venerated friend, C. Lewis Diehi, gave a greater part of his life, I assumed the position as a duty to pharmacy. I have been glad to perform this duty during the past six years and as I have worked upon the successive annual numbers I have realized as I have never realized before the great work that APhA has been performing all of these years in furnishing to pharmacy, not only of America but of the world, this pharmaceutical library in one volume per annum. Few but those in charge of the affairs of APhA realize in what high esteem the Year Book is held by pharmaceutical savants the world over. Few appreciate the sacrifices made by APhA in keeping aflame this torch of American pharmaceutical progress. In this endeavor, APhA should receive the support of all other pharmaceutical agencies of our country.

Enough, perhaps more than enough, has been said by the recipient of the third Remington Honor Medal. In closing, he wishes to give his hearty thanks to those who by their ballots selected him for this supreme honor, to those, his friends of the New York Branch who planned this delightful evening and to those from neighboring cities who have come to spend with him the greatest evening of his life. May he leave with all present the thought with which he began this address; that since the dim ages of the past, pharmacy has been a calling of unselfish service and that to-day and into the dim reaches of the future it will continue a means of service, a useful art and a valuable division of science, if we pharmacists will only rise to the possibilities of our calling. ■

1923 Remington Medalist

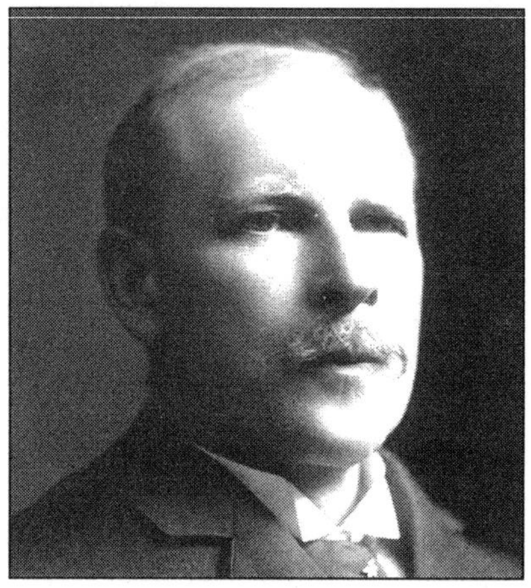

Henry Hurd Rusby
(1855-1940)

Henry Hurd Rusby was born near Franklin, New Jersey, and by the time he received an M.D. degree from the New York University Medical College in 1884, he had become a noted pharmacognosist. He headed a Smithsonian Institution expedition to New Mexico in 1880, and a Parke-Davis expedition to Arizona in 1883. Then Parke-Davis sent Rusby to Bolivia in 1885 to study the properties of the coca leaf. Rusby forged his way through South American rain-forests collecting 45,000 botanical specimens, many hundreds of which were unknown to botany.

Rusby joined the faculty of the New York College of Pharmacy in 1888, serving as dean from 1905 until his retirement in 1930. He aided Harvey Wiley's crusade to enact the Pure Food and Drug law and served as APhA president 1909-1910. But his love for exploration led him to Venezuela and Mexico in 1896, and to Colombia in 1916 to seek new sources of quinine. Rusby had just returned from his final exploration of the Amazon (1921-1922) when he was selected as the 1923 Remington honor medalist. He was introduced at the Remington award dinner by such notables as the president of H.K. Mulford and the provost of Columbia University, as well as by food and drug crusader Harvey W. Wiley.

South American Exploration

Henry Hurd Rusby

The 1923 Remington Honor Medal Lecture was presented April 16, 1923, at the Hotel Pennsylvania in New York City. Since the text of Rusby's "informal" Remington lecture was never published, the following lecture, which was "illustrated with lantern-slides" is offered to represent the explorations of the medalist, if not the actual content of his Remington lecture. It was presented to the 1922 meeting of the American Conference of Pharmaceutical Faculties, and published in the *Journal of the American Pharmaceutical Association,* volume 12, pages 52-54,January 1923, three months prior to his Remington lecture.

Let us begin with some illustrations of Indian life on the Andean tableland of Bolivia, at an altitude varying from 11,000 to 19,000 feet above sea-level, and in about 18 S. latitude. Here the climate is very cool, even in mid-summer. Although the sun's rays are very powerful at mid-day, the nights are cold, and frosts are liable to occur in any month. Trees are wanting, except for a few under cultivation, and the range ofcultivated crops is narrow. Potatoes do well. Oats and other grains are grown for the straw, but do not produce grain. The chief crop is quinoa *(Chenopodium Quinoa),* its seed constituting the staple food of the Aymara Indians. There are some cattle, with the production of butter and cheese, but sheep-raising is the principal grazing industry. Many hogs are also raised, and hens do well. The pig is a household pet, and when young, is very playful, accompanying children as do their dogs. Navigation on Lake Titicaca is by small boats, with or without sails, composed entirely of dried sedges. Mining industries are exceedingly varied and important, providing the chief wealth of the region. Some of the ranges, especially of the eastern cordillera, are perpetually snow-covered, and there are many large glaciers.

The party received valuable assistance from the Guggenheim Brothers, of New York, who own a large tin mine near the top of the eastern slope.

On the eastern slope, tree growth begins at about 11,000 feet, where the country is richly supplied with mountain streams. Travel is very difficult, owing to the numerous high ridges and deep valleys, with precipitous sides, which have to be crossed. This makes transportation the most difficult of Bolivia's problems. During the rainy season, the country to the east of the mountains is entirely cut off from the capital for months together and in the most favorable season many weeks are required to make the round trip over a route of 150 miles.

Transportation is chiefly by mules and human porters, until streams are reached which are capable of carrying rafts. These rafts are made of the wood of several species of Ochroma, in the Bombaz family, this wood being almost as light as cork. Navigation of these streams is very rough and laborious, and not free from danger. At the high altitudes, where the climate is cold, the llama, an animal in the camel family, is the beast of burden, carrying 100 pounds. Here also the alpaca is raised.

At about 5000 or 6000 feet, the cinchona trees make their appearance, both species of Calisssaya occurring in this southern district. Formerly there were large plantations of these trees in Mapiri, but oriental competition has destroyed the industry. An abundance of trees in the wild state was encountered between 4000 and 5000 feet. In the same region, the coca leaf is largely grown as a masticatory.

A few miles above the junction of the La Paz and Meguilla Rivers, forming the Bopi, the party was entertained at a large sugar-cane plantation, the cane being used in the manufacture of alcohol. In this work the bark of a Mimosaceous tree *(Piptadenia macrocarpa* Benth) known locally as Vilca, is used to hasten and increase the alcoholic fermentation of thejuice. Here also is found an abundance of the genuine matico leaf *(Piper angustfo1ium R.* and P.). This section was found to be rich in orchids, but very few were in bloom at that season. A number of interesting species of cactus were found here, one of them apparently an undescribed species, being probably the largest of tree cactuses.

A species of aroid, called Hualusa, is cultivated in this region, which the author found to yield the best potato substitute that he has known.

At the head of the Bopi, rafts were substituted for mules, and the party floated down this and the River Beni for many days, employing crews of native Indians and camping along the river when night overtook them. The weather was fine during most of the time and often it was not necessary to erect their tents. Up to this point the botanical collectors had been handicapped by the dry season, very little of the flora being in condition for making collections, but along the Bopi things were much further advanced, and large and important collections were obtained. In the cataracts of the Bopi one of the rafts was smashed and much valuable property was lost, the collections also suffering some damage. Two varieties of native cinnamon were collected here, pertaining to the genus Acrodiclidium. There was also a tree that yields a so-called "Balsam of Peru." The Bopi valley as described as a rich game country, deer, tapirs, capibaras and two species of wild hogs being frequently encountered, and excellent game-birds being very abundant. An abundance of excellent fish was found here. A long stay was made at Juachi, where the Cochabamba and Bopi Rivers unite to form the Bern. Here the party was entertained by Sr. Mostaja, a representative of the house of Denniston & Co., of New York and La Paz. Large and important collections were made at this place, the most important being the barks of the genuine and spurious Cotos. From the materials here collected the species yielding these barks *(Nectandra Coto* and *Ocotea Pseudo Coto)* were described by the author. Here also was collected a quantity of Siaya flowers, belonging to a small palm, and one of the most fragrant of known flowers. A root called Mire (pronounced mee-ray) was found that possesses strange and powerful physiological powers. Its identity could not be established, as it bore neither flowers nor fruits, but the lecturer thought it to be related to Manaca.

The next stop was at Rurrenabaque, a town on the shore of the Beni, just at the base of the Andean foot-hills. Here the party established its headquarters, and remained for many weeks. Long expeditions were made into the surrounding regions. Dr. O.E. White, of the Brooklyn Botanic Gardens, who was collecting orchids for Dr. Oakes Ames, of Harvard, made most of his collections in this region. Dr. William M. Mann, of the United States Bureau of Entomology, made very large collections of insects, especially of ants and termites. Dr. N.E. Pearson, of the University of Indiana, who was collecting fishes for Dr. Eigenmann, made important collections. The lecturer made a careful study of Cocillana and its allies, which grow in abundance in these forests. His general botanical collections at this place were very large, although he was so crippled and in such poor health that work was very difficult.

This region was described as producing the greatest variety of wild edible fruits that the lecturer had ever encountered in a similar area, and an important collection of these was preserved in formaldehyde solution. These fruits, after being botanically determined, will be placed on exhibition in the Economic Museum of the New York Botanical Garden.

An expedition was made to the little known Lake Rogugua, in central Bolivia, but the season was such that its outlet could not be traversed or explored. Early in December, the author's physical condition had become such that further work was impossible and he returned home, stopping for short periods at a number of towns en route. The rest of the party remained and continued work into the spring months. Mr. Gordon MacCreagh and his two assistants in motion-picture work ascended the Rio Negro and Manaos, and thence made their way into southeastern Colombia, where they obtained authentic information regarding, and motion-pictures illustrating the strange ceremony of Caapidrinking, and secured material of this plant for chemical and physiological investigation.

The total number of plants collected was about 2,300, represented by some 15,000 specimens and representing about 1,500 species. ■

1924 Remington Medalist

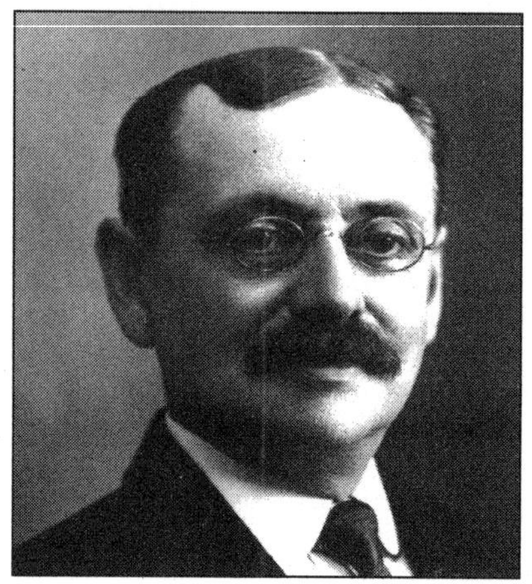

George Mahlon Beringer
(1860-1928)

George Mahion Beringer was born in Philadelphia, Pennsylvania, and after serving an apprenticeship with Bullock and Crenshaw of Philadelphia, he graduated with a Ph.G. degree from the Philadelphia College of Pharmacy in 1880. He returned to Bullock and Crenshaw for another ten years where he became manager of the laboratory, and then opened his own pharmacy in Camden, NewJersey, in 1892. He served as a trustee of the Philadelphia College of Pharmacy 1893-1921, as chairman of the College board of trustees 1910-1921, and as editor of the *American Journal of Pharmacy* 1917-1921. He was 1905 president of the New Jersey Pharmaceutical Association, director of the Camden Board of Trade, member of the City Planning Commission of Camden, and he organized the Camden Guarantee Building and Loan Association for which he served as secretary until his death.

Beringer joined the American Pharmaceutical Association in 1893, chaired the 1902 APhA semi-centennial celebration committee, served as chairman of the APhA Section on Practical Pharmacy 1902-1903, and as APhA president 1913-1914. He also served as a member of the committee of revision for both the *United States Pharmacopeia* 1910-1920 and the *National Formulary* 1908-1928.

The Influence of Association

George Mahlon Beringer

The 1924 Remington Honor Medal Lecture was presented April 14, 1924, at the Robert Trent Hotel in Newark, New Jersey. Beringer's Remington address was published in the *Journal of the American Pharmaceutical Association, volume 13, pages 460-466, May 1924.*

Custom, that inexorable master, has decreed that I must deliver an address on this occasion. Since 'custom is held to be as a law' as a law-abiding citizen I must obey the dictate even though I am well aware that public speaking is not one of my accomplishments. When the chairman of your committee on arrangements hastened to my home city to acquaint me with the honor that was to be conferred upon me on this occasion, he did not fail to present, along with his congratulations, a notice of this duty. Nevertheless, to date he has not responded to my request for a topic on which I could direct my thoughts in addressing you and so, if you are disappointed in my remarks this evening, you must lay a portion of the blame upon the broad shoulders of Professor Fischelis.

Left to my own resources, my thoughts given free reign wandered first in a reminiscent vein into the recesses of memory to some of the outstanding events in my own career and then turning from the retrospect toward the prospect attempted to peer into the future of our chosen profession with its increasing responsibilities.

When the old fellows get together, they instinctively fall into reminiscence and recall incidents long forgotten. On this evening, there is a further incentive to retrospection in the attempt to trace out a reason for this occasion to discover some *magnum opus* that justifies this distinction. With this review of the past, deeper has grown the conviction that if there have been any achievements, any success in the performance of tasks that have fallen to my lot, any meritorious services rendered that in some measure would justify this great honor, these have been largely due to the influence of those with whom I have been so fortunate as to be associated and the Divine guidance in shaping these contacts and the beneficent impressions is gratefully acknowledged.

As a product of the public schools of Philadelphia, it is fitting that the early impressions of the school should receive initial presentation. The first picture is of a little urchin, just entering his teens, a scholar in the George W. Nebinger school of that city. A prominent member of the Board of Education, at that period, was Dr. Andrew Nebinger, a brother of the man after whom this school was named. This director, from time to time, visited the school and inspired the scholars with his talks. You may call it hero worship, but we lads never had a nobler example than that worthy and leading citizen of the District of Old Southward who was universally beloved for his public spirit and philanthropy and honored for his great interest in the cause of education. In my library I still cherish, with enduring admiration for the donor though more than half a century has passed by, a copy of *The Life and Adventures of Robinson Crusoe* which I received on the eleventh anniversary of my birth as one of the prizes in competitive scholarship that he had offered that year. To me this copy is more valuable than all of the other copies of Defoe's immortal story that have been printed.

At the age of twelve, I was promoted to the Central High School, and for the next four years it was my privilege on every school day to tramp back and forth over the three miles intervening between the school and my home. In those days, a high school education was not the complement assured by the state to every boy and girl; selected students only were permitted to continue their education in this school with its renowned faculty and its academic courses in history, languages and the sciences. Athletic sports, class dances and the other forms of entertainment so popular in the high schools of today were then not recognized. The curriculum was not optional but was fundamental and each student was expected to take the complete course as mapped out with every minute of the school periods fully occupied and a measure of home studies thrown in. Each week we had to prepare at home a composition and on Monday morning as many of these as possible were read in class and criticized.

Here it was my good fortune to have a number of excellent teachers, although it cannot be said that I profited equally from all of their instruction as, despite the beautiful Spencerian copy of Professor Bartine, my handwriting is still scarcely legible. Dr. Jacob F. Holt gave us a scientific course in anatomy, physiology and hygiene that was far beyond the usual academic instruction in these branches. The professor of physical geography and natural philosophy was Edwin J. Houston, noted as an author and physicist. At this time, there was a young man in charge of the chemical laboratory who served as the assistant to the professor of chemistry and also to that of physics who was likewise an inspiring teacher that we boys greatly admired. Elihu Thomson was at that early day a mechanical and scientific genius destined to win recognition and fame. He now ranks as one of the world's leading physicists and electrical engineers, whose inventions and researches have won deserved international honor and renown and he is now an officer in the Legion of Honor and has been awarded the Rumford Medal by the Royal Society.

Graduating from the high school in February 1876, and being duly elated with the pride and roseate visions of the youthful graduate and imbued with the spirit of the centennial year and armed with an A.B. diploma and a letter of introduction from the professor of chemistry to Mr. Charles Bullock, the head of one of the leading drug firms in Philadelphia, I forthwith applied for a position to learn the art and mysteries of the apothecary. After looking me over and possibly noting my viridity as well as my earnestness, he agreed to take me on as an apprentice for a stipulated period of four years at the moderate wage then paid to such apprentices. On March 1, 1876, I engaged in the drug business as the youngest novice in the employ of Bullock & Crenshaw. I had then a latent desire to make pharmacy a stepping stone to the study of medicine which was my youthful ambition. However, the claims of pharmacy and of chemistry have so thoroughly engrossed my attention that this early intent was entirely eliminated.

The errand duties and the menial services as usual fell to the lot of the junior apprentice. The trimming of labels, hours at a time, made me sleepy and as blue as I was green. Often since have I thought of the disparagements of pharmacy and the depressing and ridiculous suggestions made to the new apprentice. An incident of this type occurred the first day of my employment. A member of a nearby wholesale drug firm came into the store, and, upon observing a new face, inquired of the manager who was the new boy? Upon being informed that I was a new apprentice he blurted out, 'My boy, take my advice, before learning the drug business you had better go right down to the foot of Arch Street and jump into the Delaware and drown yourself.' You can imagine the effect that such derisive and deprecating remarks have upon the novitiate and, doubtless, such ridicule has discouraged and deterred many a promising lad from entering upon a pharmaceutical career. Despite the advice, I stuck to the job and soon learned that the thoughtless remark was not a true index of the real nature of the speaker and in afteryears I had the satisfaction of serving him frequently and of enjoying his friendship and a measure of his confidence.

I was indeed fortunate in having as preceptors Bullock and Crenshaw. Charles Bullock was a scientist as well as a thorough pharmacist. He contributed a number of papers to pharmaceutical literature and his work on Veratrum was a notable research on an American drug. His masterly memoir of Professor William Procter, Jr., has been the basis for many of the articles that have since been published upon this eminent pharmacist whom we consider as the "Father of American Pharmacy." He gave largely of his time to the management of the Franklin Institute of Philadelphia and to the Philadelphia College of Pharmacy. The latter institution he served at, various times as trustee, secretary, vice-president and as president. His associate in the business, Mr. Edmund A. Crenshaw, was a polished, educated, Christian gentleman, a high type of business man of the old school. Thoroughly reliable and honorable in all their dealings Bullock and Crenshaw enjoyed the confidence and good-will of the entire drug trade and their wholesale and retail departments proved to be a sort of pharmaceutical Mecca that attracted many of those identified with the drug interests and many leading physicians, scientists and worth citizens. I enjoyed greatly the acquaintances thus made and the impressions gained from these contacts were deep and lasting. The sixteen years that I spent with this firm was a continuous schooling that gave me an unusually broad and varied experience.

On the day of my inception into the drug business I was introduced to Thomas S. Wiegand, who was then managing the department for the manufacture of sugar coated pills, a branch of manufacturing in which Bullock and Crenshaw were pioneers in this country. He took a kindly interest in the lonely lad and soon it became my custom to spend many of the noon hours in his company anxiously imbibing the instruction that was so freely given. Thus was commenced a friendship that cemented us closely together until death severed the tie. During his many years as registrar and librarian of the Philadelphia College of Pharmacy, 'Uncle Tommy,' as we lovingly called him, endeared himself to a host of students whose friend and adviser he was always, but to no one was he nearer or dearer than to me.

I matriculated at the Philadelphia College of Pharmacy at the period when the three members of the major faculty, Professors John M. Maisch, Joseph P. Remington, and Samuel P. Sadtler were at their prime. Fortunate were the students who were privileged to listen to such earnest, devoted and able teachers. All three have now passed to the great beyond, but, on this occasion, I must pay to their memory the tribute of gratitude that I justly owe to them as teachers and likewise in honor of the close personal friendships and associations that continued throughout the postgraduate years.

In 1880, I became a member of the college organization and for nearly forty years was actively interested in its affairs.

In 1893, on the proposal of Professor Remington, I was elected to membership in the American Pharmaceutical Association but for a number of years took no active interest in the work of the Association. It was Dr. Henry M. Wheipley, as President, who drew me out of my 'clam shell' and put me to work as chairman of the Committee on Semi-Centennial Celebration which was held in Philadelphia in 1902. To be put into some active service in behalf of an association is the best incentive and the best way to develop interest in the membership. This initial service was my introduction to the ideals and great work of the American Pharmaceutical Association and here again I am indebted to a fortunate circumstance, an historical event, for a broadened view of life and of the responsibilities of pharmacy. It brought me into friendly contact with a host of pharmacists, the leaders in the profession, through out the country and in some foreign lands. Enjoyable have been the friendships established, delightful the correspondence enjoyed and of inestimable value the knowledge of human nature as well as that of the scientific facts gained by the contact and association with such men as Maisch, Diehl, Remington, Ebert, Caspari, Sheppard, Hallberg, Oldberg, Eliel, Good, Patton, Holzhauer, Alpers, Hancock, Trumble, Dunn, Ryan, Wilbert and Francis, all of whom have answered the last call as well as those who remain as our contemporaries. There is nothing equal to an active interest in your trade or professional organization for developing one's self. It may not be possible to estimate the return by financial standards but there is a gratification, a self-satisfaction as the reward that comes from service and this is the greater if such service has been freely given without expectation of any compensation. As Penn wrote; "He who does good for good's sake seeks neither praise or reward; tho' sure of both at last."

Since my induction into the service of the American Pharmaceutical Association, I have been kept on active duty for a great portion of the time. At various times I have served upon many of its committees, as Councilor and Director, and as Chairman of the Section on Practical Pharmacy and Dispensing. In 1913, I was elected President and now comes a further signal honor and distinction in the award that is made to me this evening. Possibly, I now have 'earned the right to a rest' but I will not consider this function as an admonition to cease my labors in behalf of pharmacy as such a command will be respected only when it is issued by Divine authority that "Now the day is over."

In presenting to you some of the incidents from the gallery of memory, it is sincerely hoped that the purpose and moral that it is desired to illustrate will be perceived and that these personal narratives have not wearied you. The American Pharmaceutical Association, its ideals and the association with its members has an influence upon the career of every active member. The child forms its habits by imitating those that it sees. Each person intuitively imbibes and adopts some of the thoughts and ideals expounded in his presence so that our characters are materially affected and our careers shaped by our associations. Goethe aptly expressed the thought: "There is no teaching to compare with what we derive from intercourse with others."

The declaration of Genesis that "It is not good that man should be alone" is capable of another interpretation than that of his need for a help-mate of the opposite sex, the truth of which no married man dare deny. Equally true is the assertion that man lives not for self alone. Modern society is based upon the universal desire for association, for companionship, and the interdependence of each person upon the others.

Someone has said that pharmacy is in the melting pot. Cannot the same be said with equal certainty of every other profession? The need for refinement, for reformation in practices, has been the prime motive, the incentive that caused the formation of every pharmaceutical association. It has been the special function of the American Pharmaceutical Association, since its inception in 1852, to keep alive the refining fires of pharmacy and to mould and so shape each refined ingot that it shall serve its purpose of aiding in the scientific and ethical progress of the profession. We can point with pride to some of these achievements and to the progress made often under trying circumstances.

One dare not peer too deeply into the crystal globe or to prophesy too boldly the future of pharmacy. However we must have a vision to discern the possibilities and having discerned what is right must have the courage of our convictions and advocate the adoption. There are numerous signs in the heavens that pharmacy is finding itself and that it is assuming its rightful place among the professions. The function of this evening is one unmistakable sign. Even more so is the assumption of its proper share in scientific research and nothing has been so significant of the determination of pharmacy to recognize and maintain its appropriate place among the scientific and professional organizations than the movement for a national pharmacy building, in which the interests of pharmacy shall be housed and from which pharmaceutical research and publications shall be promulgated, that is now taking definite shape.

Pharmacy is a distinct and honorable calling and the importance of its service has been recognized from time immemorial. The most ancient records show that the practice of this art was carried on by a specially educated class of priests. The Egyptians and the Hebrews both followed such a custom. It seems strange that a practice so long established should in more recent times have become a matter of dispute and that we must now contend for the reestablishment as a principle that the compounding and dispensing of medicines is exclusively a function of pharmacy and that this service so essential to society must be performed only by those specially educated and qualified as pharmacists. It is incumbent upon each pharmacist to appreciate that he has a direct, personal and moral obligation to conduct his business and to perform his services in a strictly ethical manner so as to honor his profession. Pharmacy must shortly purge itself, by drastic methods if necessary, of those who bring discredit upon its code of ethics.

While we must recognize the interdependence of pharmacy with medicine and with chemistry in some of its aspects we must also realize that it has its own distinct fields of usefulness awaiting cultivation. The obligation to supply more exact medicines and scientifically accurate methods of preparation it is discharging faithfully. As a distinct profession, it must develop its own ideal and maintain these with honor, dignity and sincerity; it will be belittling to its standards to permit our profession to become simply a copyist and imitator of others.

One of the most serious problems confronting pharmacy at this time is the mass of restrictive laws and the volume of departmental regulations issued for their enforcement. Without properly studying or enforcing laws already on the statute books that amply control the situation, there is a fanatical propaganda for further and unnecessary legislation. There is something radically wrong when legislation destined to be beneficial and to improve the moral tone of the nation results in widespread disrespect for the law and a wholesale violation of the criminal code and with regulations, likewise, which while interfering with the necessary practices of a profession and its scientific progress stimulate, nevertheless, unethical practice and bring into the calling many undesirables whose elimination becomes an added responsibility.

On a former occasion, I addressed the New York Branch upon the possibilities of pharmaceutical research. The continual expansion of our materia medica is still further broadening this boundless field of opportunity. The introduction into medicine of new chemicals often of uncertain composition and more frequently of undetermined pharmacologic action, the application of the vitamins and of the endocrines and of the other animal organ drugs that are now becoming extensively used are but some of the newer remedies that are calling for investigation. Moreover, scarcely any article in our materia medica has been completely investigated and the scientific and commercial problems awaiting such study are too numerous for tabulation. The call for research is an appeal for the most altruistic, the highest public service that pharmacy can render. The organization of research committees and the guarantee of a thoroughly equipped research laboratory in the proposed new national building are evidences that pharmacy is awakening to this professional responsibility and field of greater usefulness. The development of the corps of workers required to till the ground is the immediate need. Each generation inherits from its predecessors an everincreasing fund of knowledge and must transmit this with its own augmentation to its successors. We are thus indebted to our predecessors and obligated to our contemporaries and to our successors.

I have already acknowledged my personal gratitude to the teacher and friend whose image is impressed upon this medal. It is especially appropriate that the name and likeness of Remington should be permanently associated with this award of honor. Faithfully he carried out his part and performed his duty as worker, teacher and leader. As a teacher he was preeminent in his ability to impart instruction in the theories and practices composing the art of pharmacy and no other man, to this day, has taught as many students in this art and so successfully impressed on them his personality. His book on this subject is the leading textbook in English. His association as coeditor in the recent editions of the *United States Dispensatory* gave increased vigor, authority and prestige to the volume. The eighth and ninth revisions of the *United States Pharmacopoeia* were prepared and published under his chairmanship and it was his genius that cast the model and made possible the scientific advancements that placed our American Pharmacopoeia in the fore rank of such national works and earned for it the title of the "autocrat of the Pharmacopoeias." At home and abroad he was hailed as the leading American pharmacist. No one wielded a stronger or more magnetic influence in our associations. His great love and interest in all matters pertaining to pharmacy continued until the final call came. The last interview that I had with him was but a few weeks before his decease. Propped up in bed, with the evidence of his serious illness showing in his countenance, his indomitable will never failed and with energy he discussed the efforts being made to create a pharmaceutical corps in the U.S. Army and he planned how he might aid in presenting the need therefor to Surgeon General Gorgas.

Each of those who have been honored by the award of this medal represents a different type of service to pharmacy. I have been endeavoring to determine to my own satisfaction how the committee appraised the services of the present recipient and in answer to queries propounded by several friends I was not able to point out any particular accomplishment of the year, any masterpiece, that would deserve this signal honor. The speakers of this evening have informed you that the award was made because I was a pharmacist. I am indeed happy to accept their judgment. Self-respect prevents me from underestimating whatever service it has been my privilege to render to pharmacy and modesty forbids my overestimating the value thereof.

It is a peculiar coincidence that the five recipients of this award are all members of the New Jersey Pharmaceutical Association and that three of these reside within the borders of the 'garden state.'

I appreciate the distinction of this occasion above all of the honors that have come to me. Cherished will ever by the memory of this evening. ■

1925 Remington Medalist

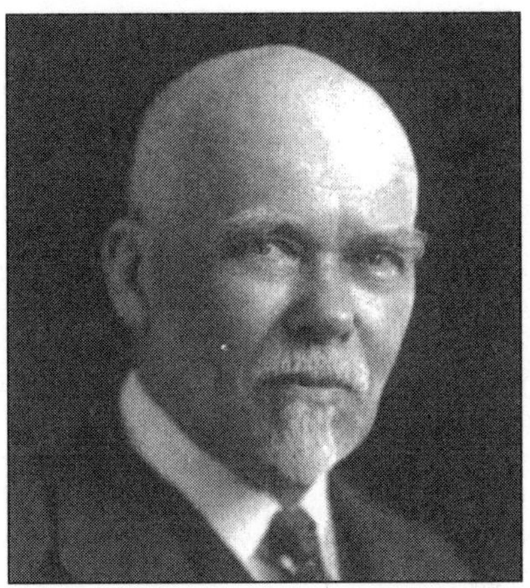

Henry Milton Whelpley
(1861-1926)

Henry Milton Wheipley was born in Harmonia, Michigan, and was an 1883 graduate of the St. Louis College of Pharmacy. He received an M.D. degree from the Missouri Medical College in 1890, and became dean of the St. Louis College of Pharmacy in 1904. His collection of Indian archeology gained him worldwide fame, and he served for more than a decade as vice president of the Archeological Institute of America, as well as president of the St. Louis Anthropological Society and the St. Louis Academy of Science. For a quarter of a century, Wheipley served as secretary of the Missouri Pharmaceutical Association.

Joining APhA in 1884, he served as secretary of the APhA Council 1902-1908 and APhA treasurer 1908-1921. As APhA president 1901-1902, he presided over the Association's golden anniversary annual meeting in Philadelphia delivering a memorable historical address. He also served as president of the American Conference of Pharmaceutical Faculties 1905-1906, and secretary of the U.S. Pharmacopeial Convention from 1900 until his death.

Traits of Human Nature

Henry Milton Whelpley

The 1925 Remington Honor Medal Lecture was presented May 25, 1925, at the Hotel Pennsylvania in New York City. Wheipley's Remington address was published in the *Journal of the American Pharmaceutical Association,* volume 14, pages 521-524, June 1925.

To explain life is as difficult as it is to define a person. As viewed today, life is the most unique and exceptional of phenomena. However, the functions of life are legitimate subjects for our study.

The biologist has so broad a purview of life and liberal conception of creation that he regards human beings as but one kind of organism in the midst of a myriad of other organisms.

In every-day routine life, few of us think in as broad terms as the biologist. We are restricted to what most concerns our momentary welfare or pleasure.

Thus it is that tonight I am impressed with the trait of human nature that encourages the recognition of real or supposed merit and the conferring of honors.

This is but an infinitesimal part of the totality of what exists. It is, however, the special prompting of the human heart and expression of the mind which has brought us together.

It is a human attribute that must have become manifest early in the life of primitive man. Certainly, it has made life worth the living for countless passive recipients of honors and many times the number of active donors.

It is often said that our present-day life tends to dull our finer sensibilities. That in the panorama of the world, modern competition and constantly feverish activities have robbed this generation of those kindly traits of character that instinctively draw people together in noble thoughts and worthy actions.

Too often does it appear true that the exalted ambitions of which our forefathers were so proud have failed to descend unto the rank and file of modern man.

Thus, it is with an intense interest and a keen sense of pleasure that I find in the establishing of the Joseph Price Remington Medal the embodiment of a precious tradition.

This award of which I am the humble recipient for 1925, carries with it tangible honor and distinction which I am sufficiently human to recognize and appreciate.

There is another fact inconspicuous in the larger aspects but full of significance to me in my nearer view.

The world will little note nor long remember what we do or say on this occasion. In my mind, however, will remain throughout the continued days of my life a deep impression made by the sentiment and atmosphere of this occasion.

The medal is made of precious metal but the association of ideas which accompany it are delightfully human and of a truly noble type.

At the present time, the medal radiates the deep and burning interest of Joseph Price Remington in pharmacy. It brings to all who knew him the same enjoyment of the expenditure of effort in our chosen profession.

In 1884, I attended my first meeting of APhA. Not having missed an annual meeting since, I am now fairly well saturated with APhA thoughts and ambitions.

Close touch in work and recreation for more than forty years with those who have determined the policy of the association has changed many of my ideals into living realities.

The officers who conducted the 1884 meeting and those elected on that occasion naturally attracted my close attention. Among them were W. S. Thompson of Washington, D.C., who was president in the chair. He was a parliamentarian of rare skill which excited by youthful admiration. When I learned that he was pharmacist to the White House, I was awed.

John M. Maisch was secretary, an office he had held for twenty years, having been elected when I was but four years old. Maisch was not a man who sought out happiness but who found pleasure in the routine of life.

It was at this meeting in Milwaukee in 1884 that I first met the Ebert-Hallberg-Oldberg trio. Albert Ebert, ever alert and usually suspicious, gave me good, fatherly advice. C.S.N. Hallberg was nearer my own age. He enjoyed oral contention and never side-stepped a debate. Oscar Oldberg, a calm, mild-mannered man who camouflaged his stubbornness and usually won out in his own way. John Ingalls, of Macon, Ga., was elected President that year. A man fortunate in his heritage and fortunate in his character. A real gentleman from the sunny south. Among others who attracted my attention were S.A.D. Sheppard, J.L. Lemberger, C. Lewis Diehl, William Saunders of Canada, George W. Sloan, Robert J. Brown, M.W. Alexander, J.M. Good, P.W. Bedford, E.H. Sargent, J.W. Colcord, L.E. Sayre, P.C. Candidus, Treasurer Charles A. Tufts, and John Uri Lloyd.

Joseph P. Remington was Chairman of the Council. This position he had held since the formation of the Council in 1880. As far as I know, J.L. Lemberger, Professor Lloyd, Professor Sayre and I are the only survivors of the 1884 meeting. Evidently, APhA past presidents have a long tenure of life. Hugo Kantrowitz informs me tonight that he also attended the Milwaukee meeting. APhA was but thirty-two years old in 1884 and the attendance small compared with recent annual meetings but at least seventeen of those present in Milwaukee had been or subsequently became presidents of the association. The ideas which animated them gave guided and controlled many in pharmacy. Those just named are only a few of the many APhA members who have lit with undying luster the history of our calling. This should not be surprising, for APhA is as broad as all Drugdom in both organization and purpose. It draws membership from every feature of the calling. Among those serving as president have been retailers, wholesalers, manufacturers, chemists, professors and last but not least ye editors.

I am tempted, yes, strongly tempted to at least enumerate some of those who are still with us and active-men who not only love pharmacy but those whole hearts and souls are in pharmacy. I hesitate because I do not know where to begin and I fear I would not know when to stop.

It is a long call from today back to the meeting in New York City in 1851 which resulted in the organization of the APhA in Philadelphia one year later. My heart is full of gratitude to those sturdy pioneers, our earnest, struggling, self-sacrificing fathers in pharmacy. They bequeathed to us of a younger generation of the fruits of their labors. They smoothed for me the pathway of a pharmaceutical career which I began in 1877.

To those who took part in this initial meeting, seventy-four years ago, belongs the glory of having set in motion the great movement which resulted in desirable pharmacy laws, state associations, NARD, ACPF, NABP, Drug Trade Conference, the improved USP, the *NF,* the *Pharmaceutical Syllabus* and many other paramount accomplishments.

To you who are young in pharmacy and likewise to us who are far past the threshold of life, APhA gives a heritage. Those who organized APhA thought in terms of future needs.

The opportunities of the present are

bent toward pharmaceutical research, the APhA Recipe Book, *A Digest* of Comments on the *USP and NF* and that most worthy and ambitious project, the Pharmacy Headquarters Building.

It is the duty of every one of us to strive to promote true pharmacy. The headquarters movement permits all to do in accordance with their ability and desire. Here is the time and place to bring out the best that is in us without a conflict between the ideal and the material.

The Remington Medalist is selected by the surviving past presidents of APhA. They constitute a living committee of living men, which has now made six awards. A new member is added each year and the expectancy of life suggests the annual passing away of a member. The personnel must change yearly. Thus, it is a living committee, ever growing but maintaining a constant of about twenty. At the present time, eighteen is the number. The members are scattered far and wide and vary in their special interest in pharmacy.

Still they have had the common experience of the APhA presidency. They all have that professional ability so desirable in judging professional ability.

The plan of award is rather unique but practical and proper. It is the idea of giving such a medal and in the name of Remington that is a concrete expression of the wide judgment, generous act and far-reaching power of the New York Branch of APhA when it provided the Remington Fund.

The Joseph Price Remington Medal was established as a token of recognition of the life and work of a man with a broad mind and vast experience in pharmacy.

One who succeeded as Professor in Pharmacy in the Philadelphia College of Pharmacy, the Father of American Pharmacy, William Procter, Jr.

Remington died January 1, 1918. How might his eyes have glistened had he seen himself as we tonight, after seven years, see him in larger stature, with fuller purpose! Remington had a satisfactory vocational success. He desired and planned to live far beyond the Biblical "three score year and ten" but the power of events is greater than the personal will.

But Remington does live in the minds and actions of many of us. The mortal touch which we have had will die with us but his work and influence will pass on unto future generations through many agencies.

Perhaps the most potent single agent of all in rich results is the Remington Honor Medal. The New York Branch of the APhA has good reason to be proud of this prompt and timely action. ■

1926 Remington Medalist

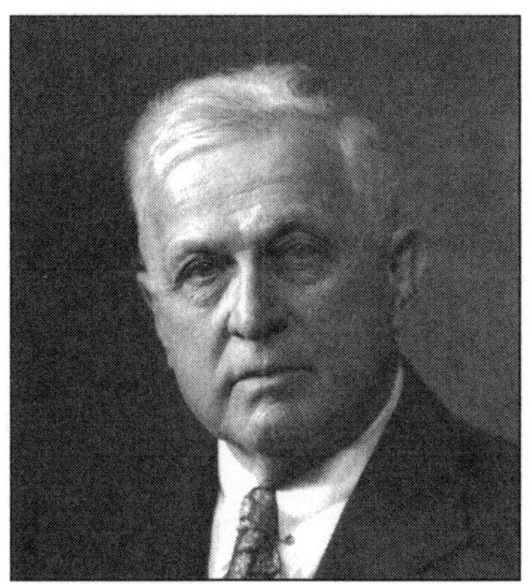

Henry Armitt Brown Dunning
(1877-1962)

Henry Armitt Brown Dunning was born in Denton, Maryland. When only 17, he joined the firm of Hynson, Wescott & Company of Baltimore, and graduated with a Ph.G. degree from the Maryland College of Pharmacy in 1897. After military service with the Fourth U.S. Volunteers in Cuba during the Spanish-American War, he took graduate work at Johns Hopkins University and Johns Hopkins Hospital. He then became part-owner of the firm whose name was changed to Hynson, Wescott & Dunning, Inc., becoming president in 1930 and guiding the expansion of the firm by the introduction of a variety of specialties. He served as president of the Maryland Pharmaceutical Association, associate professor of chemistry at the University of Maryland, a trustee of the Maryland Academy of Sciences, vice president of the Johns Hopkins University Library, and he established the science building at Washington College in Chestertown, Maryland.

Dunning joined the American Pharmaceutical Association in 1902, chaired the committee to raise funds to construct the APhA headquarters building 1924-1928, served as APhA president 1929-1930, and was the founding president of the APhA Foundation 1953-1958. The APhA flagpole memorial stands today as a lasting example of the philanthropy of Dunning.

Pharmacy Headquarters Building Assured

Henry Armitt Brown Dunning

The 1926 Remington Honor Medal Lecture was presented May 12, 1926, at the Hotel Pennsylvania in New York City. Dunning's Remington address was published in the *Journal of the American Pharmaceutical Association,* volume 15, pages 483484, June 1926.

I know that you will realize it is only natural for me to be pleased and gratified because of the nice things said about me this evening, however undeserved the commendations may be.

I can assure the Remington Honor Medal Committee and my fellow pharmacists, whom they represent, that I fully understand and appreciate the high honor which they have conferred upon men, through my selection as the recipient of the Remington Medal. There is not greater honor, in my judgment, within the gift of pharmacy and I am correspondingly grateful.

The New York Branch of the American Pharmaceutical Association is to be commended for its initiative and enterprise in establishing this splendid memorial to a great leader in pharmacy and, consequently, a great leader in the world's work. If we are kept reminded of the great work of others, we are stimulated to attempt greater things and it is only through ambition that progress results; without progress, we become decadent.

It seems to me that there never has been a time in the history of pharmacy when leadership was more needed, for the problems to be met are perhaps more difficult and intricate than ever before. It is, therefore, fitting that in honoring one of our great leaders, who gave so much of himself to pharmacy, we recognize our own obligation to give something of ourselves to the service of our calling, so that it will fulfill its proper mission and obtain the recognition which it so richly deserves. It sometimes seems to me that we pharmacists are not so self-respecting as we should be; it is only in proportion to our respect for ourselves that we impress upon others respect for us. We give, I believe, a service to humanity which is not excelled by the representatives of any other calling. I speak not only of the evident service so continuously available to the public through retail stores, corner or otherwise, distributed throughout the country, which offer shelter from rain and sun, resting places, free services, clean and wholesome surroundings, courteous attention and helpful advice, but also of the services of highly trained and technically educated, intelligent men and women who dispense potent drugs and chemicals and powerful remedial agents with the knowledge and intelligent care required to safeguard their patrons.

Until the drugless era arrives, and that does not seem to be in immediate prospect, the lives of the people of the country can be said to be in the hands of the druggists to a far greater degree than in those of any other class, profession or trade. If the public but realized that in every drug store there are constantly at hand, literally, hundreds of dangerous drugs, concerning which the druggist must have a full knowledge, not only of their individual properties, but when they are mixed together, and that druggist must be and is constantly on guard to insure the dispensing of the proper drugs, in the proper doses and under the proper conditions so that the life and health of his patrons are safeguarded, greater recognition and appreciation would be accorded pharmacy.

When I think of the great services of such men as Remington, Procter, Maisch, Caspari, Rice, and other great leaders and the service of each individual, self-respecting pharmacist, and the small recognition accorded him, I can reach but one conviction-we are poor advertisers. Let us, then, honor our great men as other professions do. Let us advertise ourselves and our service.

This brings to mind the Pharmacy Headquarters Building project and its great purpose. I have talked and written so much about this great enterprise for the benefit and service of pharmacy and humanity that I hesitate to impose upon you at this time. You know that the Pharmacy Headquarters Building is being promoted by the American Pharmaceutical Association and will be conducted under its auspices for the benefit and service of all pharmaceutical interests. It has no intention of assuming any prerogatives of the national associations, but to serve and cooperate with them, through the development of a great National Bureau, the establishment of a museum, library, and research department. The Publicity Bureau intends not only to disseminate knowledge to druggists throughout the country, develop propaganda to the public of an educational character, which will result in a better understanding of the great service which is offered and given by the druggists to their patrons, but to extend other services to all phases of drug interests, such as have been so frequently discussed that it is unnecessary to repeat them.

All of these statements which I have just offered to you represent an old story, I am quite sure, but I have some new information for your attention. It might be called an announcement. The Pharmacy Headquarters Building is an assured fact, for the Pharmacy Headquarters Building Campaign Committee has in hand sufficient funds to begin the building, enough pledged to complete it, and we are convinced that so soon as a site is selected and the building is begun, not only will the wealthier interests in pharmacy, or associated with it, come forward with sufficient additional contributions to endow its operation, but the retail druggists of smaller means, who have not subscribed, will do so. Our Campaign Committee has brought to the attention of the executive committee of the APhA Council our conclusion that the Council should recommend to the Association at the September meeting in Philadelphia, plans for voting on the location of the building, and we hope that they will take this action.

The Headquarters Building Committee, the Campaign Committee, and the Building Plans Committee are all in cooperation and in accord and all of our plans are in good shape and we are ready for action. We need more funds to represent complete success, but we have enough to justify, in our judgment, a forward movement towards our goal. ■

1928 Remington Medalist

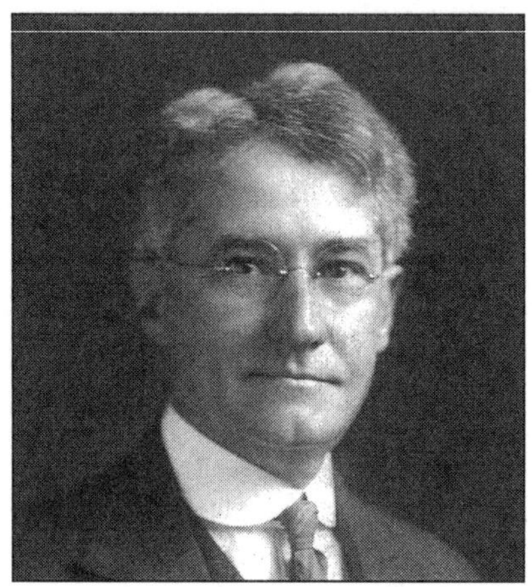

Charles Herbert La Wall
(1871-1937)

Charles Herbert LaWall was born in Allentown, Pennsylvania, served a pharmacy apprenticeship in Bloomsburg, Pennsylvania, and received a Ph.G. degree from the Philadelphia College of Pharmacy in 1893. Following employment as a chemist for Smith Kline and French Laboratories, he joined his *alma mater* as lecturer 1900-1905 when he received a Ph.M. degree, associate professor 1906-1918, and dean 1918 until his death. During this period, he served as chemist for the Pennsylvania Board of Pharmacy 1905-1912, the Pennsylvania Health Department 1906-1918, and the U.S. Department of Agriculture 1907-1912 where he worked with Harvey Wiley. He served as president of the Pennsylvania Pharmaceutical Association 1910-1911, as a member of the advisory committee on medical supplies for the War Industries Board during World War I, and as president of the American Association of Colleges of Pharmacy 1923-1924.

LaWall joined the American Pharmaceutical Association in 1896, serving as secretary 1907-1909 and chairman 1909-1910 of the APhA Section on Education and Legislation, secretary 1911-1912 of the APhA Scientific Section, APhA president 1918-1919, chairman of the APhA Council 1920-1922, and was largely responsible for the first major revision of the APhA Code of Ethics in 1922. He served as secretary of the USP revision committee 1920-1930, as an associate editor for the *United States Dispensatory* (20th-22nd editions) and *Remington's Practice of Pharmacy* (7th and 8th editions), and popularized history as author of *Four Thousand Years of Pharmacy* (1927).

Constructive Public Service in Pharmacy

Charles Herbert LaWall

The 1928 Remington Honor Medal Lecture was presented May 14, 1928, at the Hotel Pennsylvania in New York City. LaWall's Remington address has not survived, but according to *Druggists Circular*, June 1928, "Dr. LaWall made an eloquent address, in the course of which he stated that he had been born in a living room at the rear of his father's drug store which was next door to a library. These facts, he stated, were probably responsible for moulding his career as a pharmacist and author. He gave credit to his father's large and complete library in which the Remington medalist had satisfied his early desire to delve into the study and history of pharmacy."

The following address, which provides an insight into the 1928 Remington medalist, was presented by LaWall at the 1921 centennial exercises at the Philadelphia College of Pharmacy. This lecture was published in the *Journal of the American Pharmaceutical Association,* volume 19, pages 602-606, June 1930.

During the several thousand years through which the profession of pharmacy may be historically traced, it has undergone many interesting changes and vicissitudes. Its evolution has been irregular and in some respects disappointing. The reason for this is found in its lack of uniformity. It has always been heterogeneous, and its heterogeneity has been variable.

The physician-pharmacist was successively replaced by the alchemist-pharmacist, the grocer-pharmacist, the chemist-pharmacist, and later by the merchant-pharmacist.

Through all these metamorphoses there has, however, remained a distinctiveness of service which has been obscured at times, but which in its fundamentals has retained one important phase of public contact and service the preparation and sale of medicines.

From the most primitive beginnings, in which mysticism and credulity prevailed, and in which empiricism held full sway, down to the present time, when a highly specialized technical and scientific training is required by the State for the protection of the public which pharmacy serves, the dominating purpose has been to assemble, identify, select, preserve, prepare arid standardize remedial substances, which in the hands of the careless or unskilled might prove detrimental instead of beneficial.

This history of this famous art is a fascinating chapter of human progress and endeavor. It has its roots in the misty ages of the Orient and among the races of mankind contributing to its improvement were the Babylonians, Egyptians, Greeks, Romans and Arabians.

Differing in detail as to its practical application, the landmarks are shared by its practitioners in all lands and under various designations. Every civilized country has its pharmacopeia, the *vade mecum* of the pharmacist, and largely the result of his labors and researches. The *United States Pharmacopeia* now undergoing its tenth decennial revision, is the second oldest of these national authorities (the *Codex Medicamentarius* of France being the oldest), and in its technical details is a monument to American Pharmacy, which has largely been entrusted with its preparation.

Pharmaceutical education was inaugurated in America by the apothecaries of the City of Brotherly Love when they founded the Philadelphia College of Pharmacy, one hundred years ago. Since that time it has undergone many improvements and changes, as have all other fields of education, but its progress has been retarded largely because of the lack of supporting legislation in many of our States. After many years of waiting we may say with confidence that pharmacy is now on the verge of a great advance in this respect and that in the next ten years more progress will be made than has taken place in the last half century.

There has been no lack of appreciation of what has been needed, but there have been certain forces to combat and prejudices to overcome and much preparatory work to be done. In this connection, credit must be given to the constructive efforts of the American Conference of Pharmaceutical Faculties, composed of representatives of over forty leading colleges of pharmacy of the United States, which has labored unceasingly for twenty years for the adoption of higher standards and the elimination of schools operated for profit alone and not for service to the community.

There has been no failure on the part of the colleges, meanwhile, to educate the students to properly qualify under the State registration laws. The shortcomings have been in not recognizing the necessity of a broader cultural education to accompany the scientific and technical training. The pharmacist of a decade hence will be on a par as regards his preliminary education and cultural training, with the members of other learned professions and insensibly and automatically many of the inconsistencies and evils of the present practice will disappear for all time.

More and more pharmacists each year are fitting themselves for wider public service by taking special courses in bacteriology, clinical chemistry, technical analysis and sanitation, and are becoming valuable aides in public health work and analysts and experts in their respective communities. The stimulation in this direction has been especially noticeable since the close of the war, for it was during that period that many came to realize the value of scientific training and the opportunities which are open to one who qualifies along such cognate lines of study.

The interdependence of pharmacy and medicine was never more in evidence than at present, for with the introduction of biological preparations, including sera and vaccines, and the discovery of new methods of preparing and standardizing long used drugs, the physician is more than ever compelled to rely upon pharmacy for distinctive and important scientific assistance. Pharmacy and medicine have common battles to fight in combating the manufacture and sale of worthless nostrums, and in educating the public along correct scientific lines of hygiene and health conservation.

They are co-sharers, under the law, of certain compelling responsibilities which have to do with the control, regulation and distribution of drugs which are known to be habit-forming, and of alcoholic preparations. It is a gratifying fact that the large majority of the members of both professions are true to their trust and worthy of the confidence reposed in them.

When we pause to survey the new vista and see the wider horizon, we feel that the measure of our opportunities is well expressed by Rosetti:

"Nay, come up hither, from this wave-washed mound to the furthest flood brim; look with me. Then reach on with thy thought 'till it be drowned; miles and miles further though the last line be, and though thy soul sails leagues and leagues beyond, still leagues beyond those leagues there is more sea." ■

1929 Remington Medalist

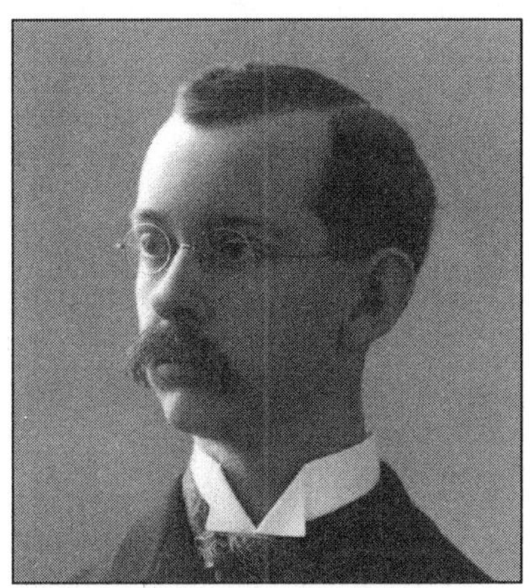

Wilbur Lincoln Scoville
(1865-1941)

Wilbur Lincoln Scoville was born in Bridgeport, Connecticut, and was an 1889 graduate of the Massachusetts College of Pharmacy. He was a member of the faculty of his *alma mater* until 1904 during which time he served as editor of the *New England Druggist* 1894-1897, editor of *Spatula* 1893-1903, and he was author of Scoville's *Art of Compounding* (1895), which went through six editions to 1936. He became chemist for Jayne's of Boston in 1904, and joined Parke, Davis & Company in 1907 serving as head of the analytical department 1924-1934.

Scoville's scientific research dealt with the study of solvents and vehicles in galenical pharmacy, and he received the APhA Ebert Prize in 1922 for his research on the extraction of cinchona. He was a member of the USP revision committee 1900-1940, and chaired the 4th revision of the *National Forinulary.*

REVISION WORK IS NEVER DONE

Wilbur Lincoln Scoville

The 1929 Remington Honor Medal Lecture was presented June 5, 1929, at the Hotel Empire in New York City during an awards dinner of the New York College of Pharmacy. Scoville's Remington address was published in the *Druggists Circular,* volume 73, pages 278-279, 302, July 1929.

First we must squarely face the fact that formulas for compound preparations are fast losing their value and influence.

When the first *NF* was prepared, formulas were a valued possession of pharmacists. Every store sold preparations of its own make, and, in some cases, the formulas were carefully guarded. The old idea that special combinations possessed special virtues still held, and private formulas were prized. Indeed the primary idea of the *NF* was to reduce the number of formulas for preparations when slight variations in color or composition made them of practically equal value therapeutically.

The tendency in medicine since then has been to decry polypharmic preparations and to apply specifics. The development of serums, vaccines and toxins, of endocrine medication, and the better understanding of the action of drugs has emphasized this tendency. Specific medication is now occupying the mind of the physician, and compound preparations are regarded mostly as placebos. Consequently he has but little interest in their formulas. The number of compound preparations that are now official is considerably less than were official forty years ago, and will probably be reduced still more in the coming revisions.

Yet compound preparations are still being prescribed in large quantities, and probably will continue to be in demand. But the physician's attention is more upon the physical attraction of these preparations than upon their medicinal combinations, and he is little concerned whether the formula is standard or not. Thus the influence of the *NF* as a formulary for compound preparations is diminishing with both physicians and pharmacists.

But when one door closes another opens, and this simply means a change in policy for the *NF.* While compound formulas are disappearing, formulas for simples are increasing. Even specific medication has its limits and with the use of mixtures of bacterial vaccines, of serum remedies, and even of endocrine products, steadily increasing, these are signs that even polypharmacy has its value and that compound preparations may sometime returnperhaps in new forms.

While the old mixtures are going out, vegetable drugs are coming back.

There is a renaissance of drugs already begun. Until quite recently we were inclined to think that unless a drug contained an alkaloid, a glucoside, a tannin or an active resinous principle and had a direct action upon some organ of the body, it could not be of much value as a medicine. But the recent studies on enzymes, vitamines and endocrine glands has shown us that while the chemical composition of vegetable or animal substances may be obscure and their mode of action not clear, yet their influence may be of great importance. We do not know what an enzyme is chemically, nor a vitamine, nor the character of most of the endocrine principles, yet the most recent medical and pharmaceutical interests have centered around the action of these indefinite bodies. We now realize that even minute traces of chemical bodies of unknown composition may exert a profound influence upon life processes. This has led to a new study of drugs, both new and old. Some of the older drugs are receiving new attention by the scientific authorities. Such old-fashioned remedies as horehound, boneset, galega, valerian, sumbul, myrtillus, etc., are being studied and new properties have been found in some.

We now realize more clearly that a direct action upon some functioning organ which can be demonstrated upon animals in the laboratory is not always adequate to determine the value of a remedy. As man is of a higher order than the animals, so some drugs have an influence upon men which is lacking with animals. This is particularly true of remedies which affect the nervous system and its congeners.

We know practically nothing about the composition or mode of action of the vitamines but their importance in life processes is universally recognized. We are beginning to realize, through them, that drugs may contain principles, as yet not understood either in composition of mode of action, which may yet be of value; that there are as yet unknown factors in life processes, and that nature synthesizes some principles in the vegetable kingdom which are necessary to the health and vigor of animals, including the *genus homo,* but which are as yet not understood. We are getting new insights into the relations of the vegetable to the animal kingdom and a new recognition of the way that nature uses the functions of the former to supply the needs of the latter. The discovery of vitamines and of the health influence of foods, as compared to their nutritive value, suggests similar conditions in drugs and opens a new field for research.

We are also learning that drugs do not act the same upon different patients, and conclusions must be achieved cautiously. As we know more about the influence of foods, of endocrine glands and of bacterial products, we shall gain new insights into drugs, and particularly those that influence the more sensitive organs. We need to know more about those drugs that act slowly but positively; that lie between the potent quickacting drugs and those of the vitamine type.

The main line of progress in pharmacy during the last two generations has been that of standardizing remedies. As the chemistry of drugs became clear, chemical means of standardization became available. Then came the biological methods, which are applicable where chemical means are not, and today there are few of the very important remedies that are not standardized.

But if the preparation is not stable, the value of standardization is so much neutralized. The dependability of a remedy must rest in the confidence which can be placed upon it at the time it is administered. When an important preparation like Tincture of Digitalis loses 25 percent of its activity in the first three months, then seems to come to a more stable condition, there is concrete evidence that we do not understand the conditions of manufacturing as we should. Even though this tincture maintains its strength after it has been aged, there remains the initial loss which but discloses our ignorance of the changes which occur and the means of preventing them. Ergot is another important drug the stability of whose preparations is uncertain. As our understanding of drug chemistry and action enlarges we shall doubtless find changes in many remedies which are preventable and which will lead to improvements in our materia medica.

As factors in securing stability we need sometimes to start with the fresh drug. Methods of collecting and drying, or of the stabilizing before drying may be the key to active preparations in some cases.

The influence of the pancreas in diabetes was known for years, and many chemists tried to extract its acting principle, but Dr. Banting was the one who proved that insulin was quickly decomposed by the enzymes of the pancreas, and needed to be extracted before those enzymes could destroy it.

European pharmacognosists have long insisted that similar conditions exist in some drugs, and that they would be valuable remedies if properly treated, whereas they have little or no value when not stabilized. They have advocated the killing of enzymes by subjecting the fresh drug to the vapor of hot alcohol before drying, with but little attention from this side of the water.

A recent article by Mr. Grier of Scotland on valerian shows that its action when fresh or properly dried and prepared is very different from the usual sun-dried drug. The odor of the stabilized drug is pleasant, whereas that of the improperly dried is not. Similar results are claimed for other drugs, such as gentian sumbul, and viburnums serpentary, hop, etc. When properly treated these drugs are said to have a very much improved and valuable action. We may need to revise our method of gathering and drying some drugs in order to secure an active preparation, and one that shall be dependable.

Another key to stable preparations lies in the menstruum used for extracting, and also in the manner of use.

We are in a rut as regards extractive methods. All drugs look alike from this angle. Because some drugs yield their active principles slowly, both the *USP* and *NF* have considered it safer, and perhaps better, to retreat all extractions on the same plan and to extract slowly. But there is much difference in drugs. Some quickly yield their active principles to solvents, and rapid extraction saves time. Still more important is the fact that a number of drugs contain antagonistic principles-sometimes chemically incompatible, sometimes physiologically conflicting. Cinchona is a type of the first and rhubarb of the second.

Now the aim of drug extraction is to separate the active from the inactive or undesired constituents, as far as possible and to get the former into a form that is convenient and pleasant to use. Where we have two constituents that are antagonistic, they may differ in their solubilities when we can separate by a wise choice of menstruum or they may both be soluble in the same solvents, but differ in the rate of solubility. Some of our drugs belong in the latter class, and the desirable principles are more quickly soluble than undesired. These drugs are more profitably treated by rapid extraction. Wild cherry is an example. We can get a preparation of better flavor, less likely to precipitate or with a smaller amount of precipitate, and with fewer incompatibilities by a rapid extraction than by slow. The same is true of some other drugs.

Some study of individual drugs is needed on the rate of extraction.

The temperature at which extraction is conducted is a factor of some importance in some cases. Since solubility is influenced by temperature, the reason for this is obvious. Extremes of temperature are probably not desirable, and the number of drugs in which relatively small changes in temperature make a pronounced effect is probably small. Yet the subject is worthy of study.

Hot extraction has not given the results that had been hoped for, except in a few cases, but a moderate warmth-perhaps 100 deg. to 120 deg. F. is often helpful. Yet even here the problem is complicated by the fact that changes in menstrua sometimes gives similar advantages.

The menstrua used in extracting need better study. For our official preparations twenty different strengths of alcohol are used as menstrua. Some of these differ by only 1.5 to 3 percent. It is very improbable that these slight diferences are at all necessary. These twenty menstrua are the result of chance in many instances, individual revisors selecting arbitrarily a mixture without first asking the time-honored question, “Isn't there something else just as good?” The next revisions can well cut down the number of menstrua to perhaps half.

The value of 95 percent alcohol as a menstruum may be questioned. In extraction we have to consider penetration, as well as solubility, and there is evidence that the very strong alcohol does not penetrate drug cells well. Europe uses 90 percent as its strongest alcohol, and perhaps gets better results. Resinous and oily extractives are mostly soluble in 90 percent alcohol, and the extraction is facilitated, in some cases at least.

In assay methods it is found that when drugs are extracted with even such a thoroughly immiscible a solvent as petroleum ether, a preliminary moistening of the drug with water increases the solvent action of the ether. We prefer a 90 percent alcohol for capsicum, but have not tried it for other drugs on which there is promise of advantage.

On the other hand, we have yielded to a suggestion that the alcoholic strength of some preparations can be reduced without first ascertaining whether they will also be reduced in value or stability. A number of our preparations suffer from hydrolysis because the alcohol is not strong enough to prevent this.

The European diluted alcohol is 70 percent, ours is 49 percent. In some preparations there is already good evidence that the stronger alcohol is needed for stability.

We have been judging our preparations almost entirely by physical appearance. If a liquid preparation remained clear, it is taken as evidence that no change has taken place. That is an unsafe assumption. Important changes in composition and action may take place without being shown by physical appearance. Some of these can be proved now; others may need further developments in methods and in our knowledge of constituents and action before we can get satisfactory evidence of a change of importance. In some drugs we already have good evidence of a need of change in menstruum.

There are also few cases of inconsistencies in menstrua: the fluid extract being made with one strength, the tincture with another. There is no good reason apparent for such differences.

A fourth method of stabilizing liquid preparations is by means of added stabilizing agents, or by special adjustments.

We have used glycerin for many years, and often with good success, for stabilizing fluidextracts and tinctures, but we have been using it as a menstruum, in which character it is not a success, except for the astringent drugs. It hinders extraction in many cases. It should be used in finishing the product rather than in beginning its manufacture.

Its function appears to be largely that of preventing hydrolysis, and preliminary experiments have indicated that its place can be taken by sugar to equal advantage.

Acids are used, in some cases with excellent results. The alkaloidal drugs particularly respond to acid, both as a solvent and as a stabilizer. As a solvent they have a place in the menstruum, in which they are commonly used. But their function appears to be quite as much a stabilizer as solvent. With the alkaloidal drugs they may hinder the extraction of some other constituents that are prone to precipitate.

The kind of acid used is undoubtedly a factor in some cases. Hydrochloric acid, or an inorganic acid, seems best in the cases of cinchona, conium, ipecac and sanguinaria, while organic acids are used for aconite, hydrastis, ergot, nux vomica and lobelia. For aconite tartaric acid has been preferred. This suggests another action which I do not think has been studied. Since the optical rotation of most alkaloids is an important property in their action, one wonders whether tartaric acid may have an influence in maintaining the natural rotation of the alkaloids. Its preference in aconite suggests this. This is a field that may prove of importance.

Alkalis are still used in a very few drugs-as ammonia water in senega and potassium carbonate in rhubarb preparations. We thought for years that it was necessary in licorice preparations, but have lately learned better. In cascara preparations alkalis are used to destroy the bitter principle, but they also reduce the activity. The general indications are that alkalis are more detrimental than helpful, hence they are of questionable value as stabilizing agents.

The later interest in hydrogen concentration, usually stated as pH value of charming mystery has suggested that a dose adjustment of the reaction may be of value. There is a witchery about the methods and phases of this line of work that wins a glamour of its own and expects greater things than sober reasoning might warrant.

But there is a great interest in this phase of study, many are engaged in it, already it has shown value in some cases. It is being studied on most drug extracts and we shall know more about it soon.

Another field that merits attention is the effect of catalysts in industrial work has progressed tremendously of late, and has produced remarkable changes in some products. A review of the nature and use of catalysts as used in other lines may lead to an application of this principle to some pharmaceutical preparations.

This work needs to be done by workers who are posted on physicochemical methods and are able to apply the needed technique. Whether it may accomplish much for pharmacy is an open question, but at least it is worth some study. We cannot afford to ignore any line of chemical development, for any phase may prove adaptable to pharmaceutical problems.

We realize more clearly the need for supplementing standardization with stabilizing, and all the latest resources of chemistry may need to be applied to this line.

These are some of the problems which the next revision committee should consider. And they include only one phase of the work. There are chemical problems, botanical problems such for instance as how to spell xanthoxylum-assay problems, pharmacognostic problems, posology problems and pharmaceutical problems as well. Certainly the next revision committee will have no lack of problems.

And this is not our legacy to them. The legacy of revision comes from the future, rather than the past. It is preparation rather than record. It looks to the present for information and tools, and applies them to the future. Its work is always ahead.

And that adds another problem how best to develop and maintain continuous revisioh work, For such problems as I have suggested are not to be solved in the short time of revision. Some are life problems. If treated spasmodically their solution is far in the future. If treated systematically future revisions will soon be on a more sound scientific basis.

Revision work, like woman's work, is never done. ■

1930 Remington Medalist

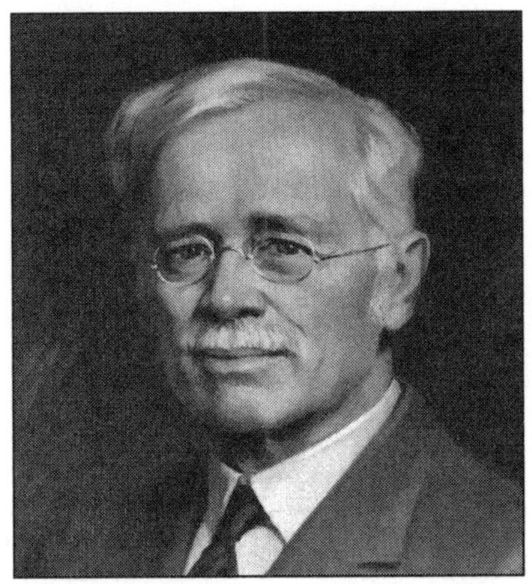

EDWARD KREMERS
1865-1941

Edward Kremers was born in Milwaukee, Wisconsin, and received a Ph.G. in 1886 and M.S. in 1888 from the University of Wisconsin. He then travelled to Germany where he earned a Ph.D. from the University of Goettingen in 1890. He returned to Madison as instructor 1890-1892 and director of the course in pharmacy 1892-1935 at the University of Wisconsin where he introduced the first four-year course in pharmacy in the U.S., the first Ph.D. course with a major in pharmacy, and the first course in the history of pharmacy. He served as editor of the *Pharmaceutical Review* 1896-1909 and *Pharmaceutical Archives* 1898-1903, and as co-editor of the *Standard National Dispensatory.* He served on the USP revision committee 1900-1910, president of the American Association of Colleges of Pharmacy 1902-1903, and president of the Wisconsin Pharmaceutical Association 1930-1931.

Kremers was recipient of the American Pharmaceutical Association Ebert Prize in 1887 and 1900, served as chairman of the APhA Scientific Section 1897-1898, APhA historian 1902-1912, during which time he initiated the formation of the APhA Historical Section, and as APhA honorary president 1933-1934. Many will remember him as the co-author (with George Urdang) of *Kremers and Urdang's History of Pharmacy* (1940) in which he declared in the Preface that Madison, Wisconsin, is "the natural birthplace of the history of American pharmacy."

A Self-Made Man Is a Man To Be Respected

Edward Kremers

The 1930 Remington Honor Medal Lecture was presented May 6, 1930, at the Hotel Emerson in Baltimore during the banquet of the 78th American Pharmaceutical Association annual meeting. Kremers' Remington lecture has not survived, but the following address which he made four days later at the University of Maryland School of Pharmacy captures his views of the reform in American pharmaceutical education and is published in *The First Century of the Philadelphia College of Pharmacy* 1821-1921, Joseph W. England, editor, pages 319-322, 1922.

When Peter Lehmann in 1821 told his fellow druggist, Henry Troth, of Philadelphia: "Henry, this won't do, the University has no right to be taking our boys away at noon to make them M.D.'s" he sounded the note of independence of the apothecary from the physician so far as the education of his apprentices were concerned. But he seems also to have struck the death knell of a pharmaceutical curriculum by the old colleges of the east. In 1893 the late President Elliot visited Wisconsin. Doctor Adams introduced your speaker to the veteran educator of Harvard as the "Dean of Pharmacy," a compliment that was cheaper than a corresponding salary. "As yet we have not undertaken to teach that subject" was Elliot's reply. To speculate on how different the history of pharmaceutical education in this country might have been, had Harvard, Yale, Princeton, not to include Johns Hopkins of more recent date, taken upon themselves to teach pharmacy, may be useless at the present time.

This much, however, we know: the druggist of Philadelphia, who had declared home rule in 1821, as soon as they began to look about for lecturers, realized their dependence upon medical men as teachers. We also know that for half a century, the "school" was but a "fortbildungsanstalt," a continuation school. What the apprentice and clerk had learned behind the prescription counter and in the laboratory during the day, the lecturer attempted to systematize for them in several evening lectures during the winter months. To the credit of the Philadelphia College of Pharmacy be it said that it always took its "school" seriously, whereas some of the other colleges accomplished but little in this direction, or nothing at all.

For half a century the lecture system was about the only means of instruction used. It certainly was the cheapest. Moreover, it was justified by those who employed it because the student's real school was the drug store. The lecture summarized and supplemented the knowledge and experience there acquired. Whatever may be said about the classics and the humanities generally during this period scientific education and with it, the professional education of the engineer, the chemist, the physician, did not stand still. The shop of the engineer and the office of the physician had been replaced in large part by college laboratories. Pharmacy was reluctant to follow. The drug store was still looked upon as the essential mans of instruction. Moreover, laboratory instruction was costly and the old line colleges, being without endowment, where dependent almost entirely upon students' fees. It was Michigan that took the first step to substitute systematic laboratory instruction for the apprenticeship system which, for the most part, never had any great educational value for the simple reason that the average druggist of this country has never been an educated pharmacist. There were a few preceptors with whom an apprenticeship meant a liberal education, but they were few and far between.

When Michigan made application to membership in the old Conference of Colleges, she was refused admission because she did not demand drug store experience for graduation. Nevertheless, the example of Michigan was followed by other state universities. Moreover, the trend away from apprenticeship became more marked with each year. When, therefore, in 1900 the second Conference was organized, not one of college organization, but of pharmaceutical faculties, the stone that had been rejected in the seventies was made the cornerstone, and Prescott was elected the first President of the Conference. But even before this another step had been taken, which, so far as it did not remain unnoticed, received little else than ridicule. Thus the Dean of Northwestern, who, in the name of efficiency, had concentrated the former so-called two-year course into one calendar year, suggested that someone might be crazy enough-though he did not use this word to offer an eight-year course. This criticism amused. But it did not hurt when Professor Prescott replied to a question as to what he thought of the step: "It will do no harm." The young innovator had looked up to his venerable colleague for encouragement and had received a shrug of the shoulder. This was in 1893. Soon thereafter, President James, then of Northwestern, left his Evanston Campus to address the pharmacy students in Chicago. He told them that every boy and girl aspiring to become a pharmacist should take a four-year course at college. It was also a few years later that Professor Prescott wrote: "We are contemplating giving a four-year course. What has been your experience?" When, in 1892, President Chamberlin asked me how many students I expected in the proposed four-year course, I replied: "Mr. President, I am not concerned with numbers, but with an ideal." Today this ideal has become the practical. Georgia, Iowa, Minnesota, Michigan, Washington, and possibly others, have gone Wisconsin one better by making it the only undergraduate course. In a few years it will be the only course offered by the members of the American Association of Colleges of Pharmacy.

If Wisconsin allowed some of her sister institutions to take this final step first, for reasons that were local and need not be discussed here, she did not rest content with this beginning that placed pharmacy on a par with the other college courses on the campus. For it was but a first step to place the pharmacy course on the same academic footing with other courses leading to the A.B. and B.S. degrees. The graduate of the pharmacy course was no more to be looked upon as a full-fledged pharmacist than the graduate of the engineering course was accepted as an experienced engineer. As Dean Johnson put it so aptly: "Our graduates are not engineers, but men with a capacity to become engineers." So our graduates were not turned out as pharmacists, but as men and women with a capacity to become pharmaceutical practitioners.

If we had succeeded in laying a foundation, broad and strong, the next step was the erection of the superstructure. This meant graduate, not post-graduate work. Graduate, not post-graduate study, implied the capacity to do independent work. This could best be taught by research. At first we were permitted to give the degree of Doctor of Philosophy with Pharmaceutical Chemistry as major. Pharmaceutical Botany under Dr. True, a recent disciple of Pheffer, the noted plant physiologist at Leipzig, followed. When, however, we offered Pharmacy as major, a battle was on, a battle of which your present Dean can tell a story. Pharmaceutical chemistry, after all, was chemistry, and pharmaceutical botany was, but pharmacy, God forbid!

If his colleagues of the Philosophical Faculty at Giessen had accused . Liebig of introducing the methods of the kitchen into academic procedure, we were accused of doing something equally abhorrent or even worse. Had not a few years before a superintendent of public instruction, in his biennial report to the Governor, made the statement that the University would be justified in teaching how to make boots and shoes if she persisted in giving instruction in butter making and pharmacy. Well, strange things have happened educationally since the days of Liebig a hundred years ago. Not only did we win the fight but in 1926 the Department of Pharmacy had six successful candidates for the doctorate, five of whom took it with pharmacy as major.

Thus the highest degree given in course by any university is now being given without question to students who have pursued the graduate triennium in pharmacy.

But what of the practical results of this academic achievement? Without going into details, let us consider a few typical cases.

1. A Maisch could wait on the customers of his drug store during the day and lecture on botany and materia medica in the evening. During the winter months he attended to his duties as Dean of the Philadelphia College of Pharmacy and during the summer months to those as Secretary of the APhA. In addition, as editor, he published monthly issues of the *American Journal of Pharmacy.* Today these offices are filled by five men. Not that the capacity of these five men had deteriorated. The offices call for different types of specialization. The good old times when a well-posted retail pharmacist with an itch to teach could be made a college professor by his friends have passed. The practice of pharmacy calls for one kind of training; the duties of the teacher demand a different kind of experience as well as a deeper and broader education.

2. There exists in this broad country of ours a college of pharmacy in a large industrial community. The pharmaceutical industries of that area have innumerable problems to be solved. However, the directors of these industries do not, for the most part, go to their college of pharmacy with their scientific difficulties. They go to the chemical laboratories of local and even distant universities for solutions of their larger research problems. Needless to state, that particular institution is still continuing exclusively along the older lines of undergraduate instruction.

3. The third attainment, if such it may be called, is even more negative in character. At the Indianapolis meeting in 1917 the perennial question of the status of the pharmacist in the Army and Navy was up for consideration. I ventured to suggest that, in order to give pharmacists in Government service a status before the Civil Service Commission, an educational requirement of a four-year course leading to one of the accepted bachelor's degrees be demanded as prerequisite. Unfortunately for my suggestion, none of the eastern colleges at that time offered such a course, yet they were most interested in supplying prospective candidates for these positions. Today the higher ranks of Navy pharmacists are again up for discussion before Congress. Interested as I am in advancing the position of the pharmacist in the Government, be it in its civil or military branches, I can but express my regret that those who are most ardently seeking to bring about this advancement, did not see fit to go a step farther. The pharmacist in Government service cannot expect full recognition until he presents himself with an educational background equal or superior to that of professional men in medicine, an educational background equal or superior to that of professional men in medicine, engineering, chemistry, botany. Your own dean, when in the Hygienic Laboratory doing the duties of pharmacist, not in the official but in the real sense, was listed in the civil service as pharmacologist. The official pharmacists were store keepers and, I am told, are such today. So long as this condition lasts, pharmacists in Government Service will not receive that recognition which we so much desire. To our Government we must offer the very

best educated of our young men and none else.

Please do not misunderstand me. The socalled self-made man, though he be not as common today as he was in the past, is still a man to be respected if not always admired. As the late President Roosevelt once put it: "The college graduate is not necessarily better than the non-graduate. He should, however, be better than he would have been without his four years of under-graduate experience on the college campus." The doctor of philosophy, as a German professor once put it, at least in a story told by the late President Ira Remsen of your Johns Hopkins University, may be nothing but an "Esel." Nevertheless, the bachelor and the doctor of our American colleges and universities have captured for themselves places, not only in our social fabric, but in industry, even in commerce. Medicine, law, engineering, journalism, chemistry, teaching, are no longer satisfied with the education and training characterized by the bachelor's degree, but demand that which is the equivalent of the master's degree and in not a few instances that which is the equivalent of the doctor's degree.

If there are the "asses" among our doctors of philosophy, this fact has not changed the trend of the times. Pharmacy, it must be confessed, has not kept fully abreast with this change. However, the endowments which some of our older colleagues have acquired, or the support which some of them, like your own, are now receiving from the state, are making possible this important change so far as our educational institutions are concerned. When once this change has become general, it will be translated into universal practice, though that may require a generation and more before it can be fully accomplished.

In this transition stage, the old Maryland College of Pharmacy with its fine traditions of a Caspari, a Simon, a Culbreth, and with its present status as an integral part of the University of Maryland, endowed with two millions of tax payers to borrow a phrase of the late Governor Peck of Wisconsin, better known to most people as the author of Peck's Bad Boy's bound to play an important role. The fine building, the dedication of which we have come to celebrate, will afford an admirable physical background for the work it is to accomplish. Its faculty is full of promise of the right spirit to bring to a successful accomplishment the new undertaking. Its alumni and friends, while true to the memory of the past, will, no doubt, enter into this new spirit of enthusiasm. I am convinced that this new institution, the cornerstone of which, figuratively speaking, we have laid today, will develop into an educational structure the influence of which will be felt not only in this good city of Baltimore, not only in this great commonwealth of Maryland, but throughout the length and breadth of this our native land. ■

1931 Remington Medalist

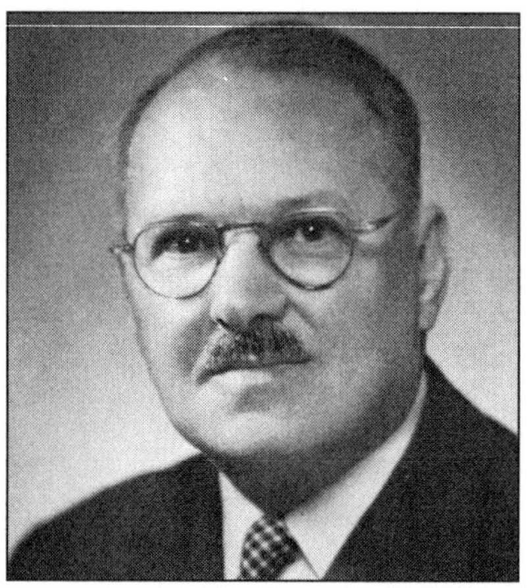

Ernest Fullerton Cook
(1879-1961)

Ernest Fullerton Cook was born in Lionsville, Pennsylvania, and after serving an apprenticeship with Mentzer and Clugston of Waynesboro, Pennsylvania, he received a PD degree from the Philadelphia College of Pharmacy in 1900 while working at the pharmacy of George M. Beringer in Camden, New Jersey. He joined his *alma mater* as assistant to Joseph Remington working on the U.S. *Pharmacopoeia* (8th revision) and *Remington's Practice of Pharmacy* (4th to 6th editions) while experimenting on galenical preparations. He also assisted in the establishment of a dispensing laboratory at the College where he served as professor of operative pharmacy and business administration. He was elected as a member of the USP revision committee in 1918, and served as chairman of the USP revision committee 1920-1940.

Cook took an active role in international drug standardization after graduate work at the University of Berne, Switzerland 1926-1927, serving as a member of the International Commission of Pharmacopoeial Experts 1937-1954, and as a co-editor of the *International Pharmacopoeia.* He served as American Pharmaceutical Association honorary president 1954-1955.

PHARMACY, REMINGTON, AND THE *USP*

Ernest Fullerton Cook

The 1931 Remington Honor Medal Lecture was presented November 16, 1931, at the Hotel Pennsylvania in New York City. Cook's Remington address was published in part in the *Journal of the American Pharmaceutical Association,* volume 20, pages 1264-1267, December 1931. Cook's entire Remington address is published here for the first time from an original manuscript because it includes a vivid insight into the life of Joseph P. Remington.

The Award of the Remington Medal brings vividly to mind the personality and accomplishments of Remington himself. That such a medal should have been established and regularly presented for more than a decade is a recognition of qualities of mind and spirit which have inspired many who counted him their friend and which, in review, should offer stimulation and an ideal to many young men who were not privileged to know him personally.

Through his boyhood he lived in an atmosphere of implicit faith in Divine guidance as touching every activity of life. He was taught and guided in principles of honor, honesty and morality by a loving mother of rare test; his daily contact was with a spirit of humanitarian service which his physician father practiced, and yet he was early in life thrown upon his own resources and subjected to conditions which developed self reliance and character.

Throughout his life he retained this simplicity of faith and before making momentous decisions always placed himself in a reflective mood, and as he expressed it, "listened for the voice."

His brothers and sisters had been sent to the Friends' School at Westown but after his father's death, economy was necessary and he entered the "Central High" and was always proud of his graduation from that justly famous school.

Remington knew his own mind and it was his decision that he would study pharmacy. He was fascinated by chemistry and the sciences when in high school and had a practical and inventive mind and pharmacy made a strong appeal.

Now came a series of new impressions to stimulate and mould his character and life. Was it a more coincident that this Quaker boy, quiet, modest and without special influence, should have associated during the next few years with the most forceful personalities in the American Pharmacy of his generation, yes, of this century?

His first drug store experience was an apprenticeship with Charles Ellis, the head of a firm of wholesale manufacturing and retail druggists and also at that time the president of the Philadelphia College of Pharmacy. Here he came into friendly and helpful contact with Mr. Ellis. Often, when in a reminiscent mood, Remington told of his observations and experiences during these four years of apprenticeship. Mr. Ellis, a Friend, always wore "plain clothes" and although the business was largely wholesale, Mr. Ellis frequently was present in the retail store and personally met many customers.

One story Remington often told to illustrate quick thinking and wit, pictured the retail section of the Ellis pharmacy with Mr. Ellis hurrying to the front to meet several Quaker lady customers; he described and illustrated his manner and greeting, dignified but cordial, and then his showing them a beautiful sample of gum arabic just received, which he displayed on dark blue paper, when suddenly from the trap-door over head a shout "Look out below-here comes the precipitated chalk," and a mass of native English chalk, several hundred pounds in weight, comes tearing through the hole in the ceiling, smashes into a pyramid on the floor, and scattered like a thousand comets in every direction. One of the boys had placed a rope around a lump of chalk just imported and hauled it through the series of trap doors toward an upper floor and on the way it had crumpled and smashed to the floor of the store. The rules had been broken for the platform with rope at the corners should have been used, but fortunately no one was hurt and Mr. Ellis forgave the culprit.

Many preparations were made in the laboratory and a firsthand knowledge of crude drugs and milling and manufacturing was the opportunity offered. One of the few youthful pictures of Remington was taken from the street in front of the Ellis store with young Remington standing at a second story window, resting his hand on a large spatula. He used to relate that he had just come from working at a crude plaster machine, which in later years was at the College. The hot plaster was poured into a hopper about fifteen inches long and was then pressed through a slit at the bottom on to muslin or cloth pulled along beneath.

The next step in his growth must have been definitely planned and with a keen appreciation of its opportunities, for in 1876, now a graduate of the Philadelphia College of Pharmacy and with four years of unusual practical experience, Joseph Remington entered the employ of Dr. E. It Squibb, who enjoyed at that time a nationwide reputation as a manufacturer of pharmaceuticals and chemicals.

In later years he kept in the closet of the work shop at Longport, a little leather bag, about ten inches square, attached to a long strap, which he prized because it had carried his personal belongings when he made that first trip to Brooklyn.

He often talked of this period and considered it one of the greatest and most influential experiences of his life. Dr. Squibb must have looked upon Joseph and loved him for his many splendid qualities for he took him into his home as a son, walked with him to and from the laboratory daily, discussed with him his experiments and processes and stimulated his love for the science underlying pharmacy. But more than this, Dr. Squibb left a tremendous impression upon this young mind concerning the all-importance of truth and honesty, principles of conduct which governed every act of Dr. Squibb. Remington loved to tell an incident in illustration of the inflexible character of this famous man. Together they were inspecting some laboratory operations when Dr. Squibb discovered that a trusted workman had unintentionally used an incorrect percentage of alcohol in the menstruum for a Fluidextract of Cinchona. The amount was relatively large, something like a barrel, and cinchona in these days was costly. However, without a moment's hesitation, Dr. Squibb ordered the man to pour it all into the sewer.

Afterward young Remington protested and suggested that they could have recovered the alkaloids but Dr. Squibb replied: "Joseph, the influence on that man is worth the cost, he will never again make a mistake."

Remington often spoke of the mental struggle he experienced in deciding to leave Dr. Squibb. He reveled in the spirit of the man and in his scientific achievements and always regretted that he had not been able to continue in this field, giving his time and energy to research. He often resented the pressure of many executive duties which kept him from his beloved laboratory; but he accepted these as uncontrollable, and as his job, and put into every activity his best thought and service.

His future steps were not blindly followed. It was with Dr. Squibb's approval that he returned to Philadelphia and placed himself in line for teaching. Determined to obtain the broadest foundation he arranged for a position at the chemical plant of Powers and Weightman, where again his personality and ability won for him an intimate contact with those outstanding men of the period. One incident of this time dealt with a business principle and was impressed upon him by Mr. Powers. He often told it with a recognition of its amusing features.

One of the retail accounts was overdue and repeated billing had no response. The amount was not large, something like $28.02 and Mr. Powers called young Remington in one day and told him to go to the pharmacy and collect the bill. Remington said he went with some hesitation but to his delight the customer paid the bill, at least paid him $28.00. He returned to the plant, and, with an evident sense of pride, handed the money to Mr. Powers. Mr. Powers counted the money, looked at the bill, again counted the money and then said, "But I only find $28.00; how about the 2 cents?" Remington replied that he supposed that it would be all right to get the $28.00 and forget the 2 cents, and even offered to pay this himself but Mr. Powers said, "Joseph, Mr. — owes us that two cents just as much as the $28.00 and he must pay it. Now go back and get the balance."

While still working with Powers and Weightman during the day, he became associated with Professor Edward Parrish who was then (in 1871) Professor of Pharmacy at the College. Many here know of Professor Parrish, at least by reputation, for *Parrish's Pharmacy* was the one text book in Pharmacy in America for many years and Professor Parrish himself was a man of culture and education and of exceptional ability. Remington often spoke of him and always with the greatest respect and affection. One feature with which he was especially impressed was his capacity as a lecturer, and I have heard Remington say that the College of Pharmacy never know a more polished or accomplished speaker than Professor Parrish.

But Remington had definitely in mind, as his goal, the Professorship in Pharmacy at the College, and realizing that a prerequisite was a retail drug store contact he opened his own drug store, in 1872, at 13th and Walnut Streets, Philadelphia, a corner opposite the large and exclusive Philadelphia Club and in what was then an excellent section in the neighborhood of many physicians' offices.

In this same year Professor Parrish died and Professor Procter, although he had retired from active teaching, again took up his teaching and kept young Remington as his assistant. This contact must have made its impress upon him, for even then Procter's place as the "Father of American Pharmacy" was established, but the one memory which came to the fore in later years was the indefatigable energy of Proctor in his own drug store in experimenting continuously with drug extraction.

Two years later Professor Procter died and, as opportunity beckoned, Remington with his remarkable preparation was ready to respond.

I have often heard him say that a young man must not be impatient, for it usually requires about ten years of hard work and preparation to be ready for worth while things. This coincided with his own life record, for his apprenticeship in pharmacy began in 1863, and, after a rich experience, he is elected to a full Professorship in 1874. Again about ten years went by, full of activity in varied fields of pharmacy. He was Chairman of the Committee on Pharmacy for the Centennial Exhibition of 1876, established the Operative Pharmacy laboratory at the College, helped to found the Pennsylvania Pharmaceutical Association, became in 1879 an associate editor of the *US. Dispensatory*, was a member of the 1880 Pharmacopeial Convention and elected to the Revision Committee and actively participated in the meetings and affairs of APhA. By the close of this second ten year period, he was ready to write his text book *Remington's Practice of Pharmacy* which, probably more than any other one activity, gave him nation-wide and international recognition.

An incident of this period illustrates the

standard of accomplishment which Remington strove to reach in every undertaking. He had just completed the *Pharmacy* text and had so exactingly checked every statement and figure that he was positive no errors would be discovered. In a few days, however, someone pointed out several typographical mistakes and in disappointment and chagrin, Remington took to his bed, actually physically sick. Mr. J.B. Lippincott, Senior, had taken great interest in the young author and heard how Remington was feeling and to cheer him sent a note in which he stated that he, Remington, should not be so downcast, that his was the common experience of all authors, that even Webster's first *Dictionaiy* went to press without including the word "dictionary." However, this did not lessen his vigilance and care and nothing gave him greater annoyance than to discover an error in his own work or in that for which he was responsible.

The master passion of his life, however, was his pride in Pharmacy and his confidence in its future. He gave to its development all of his own great powers and cooperated with every sane movement of his day which promised the advancement of the art and science he loved. He clearly foresaw that pharmaceutical education must advance with medicine if pharmacy was not to lose its place as an associated medical specialty and in 1895 he took the initiative in advancing the courses of pharmacy in his own Alma Mater so that at that time they paralleled the scope and hours being required for the majority of medical students in the United States.

These glimpses of Remington the pharmacist and Remington the man, are due his memory and they should be an inspiration to younger men in pharmacy. They are offered in remembrance of the years of close association and inspiration, in his company. He was exacting in his demands upon his associates, but he also won and held their loyalty and affection. He gave liberal recognition to their part in joint projects and continuously urged upon them, as a duty and an opportunity, participation in Association and College activities for the advancement of the profession.

There is no intention that I should here present a biography of Professor Remington; I have had in mind only a review of the remarkable combination of circumstances which influenced the character and personality of the man whom we rightly honor tonight through the perpetuation of his memory, and the recollection of the sterling qualities which he possessed.

As he advanced in experience and in years, he received now opportunities continuously and many new honors came to him at home and abroad. Where pharmacy's problems were discussed, he was called into conference for more than a quarter of a century and increasingly regarded as the friend and wise counsellor of every group in pharmacy. This high regard was mutual, for he inspired confidence and genuine affection by his fairness and tact and by his skill in leading his associates into a course of action which reflected credit upon all.

But this brings my thought squarely up to the pharmaceutical situation in 1931 and it leads me to wonder how Remington would have reacted to today's problems. Pharmacy has always had a broad application. Hundreds of years ago it linked the primitive gatherers of herbs and roots in jungle, desert or mountain with the medieval mystic searching for the Elixir of Life or the Philosopher's Stone. As the medical sciences have developed pharmacy has always been associated in the gathering, experimenting, preparing and dispensing of medicines and therapeutic aids to treatment. Today pharmacy serves as a bond between the most intricate researches of the medical sciences and the practical application of these to medical use. This is still the major field of pharmacy and there is no limit to the opportunities presented.

To the unprecedented of the last half century the medical sciences have contributed their share, and the intense activities of chemists, physicists and bacteriologists in health promotion are reflected in both medicine and pharmacy. In this constant search for facts we naturally see two trends. One of these is the discrediting and misuse of some of the older remedies and methods. The other is the discovery and introduction of the new. This situation is revolutionizing pharmaceutical service in everyone of its phases, but it is not destroying pharmacy itself, for many with ability and understanding have foreseen and are meeting the developments as they arise.

It is fully realized that the pharmacist graduating today must be thoroughly grounded in the principles and facts underlying pharmacy and then must specialize either in the sciences or in business, as personal plans for the future may demand. Pharmacy colleges are now equipping and organizing to take their part creditably in this advancing program.

Pharmacy is not worthy of survival as a profession if it cannot recognize and honestly face the new situations of this progressive and searching age. True it is disturbing to be jostled out of one's complacency and discover that entirely new circumstances must be met. Are they, however, less interesting, or are the service opportunities less definite than in the past arid is there not an adequate reward?

To stand still is to perish; pharmacy must awake or the opportunities will go to others more progressive and with a clearer vision.

What are some of the new conditions?

The manufacturing of chemicals and intricate pharmaceutical products are of necessity in the hands of large and modernly equipped organizations. Pharmacists rightly find abundant and profitable opportunity in these organizations. As technical experts in the many pharmaceutical operations, as analytical and research chemists, as managers, officers, and frequently as owners, as salesmen, advertising experts, and as "detail men," they are the back-bone and brains of those organizations, great and small.

No training in the sciences can be too advanced for the pharmacist who would make his place in those business and professional groups. No one can deny that here is scientific pharmacy as never dreamed of in any previous period and with a fascination and a future so large that it has only been touched.

Think of the developments of the past few years; insulin, liver extract, biologicals, the vitamins, arsphenamin, the barbital group, local anesthetics, and new antiseptics. The number is legion and some of these new substances are notable contributions to the maintenance of health and the cure of disease. The medical sciences are absolutely dependent today upon pharmacy's contributions to medical practice and there is no danger that this need will lessen, for the field is expanding and the opportunities are only restricted by the limitations of the pharmacists entering this phase of practice.

As one reviews even the past twenty-five years it is difficult to believe that so great an advancement has been made in so short a time. In this period two legislative measures have brought about a revolutionary change in the programs and established policies of the nation in the matter of truth and recognized responsibility.

The Harrison Act controlling the sale and distribution of narcotics and the Food and Drug Act requiring a true statement of fact concerning foods and drugs, have to their credit been incorporated as the foundation policy of all great pharmaceutical organizations and insure their perpetuation and success. Let it not be forgotten that both of these measures were promoted and made law largely through the initiative of pharmacists.

The activity of Governmental enforcement officials turned in the beginning, about twenty-five years ago, much more energetically toward the food situation, as there was the greatest need. In this field today the results are phenomenal, for cooperation is the policy of the large food distributors and almost universal compliance with food regulations is the result.

In the medical field the problems are far more difficult than when dealing with foods, but tremendous advances have been made and the policy of most producers today is entirely in harmony with the declared principles of the Food and Drugs Act.

It is believed that more and more the wise business heads, working with the professionally trained scientific groups responsible for the creation and production of medicinal products, will recognize the wisdom of a policy which avoids a constant clash with enforcement officials and will expand the program, so ably begun by the "Contact Committee," whereby the manufacturer, who is honestly trying to maintain the ethical ideals of his profession, cooperates with the officials of the Government in a solution of the scientific questions involved, in the interpretation of terms and in the development of methods of analysis, fair to all.

But the retail pharmacist, what is his future?

Dispensing doctors, group practice among physicians, the clinic, the hospital, the expansion of drugless therapy, the abandonment of therapeutic teaching in many medical colleges, the growth of specialties, the chain store and cut prices. These are problems enough to discourage the most optimistic among the older professional pharmacists. There is no panacea for those ills; pharmacy or no one group is responsible for this appalling array of problems facing the retail pharmacist of today.

Each difficulty, however, has its solution and leadership in pharmacy is arising, ready to grapple with each problem in turn and furnish the answer. The dispensing doctor is largely an economic development. The Committee on the Cost of Medical Care intimates that up to a certain point this is justified but beyond it, the doctor must turn for help to the skilled dispensing pharmacist.

Certain it is that this development has given many pharmacists an opportunity to manufacture the products used and to detail and sell them to the doctor. If the retail druggist is alert to his opportunities he may often be the one to supply the doctors of his neighborhood with the drugs they dispense. Retailers often overlook this opportunity. Often it is the chance to do some manufacturing. Here especially the retailer has the advantage if he uses it, of supplying doctors with products which are free from the danger of subsequent proprietary exploitation, after the doctors have sufficiently introduced them. Physicians are becoming increasingly conscious of the use to which they have been put in this respect in the past.

"Group Practice" offers real scientific opportunity to highly trained pharmacists. Every such group needs a well-equipped professional pharmacy as a unit in the organization. Here is no loss to pharmacy but a new field for development-pharmacists entering the medical colleges of this country. True the new departments of pharmacology were expected to supply this need and perhaps so drastic a move was necessary to free the schools from the continuance of teachings no longer accepted by the new group who demanded physiologic evidence of every therapeutic claim.

Happily this extreme view is passing; more tolerance and greater wisdom has come and medicine still accepts a large and important group of therapeutic agents and is teaching the doctor how to use them scientifically and with results.

Pharmacy also has a real lesson to learn from the doctor; unless it is learned the future pharmacist, however thoroughly trained today, will soon find himself out of step with the times. Medicine has intensively adopted the policy of keeping up-to-date by means of graduate schools, short courses in the latest developments of medicine, unbelievably helpful lectures and demonstrations at every Association meeting, local, state and national, and almost one hundred per cent membership and attendance. When is pharmacy ready to adopt a similar program? It is the answer to many of pharmacy's problems of today.

How about the "specialty?" These must not be condemned as a class. Many of the most dependable remedies of today were developed through the stimulus and the financial return made possible by the "specialty." Other so-called "specialties" however, are a menace to medicine and pharmacy and again the solution is largely in the hands of the retail pharmacist. He is supplied with the *Pharmacopeia* and the *National Formulary;* these are intended to provide standard remedies of every type, up-to-date, complete, efficient and palatable, a reliable preparation for practically every therapeutic need. Every recent survey of prescriptions and a study of the formulas and catalogues of physicians' supply houses prove that the official substances are still used far in excess of any other therapeutic agents.

If every retail pharmacist, or if 25 percent of them, were awake to this situation, they would be detailing the doctors of the country with official preparations and samples and "specialties" would be less a factor.

As to "chain stores" and "cut prices" I believe the answer is sound business education. The independent pharmacist, adding personality to a business efficiency equal to that of the "chain," need have no fear of competition.

The future of pharmacy is bright if we are willing to pay the price. Integrity, thorough training, happiness in the service of humanity, and willingness to work. This combination will insure a successful future to any pharmacist.

As the recipient of the Medal this year, I am not unmindful of the honor it conveys but much more am I impressed by the sense of added obligation it places upon its recipients. To justify the judgment of friends, to lend distinction to the memory of a great man, and to serve pharmacy as he served it, is a goal and a stimulus for intensified effort. ■

1932 Remington Medalist

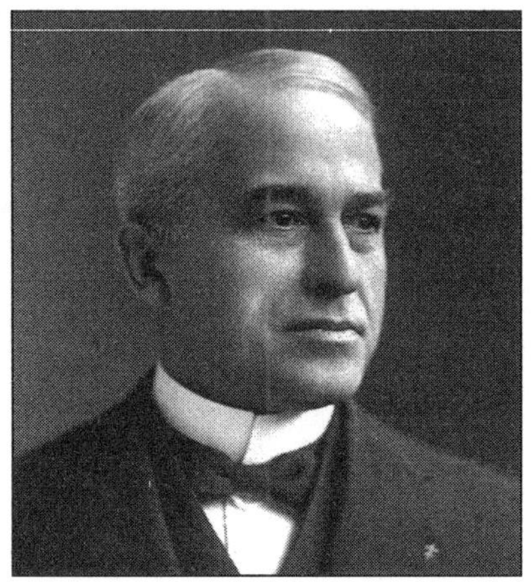

EUGENE GUSTAVE EBERLE
(1863-1942)

Eugene Gustave Eberle was born in Watertown, Wisconsin. After graduation from the Philadelphia College of Pharmacy in 1884, he returned to Wisconsin to practice pharmacy in Madison, but soon moved to Texas to continue in practice. He was employed in 1894 by the Texas Drug Company in Dallas, a position he held until 1900 when he became professor at the University of Dallas department of pharmacy. When the pharmacy department merged with Baylor University in 1903, Eberle became dean of the new school of pharmacy serving until 1915. During this period, he also served as president 1901-1902 and secretary 1910-1914 of the Texas Pharmaceutical Association, and he founded the *Southern Pharmaceutical Journal* in 1903, serving as its editor until 1915.

Eberle joined APhA in 1896, serving variously as chairman of the APhA Section on Education and Legislation 1901-1902, secretary of the APhA Section on Historical Pharmacy 1906-1909, APhA second vice president 1902-1903, APhA first vice president 1908-1909, and APhA president 1910-1911. In 1915, Eberle was selected as the first full-time editor of the *Journal of the American Pharmaceutical Association,* a position he held until his retirement in 1938. The fact that the APhA journal assumed a predominant position among professional journals under his 23-year tenure is a lasting tribute to the 1932 Remington medalist.

Beyond the Four Walls

Eugene Gustave Eberle

The 1932 Remington Honor Medal Lecture was presented October 12, 1932, at the Hotel Emerson in Baltimore at a joint meeting of the New York and Baltimore APhA Branches. Eberle's Remington address was published in the *Practical Druggist,* November 1932.

The Committee has given me the high privilege of being one of a number heretofore selected for the honor represented in the award of the Remington medal and I accept the distinction with a feeling of added responsibility.

I thank all who are here tonight, those who have encouraged me by their letters and messages and heartened me by their friendship to accept the honor.

We reveal to one another what we are by what we do. I lack words which would express to you, my friends, the feelings that possess me. Some of you have known me personally for many years; the acquaintance with others is through my humble efforts in your service. Your commendations impress me more than ever that to err is human, and my determination is strengthened that with your help I will be more watchful and careful than ever in my work.

In a happy vein, the better half of a Texas relative told me in his presence of one of his shortcomings; his reply was that once he didn't do as charged, but he was not credited with that one time. The speakers have reversed the application but perhaps I should be thankful that the spokesmen did not consult with Mrs. Eberle regarding what might be said of me.

Professor Remington was known to me before my student days at the college of pharmacy through my brother, who completed the pharmacy course in 1873, soon after Professor Remington became a member of the faculty. After my college years and going to Texas I heard from him occasionally regarding matters applying to the *Pharmacopoeia,* the College and the Association. Later, it was my pleasure to have him as my guest, when he made the personal acquaintance of many Texas pharmacists. The relationship of a student developed into that of a friend and coworker. I recall visits on a number of occasions at his home when he was the happy host. Sadness tinctured the visits to him during his last illness. On one occasion he said, "Eugene, the end of my days is approaching, my work is finished and I must be ready to go." This view he supported by references to a number with whom he had been associated and who had passed on.

During the years of his active pharmaceutical life Professor Remington held a commanding position and was influential in all matters pertaining to pharmacy. Alumni remembered him even though they never met him after school days his name was the word of introduction among them.

The recipient of the Remington Honor Medal last year who for more than a decade worked with Professor Remington, sketched his teacher by weaving into the warp and wool of his address life stories of his tutor, as told by him during the intermissions of working hours, and the experiences of close association. Other recipients of this honor have spoken of different relations and attributes of the one in whole memory the medal was established.

I am responding to a request by bringing into my address brief references to some who have achieved great things in pharmacy or, after leaving pharmacy, rendered worthwhile services that memorialize them, and also to bring here for your inspection a few books, papers and other historical material of which mention will be made in my remarks. No special groupings, periods or sequences are followed.

Throughout the ages nations have vied with each other in the acquisition and application of knowledge; individuals have risked life and fortune in the search to add to their own information and the common store of knowledge. These researches were prompted and promoted because of the native desire to gain something that the other had not, to measure up to the advantages possessed by them, or acquire opportunities for a community, a nation or the world. Multiplied or divided this gives rise to groups who are better informed or qualified for doing certain work or carrying on specific studies. Investigation, experimentation and application are necessary for gaining knowledge, developing the mind and means of progress, directing thought for the welfare and health of mankind.

Pharmacy has many and varied points of contact, many divisions through which service is rendered and as a result its search for supply and demand has developed other activities and qualified its votaries to be helpful in many directions; it has stimulated thought, and energized action.

Not infrequently the statement is made by individuals who have had experience in drug stores or studied pharmacy that they were able to apply the experience or knowledge thus obtained in other activities they engaged in, often quite foreign to pharmacy, which had been the stepping-stone to other opportunities, and enabled them to render service otherwise than in the applied field of pharmacy for longer or shorter periods. Newton as a youth served Clark, the apothecary in Grantham, and professed to have benefitted by his work with mortar and pestle. Thomas Huxley's thoroughness as an apprenticed pharmacist won him a place in Charing Cross Hospital; honor followed honor to the end of his days, with the earnings of many titles and degrees. In his address at Johns Hopkins in 1876 he evidenced his knowledge of pharmacy. Davy was apprenticed to an apothecary of Penzance, Bingham Borlase, by name, but his experimentation was disturbing to the quiet habits of the apothecary. They parted company and Davy was lost to pharmacy. Hans Christian Oersted was the son of the Danish apothecary and served in his father's apothecary shop and managed for a time the Manthe Apotheke in Copenhagen. This was the beginning of his world service his laboratory experiments in search of some connection between magnetism and electricity and these, according to Arthur E. Kennerly, "have profoundly affected the conduct of civilized life."

While John Uri Lloyd's contributions to the American Pharmaceutical Association in the 70's were considered primarily pharmaceutical they had a further important significance. Dr. Wolfgang Ostwald, foremost colloidal chemist, said that "to colloidal chemistry, as far back as a half century ago, your veteran member, John Uri Lloyd, made contributions of fundamental importance." He said it seemed to him that the public recognition of the science by the American Pharmaceutical Association is coincident of an unusual degree of acumen and scientific farsightedness.

J.H. Breasted, noted Egyptologist, is a graduate in pharmacy and Sir Henry Wellcome is not only outstanding in pharmaceutical and medical researches and promotions but for researches into the earth's secrets as an antiquarian.

Sir Hans Sloane obtained his pharmaceutical education at Apothecaries Hall and Chelsea Physic Garden which he later purchased and presented to the Apothecaries' Society. His library and other collections formed the nucleus of the British Museum.

The premier colonist of Canada, Louis

Hebert, was born in Paris, son of the apothecary to the court of Catherine de Medici, and Louis was trained in the same profession. The apothecary had the advantage of knowledge which aided him in his agricultural work, for as a student and with a desire for service, everything was to him a matter of serious study and, hence, the results of his work contributed largely to the development of Canada.

Henrik Ibsen was apprenticed to a pharmacist, Jene Aarup Reimann, at Grimstad, in 1844, and remained with his successor, Lars Nielsen, until April, 1850. The original pharmacy in which Ibsen spent six years has been replaced by a new building and is known as the "Ibsen House;" the fittings of the old pharmacy have been retained in the new premises. Ibsen wrote "Katilina" before discontinuing his pharmaceutical work.

0. Henry was an apprentice in the pharmacy of his uncle, Clark Porter, in Greensboro, N. C. and, later, was employed for a time in a pharmacy at Austin, Texas. It was in Dr. Pinckney Herbert's office in Asheville that 0. Henry wrote his last complete story, namely, "Let Me Feel Your Pulse." He rests in Riverside Cemetery, Asheville, N. C. It is now proposed to convert the jail which for a time held Sidney Porter a prisoner in Austin, into a memorial library to 0. Henry. The suggestion originated, it seems, with Steve Pinckney of Houston, Tex., whose father worked side by side with Porter in the old Land Office in Austin.

Pierre Pomet, chief pharmacist to the King of France, was born in Paris, 1658. After completing his apprenticeship he traveled extensively in England, Italy, Germany and Holland. On the different voyages he acquired an intimate knowledge of medicinal substances and in due time opened a pharmacy in Paris. His talents and honesty won him the esteem of the most skillful physicians and it was at their invitation that he undertook at the "Jardin des Plantes" a demonstration of the drugs that he had collected at great expense from all countries with which France had relations at that time. He was occupied with a description of the rare specimens in his cabinet at the time of his death in 1699, at the age of 41 years. On the same day he was sent a pension which Louis XIV had granted as a reward for his services.

Pharmacist David Waldie suggested the use of chloroform to Sir James Y. Simpson, noted surgeon, who made the first surgical use of chloroform. A bronze of David Waldie marks the "Chloroform Pharmacy."

Physician pharmacist Crawford W. Long's statue has been placed in Statuary Hall in the Capitol, as the first to employ ether anesthesia in surgical operations.

Sir Joseph Wilson Swan, pharmacist, was former president of the British Pharmaceutical Society and also of the Faraday Society. His work was the basis of a form of photoengraving and his name is widely known in connection with the development of incandescent electric lighting. He preceded Edison in several discoveries and was associated with him in a number of patents.

John Walker, pharmacist of Stockton, England, invented the friction match. So it can be said "that pharmacists brought light to them that sat in darkness."

Liebig and Wöbler were associated with pharmacy, likewise Louis Pasteur. Louis Thenard, while without financial means, secured the opportunity of studying under Vanquelin, director of the Paris School of Pharmacy, because the director's sister wanted a boy to help her in the kitchen. Thenard discovered Hyrodgen Peroxide; he became a peer of France. Otto Unverdorben, Erfurt pharmacist, and Friecffieb F. Runge of Breslau led the way to A. W. Hofmann's discoveries of dyes and medicinals of coal tar. Unverdorben soon entered the mercantile field but Runge remained in pharmacy during the greater part of his life. Hermann Frasch served pharmacy before developing sulphur mining in Southwestern United States.

A multitude of names could be added of those who served pharmacy for a brief period, or during their life-time, and rendered other conspicuous services to their profession or in other fields.

If an excuse should be needed for featuring these relations in my address a paraphrase of Charles Dawes' creed-applying it to pharmacy is my answer-"If you work in a profession, in Heaven's name work for it. If you live by a profession, live for it. Help advance your co-worker. Respect the great power that protects you, makes it possible for you to achieve results. Speak well for it. Stand for it. Stand for its professional supremacy. Do not belittle it."

The Washington Bicentennial Celebration brings to mind historical events and associations of the activities of that period. Pharmacy points out that General Mercer, one of Washington's most intimate friends, was an apothecary and that the building in which he practiced his profession is still standing and contains some of the bottles and shelving belonging to that historic apothecary shop, and in it General Washington had a desk for his personal papers and correspondence. The Leadbeater Pharmacy in Alexandria has records of purchase by Martha Washington, and no doubt, the General made purchases at "Die Apotheke" in Bethlehem, Pa., during his campaigns.

Dr. William Brown prepared a military pharmacopoeia for the American Army. Dr. Lyman Spalding is the father of the *United States Pharmacopoeia* of which the 11th revision is nearing completion. He is entitled to a place in the Hall of Fame; his name should be memorialized by physicians, pharmacists and chemists.

This celebration, therefore, will in some localities be featured in pharmacy windows. Pharmacy Week was chosen as the time for this presentation, when pharmacies carry the message of pharmacy, of which the President of the United States has said, "On the development of drugs and their uses depend to a considerable degree the health and welfare of the people of the world. Daily our laboratories are engaged in the pursuit of newer knowledge which will make constantly more effective the unending combat against illness and disease. The pharmacists of our country are indispensable allies of the physicians. It is fitting, therefore, that each year we should formally acknowledge our indebtedness to them. I am glad to extend to the pharmacists of the nation the good wishes of all our people."

Governor Albert C. Ritchie, of Maryland, has emphasized the importance of pharmacy in Public Health work, and named the latter as one of the essential activities of the State. He admitted the difficulty of evaluating one undertaking of the state above another, which, according to conditions, might vary in importance. However, if it became necessary to make a choice between what the State must carry on and some other undertakings, then the Public Health and Educational program would have to be included among the essentials. He valued pharmacy as an essential activity of Public Health Service.

The public as well as pharmacists should see to it that pharmacists are placed in positions requiring pharmaceutical experience-in Government service, hospitals, and other public institutions.

As you know, the idea of Pharmacy Week was presented by the late Robert J. Ruth at the Buffalo meeting of the American Pharmaceutical Association in August, 1924, in his address as chairman of the Section on Practical Pharmacy and Dispensing. The underlying motive was the education of the public relative to the mission and service of pharmacy. From this beginning the celebration of Pharmacy Week has spread throughout the United States, Canada and distant parts of the world, as well. It is a matter worthy of favorable comment that the thought which was uppermost in the mind of the founder has been carried forward and the educational features have developed to such an extent that libraries and schools are making use of them. Hearty support has been given by national and state associations, the pharmaceutical publications, and the daily press, strengthened by the cooperation of clubs and chambers of commerce and other organizations.

The story of pharmacy has been published in book form under the title of "Fighting Disease with Drugs." The purpose of the symposium is to bring to the attention of the lay readers and the members of allied professions the story of pharmacy as it is related to the preservation of life and the alleviation of pain and suffering, an important part in the world's activities and history.

A story of the world's history and of the developments which came as a result of voyages for making discoveries created trade routes and established commercial relations between nations. The search for drugs has been of great importance because of their pharmaceutical and medical application, supplying the means for protection against disease and conservation of health, and in varied other uses-foods, in manufactures, and arts.

The control of yellow fever, malaria and other afflictions, and the building of the Panama Canal are examples of these contributions to the health and wealth of nations.

While the quest for gold stimulated most of the early ventures searches, pioneering and travel into foreign lands many of the undertakings had as motives the possibilities of finding new drugs, spices, perfumes, and of learning from other people something that would add to the industries, wealth and information of their own people. Few professions have a more thrilling or romantic history than pharmacy, and its discoveries have increased the opportunities of other professions, sciences and industries. Time will not permit a discussion of the results of these voyages and travels, but brief references to discoveries made by several pharmacists in the study of a few very important drugs may be of interest.

The discovery of morphine presents several phases which testify to the service of pharmacy. Physicians and surgeons can hardly do without morphine in their practice and it has not only contributed to the advance of pharmaceutical chemistry but pharmacology and therapeutics. Like many boons of mankind this narcotic has the power of doing harm. Opium has been a troublemaker among nations, and a large Far-East population is held in subjection because of habituation to the enticing narcotic. Pharmacists realizing effects have persistently and consistently studied and supported means for safeguarding the public against narcotic addictions, and the same may be said regarding their attitude to other habit formers and ill-advised use of them, showing that they do not permit gain thereby to enter into such questions. In 1803, at the age of twenty years, Wilhelm Adam Sertürner, separated morphine from opium, while engaged in Cramer's Pharmacy at Paderborn, Germany. The first announcement of Sertürner's work with opium was made in 1805 in Tromsdorffs *Journal der Pharmazie.* Three pharmacists, independently of each other, discovered morphine, but to Sertütner belongs the credit of having recognized its basic properties, entitling him to the distinction of founding alkaloidal chemistry. It was not until 1817 that Sertürner received full recognition for his work. After Gay-Lussac read a translation of the discoverer's work, the Institute of France voted him a prize of 2000 francs. Scientific societies in Hamburg, Berlin, Paris, Batavia, St. Petersburg and Lisbon elected him to honorary membership. This is an example of drug store research.

The first authentic record of the use of Cinchona bark dates back to 1630 when Francisco Lopez de Canizares, Corregidor of Loxa, was cured of the fever by its use; the wife of the Spanish Viceroy of Peru, Countese Ana of Chinchon, about ten years later, brought some of the bark to Spain; the first general introduction of the drug into Europe was by the Order of Jesuits. These references give us four names applied to Cinchona -"Peruvian Bark," "Loxa Bark," "Jesuits' Powder," "Cinchona." About 100 years after the experiences referred to, the source of Cinchona became known through Charles Marie de La Condamine, a French scientist who had gone to South America with Pierre

Bouguer and Louis Godin for an entirely different purpose; namely, to measure an arc of the meridian on the plain of Quito. Aside from bringing back specimens of the cinchona tree, which he described, he made the rubber tree known in Europe.

In 1820, Pelletier and Caventou, Paris pharmacists, studied the constituents of Cinchona and showed that the cinchonine of Gomez was a mixture of two alkaloids; to one of them they gave the name of quinine. They were awarded the Prix Monthyon of 10,000 francs for their discovery of quinine and this was the only reward they obtained for their cinchona researches, for they took out no patents. A monument has been erected to them in the Boulevard St. Michel, Paris. Without quinine the building of the Panama Canal would have been impossible.

In one of the addresses at the Cinchona Tercentenary it was said that the discovery of quinine, important therapeutically as that was, marked but the beginning of the chemical researches conducted in connection with this drug, a most valuable contribution by South American Indians to our European and American materia meclica. Thanks to the manufacture of quinine on a large scale, also thanks to the purity standards demanded by the several pharmacopoeias of civilized countries, the by-products which accumulated became the objects of further research. Today more than twenty alkaloids are known to exist in cinchona barks and the barks of related genera of trees. Some of these have been used as specifics in modern medical practice. One might say with little exaggeration that Dr. John Sappington, who, by the way, is said to be of Maryland ancestry, made the Missouri Valley habitable.

The Gustavian is one of the notable epochs of Swedish history, which includes Linne, Swedenborg and Bellman. Apothecary Carl Scheele ranks as one of Sweden's greatest sons; perhaps no one stands above him as chemist and but few beside him.

The House of Christian Charity, founded by the will of the French pharmacist, Nicholas Houel, in 1584, stipulated that it be a school for orphans to be instructed to serve and honor God, to acquire good literary instruction and to learn the art of the apothecary. Later, this institution became the Paris School of Pharmacy. Among a large number of French pharmacists whose researches are outstanding, in addition to those named are: Baumé, Parmentier, Pelletier. Germany produced many noted pharmacists sketched in Brugg's *Buch der Grossen Chemiker.* Among them Klapproth, discoverer of four elements and one of the compilers of the Prussian Pharmacopoeia; Hermann Thoms, before his death, completed his comprehensive work on pharmacy to which he, with cooperation of about one hundred co-workers and specialists, had given more than ten years of study.

The brief remarks of this address are necessarily incomplete; in fact they are little more than references without any intention to make censorium critical comparisons of the pharmacy of different periods, different countries or the accomplishments of individuals, but deemed sufficient, perhaps, which is a purpose, to impress that pharmacy has a history which is fundamental in contributions to human welfare and progress.

It would please me if time permitted to speak of the founders of pharmaceutical and chemical manufacturing establishments who have added greatly to the industries and to wealth and to improved health conditions who came from the ranks of pharmacists, of the number of those who rendered essential services to their communities, always loyal to them and often unmindful of self.

Looking back and forth and into the present developments one cannot fail to recognize the importance and possibilities of pharmacy, and in this work the retail pharmacies and other divisions of the drug industry share in the medical research. It is true that the facilities and purpose of the clinical, research and manufacturing laboratories are outstanding, but those who know pharmacy are aware that in the pharmacies of today, as in the times of

Scheele, Liebig, Caventou, and many others, discoveries have been made and are being made that add to the common fund of medical research and science, and the sources are often forgotten or credited elsewhere.

Perhaps everyone will admit that if pharmacists magnified their profession to the fullest, there would be developed a relatively greater appreciation of it; and, as a result, its opportunities would be developed to a greater extent, and the public could have a better understanding of its worth. There are few industries to which pharmacy has not directly or indirectly contributed; in most of the divisions of science and art pharmacy has a part and has contributed very largely to the achievements of medicine.

American and European recognitions were given to Dr. Frederick Power in the awards of the Ebert Prize, the Flueckiger Medal, the Hanbury Medal, two diplomas of honor, five gold medals and one silver medal. He is remembered for his work on chaulmoogra oil and many other researches that have memorialized him.

Albert E. Ebert's interestedness and loyalty to pharmacy is evidenced by his will, whereby he gave all he had in worldly possessions to the American Pharmaceutical Association.

As you know, American Pharmacy has under way a Pharmacy Building in Washington. Liberal donations have been made but endowments are needed; it presents an opportunity for making the public better acquainted with pharmacy and the service it renders.

Permit me to thank you for your consideration and again express my appreciation for the honor of this award, which I prize highly because it is a memorial to by beloved teacher, Professor Remington, and testifies to your valuation for the work I have endeavored to carry on, and your friendship which I greatly esteem. ■

1933 Remington Medalist

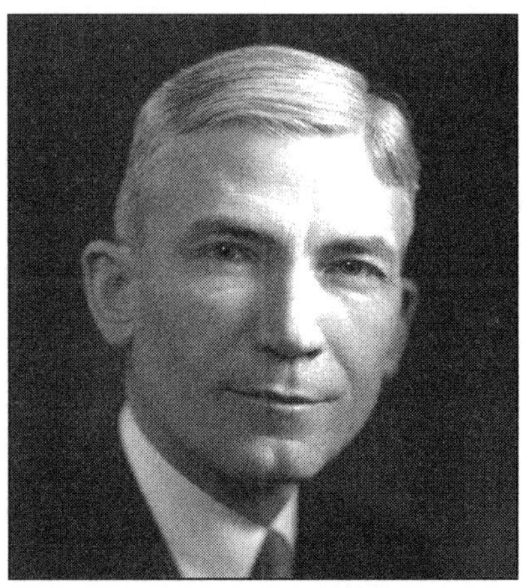

EVANDER FRANCIS KELLY
(1879-1944)

Evander Francis Kelly was born in Carthage, North Carolina, and first became interested in pharmacy when a pharmacist relative asked Kelly to come to Green Cove Springs, Florida, to manage his pharmacy. After two years in Florida, Kelly entered the Maryland College of Pharmacy, graduating in 1902. He was employed by Sharp & Dohme from 1902 to 1911 as manager of the manufacturer's laboratory stock room. He also joined the faculty of the Maryland School of Pharmacy in 1903 serving variously as assistant in the pharmacy laboratory, associate professor 1906-1916, and professor of pharmacy and dean from 1916 to 1926. He also served as professor of chemistry at the University of Maryland Dental School 1918-1926, and as a lecturer in pharmacy at the Johns Hopkins Medical School. He served as secretary of the Maryland Pharmaceutical Association 1907-1942, a member of the *U.S. Pharmacopeia* Revision Committee 1920-1930, chairman of the USP Board of Trustees 1940, and vice president of the American Association of Colleges of Pharmacy 1921-1922. Among his many contributions to the pharmaceutical literature was the 1930 revision of *Caspari's Treatise on Pharmacy.*

Kelly joined the American Pharmaceutical Association in 1905, first helping to organize a local branch in Baltimore, serving two-year terms each as secretary and president. He served as vice chairman 1918-1923 of the APhA House of Delegates during which time he provided the leadership in reorganizing the House into an effective APhA legislative body. He also served as APhA treasurer 1921-1925, and in 1926 was elected APhA secretary serving until his death in 1944. Standing as a tribute to Kelly's leadership is APhA's headquarters building, the American Institute of Pharmacy, which was funded and constructed during his 18 years as APhA's chief executive officer.

A Considerate Professional Mistress

Evander Francis Kelly

The 1933 Remington Honor Medal Lecture was presented on October 11, 1933, at the Pythian Temple in New York City. Kelly's Remington address was published in the *Journal of the American Pharmaceutical Association,* volume 22, pages 1149-1152, 1933.

It has been my privilege to have been connected with pharmacy for nearly thirty-five years and, during that time, to have served in almost every division of it. It has been my privilege, also, to have known a large number of the men and women associated with pharmacy, including many of the leaders in both the profession and the industry. It was my good fortune to know the distinguished pharmacist in whose honor this award is named.

With very few exceptions, mine has been a pleasant experience and a profitable one, not so much in material gain as in the splendid contacts and rich friendships that have been made possible for me and which are life's greatest rewards. My entry into pharmacy was entirely accidental on my part and was intended to be but brief. The work and the prospects were soon found to be so interesting as to lead to the adoption of pharmacy as a life's work, a decision which, so far, there has been no regret. My apprenticeship was spent in a well-conducted pharmacy under a good preceptor, in pleasant surroundings and among delightful people, one in particular. It later became possible for me to enter upon a course in pharmacy in the Maryland College of Pharmacy, now the School of Pharmacy of the University of Maryland, and in this institution, then an organization of pharmacists with a teaching faculty, to come under the instruction and influence of a truly remarkable group of pharmacists. Among them were such leaders as Caspari, Simon, Cuibreth, Hynson, Base, Schmidt, Piquett, the Dohmes, Hancock, Elliot, Mansfield, Frames and many others who impressed me by their ability, their love of the profession and their code of ethics. This circle of friends and advisers has steadily widened in the intervening years, I am happy to say. Their guidance and support have made it possible for me to do the work in which I have been interested, and they contributed to such progress as has been possible to me. The lack of time and my inability of expression make it impossible to name all of them and to pay the tribute to these friends that they deserve. I am glad to thus briefly acknowledge my great indebtness to them.

You will, I am confident, understand a special reference to one of this group. Charles Caspari, Jr., influenced my life by precept and by example more than any person outside my family and it is a privilege to pay this tribute to his memory.

As our British cousins express it, Mrs. Kelly associates herself with these statements and joins me in sincere thanks to those who, in cooperation with our friend, Dr. Schaefer, established this medal, to those who awarded it to me, to those who have spoken so kindly tonight and to those other good friends who by their presence here or by their messages or otherwise have made this a memorable occasion for us and for our children.

The receipt of such an honor is a high

mark in any pharmacist's career and it has led me, with other events, to a rather searching appraisal of myself and of the calling to which my working life has been given. The self appraisal is of no interest here other than to mention that it has occurred with greater frequency as the years have passed and with increasing concern to the oppressed. Certain comments about our profession may be of interest as your working life or that of those dear to you have also been devoted to pharmacy.

The working life of the individual is, at the best, but a comparatively short period of time. To those who live with purpose and effect, it seems entirely too short: to those who merely live, time is of but little importance. During this brief period, we make our entire contribution to human progress. There can be no repetition, no opportunity to correct omissions or mistakes. From the standpoint of the general welfare, the working life is the most precious possession that the individual can give to any cause and, by the same token, it is the most valuable contribution that any cause can receive from the individual. The sum of the working lives of the individuals is the total of human progress.

The choice of the activity to which our working lives is to be given is, probably, the most important decision of our lives. A few changes from the first choice, frequently the first choice leads into other fields of endeavor, but the large majority follow the original selection. Despite its importance, the selection is usually accidental or is influenced by circumstances and surroundings. Possibly, this procedure is Nature's way of maintaining the balance, but the result might, at times, lead to the conclusion that progress is made in spite of rather than because of our own efforts. The selection of those who enter our profession is a question of primary importance to its future.

The success and future progress of a profession depend in large measure, it seems to me, upon four conditions: its necessity to human welfare and comfort, and its contribution to the general good; the ethics and restrictions under which it is practiced; the attitude to the profession of those who practice it; and, lastly, the surrounding conditions.

It appears to be well established that pharmacy was an organized activity when recorded history began, and that it has had a continuous existence since that time. Its history, despite the dark spots that mar the record of all human activities, is creditable and indicates that pharmacy has kept reasonably abreast of progress in other fields. In addition to its own development, pharmacy has contributed to human knowledge and to the progress, even to the establishment, of others. Unless it had been a necessary service, it would long ago have disappeared as an organized division of society. Pharmacy has earned recognition as separate and important division of medical care, through its long service and through its contribution to public health and to human welfare.

Although it has been led astray at times and lent itself to practices contrary to and outside of its purposes, the course, in general, has been so true as to be a source of pride and inspiration to every pharmacist, especially when the responsible character of its work and the dangerous properties of many of the substances it employs are considered. If the past is a guide to the future, the permanency of pharmacy as a public health profession is assured as far as any assurances can be understood.

The code of ethics, and the governmental as well as voluntary restrictions which pharmacy has developed and accepted for its own regulation, are in accord with its aim and purposes, and reasonably bear comparison with those of other public health professions. The training and educational process for entry, the tests imposed for registration, and the restrictions on the practice of pharmacy, are designed to develop a responsible citizen and a dependable pharmacist and to provide adequate service and reasonable protection for the public interest. The approved ethics and standards indicate a rather high purpose for the calling and that its practitioners accept pharmacy as a profession with a clear recognition of the responsibilities and limitations imposed and accepted. It must be evident, however, to anyone who makes himself acquainted with present-day conditions, that pharmacy has not had legal protection, in its file, commensurate with these responsibilities arid limitations, and in keeping with the public interest. Drugs and medicines, because of their nature, cannot be dealt with as ordinary articles of commerce, and public welfare demands that they be dealt with on a different basis.

Two unfortunate conditions contribute to this situation which should be recognized as dangerous to our future. Pharmacy is required to furnish articles as well as professional service and advice and is, therefore, subject more than other professions to certain influences of a commercial rather then a professional character. In the present tenancy to distribute anything and everything, and in the apparent lack of a definite objective, the public sees the widest variations between our professional ideals and our actual practice. Recent developments in government procedures have brought pharmacy face to face with the dangers of over-commercialization and with the necessity for a decision as to whether it shall be primarily a profession or a business.

The second condition is that, while the registered pharmacist is strictly regulated in his practice, those not registered are permitted to engage indirectly in practice. A similar evasion is possible in other legally controlled professions but not to such an extent as in pharmacy. Many institutions, some of which are manifestly distributing agencies in the main, are permitted to operate under the name and reputation of pharmacy without the restrictions imposed on qualified pharmacists. They are frequently owned and operated by those who have no basic training in pharmacy, who are unacquainted with its service or ethics, who know but little about the dangers involved for the public, and who are in the very nature of the case interested principally in the possible profits. Such persons have a useful place in commerce but have no place in a profession dealing so intimately with life and death.

There can be no reasonable criticism of business or of those who engage in it. Business is as necessary to human welfare as the arts, or the sciences, or the professions. Every profession must have a business background and be conducted on sound economic principles. The pharmacist must buy and sell. But he cannot long expect the status and the advantages of a professional man without giving the professional requirements his major thought and attention. He cannot hope to escape the classification of a merchant if he makes business activity and retail distribution his major concern. The law of cause and effect works in our activities as inevitably as in all others. The attitude of pharmacists to their profession must decide this issue.

The general conditions surrounding the practice of pharmacy in our land are probably as favorable as those of other professions. The pharmacist is accepted as a useful and respected member of society. The drug store or pharmacy is recognized as an important institution in every community and has made a useful place for itself in the lives of the people. The jokes poked at it recently indicate that the public realizes how far many pharmacists have wandered from their real function and not that confidence has as yet been lost in pharmaceutical service or in the integrity of the pharmacy as an institution. The Chief Magistrate of the Nation has recently recognized pharmacists as professional persons -and our national and state governments, in connection with matters of great importance, have repeatedly shown their confidence in the profession by trusting to it certain very responsible duties. Recent intensive surveys, conducted by those outside of our profession, have shown beyond question that pharmacy continues to be a necessary public health profession and that in personnel and in extent and character of service, it occupies a position of importance in our social organization. Its ethics, its self-imposed standards, its educational requirements and its equipment are being steadily advanced. Contrary to the statements of its critics and of those who see it as a vanishing profession, pharmacy has made progress in recent years, has improved its service and has strengthened its position as a profession. A keen student of the situation has recently said that one weakness of pharmacy, as we see it today is the failure of the public to recognize the part it plays in the modern treatment of disease. He might have said that the weakness of pharmacy is its own failure to realize it fully discharge its part in public health. The public cannot be expected to recognize what it cannot see and it must be evident that in recent years pharmacy has studiously hidden its public health service, splendid as it is, from public view. Our programs, our papers and our publications have emphasized almost everything else except our public health service and connection, which are, evidently the reasons for our existence and the very basis of our strength. The principal effect of Pharmacy Week, which we celebrate this week, has been to emphasize professional pharmacy to pharmacists.

In the present century, our nation has undergone a voluntary social revolution of the most fundamental character and of the widest scope. Our theories of living, of government, of religion, of ethics and even of thinking have been radically changed. One of the outstanding changes is in the public attitude to health and physical wellbeing. Public health is today probably the most powerful social force next to education and possibly to the church. People are health conscious and health anxious. They no longer look on health as an accident of birth or condition but as something to be won and controlled. Those who minister to health are no longer mysterious and to be consulted only in emergency, but are valued as among the most important public servants.

Pharmacy's part in the treatment and prevention of disease and in the presentation and improvement of the public health is important and creditable. The Charter's Report said "A well-informed pharmacist is the best single individual to disseminate information about public health." The Committee on the Cost of Medical Care reported that "Drugs, medicines and medical-supplies are essential to an adequate medical service, both therapeutic and preventative."

It is nevertheless true that pharmacy has neither recognized its opportunity nor fully discharged its responsibility in the public health movement-as these reports also indicate. Its sixty thousand pharmacies should be looked upon as so many public health situations by the public. In this respect, the attitude of the members of our profession and even of its leaders, has been unfortunate. For its own welfare and future progress, pharmacy should emphasize its present contributions to public health and should increase them to the extent of its capacity. With its personnel, its organization, its equipment and particularly in its intimate contacts with the people, pharmacy could be and should be one of the dominant forces in public health. Now it is considered by many only as a distributing agency and, at that, of many articles of doubtful value to public health.

We should realize, too, that the public have not only become interested in public health but also critical of those whom they have licensed to protect and control it. The existence of a Committee on the Costs of Medical Care, its title and the character of its final report are extremely significant to the public health professions. The serious proposal to even partly socialize medical care carries its own message. Developments in other countries show that it cannot be lightly dismissed.

I have no fear that pharmacy will disappear because of the profound conviction that it is a necessary and indispensable public health service. There can be a question as to how and by whom the service will be rendered in the future. Fortunately, the answer is, to this time at least, on our hands. We cannot, however, give our major thought and attention to there matters and expect this all important question to answer itself in our favor. With a little organized thought and effort, the public attitude could be changed and self-control in our field assured us.

The history of pharmacy, the professional obligations that pharmacists assume on accepting registration and the soundest economic judgement, leaving ethics entirely aside, should influence them to take their proper and responsible part in public health, to contribute their full share in its advancement and to receive the recognized professional status and the return to which they would be so richly entitled. It is difficult to conceive of a greater opportunity or a deeper satisfaction than to contribute to the health and physical well-being of people.

Pharmacy has been a kind and considerate professional mistress to me. It has given me the opportunity to live a full life in a worth while calling. It has honored me and I have thoroughly enjoyed my life. If a text had been a part of these remarks, the following would have been my choice:

Wherefore I perceive that there is nothing better, than that a man should rejoice in his own works: for that is his portion: for who shall bring him to see what shall be after him?

I like to paraphrase St. Paul's statement to read, "They are members of no mean profession."

Pharmacy and those who practice it, have had and will have my fullest confidence and support so long as it is permitted to give them. ■

1934 Remington Medalist

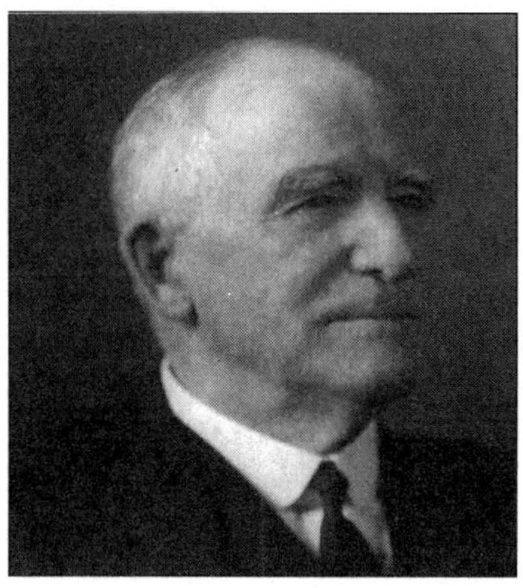

HENRY SOLOMON WELLCOME
(1853-1936)

Henry Solomon Wellcome was born in Almond, Wisconsin, and apprenticed as a pharmacist in Garden City, Minnesota. He was employed in pharmacies in Rochester, Minnesota, and Chicago, Illinois, where he attended the Chicago College of Pharmacy until it was destroyed by fire. He then enrolled at the Philadelphia College of Pharmacy where he graduated in 1874. Alter two years with Caswell, Hazard & Co. in New York City, he joined McKesson & Robbins to embark on missions to South America to study the native cinchona forests. Silas M. Burroughs invited Wellcome to England, and in 1880 they established Burroughs, Wellcome & Co. in London. When Burroughs died in 1895, Wellcome assumed entire responsibility for the firm's future. In 1901 he founded the Wellcome Tropical Research Laboratories in Khartoum, Sudan, where he discovered several prehistoric Ethiopian archeological sites; in 1913, he established the Wellcome Historical Medical Museum in London, providing a home for the treasures he had collected in his world travels. U.S. Secretary of War J.M. Dickinson appointed Wellcome to visit Panama to survey the sanitary conditions in the Canal Zone; Wellcome's report resulted in greatly increased government support for General Gorgas to continue his monumental sanitary work in Panama.

A member of the American Pharmaceutical Association since 1875, Wellcome served as APhA honorary president 1931-1932, and he took an active role in the establishment of APhA headquarters building. He became a naturalized British subject in 1910, and was knighted by King George V in 1932.

A Notable and Worthwhile Project

Henry Solomon Wellcome

The *Journal of the American Pharmaceutical Association* (volume 23, pages 490-498, 1934) reports that in Washington, D.C., during the 82nd APhA annual meeting banquet, "Sir Henry S. Wellcome briefly and feelingly acknowledged the honor, referring to Professor Remington as a member of the faculty of the Philadelphia College of Pharmacy when he was a student of that institution. He also paid tribute to William Procter, Jr., John M. Maisch, Robert Bridges, and other pharmaceutical educators of that period. He concluded with words of thanks and appreciation, and accepted the Medal as a distinct honor." Wellcome's full remarks have neither been published, nor has an original manuscript been located.

Wellcome addressed the 1930 APhA annual meeting, and his remarks that follow appeared in the *Journal of the American Pharmaceutical Association* (volume 19, pages 676-679, 1930).

I much regret that in recent years it has not been possible for me to attend the Annual Meetings as often as I wished. However, as a life member for many years, I have never ceased to feel a deep interest in the development and progress of the Association and have followed closely its admirable work.

It is very encouraging and gratifying to observe the increased progressive spirit manifested in the activities since my last attendance four years ago. It is, indeed, refreshing to see so many virile young men taking a part in the work of the Association.

President Dunning has requested me to make some remarks and offer suggestions regarding the projected American Institute of Pharmacy and the headquarters building. The plans proposed are, to my mind, practicable and most admirable. Furthermore, we owe Dr. Dunning a deep debt of gratitude for the splendid efforts they have made to finance this proposition. Their success in raising funds for carrying out this scheme is remarkable, especially when we consider the financial conditions which have prevailed during the past several years. I beg you, however, not to forget that still more funds are urgently needed for properly completing this most important undertaking, and to complete it in a manner worthy of our great purpose.

I hope most earnestly that every member of the Association will realize and appreciate the immense benefits to be derived from the consummation of these plans. The lofty aims of this project should commend it to every pharmacist, for its success will mean the regeneration of the practice of pharmacy as a scientific profession, based on ethical standards. Such regeneration will secure to professional scientific pharmacists proper recognition amongst the learned professions.

Today the world appears to be at the beginning of a new era, with amazing discoveries and new developments in every branch of science. On every hand we see marvelous inventions in mechanics, notably air flight, radio, and television, all leading to anticipation of still greater discoveries in the near future; but, in participating in this great advance, we are most concerned in the recent wonderful scientific discoveries associated with the healing art such as medicine, surgery, chemistry, bacteriology, and pharmacy.

This great awakening of the mental faculties of man, unraveling for us the infinite secrets of nature, indicates unlimited possibilities of continuous advancement. These marvelous achievements should arouse and inspire us to use wisely the talents God has given us-that we may win the goal and accomplish much in our field of operations for the betterment of mankind.

In these days no one can afford to stand still with closed eyes. All departments of science are in the race, and we are merely at the beginning.

All pharmacists are deeply concerned in the possibilities of these scientific developments, and should realize the vital importance of keeping abreast of this mighty wave of progress. Those who are inspired with lofty ambitions must qualify themselves for the attainment of higher scientific standards, and will thus deserve and secure due recognition by the medical profession and the scientific world generally.

The government officials in Washington who are responsible for advising on the allotment of sites in the specially reserved locations, have assured us that they realize the national importance of the activities of the American Institute of Pharmacy for the advancement of science and the raising of the status of professional pharmacy. They also manifest appreciation of the advantages of having the headquarters building with permanent officials located in Washington, as this will facilitate intercourse with government departments in respect to legislation and other important official matters affecting the interest of pharmacists.

The location selected for the proposed building is unique and certainly one of the most beautiful sites in Washington, being situated close to the Academy of Science and directly facing the Lincoln Memorial. The authorities are favorable to this project, but they require that the building on this selected site must be architecturally imposing and worthy of being grouped with the Lincoln Memorial and other stately buildings which surround it.

For generations this building will remain a noble temple of scientific pharmacy. Therefore, it should be adequate to provide for future developments, Incidentally, I might mention that this site provides solid surface rock foundation which will greatly lessen the cost of construction. Washington has become a Mecca to which people make pilgrimages from all parts of America and of the world, and the home of the Institute should be one to compel attention and command respect.

President Dunning has requested me to make some suggestions regarding a museum in the headquarters building. The dimensions of the building indicated in the tentative sketch design are, I believe, inadequate, especially when we look to the future. I believe it to be of great practical and scientific importance that adequate space should be set apart for two museums.

One museum should contain a complete collection of materia medica specimens of the highest grade to serve as standards of quality for the purpose of comparison and test; and as complete a collection as possible of specimens of lower grades of materia medica of inferior quality and specimens that are adulterated or sophisticated, also for the purpose of comparison and test. A collection of standardized medical, chemical and pharmaceutical products would also be of great value for the purpose of comparison and test.

Such a museum of materia medica, medicinal, chemical and pharmaceutical products, for comparison and test, would be invaluable to research workers and to pharmacists generally. I have no doubt the materia medlica department of the colleges of pharmacy throughout the United States would be glad to cooperate and perhaps present these specimens to the American Institute of Pharmacy.

As to the second museum, I suggest that the American Institute of Pharmacy should have an historical pharmacy museum in the headquarters building. There is in America a rare opportunity to secure historical pharmacy material connected with the practice of pharmacy from the time of the earliest settlements in the new world. Such opportunities do not exist in the countries of Europe where history goes back for thousands of years, and where comparatively few objects from the most ancient periods have been preserved. You have here a chance to make collections of historical objects of surpassing interest. The ideal place for such a museum is in this building.

The Library of the American Institute of Pharmacy should be as complete as possible in technical and historical works relating to pharmacy, chemistry and allied subjects, and would be one of the most important features of this institution. The educative value of such a library cannot be overestimated.

In regard to the museum and library great care should be taken to avoid exposure to the direct rays of the sun. Manuscripts, printed books, materia medica and other museum specimens are liable to be seriously damaged and even destroyed if strict precautions are not taken in this respect.

I want to make this suggestion: that in this museum there should be a gallery where the portraits of those who have done great things in the development of pharmacy and to whom we owe so much should be placed after they have passed away. None should be placed there by special favor, but only for real merit and beneficial service to mankind.

Practical Research laboratories with up-to-date equipment are not only desirable but necessary in association with such an institution as this. For various practical reasons they should not be housed in the main building, but should be completely isolated. The preferred practice now in buildings for such purposes as the American Institute of Pharmacy is to have the laboratories, chemical and bacteriological, in an isolated building, thus avoiding fumes and danger from combustible and explosive material, as well as infection from bacteria.

This is a noble and worth-while project. I earnestly appeal to the members of the Association to wholeheartedly support Dr. Dunning by contributing liberally to this fund. You cannot carry out a scheme like this without money.

Every individual member of the American Pharmaceutical Association should feel a deep personal interest and pride in this project, and should do his utmost to assist the committee in raising the necessary funds. The membership of the American Pharmaceutical Association today is very large and represents vast assets in capital and income which are increasing year by year.

The population of the United States today is more than one hundred and twenty million. Soon the population will be doubled, and it is not difficult to vision the time when it will be trebled and even quadrupled. While the population and wealth of the nation increases, the number of pharmacists will certainly be quite as rapidly multiplied. From the practical business side of pharmacy, I believe that every cent contributed to this undertaking will yield many fold in helping to translate our ideals into actualities.

Unless there is a regeneration and a real advancement in the practice of pharmacy along ethical, scientific and professional lines, there will be little hope for young men of intellect who have healthy ambitions for pharmaceutical careers.

The success of the project of the American Institute of Pharmacy will beautifully meet the demands of the situation. ■

1935 Remington Medalist

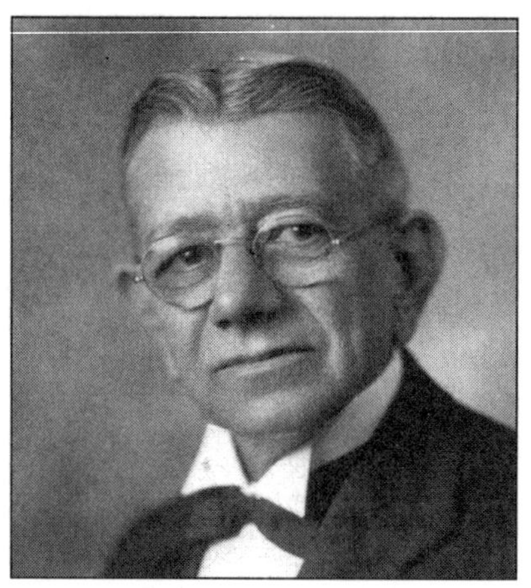

SAMUAL LOUIS HILTON
(1866-1944)

Samuel Louis Hilton was born in Washington, D.C., and was a 1888 graduate of the National College of Pharmacy. Following graduation he opened his own pharmacy in the nation's capital, which he operated for 46 years Here he prepared medicines for Chief Justice William Howard Taft and other notable personalities and he operated a well-equipped analytical laboratory on the second floor. He also served for five years on the faculty of his alma mater as professor of analytical chemistry and later served a two-year term as college president. He served a three-year term as president of the City of Washington Retail Druggists' Association, as president of the City of Washington APhA Branch, and as secretary of the Board of Pharmacy for eight years.

Hilton first served as a delegate to the Pharmacopeial Convention in 1890, and was elected treasurer of the U.S. Pharmacopeial Convention in 1910 and again in 1920. He served as chairman of the APhA House of Delegates 1919-1920, APhA president 1921-1922, and chairman of the APhA Council 1925-1940. And it was Hilton, the 1935 Remington medalist, who inaugurated the movement to build the American Institute of Pharmacy, headquarters of the American Pharmaceutical Association.

SAND, MORTAR, AND STONE

Samuel Louis Hilton

The 1935 Remington Honor Medal Lecture was presented October 19, 1935, at the Mayflower Hotel in Washington, D.C. Hilton's complete Remington address has not survived, but the following accounts of the ceremony are recorded in the *Journal of the American Pharmaceutical Association,* volume 24, pages 925-927, October 1935.

APhA secretary Evander Kelly introduced the 1935 Remington medalist whose sterling qualities contributed largely to the success of the [APhA headquarters] building project, and credited the medalist with the performance of essentials that resulted in the beautiful structure. When the time came that work could be started on the foundation of the building, the knowledge possessed by "Sam Hilton," who as a lad played in this section on the very grounds now occupied by the Institute of Pharmacy, was of great value. From the time that the first stone was placed, day-by-day, as the structure took shape, this enthusiast visited the site. Of no other person can it be said that he has as intimate an acquaintance of the location, ground, sand, mortar, stone, and equipment as the guest of honor. In his introductory remarks, the Remington medalist acknowledged the honor of being deemed worthy of the award and extended thanks. He referred to the thought which resulted in the memorial to a leading American pharmacist and the plan by which it is perpetuated.

Continuing, Hilton spoke of his early acquaintance with Professor Remington in 1890, and [how] the friendship formed was strengthened on the journey to New Orleans in 1891 when he attended his first meeting of the American Pharmaceutical Association. He mentioned a conference on pharmacopeial matters in Washington when the hours of the delightful evening ended at 4 o'clock in the morning.

On many occasions thereafter, it was his pleasure to be with Professor Remington in the classroom, in the home, and at the annual meetings of the Association. He spoke of Remington's outstanding qualities of leadership and happy conversations; his ability to adjust to difficulties and promote successful organizational work whereby improvements were made effective by the Association. He spoke favorably of his [own] chairmanship in pharmacopeial revision and authorship.

In concluding his remarks, the medalist referred to his happiness as a result of work and again expressed thanks and appreciation for the honor conferred. Moments of visitations among friends closed the evening's ceremonies. ■

1936 Remington Medalist

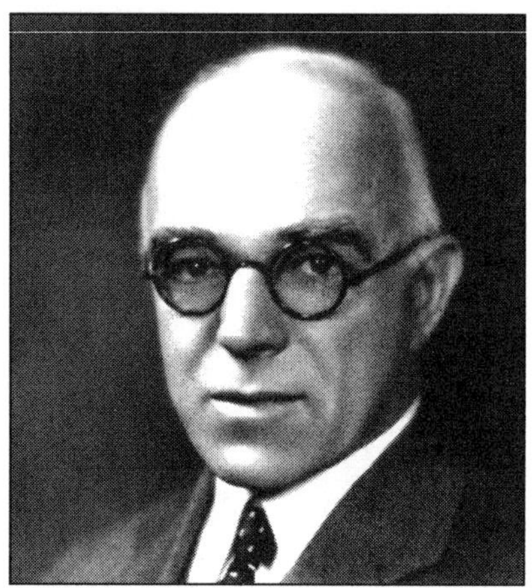

EDMUND NORRIS GATHERCOAL

(1874-1954)

Edmund Norris Gathercoal was born in near Sycamore, Illinois, and he commenced his apprenticeship in the Chicago pharmacy of Thomas W. Sollitt at the age of 17. He graduated from the Chicago College of Pharmacy in 1895 receiving a microscope as a prize for his proficiency in pharmacognosy. After two years study at Rush Medical College, Gathercoal opened his own pharmacy in Wilmette, Illinois, which he operated for eight years. In 1907, he disposed of his pharmacy to accept a full-time teaching position at his *alma mater,* whose name had become the University of Illinois School of Pharmacy.

Gathercoal continued to conduct research in pharmacognosy, authoring a widely used textbook on the subject, and in 1915 he received the APhA Ebert Prize for the pharmacognosy of medicinal Rhamnus barks. He was assistant editor of *Botanical Abstracts,* a member of the Revision Committee for *USP X1* and chairman of the committee of revision for *National Fonnulary VI*. He served for 15 years as secretary of the APhA Chicago Branch, chairman of the APhA Scientific Section 1919, president of the National Conference on Pharmaceutical Research 1929, APhA first vice president 1923, and APhA president 1937-1938.

Achievements of the Past: Prospects for the Future

Edmund Norris Gathercoal

The 1936 Remington Honor Medal Lecture was presented October 19, 1936, at the Hotel Pennsylvania in New York City. Gathercoal's Remington address was published in the *Journal of the American Pharmaceutical Association,* volume 25, pages 1028-1036, November 1936.

Research, as defined by Boyd, consists merely of searching for new knowledge or of trying to prove something. It is elemental and universal. It is applicable to any field of human endeavor. It is essentially experimentation-experimentation under conditions that are carefully controlled.

Research by the detective leads to evidence; by the reporter, to news; by the politician, to new taxes. Research by the agronomist leads to improved or new crops; by the cook, to finer meals; by the dietitian, to fewer dyspepsia remedies. Research by the educator leads to clearer thinking; by the sociologist, to improved living; by the *USP* and *NF* Revision Committees, to better health.

Every one, no matter what he does, should understand the principles of research. Nothing so increases one's fund of knowledge as consistent research, even though on a small scale. According to Emerson, knowledge is power. Unfortunately, statements are often matters of opinion rather than of knowledge. For instance, the ten-year old brother, who has just come from the pump with a pail of water for dinner, says that it is half a mile from the kitchen door to the pump, but his elder brother says it is but thirty feet; Dad, who set the pump some years before, has never measured the distance, so he gets the tape and he and the boys carefully measure it. They proudly announce to the family at dinner that it is fifty-six feet, five and one-quarter inches from the center of the kitchen door sill to the center of the pump cylinder. The boys can tell you, nearly fifty years later, what that distance was. They know it, because they experimentally determined it.

As research is concerned with new knowledge and new things, the question sometimes arises: What is new knowledge or a new thing? One of the wisest of men has written: "There is no new thing under the sun" (Eccl. 1:9). However, the infant starting out in life at one day old has no knowledge. All things and all facts are "new" to him. Perhaps we should distinguish between "private" research and "public" research: the former for the private knowledge or use of the individual; the latter for publication to the world. Each person acquires a goodly part of this knowledge by experiment. The young child learns that when he touches fire or the hot stove his fingers are "burned." It is "new" knowledge to him, but not "new" to the world. The distance from the kitchen door to the pump was "new" knowledge both to the family mentioned above and to the world; it was of interest to the family but would not be of interest to the world. "Private" research along any line of knowledge should never be discouraged, but the publication of the results of research should be carefully considered from the point of previous publication and from the point of public interest; also, from the point of private interest, which sometimes, because of the desire of private gain, prohibits publication of research results of great value to the world.

Pure and applied research are frequently distinguished. C.E.K Mees says that the difference is "merely one of intention." The intention of one who enters "pure" research is simply to advance human knowledge, while the worker in "applied" research seeks to discover new knowledge or new things that may be applied in a practical way to useful purposes. It is frequently the case, however, that the worker in "pure" research makes discoveries that have a very practical application, and, on the other hand, the worker in "applied" research may develop some of the most fundamental and important truths of science. Mendeleeff developed the periodic classification of the chemical elements by "pure" research. This periodic table has since become of great practical importance to all workers in chemistry, particularly in "applied" chemistry.

The varieties of research are almost innumerable. Every science and profession and practically every industry is actively engaged in research at the present time. There are underlying principles common to all of these varieties of research, yet each has some peculiarities of its own. Allied researches form such outstanding groups as medical research, industrial research, agricultural research, sociological research, mathematical research, etc. These groups are largely made up of scientific researches, such as chemical, physical, biological, mechanical, psychological, educational, astronomical and so on ad infinitum. Each general science, each philosophy, each industry, is split up into specialized sections or divisions, and in each of these divisions several named varieties of research are known. The total number of named varieties of research may run into the thousands.

Medical research comprises a large group of scientific and sociologic researches, and is of outstanding interest to the whole world because of its humanitarian accomplishments in the relief of pain, the mitigation of disease and the lengthening of the span of life. In 1800 the average length of human life in civilized countries was 27 years; today the average is 57 years. An increase of 100 percent in the average span of human life is perhaps the outstanding research achievement in all history.

Pharmacy for more than a century has played an important part in medical research. The discovery and improvement of the extraction of vegetable and animal drugs; the extraction and purification of the active principles of plants; the discovery and development of dosage forms of medicine, such as coated pills, capsules, cachets and ampuls; the development of masking agents and pleasant vehicles for disagreeable medicines; and the discovery of new medicinal plants, chemicals and biologicals are all important pharmaceutical contributions to medical science during the past century and particularly the last half century.

USP and *NF* research is pharmaceutical research concerned with the standardization of medicines. It endeavors to present new types of standards, new standards within established types and the improvement of established standards.

The creed of the research laboratory, according to Dr. George D. Beal, is as follows:

1. To provide the specialist with ample opportunity for expression.
2. To make available to industry and to civilization the best of scientific knowledge.
3. To add, through industrial development or scientific achievement, something to the sum total of human knowledge that will benefit mankind.

Research is as ancient as man. Historically it appears to have flourished in ancient Egypt and Babylonia, and in the Grecian and Roman golden ages. It was particularly dormant during the Middle Ages, but began to revive with the great awakening in art and literature at the Renaissance. Beginning with the nineteenth century it developed more rapidly in Europe and especially in the young United States. During the last half century its development has been much accelerated, until today its accomplishments are so numerous that the individual mind cannot comprehend them. The early experimenters worked mostly alone, usually in great need, sometimes in dire hardship. If they had money or income they poured it into their work, until perhaps they were poverty stricken and in debt. They usually had but little encouragement from friends and advisors frequently obstacles and ridicule. They had few of the mechanical and technical aids of today, but were forced to prepare their own apparatus and instruments. Morse prepared every foot of insulated wire that he used with the telegraph, winding it with cotton by hand. Leewenhoek was a small town drygoods merchant, but he ground the lenses and made the microscope with which he saw microorganisms as minute as bacteria, and became the first to describe them. Marie and Pierre Curie toiled unceasingly to separate radium from vast quantities of earth. Scheele in his meager laboratory at Upsala or in his apothecary shop at Koping discovered many important medicines.

As Longfellow, in Keraxnos, writes: "Thine was the prophet's vision, thine The exultation, the divine Insanity of noble minds That never falters or abates, But labors and endures and waits Till all that it foresees it finds Or what it cannot find, creates!"

These "lone-handed" experimenters brought to the world some of its most important discoveries. From the dawn of history to the beginning of the present century, their names constitute a long and remarkable roll. As examples, we mention just seven almost at random: Hippocrates (460 B.C.), the father of medicine; Archimedes (260 B.C.), the discoverer of fundamental laws of mechanics; Galileo (1600 A.D.), the founder of astronomy; Leewenhoek (1650 A.D.), first to use the microscope and discover bacteria; Sir Humphry Davy (1800 A.D.), a great chemist; Michael Faraday (1820 A.D.), the founder of electrical science; and Pelletier (1820 A.D.), a pharmacist and the discoverer of many alkaloids.

The earlier pharmacopoeial revision committees depended for the improvement of the book almost entirely on the published results of research pertaining to the standardization of medicines. Such publications in 1820 and even up to 1860 or 1870 were few. As the pharmaceutical literature improved and became more voluminous, scientific progress in the *Pharmacopeia* became more marked. Some research, no doubt, was carried on by individual members of the several revision committees from the very beginning of the *Pharmacopeia,* but evidence of this is difficult to obtain from the history of the *Pharmacopeia.* About the middle of the nineties of the past century, Dr. Charles Rice, Chairman of the USP Revision Committee, established a USP fellowship at the University of Wisconsin. With the eighth decennial revision of the *Pharmacopeia* (1905) and the third edition of the *NF* (1906), research by the individual members of the revision committees became more evident.

The preparation of the chemical and plant drug monographs, introduced into the fourth edition of the *NF* (1916), was a huge task and involved much research. The research accomplished by Dr. E. L. Newcomb and his collaborators on the ash-content of drugs (1920-1925) involved more than 10,000 ash determinations. The results of this work have never been published, though they have been extensively utilized in the *Pharmacopeia* and the *NF.* The microscopic measurement of tissue elements and of starch grains and crystals in plant drug powders by Fischer and Newcomb involved more than 100,000 figures. The results of this work were extensively incorporated into the Pharmacopeia and the *NF* and markedly increased the scientific standing of the plant drug monographs in both of these books. All of this research was of the "lone-handed" type, poorly financed, ridiculed by some, unappreciated by others, unpublished and largely unrecognized. In the production of the eleventh revision of the *Pharmacopeia* and the sixth edition of the *Formulary,* research has been much further developed, collaborative work has been undertaken on a large scale and more publicity has been given to it.

Since the beginning of the present century, organized research has gradually replaced the lone-handed experimenter. A research organization of today usually implies a separate laboratory or laboratories, extensive equipment, suitable apparatus, a large library, liberal financing and highly qualified personnel. It gives the experimenter assurance of a living salary, comfort in his work and the assistance he needs. It means systematic, well-directed coordinated effort. It results in more prompt, accurate and numerous accomplishments, in a followup of new ideas, and in a quicker, more extensive utilization of the new knowledge. It is the underlying cause for the marked growth of research during the present century.

It is now time that *USP* and *NF* research be organized. This research should be centered in a suitable laboratory, be provided with equipment, apparatus and library and be in charge of an efficient personnel. It needs to be adequately financed and publicly recognized. The *Pharmacopeia* and the *Formulary,* as legal standards for medicines, have advanced in public esteem during the last five years,and a high degree of scientific accuracy is now required of them.

Chairman E. Fullerton Cook of the USP Revision Committee clearly set forth in his report before the American Pharmaceutical Association at Dallas this year, the need of continuous revision. The day of the decennial revision is past. This Committee has made definite arrangements to issue annual supplements to the *Pharmacopeia* and these will soon become annual revisions of the *Pharmacopeia.* These annual revisions, however, cannot depend exclusively upon published research. It is necessary to check standards and where these fail, their improvement is demanded. Entirely new methods of standardization are constantly required. We can no longer wait until individual initiative has produced these methods. Furthermore, research in the pharmaceutical industrial field, as also in the several scientific fields on which pharmacy is based, is tending more and more to monopolize its results and prohibit their public use. This means that some of the really great advances in pharmacy cannot be utilized in the legal books of drug standards until years after they have been discovered. The revision committees cannot expect their chairmen to serve as directors of research, or their sub-committee chairmen to serve as departmental research heads. Finally, the whole subject of research in connection with these legal standards must be brought under one head and handled as one great section of pharmaceutical research, if the best results are to be had.

C.E.K. Mees classifies organized research as follows:

1. University Research Laboratories
2. Government Research Laboratories
3. Foundation Research Laboratories
4. Industrial Research Laboratories, maintained by individual firms
5. Industrial Association Research Laboratories
6. Industrial Fellowship Laboratories
7. Private Consulting Research Laboratories

1. Almost every American university now has one or more buildings and separate staffs devoted to research. Dr. Karl T. Compton, President of the Massachusetts Institute of Technology, stated in his address at the semicentennial of Sigma Xi: "Educational institutions have always been the places where the great bulk of new discoveries are made and ideas formed, and this will continue to be so, since there exist no other organizations where such studies can be similarly pursued." Dr. Roger Adams, when president of the American Chemical Society, said, "The basic and fundamental information for more than 95 per cent of the industrial processes has been originally discovered and described by the university investigator."

Many of the colleges of pharmacy take an important place in the graduate faculties of their universities and contribute extensivelyto their research accomplishments. The earliest thesis under the direction of an American pharmaceutical faculty offered in connection with the granting of the degree of doctor of philosophy of which we have knowledge is that presented by Oswald Schreiner at the University of Wisconsin in 1902. The pharmacy colleges of the Universities of Florida, Maryland, Washington, Michigan and Wisconsin are especially noted for their research achievements.

2. The Government Research Laboratories include those in the U.S. Bureau of Standards and the U.S. Bureau of Mines, as well as the U.S. Food and Drug Administration Laboratories, and many others.

3. The Rockefeller Institute for Medical Research is an outstanding research foundation; also, the Bartal Research Foundation of Franklin Institute, and the Laboratory of the American Medical Association are of this type. The new laboratory of the American Pharmaceutical Association at Washington, which eventually will be well endowed, belongs in this group. The *USP* and *NF* research activities should center in this APhA Laboratory.

4. The Laboratories of the General Electric Company, the General Motors Corporation, the Eastman Kodak Company and sixteen hundred others, according to Bulletin 91 of the National Research Council issued in 1933, belong in the Industrial Group. Especial mention should be made of the great pharmaceutical research organizations of Parke, Davis & Company, Eli Lilly & Company and others. Research organizations on a somewhat lesser scale are important in many of the pharmaceutical manufacturing houses, including many firms producing proprietary medicines only.

Parke, Davis & Company began research on Cascara in 1877. In 1885 the firm sent Dr. H. H. Rusby on an extensive trip into South America to obtain scientific information about new plants and samples of them for investigation. In 1879 the first work was done on the chemical assay for the standardization of drugs. The first development of biological and physiological work was begun in 1894 and in 1902 the first separate large building was erected to house the biological and scientific work. The present research personnel includes about eighty people working in twenty-eight divisions of the work.

5. The National Canners Association, the American Institute of Baking, the Portland Cement Association and other industrial associations maintain cooperative research laboratories.

6. The Mellon Institute of Industrial Research and the Battelle Memorial Institute are outstanding examples of industrial fellowship laboratories.

7. Arthur D. Little, Inc., of New York, the Miner Laboratories of Chicago, the LaWall and Harrisson Laboratories of Philadelphia and many others belong in the group of private consulting research laboratories.

The housing of research is an important item from the physical standpoint, even though Boyd, says, "It is not really in a laboratory that problems are solved." Charles F. Kettering has said, "They are solved in some fellow's head. All the apparatus is for is to get his head turned around so that he can see the thing right." The general discussion of housing is beyond the province of this address; however, we would mention that *USP* and *NF* research can be located in the present American Pharmaceutical Association building the Institute of Pharmacy in Washington. The rooms now available for laboratory purposes are ample to accommodate a laboratory with annual maintenance cost of twenty-five thousand dollars. When research income becomes greater than this, larger quarters will be needed, though the laboratory probably never will be large enough to require a separate building of its own.

A new building to be located on the area of ground back of the present APhA building at Washington has been suggested. Such a building, suitable for housing many APhA activities will eventually be necessary, and immediate steps should be taken to obtain the land. However, a single section or wing of a building suitable for this location would be ample for a laboratory expending a hundred or two hundred thousand dollars annually.

"Senses supplemented" is the phrase

used by Boyd to indicate the use of instruments: our physical senses are so restricted that without senses-supplementing instruments, modern research would be impossible. We need no more than mention as aids to sight, the fluoroscope with which our very bones may be seen, the stroboscope for observing periodic motion, the spectroscope, the microscope and the telescope; as aids to hearing, the telephone, the radio and sound amplifiers that make audiblein-finitely faint sounds; as aids to the touch, the thermometer to detect the changes in temperature more accurately and delicately than can be done by touch, the thermopile to estimate heat radiation, and the balance to determine the weight of objects more accurately that by "hefting" them; as aids to taste, acidimetry to determine sourness accurately and saccharimetry to determine sweetness, or the amount of sugar present; as an aid to smell, the automatic carbon monoxide "smellers" to detect the gases from auto exhausts.

As instruments and apparatus of precision and high quality are invaluable aids in research, steps are now being taken to furnish and equip the APhA Laboratory in Washington.

The library, so useful for "paper exploration" as Boyd terms it, is frequently the laboratory where each research project receives its first study. Certainly before any research is undertaken for publication, it is most important to know what everybody else has done in the matter. Likewise, a clearly defined conception of a problem is frequently made in the library. The library in the American Institute of Pharmacy will be a valuable adjunct to the APhA Laboratory and to research that is conducted there.

The financing of research is always a problem. It has been estimated that the annual cost of research in the United States is not less than two hundred million dollars, or one four-hundredth of the total normal income of the United States.

A. F. Woods of the U.S. Department of Agriculture has stated that the individual states and the United States together spend about thirty million dollars annually in the development of agricultural industries; this is equivalent to about one twenty-five-hundredth of their total value or one fourhundredth of their gross income.

The recent survey of the National Research Council indicates that the annual expenditure on research by the 1600 industrial organizations which maintain research laboratories is 1.3 percent of the capital invested. This figure is very conservative. The cost of organized research in the chemical industry is estimated to be about 3 percent of the invested capital. While the cost of research in the great pharmaceutical industrial establishments cannot be ascertained, it probably runs at least as high as in the chemical industry. The American Medical Association Laboratory, devoted largely to the research problems of the Council on Pharmacy and Chemistry, requires about ninety thousand dollars annually for its maintenance.

The combined annual income for the *USP* and *NF* may be conservatively stated as more than fifty thousand dollars. Of this income, not less than one-half should be set aside for research purposes. A large part of this appropriation should go directly into the laboratory. The laboratory should also have an independent endowment that would yield not less than thirty thousands dollars annually.

The *USP* and *NF* research income should also provide research facilities and guidance in the APhA Laboratory to graduate students from colleges of pharmacy and other institutions, who desire to complete their practical work in research on *USP* and *NF* problems.

Also out of the *USP* and *NF* research income, partial support should be provided for research on *USP* and *NF* problems in the individual colleges or institutions. For instance, the valuable research on vegetable drug extraction, partially supported for three years by the APhA Research Fund at the University of Florida College of Pharmacy would have taken a sizable slice from even a fifty thousand dollar annual income, if it had been conducted entirely in the APhA Laboratory. The *NF* Research Fund now partially supports ten distinct items of research conducted in about as many colleges of pharmacy.

Even with these methods of advancing *USP* and *NF* research, it cannot be properly accomplished in a single laboratory. This research must be very largely of a cooperative, collaborative or referee character, and must be supported in a collaborative way by the colleges of pharmacy and the pharmaceutical industrial institutions.

The preparation and standardization of Reference Cod Liver Oil is a fine example. The USP Revision Committee arranged for a vessel and crew to catch the fish and carefully separate the livers under almost aseptic conditions. These livers were then brought into the E.L. Patch Company factory, which had been thoroughly cleaned, cleared of all cod livers and cod liver oil, and rented by the Committee for several days. With great heed to cleanliness, the oil was extracted, clarified and bottled in ounces under nitrogen gas. About twenty laboratories collaborated in the vitamin assay of this oil at a cost approximating one thousand dollars each. The production of the oil costs seven thousand dollars. It is now being distributed as a reference standard to laboratories throughout the world.

Such extensive and valuable researches as are now being advanced by the USP Revision Committee on the vitamin assays, the digitalis and ergot assays, and the standardization of products for anemia could never be satisfactorily completed in a single laboratory nor be financed exclusively by the *USP* and *NF* organizations.

As in the past revisions, the recent revisions of the USP and *NF* have drawn upon the research accomplishments published in the literature pertaining to pharmacy, medicine, chemistry, botany and other allied fields. It is essential for the proper growth of the *Pharmacopeia* and the *Formulary* that this literature should be constantly reviewed with the single thought of utilizing the new methods of drug standardization that are presented. On the other hand the *Pharmacopeia* and the *Formulary* should return the favor with a rich research literature of their own.

The personnel of the research laboratory, in connection with any institution, should be headed by a director of both executive ability and scientific training. The director should have associated with him a few persons of varied scientific training who have originality, vision and the courage of the true pioneer. This small group should be supplemented by suitable assistant and routine workers. Two-thirds to three-quarters of the cost of research is in salaries.

Arthur D. Little says that our up-to-date explorers are "those having the simplicity to wonder, the ability to question, the power to generalize, the capacity to apply." Among pioneers, youth has always been prominent. Therefore, perhaps one of the really desirable qualifications for the experimenter in the research laboratory is youth. A list of the discoveries by men who had not reached the age of thirty is most astounding. The staffs of the research laboratories of today consist largely of young men and women; this is true because of the qualities of youth for such work and because the price of youth is not high, relative to the quality of service it can render.

Among other qualities of the true experimenter, Boyd lists as chapter heads the following: Curiosity, Imagination, Experimentalism, Enthusiasm, Patience, Persistence, Faith, Courage, Common Sense, Honesty and Modesty.

The accumulated knowledge of the human race represents the achievements of research. Perhaps it is not quite fair to say that all knowledge is entirely due to research. It is true that rather frequently new knowledge is developed or new discoveries made without definitely controlled experimentation. "Accident" and "luck" are often mentioned in connection with research, but it is worthy of note that the "accident" usually happens, or the "luck" comes, to the person who has studied and thought and experimented.

In connection with the U.S. *Pharmacopeia,* it is only necessary to compare the first *Pharmacopeia,* that of 1820, with the most recent *Pharmacopeia,* that of 1936, to note the vast changes, enlargements and improvements due to research. In the first *Pharmacopeia,* we find the crude drugs and chemicals listed by name. The only information given in connection with the 235 plant drugs is the part of the plant that constitutes the drug and the name of the plant that yields the drug. Forty-six of the chemical drugs are named only, except that three of the acids have specific gravity figures. Sixty-five items that would now be classed as chemicals are in the section of the book devoted to preparations, and directions are given for their manufacture, but no standards to determine quality and purity are given. In the most recent *Pharmacopeia* the vegetable drugs are scientifically described both macroscopically and microscopically, and in powdered form. Standards as to water content, ash yield and percentage of active constituent are frequently given. Many tests and assays to determine the identity, quality and purity of the drug are included in the chemical drug monographs.

Chairman Cook says, "It is no exaggeration to say that within the covers of the *Pharmacopeia* (USP XI) there are hundreds of thousands of factual statements, every one of which is expected to be correct. Many of these combine to make up the enormous number of tests which prove the identity and purity of official products. These tests and assays have been evolved through many decades and are often accepted as theoretically correct from one *Pharmacopeia* to another, simply because no occasion has arisen to subject them to the 'acid test' of a case in court."

No one dare say that human knowledge in any line has reached its ultimate limit, or that anything has attained perfection. Every scientist realizes that in his own particular specialized field the known is but a small island in an illimitable ocean of the unknown. Professor Frank R. Lilly of the University of Chicago, in his address at the semi-centennial of Sigma Xi, said: "It is at least arguable, certainly in biology, that the progress of research creates more problems than it solves; that the faculty of imagination, which is at the bottom of all creative research, is not satisfied with its diet of results, but is on the contrary stimulating new growth. Thus while we can clearly perceive that we are mere beginners, there is no way of anticipating the future of research nor the evolution of human intelligence."

When we look at US. *Pharmacopeia XI* and *NF VI,* they do appear to be very fine books. Certainly we have put into them the best that we had. However, when we note the volume of criticisms calling attention to the "errors" in the books, our pride hasteneth to a fall.

We know not what the future holds for the *Pharmacopeia* and the *Formulary,* but the sign-posts definitely point to at least three well-defined issues of the immediate future, viz.:

First.—Revision will be necessary and will continue at a greatly accelerated pace.

Second.—Revision now demands intensive well-organized research. This research covers essentially the same fields for both the *Pharmacopeia* and the *Formulary.* There is no reason why *USP* research should be separated from *NF* research.

Third.—There should be a marked difference in the scopes of the two books. The *Pharmacopeia* should standardize the "simples," i.e., the plant, animal and chemical drugs; the *Formulary* should standardize the required preparations of the drugs official in the *Pharmacopeia.* The great advantages of this arrangement to the *Pharmacopeia* would be that it would then control the simple therapeutic agents required and used in medical practice and that the Revision Committee could concentrate on the standardization of those agents most amenable to strictly scientific control. Such an arrangement would give the *Formulary* a sound therapeutic foundation, and enable its revisers to concentrate on the standardization of the preparations. It would give each book a distinctive sphere, would remove any cause for conflict, and would bring about greater efficiency. ■

1937 Remington Medalist

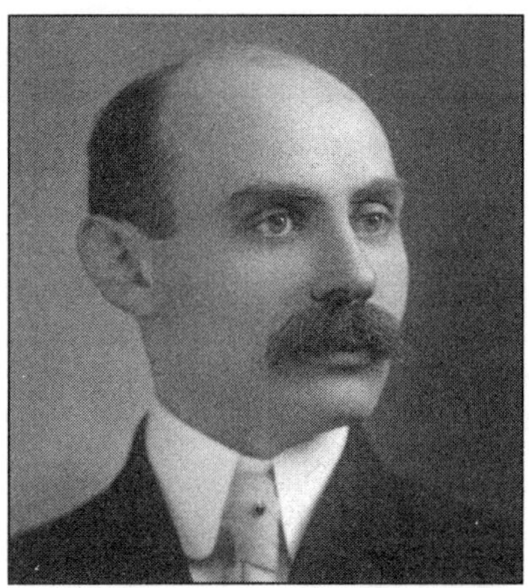

J. Leon Lascoff
(1867-1943)

J. Leon Lascoff was born in Vilna, Lithuania (then part of Russia), and obtained his pharmaceutical education in Russia. He immigrated to the U.S.A. in 1892 and commenced working as a pharmacist for David Hayes and Sons of New York City. He purchased his own pharmacy in 1899, moving to Lexington Avenue at 82nd Street in New York City in 1931, where with his son, Frederick D. Lascoff; they limited their practice to dispensing prescription medication. In 1910, he was appointed a member of the New York State Board of Pharmacy, serving as president 1914, 1921, and 1929. He was founder and past president of the New York County Pharmaceutical Society, founder and treasurer of the New York Veteran Druggists Association, and a longtime trustee of Columbia University College of Pharmacy. In 1936, Lascoff was honored for dispensing one million prescriptions, and he became known as an authority on prescription incompatibilities.

Joining the American Pharmaceutical Association in 1903, Lascoff served variously as APhA Section on Practical Pharmacy and Dispensing secretary 1911-1912 and chairman 1912-1913; chairman of the APhA committee that compiled the first edition *of The Pharmaceutical Recipe Book* (1929); APhA first vice president 1936-1937; and APhA president 1938-1939. During his term as APhA president, Lascoff brought together at the 1938 APhA annual meeting a group *of* prescription pharmacists that provided the germ of an idea for the creation of the American College *of* Apothecaries in 1940. Upon Lascoffs death, ACA established the “J. Leon Lascoff Award” to memorialize his contributions to the advancement of professional pharmacy.

LET US HAVE FAITH

J. Leon Lascoff

The 1937 Remington Medal was presented October 25, 1937, at the Hotel Pennsylvania in New York City. The *Journal of the American Pharmaceutical Association* (volume 26, page 942, 1937) reports that Lascoffs Remington address reviewed "his experiences as a practicing pharmacist," and expressed "the conviction that professional pharmacy has a bright future." Lascoff's Remington address was never published, and his manuscript has not survived. The following excerpts from Lascoff's 1938 APhA presidential address (*Journal of the American Pharmaceutical Association,* volume 28, pages 766-775, 1938) appear to mirror the views he probably presented in his Remington address.

I came to this country in 1892, at the age of twent-five, and at that time had had six years practical experience and had completed my pharmaceutical education. I am somewhat shocked by the realization that forty-seven years have passed since then and, yet, the length of time rather eases me because for that entire period, I have been privileged to practice Pharmacy in this country and to do what I could to interest others in Pharmacy from a professional point of view.

I became a member of the American Pharmaceutical Association in 1903. The first annual meeting that it was my privilege to attend was in New York in 1907, at the then "new" Hotel Astor, and the first paper that I ever presented before the American Pharmaceutical Association was before the Section on Practical Pharmacy and Dispensing at that meeting. In 1915 and 1916 I served as president of the New York Branch of the American Pharmaceutical Association. I think I have attended most of the annual meetings of the American Pharmaceutical Association since I first joined and I served as chairman of the Section on Practical Pharmacy and Dispensing in 1913.

In the chairman's address that year, the conditions confronting Pharmacy were reviewed. Even at that time, the prophecy was being made that we should have two types of drug stores-one dealing with the purely professional aspects and the other, the more or less commercial institution. I made the plea, "Let us have more pharmacies and fewer drug stores." I mention this in the name of consistency, as the feeling which I had then, I have now. I believe there is need for more pharmacies conducted by professionally-minded men, conscious of their professional obligation to the public, and endowed with a deep-seated determination to give Pharmacy its proper place in the professional world.

I hope you will condone these more or less personal references to myself. However, I am speaking not only to the group assembled here, but I have before me as I speak, the pharmaceutical body of this country, and I want them to know that the principles which I announce and the precepts which I seek to emphasize are more than lip service and that I am crystallizing, in a few statements, that work which has been the heart and soul of my existence.

From the beginning of my career in Pharmacy, I have been imbued with a deep love for my profession and I have earnestly tried to make use of every opportunity for making Pharmacy mean more, not only to me, but to my fellow pharmacists, to the other public health professions, and to the public at large. I do not know how well I have succeeded, but I can say, with the deepest personal satisfaction, that I have at least done my best.

I am sure you will pardon me for making a reference to the *Recipe Book.* This is one of the important undertakings of the Association and one which I really believe can be made of much greater value. I became chairman of the *Recipe Book* Committee in 1920, and am still serving in that capacity. The first *Recipe Book* was issued in 1929 and the second in 1936. About eight thousand copies of *Recipe Book II* have been sold and this I take to be a substantial endorsement of what the *Recipe Book* attempts to do. I have interpreted the function of the *Recipe Book* to be that of furnishing workable, dependable and practical formulas for many drug, chemical toilet and similar preparations, for which the pharmacist has frequent calls, but which, for some reason or another, are not officially recognized either in the *Pharmacopeia* or the *National Formulary.*

Anyone with experience in the retail drug business knows that there is an actual demand for a work of this kind and it is in recognition of this demand that the *Recipe Books* of the Association, have been edited and compiled.

It is my feeling that the sale of the *Recipe Book* can be greatly expanded. The Book should be advertised, retailers and manufacturers should be aware of its use, and if this were done, I have not the slightest doubt that it can be made of still greater value to pharmacists and the drug industry.

We hear a great deal today of the socialization of Medicine. I am much impressed with the belief that this term is used by many who have not gained a sound understanding of what is involved but, as a pharmacist, I know that if there is to be any further socialization of Medicine it is bound to involve the socialization of Pharmacy.

I believe that the Association should continue to give close study to the conditions under which socialized Medicine is practiced in England, Germany and other countries of Continental Europe. With accurate information with respect to the status of Pharmacy under these socialized services we would be in position to more satisfactorily decide which of the developments are helpful and which are to be avoided.

I do not know, nor do I claim to know, just how socialization will proceed. I am not altogether convinced that there is need for any widespread, sweeping changes in the conditions under which medical services are furnished. I am far from being assured that the government, either federal or state, or both, is suited to administer the medical facilities of this country, and I should urge the policy of watchful waiting.

The surest means, in my judgment, of protecting the interests of Pharmacy under the present system, is closer cooperation with Medicine and other public health professions. Necessarily, Medicine and Pharmacy have much in common. It would seem that each of them would be in a better position to meet their problems and to discharge their obligations to the public if they worked in closer harmony. The American Pharmaceutical Association could serve in no better way than to bring about a more effective relation and a reasonable understanding between Medicine and Pharmacy, so that a constructive, socially-minded and practical program might be developed.

Another essential in maintaining the proper place for Pharmacy in the changed conditions which will come about is to have Pharmacy recognized by actual membership on state and municipal boards of health. While much headway has been made in this respect, there has been no real organized effort behind it. Pharmacy is now recognized on the boards of health of several states and some advance was noted this year. Legislation was passed in Oregon and in NewJersey authorizing a pharmacist on the Boards of Health, and legislation in New Hampshire, while not specifically specifying Pharmacy, was, nevertheless, passed with the understanding that a pharmacist would be given membership on the Board of Health of that State.

I emphasize this as one of our professional objectives because Pharmacy cannot occupy that place in the public health scheme to which it is entitled, unless it is given a voice and a responsibility in public health administration. I urge that the American Pharrnaceutical Association continue its interest in this subject and that legislation providing for a pharmacist on the boards of health of every state be made one of its major objectives.

I think, too, that we should show greater interest in the development of hospital pharmacy, as, necessarily, the hospital pharmacist will come into close contact with Medicine and other medical specialists and will be in position to interpret Pharmacy to them in a basic and fundamental way.

If the law of every state requires that a registered pharmacist must be in charge of a public pharmacy, then there are indeed strong reasons why the dispensing of medicines and poisons in a hospital should be equally supervised and controlled. It is because of the unusual character of the work which the hospital pharmacist is called upon to do that hospital pharmacy bids well to become a basic factor in our field.

There is much to indicate that medical practice will bc centralized more and more in hospitals, particularly under voluntary sickness insurance and other insurance plans. I am glad that the Association has instituted a section on hospital pharmacy and I urge that the members support it to the fullest extent.

Pharmaceutical education is basic to the professional standing of Pharmacy. Our educational standards must compare favorably with educational standards in other public health fields if Pharmacy is to occupy a reasonably satisfactory place in the professional scheme. It is for this reason that we should give active support to the work of the American Council on Pharmaceutical Education.

The Council was set up, as you probably recall, by the American Pharmaceutical Association the National Association of Boards of Pharmacy and the American Association of Colleges of Pharmacy. Membership on the Council consists of three from each of these groups, together with one from the National Council on Education.

The work of the Council has progressed reasonably well and I look upon it as one of the most constructive things ever undertaken in our field. It is certain to better our teaching institutions and is bound to produce better educated and thus better qualified pharmacists. These factors are fundamental and are certain to result in elevating the standards throughout our field.

While we all recognize that the drug store is under tremendous economic pressure, and that competition, in a commercial sense, has become extremely intense and severe, this is all the more reason why we should do our best to develop Pharmacy along professional lines. While I do not hold the hope that retail pharmacy will ever be free from commercial difficulties, I believe those difficulties will be minimized by advancing its professional standing. It is from this point of view that I have developed my own work in Pharmacy and it is to this point of view that I would attract the attention of pharmacists in general.

I know it is frequently said that, there is not enough professional work in this country to support a great number of professional pharmacists, but I also know that no one can vouch for the accuracy of this statement, as no real attempt has been made on the part of Pharmacy in general to increase professional work. The advance in pharmaceutical education, the advance in the medical sciences and the advance in public health needs, are opening up new opportunities for men and women trained in the sciences upon which public health depends. I am convinced that in this new order of things, many new opportunities will be opened up for pharmacists if they themselves are willing and able to grasp them.

I have confidence in the future of Pharmacy. I have faith in its integrity, and know that it serves an absolutely essential purpose. As I look back over my fifty years as a practicing pharmacist I am filled with that sense of satisfaction which comes from having done the job as best I could. I am concious of that warm feeling which comes from having done one's best to reach the realization of one's ideals. I can do no more than to express my own personal faith in Pharmacy and to give you every assurance within my command that if I had my years to live over, I would pursue exactly the same path and adhere to exactly the same prinicples. And so, in the words of imortal Lincoln: "Let us have faith that right makes might and in that faith let us, to the end, dare to do our duty as we understand it." ■

1938 Remington Medalist

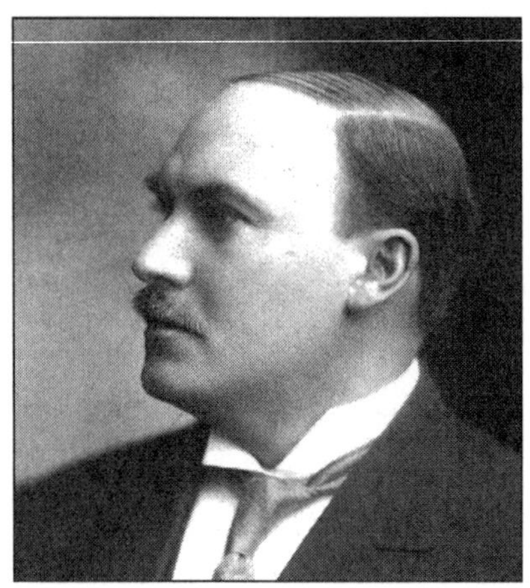

Henry C. Christensen
(1865-1947)

Henry C. Christensen was born in Union Grove, Wisconsin, and raised in Kearney County, Nebraska. He apprenticed as a pharmacist in Minden, Nebraska, and graduated from the Northwestern University School of Pharmacy in 1893. He then opened a pharmacy in Chicago which he operated 1893-1911. He served as a member of the Illinois Board of Pharmacy 1907-1921, and was a founding member of the Inter-State Association of Boards of Pharmacy in 1908. He was appointed chairman of the advisory examination committee of the National Association of Boards of Pharmacy in 1913, and the following year, he was elected as the first full-time NABP secretary, opening an NABP office in his Chicago apartment. During his term as NABP secretary, from which he retired in 1942, he established NABP districts in 1920, moved NABP into its first suite of offices in 1922, initiated the *NABP Bulletin* in 1936, and served as NABP honorary president 1943-1944. During this period, he also served as vice president of the National Drug Trade Conference and secretary-treasurer of the Drug Trade Bureau of Public Information.

Joining the American Pharmaceutical Association in 1906, Christensen served on a number of APhA committees, as a member of the APhA Council 1927-1942, and as APhA president 1930-1931. He subsequently was responsible for developing a pharmacy exhibit at the Chicago "Century of Progress" World's Fair 1933-1934.

The Dual Nature of Pharmacy

Henry C. Christensen

The 1938 Remington Medal was presented November 30, 1938, at the Hotel Pennsylvania in New York City. The *Journal of the American Pharmaceutical Association,* volume 27, page 1197, 1938, reports that the 1938 Remington medalist presented "an informal address expressing appreciation for the award and for the cooperation which had made this possible. Dr. Christensen spoke of the future of Pharmacy with optimism and urged that the education and training of future pharmacists be advanced in keeping with the progress of the other public health professions." Christensen's full Remington address was not published, and the original manuscript has not been located.

The following text consists of excerpts of Christensen's 1931 APhA presidential address as published in the *Journal of the American Pharmaceutical Association,* volume 20, pages 795-806, 1931.

For over three-quarters of a century, the American Pharmaceutical Association has been guiding the destinies of pharmacy in the United States and its dependencies. In all that time, there has never been a greater need for stressing the professional side of pharmacy than there is today. During the evolution of our profession on this continent, it has passed through many phases. From almost purely professional work, it has passed at times and in places into almost purely a merchandising business. The retailer, in many cases through necessity, has developed into a dealer in toys, a purveyor of food, and vies with the tobacconist, usurps part of the clothier's business, competes with the confectioner, aids in the postal business, weighs you for a penny, rents you a book to read and conducts a free information bureau. So conspicuous have these activities become, that the retail pharmacist has crept into the cheap jokes of the press and stage.

Some contend that this situation will lead to two classes of pharmacies in the future, the so-called "drugless" drug store and the exclusive prescription pharmacy. The field for the latter type is strictly limited to large centers and particular locations, where the demand is sufficient to support such a venture. I disagree with those who contend that this separation into two types is necessary. The majority of stores throughout the length and breadth of this country are compelled to do a certain amount of merchandising in order to provide the community with the trained pharmaceutical service necessary in protection of the public health and welfare. But they should remember that they are pharmacists first, and merchandising should be secondary in place.

Pharmacy from its very beginning in this country has been dual in nature the professional coupled with merchandising. But the dignity of the profession should be upheld. Pharmacy is the only excuse for the existence of the so-called drug store. With the drug sign down, how much merchandising can be done. If the atmosphere is that of a department store, how much prescription business will be attracted? The law gives to the pharmacist certain rights and privileges denied to others who do not have his qualifications and training. Why should he neglect these opportunities in favor of fields where competition is unlimited?

The problem confronting pharmacy today, therefore, is to discover the happy medium between the professional and the merchandising trends. The American Pharmaceutical Association is peculiarly fitted to lead the "Back to Pharmacy" crusade. The first step, perhaps, is to convince the pharmacists themselves of the opportunities they have been overlooking. Even a merchandising pharmacist can succeed better by stressing the professional aspect of his business. The second step is to counteract the loss of prestige with the public as a result of the era of over-merchandising. Only a thorough going publicity campaign by an expert in public relations can accomplish this.

No one denies that there is a crying need for more publicity of the right kind for pharmacy. We quite frequently receive attention in the cartoons and on the joke page, but that type of publicity should be suppressed instead of encouraged.

Henry Ford's theory early in his career was that the more often a Ford car was mentioned, regardless of what was said about it, the more free publicity it received. Soon, however, he discovered that a large number of middle class people with buying power were selecting other cars, because they did not wish to be embarrassed by Ford jokes. How long has it been since you have seen a Ford joke in print? Mr. Ford decided that such publicity was undesirable and had it stopped.

The first question that comes up relative to publicity is financial. We cannot limit expenditures to $1000, the amount contributed to the Drug Trade Bureau of Public Information during the past year, and expect to get $25,000 worth of results. We usually reap returns on investments in direct ratio to the amount of money invested, be it publicity or otherwise. Until pharmacy is ready to provide the budget for a trained publicrelations man as other professions and trades are doing, we cannot expect to get the newspaper mention and other publicity they get. Only a man with newspaper training knows how to write the copy so that it will receive the editor's OK for publication.

The time for giving careful consideration to this whole problem of public relations is now, as we shall, doubtless, have much news of public interest breaking during the 1933 Chicago World's Fair and we should be in position to derive some benefit from it.

The trite saying, "a river rises no higher than its source," is applicable; pharmacy will rise no higher than the men who feed the stream at its source. Although I am one of the older generation of pharmacists, I do not apologize for the men of my time. They fulfilled their mission in a creditable manner.

However, I am not so short-sighted as to overlook the fact that the graduates of the four-year course will make a higher grade of pharmacist than the man who graduated from the two-year course, with perhaps only two years of high school, to say nothing of the man who became licensed without any college training. Thus, as more of these better educated pharmacists slip into the stream of pharmacy, we can expect to reach a higher level in accomplishment.

There can be no question that the agreement between the National Association of Boards of Pharmacy, the American Association of Colleges of Pharmacy, and the American Pharmaceutical Association to establish the four-year course in pharmacy in 1932 has been very helpful in securing a broader recognition of pharmacy as a profession. This is especially true in governmental and educational circles where the sciences and arts and professions are expected and required to give standard collegiate courses of an approved content arid length.

If there are any who oppose the four-year college requirement in pharmacy, they overlook the fact that we are compelled to choose between being a trade or a profession. If we are a trade, then no educational requirement whatsoever is necessary. If we are to be rated as a profession, then we must enforce professional standards and have no right to advocate any standard below the collegiate course of four years.

As Dr. J. H. Beal has so aptly stated: "If the commercialists succeed in eliminating pharmacy entirely from the retail drug store, there will no longer be any means of placing any restriction upon those who desire to engage in the sale of drugs and medicines. In other words, the little bit of pharmacy which remains should be treated as a most precious possession. It is the basis of our franchise from the state when a license to practice pharmacy is granted." This is the factor which has been overlooked by those who desire to hold to lower standards, thus making pharmacy a trade. So long as we desire to hold to the rights of professional men, we must be willing to qualify by meeting the requisite standards for practicing a profession. The only reason pharmacy has been granted only half-professional recognition in the past is that we have been unwilling to meet the full professional prerequisites.

We may as well admit that up to the present, most of the research work on medicinal preparations has been done either by manufacturing firms or by or in the medical schools. However, with the advent of the four-year course in pharmacy, we shall have better trained men in our own ranks. We shall discover some with a flair for research work, and we must develop within the field of pharmacy, per se, a corps of research workers. I realize that little research work can be done by the undergraduate, but wherever graduate work is being offered the colleges should make every effort to encourage research. There are many fields in which this could be carried on.

Let me take one single illustration, and that is the stability of drugs after they are manufactured either by the pharmacist or his source of supply. Is Tincture of Aconite as potent one year after manufacture as it was at the time it was made? Manufacturers are constantly working on some of their special products to develop such stability. But on the great bulk of medicines, chemicals and galenicals which a pharmacist dispenses, we have little authentic information as to the period of their effectiveness. Here is the opportunity for the colleges with graduate schools. If these institutions were to set up certain problems of this nature to be worked out during the year, publishing the results, I can foresee a wholesome rivalry and desirable competition growing up that will redound to the prestige of pharmacy. By building up such a corps of researchers, work of inestimable value to pharmacy will be accomplished and we shall enjoy a scientific atmosphere that will be priceless to our profession.

The movement in this country to reestablish and emphasize professional pharmacy is reflected in the greater use of the *U.S. Pharmacopeia* and the *National Formulary* both by physicians and pharmacists. In the Chicago area, particularly, a definite drive is being made to induce physicians to prescribe the preparations of the *USP* and *NF,* by drawing their attention to the fact that for every "proprietary" they prescribe, there is an equally good or better product in the *Pharmacopeia* or *Formulary.*

Physicians are beginning to realize that the hope of every manufacturer, even though he may profess to be vending exclusively through the medical profession, is that the time will arrive when customers will ask for these products by name over the counter. Every pharmacist in his contacts with physicians should show them that it is to the doctor's and patient's advantage to prescribe *Pharmacopeia* and *Formulary* products. In order to do this intelligently, the pharmacist must keep posted on the official preparations and their uses. Pharmacy's interest is primarily the welfare of the public.

The pharmaceutical service in hospitals is still unsatisfactory and remains one of the most important pharmaceutical questions to be solved. I recognize that it will require careful consideration before definite requirements can be laid down governing this function of a hospital. However, I hope that before long a requirement governing the hospital pharmacy and the service it renders will be included among other requirements of an approved hospital and will thus become effective in every section of the country. Pharmaceutical service in hospitals should be as carefully regulated and made as safe for their patients as is the pharmaceutical service in pharmacies.

More and more national boundary lines are being wiped out, particularly so far as science is concerned. Heart disease in Germany differs but little from similar ailments here, and digitalis acts on a Frenchman's heart in the same manner as it does on that of an American. By close contact, we benefit by the progress of other nations, and the advances in American pharmacy thereby become more effective and influential in foreign lands.

While the American Pharmaceutical Association is more particularly concerned with promoting the professional side of pharmacy, we must not lose sight of the fact that retail pharmacy, the root and foundation of all pharmaceutical activities, also has its economic phases which require consideration. The Association is therefore well within the scope of its many useful activities in aiding in the survey of the drug business which is being conducted in St. Louis under the direction of the U. S. Department of Commerce and which will, no doubt, result in making available information of great value to retail pharmacy.

A number of other surveys are being carried on in cooperation with the revision committees of the *U. S. Pharmacopeia* and the *National Formulary,* to determine the extent of prescription practice, and the drugs and preparations used in prescriptions so that those standards may fully serve their purposes to the professions of pharmacy and medicine.

More recently, W. Bruce Philip of California is conducting a survey with the object of correcting unfair and dishonest trade practices. Mr. Philip contends that, there must be a legal, fair and honest way to correct the evils of unfair and dishonest merchandising conditions which have demoralized the drug business up to a danger point, both for the consuming public and the profession of pharmacy. The evils of predatory price cutting, unwarranted and misleading advertising, manufacturers' deals, quantity discounts, quantity buys and hidden demonstrators, are destroying the legitimate business of national advertisers.

He says, "It would be ridiculous, if it were not so tragic, that a mere handful of predatory price cutters, who care nothing for the sick, the retailer, the wholesaler or, the manufacturer, can destroy fair and honest merchandising. There must be a legal and honest way to right these conditions, and I and those who are willing to aid me and are aiding me will find it. To that purpose, a survey of actual conditions has been made throughout California and one is being started by me to cover the whole United States. Facts are being accumulated and the drug world has started real thinking. One of the biggest successes so far in this survey is the bringing closer together of those of the profession and letting one another know what the other is doing or has done. It is made in the interest of the retail pharmacist and the public."

The Committee on the Costs of Medical Care, on which pharmacy fortunate is represented, as it should be, is now in the fourth year of a five-year fact-finding study to determine the basic principles underlying the costs of medical care. This is not a governmental organization but is financed entirely by private funds.

In closing, I want to express my appreciation for the very whole-hearted manner in which I have been supported. This spirit of cooperation has been invaluable to me in doing what I could to further the interests of pharmacy as a whole. ■

1940 Remington Medalist

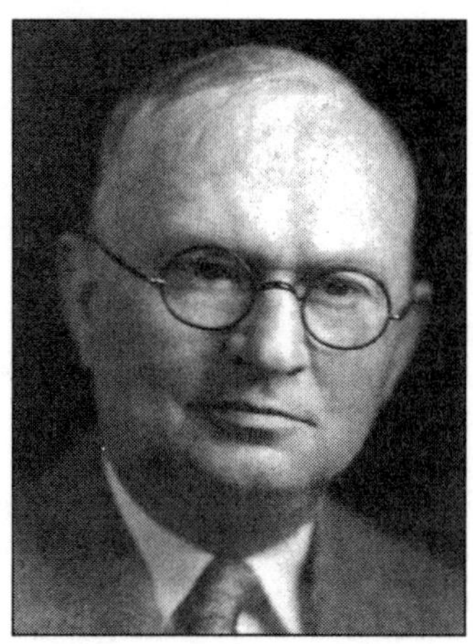

Robert Lee Swain
(1887-1963)

Robert Lee Swain was born in Redden, Delaware, and graduated with a Pharm.D. degree in 1909 and an LL.B. degree in 1932, both from the University of Maryland. He operated a pharmacy in Sykesville, Maryland 1909-1928, after which he served as a member 1920-1940 and secretary 1925-1940 of the Maryland Board of Pharmacy; Maryland deputy food and drug commissioner 1922-1939; and president 1937 of the Maryland Pharmaceutical Association. He served as founding chairman 1929-1939 of the National Conference of Law Enforcement Officials, and director of education 1930-1932 and president 1938 of the National Association of Boards of Pharmacy. Through his columns in *The Maryland Pharmacist* which he edited 1925-1940, he gained a reputation as a commentator on the pharmaceutical scene. In 1933, he became pharmacy editor of *Drug Topics,* and in 1939, vice president of Topics Publishing Company as well as editor-in-chief of both *Drug Topics* and *Drug Trade News* until his retirement in 1960.

Swain joined the American Pharmaceutical Association in 1909, serving as chairman of the APhA House of Delegates 1929-1930, member of the APhA Council 1933-1951 and 1953-1959, and APhA president 1933-1934. As chairman of the APhA Committee on the Modernization of Pharmacy Law, he led the movement to revise state pharmacy laws.

Basic Principals of Pharmaceutical Legislation

Robert Lee Swain

The 1940 Remington Medal was presented November 28, 1940, at the Hotel Pennsylvania in New York City. Swain's Remington address was not published, and the original manuscript has not been located. The following text was authored by Swain as chairman of the APhA Committee on the Modernization of Pharmacy Laws and published in the *Journal of American Pharmaceutical Association, Practical Pharmacy Edition,* volume 1, pages 399-402, 1940.

In determining upon a pharmaceutical legislative program, the one important matter to decide is the legal status of drugs and medicines. Are these products to be considered as mere articles of merchandise, or should their character as merchandise be merely incidental to their broader and more essential function in the treatment of disease and the conservation of health?

The APhA Committee on the Modernization of Pharmacy Laws has proceeded on the latter basis, as it would be impossible for pharmaceutical legislation to afford the public that kind and degree of protection which is needed in the production and distribution of drugs arid medicines if they were considered simply in the light of their commercial attributes, and this article will be devoted largely to a further discussion of this subject.

The so called Model Pharmacy Act as drawn by the Committee proceeded upon the belief that pharmacy is an essential public health profession, and that the production and distribution of drugs and medicines is essentially a professional function and should be subjected to public regulation and control. Therefore, the Model Act as drawn limits the production and distribution of drugs and medicines to persons and concerns operating under permits issued by the Board of Pharmacy. This applies to manufacturers, wholesalers, retailers, dispensing practitioners in the fields of medicine, dentistry, veterinary medicine, etc., dispensaries, clinics, hospitals and empowers the Board of Pharmacy to designate those drugs and medicines which in its judgment may be safely distributed by others than registered pharmacists, but even in these instances limiting the privilege to those persons to whom a permit has been issued.

The Pharmacy Act as drawn by the Committee on the Modernization of Pharmacy Laws has been criticized on the ground that it is too comprehensive and far reaching to have hope of adoption by the state legislatures. The Committee admits that there is some basis for this criticism, but the Committee proceeded on the belief that it could serve pharmaceutical legislation best by making available a draft embodying provisions which were theoretically desirable, leaving to the various states the task of seeking to secure the enactment of the Act as drawn or else permitting them the opportunity of modifying it in the light of what they considered the practical necessities. However, the Committee feels that an understanding of the theory and philosophy of the model draft is essential to an understanding of pharmaceutical legislation, and that the bill should be carefully and earnestly studied before any legislative program is embarked upon.

Simply because of their bearing upon this discussion, we should like to call attention to the preceding reports by the Committee on the Modernization of Pharmacy Laws. These were published in the November 1937 and November 1938 issues of the *Journal of the American Pharmaceutical Association* and represent several years of earnest study of the subject.

One of the reports constitutes a comprehensive survey of existing pharmacy laws and should be carefully read by all who really seek an authoritative understanding of the field. In making its study of existing pharmacy laws, the Committee was early impressed with what it considers a serious defect, namely, the absence of basic definitions. While the pharmacy acts operate exclusively upon drugs and medicines, the terms "drugs" and "medicines" are very infrequently defined, and such definitions as do occur are themselves much too limited to serve the purpose for which pharmacy laws are intended.

The Committee has recommended that in the event it is not considered desirable or feasible to rewrite the existing state pharmacy act, the act should be amended so as to provide workable definitions for the main subject matter which the act is intended to control and regulate. Proof that the Committee recommendation is sound is to be found in the recent cases in which Boards of Pharmacy sought to convince certain Courts that vitamins are drug products. One reason why the Boards failed to maintain their position, as pointed out in one of the decisions, was that "the statute does not specifically define either drugs or medicines." In both cases the Boards of Pharmacy endeavored to persuade the Courts to adopt for the purpose of the Pharmacy Act the definitions of the term "drug" as set forth in the Food, Drug and Cosmetic Act. In one case the Court stated: "These definitions apply to the federal act, which was adopted for different and other purposes than those moving the state pharmacy statute, and cannot, in my opinion, govern the construction of the state legislation."

While the Courts in these respective States did not give the basis for their conclusions, they probably had in mind the very point emphasized in the reports of the Committee on the Modernization of Pharmacy Laws, in which it was stated that the definition of the term "drug," as used in the Food, Drug and Cosmetic Act, was not suited to the needs of a pharmacy law.

In order to make this clear, a careful reading should be given the definition of the term "drug" taken from the federal Food, Drug and Cosmetic Act: "The term 'drug' means (1) articles recognized in the official *United States Pharmacopeia,* official Homoeopathic Pharmacopoeia of the United States, or official *National Formulary,* or any supplement to any of them; and (2) articles intended for use in the diagnosis, cure, mitigation, treatment or prevention of disease in man or other animals; and (3) articles (other than food) intended to affect the structure of any function of the body of man or other animals; and (4) articles intended for use as a component of any article specified in clause (1), (2) or (3); but does not include devices or their components, parts or accessories." A study of this definition will show that it is admirably suited to the purpose of the Food, Drug and Cosmetic Act, which is to prohibit the movement in interstate commerce of adulterated and misbranded food, drugs, devices and cosmetics.

The Pharmacy Act, however, has an entirely different function, and deals primarily with the production and distribution of drugs and medicines. When considered from the standpoint of the Food, Drug and Cosmetic Act, water might well be a drug or a food, as there is every reason why adulterated water should not be sold and equally good reason why the label on a container of water should not contain untruthful and misleading statements. It will be seen at once that water could not be considered a drug under the pharmacy acts if it were to be subjected to the limitations in production and distribution which pharmacy acts contemplate. The same observation could be made of sugar, lard, salt, baking soda and a number of other products which are officially recognized in the *Pharmacopeia* and for which there exists good reason why they should not be sold in adulterated or misbranded form.

It was for this reason that our Committee has suggested that when the term "drug" is defined in a pharmacy act the definition as given in the Food, Drug and Cosmetic Act be modified as follows: "The term 'drug' means (1) all articles recognized in the official *United States Pharmacopoeia,* official *Homeopathic Pharmacopoeia of the United States,* or official *National Formulary,* or any supplement to any of them which are intended for use in the diagnosis, cure, mitigation, treatment or prevention of disease in man or other animals; and (2) all other articles intended for use in the diagnosis, cure, mitigation, treatment or prevention of disease in man or other animals; and (3) articles (other than food) intended to affect the structure or any function of the body of man or other animals; and (4) articles intended for use as a component of any article specified in clause (1), (2) or (3); but does not include devices or their components, parts or accessories."

It is our feeling, too, that the word "prescription" should be defined. Here, also, a few state acts attempt to define this term, and again such definitions as do occur are inconclusive all thoroughly unsatisfactory for a modern pharmacy law. These definitions seem to be concerned exclusively with the status of the order for drugs and medicines which the pharmacist receives, and necessarily have no bearing unless the order is received. The time has come, in the judgment of our Committee, when the term "prescription" should be defined in such a manner that it must be sent on to the drug store, and that violation of the pharmacy act would take place when certain drugs and medicines were dispensed in any other manner. In other words, our Committee is not nearly as much concerned with the nature of the order which may be sent to the drug store as we are in assuring ourselves that the order will be sent to the drug store.

It will be recalled that under Section 502(j) of the Food, Drug and Cosmetic Act a drug is misbranded "If it is dangerous to health when used in the dosage, or with the frequency or duration prescribed, recommended or suggested in the labeling thereof." Proceeding under the authority of this section the Federal Food and Drug Commissioner has declared certain well known drugs to be dangerous and has limited their distribution to physicians' prescriptions.

In order, however, to give effect to the ruling of the Commissioner, it must be assumed that the Food, Drug and Cosmetic Act has intrastate jurisdiction. We have no disposition to argue this point here and will not do so other than to state that there is strong legal opinion in support of the belief that the Federal Food, Drug and Cosmetic Act does not have intrastate effect.

Quite aside from which is the correct point of view, the mere fact that a difference of opinion exists is sufficient reason for meeting the situation by amending our pharmacy laws in such a manner that all drugs declared to be dangerous by the Food and Drug Commissioner may be dispensed only on physicians' prescriptions. This would serve the purpose of the federal act and would remove all question of legality, as certainly the state may, if it so desires, limit the distribution of dangerous drugs in this manner.

But, concurrent with this amendment to the pharmacy act should be another amendment defining the term "prescription." Prescriptions should, in our judgment, be defined as an order for drugs and medicines written by a legally competent practitioner of medicine, dentistry or veterinary medicine to be compounded and dispensed by a registered pharmacist in a duly registered pharmacy (in those states requiring store registration under the pharmacy law) and to be kept on file a designated period of years.

This will be seen as of still greater importance when we recall that there is a tendency to limit potent drugs and medicines to physicians' prescriptions. This is well illustrated in the state legislation so limiting barbituric acid compounds; and in some states, notably Pennsylvania, this includes weight reducing preparations and perhaps others.

Unless the term prescription is defined so as to limit it to the practice of pharmacy in a duly registered pharmacy, we may find that we have unwittingly centered the distribution of many important drug products in the hands of the dispensing doctor. This statement is not meant as a slap at the dispensing practitioner, but in fairness it must be contended that pharmacists have been trained for the practice of pharmacy while medical men have had virtually no training in this field.

Pharmacy acts should also include workable definitions of the terms "pharmacy" and "drug store," and here, too, we find that by and large the state pharmacy acts attempt no such definitions. The term pharmacy should be defined both as the profession and the place where the profession is practiced. A reading of the pharmacy acts as now in effect will disclose that there is a great doubt whether their provisions were meant to include the hospital pharmacy, the clinic pharmacy, the dispensary or other places where drugs and medicines might be compounded and dispensed.

In explanation of this somewhat glaring omission, it might be said that our pharmacy acts more or less generally conform to the legislative pattern first established about 1870 when the states first began to enact pharmacy laws. At that time the task was to bring the retail drug store within the purview of the pharmacy act, and this provoked opposition enough without attempting to give the pharmacy acts a wider application by giving them authority over hospitals and other places where drugs might be compounded and dispensed. True, the early pharmacy acts have been amended from time to time, but even so they have not met the situation which now confronts us, namely, extending the authority of the board of pharmacy over all places, irrespective of kind, where drugs and medicines are compounded and dispensed. The rapid development of hospital pharmacies and the inclusion of a well-operated pharmacy as the basis for recognition of a hospital by the American Hospital Association have given pharmacy a higher status in hospital practice and make it imperative that the pharmacy in such institutions be in the hands of professionally and legally competent persons.

It would, of course, be possible to extend this discussion at great length, as a study of our pharmacy laws might well show that they need to be amended so as to provide basic definitions other than those which have been discussed here. However, my purpose has been to emphasize the imperative need of incorporating basic definitions in our pharmacy laws, and I hope that what has been said here has served that purpose. ■

1941 Remington Medalist

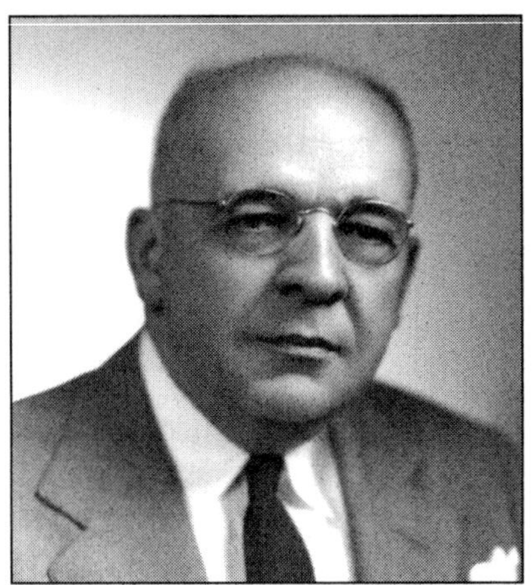

George Denton Beal

(1887-1972)

George Denton Beal was born in Scio, Ohio, son of the first Remington medalist, James Hartley Beal. He received a Ph.C. degree in 1906 and a Pharm.D. degree in 1907, both from the Scio College of Pharmacy, after which he earned a 1911 Ph.D. degree in chemistry from Columbia University. He then joined the faculty of the University of Illinois as instructor in chemistry 1911-1914, associate 1914-1918, assistant professor 1918-1920, associate professor 1920-1924, and professor 1924-1926. In 1926, he joined the Mellon Institute of Industrial Research in Pittsburgh, Pennsylvania, first as assistant director and then as director of research. He also served as a director of the Pittsburgh College of Pharmacy, a trustee of both Mt. Union College and the Philadelphia College of Pharmacy and Science, national president of Phi Lambda Upsilon, a member of the National Research Council 1922-1927, and a member of the USP Revision Committee 1920-1945.

A longtime member of the American Pharmaceutical Association, Beal served as APhA first vice president 1934-1935, as APhA president 1936-1937, and was largely instrumental in the establishment of the APhA Drug Standards Laboratory, personally supervising the development and assisting in raising funds to make the laboratory a reality.

PHARMACEUTICAL EDUCATION AND RESEARCH

George Denton Beal

The 1941 Remington Medal was presented December 4, 1941, at the Hotel Pennsylvania in New York City. Beal's Remington address was not published, and a copy of the manuscript has not been located. Two notable lectures by George Beal have been published. One is his 1937 APhA presidential address published in the *Journal of the American Pharmaceutical Association,* volume 26, pages 1007-1016, 1937. The other, entitled "Pharmaceutical Education and Industrial Research," presented on May 15, 1947, at the University of Illinois College of Pharmacy appears in the *American Journal of Pharmaceutical Education* (volume 11, pages 373-389, 1947). Both reflect views that were probably included in Beal's 1941 Remington lecture. We have selected a slightly abridged version of the 1947 lecture as more representative of the broader scope of activities and interests of the 1941 Remington medalist.

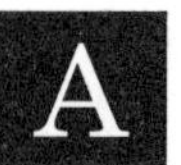
A properly designed, properly administered curriculum in pharmacy provides a sound basic training for persons who plan to devote their lives to industrial science. In order to determine whether this is true, it would be well to consider this educational program from the standpoint of the function of pharmacy. Does the profession of pharmacy, in its several branches, parallel the principal functions of industry? Viewed in all its departments, there seems to be the required similarity.

The similarity is probably not apparent to the casual observer. That which meets the eye of the man on the street is the corner drug store. In the public eye the practice of pharmacy is a retail business. According to location that business extends from the purveyance of medicinal agents, health goods, and sick-room supplies, through the distribution of cosmetics, toiletries and tobacco to a very general confectionery and lunch-room business, with a news-stand on the side, until in many instances the operations are those of a general merchandising store.

When the general public or even members of another profession fail to recognize the professional role of pharmacy, it is because their eyes have been filled and their minds confused by the restaurant and racket-store features. Pharmacists speak of this and that having been taken out of the hands of pharmacy. What they should say, and what too many will not admit, is that a segment of the profession has lost its grip on something through inattention. They blame others for grasping, whereas they should chide themselves for negligence.

During the past fifty years a very large part of the retail pharmaceutical trade has been devoted to the promotion of wholly unrelated miscellaneous lines, each added as a potential profit maker. Miscellaneous manufacturers and wholesale distributors have encouraged this, they having in mind the long hours during which pharmacies remain open, thus extending the time during which their products are available to the casual shopper homeward bound from the movies or the careless shopper in the residential neighborhood. Even all-night lunchrooms have closed because they could not meet the competition of the lunch features of the drug store soda fountain. And, to a large extent overlooking the fact that they were first of all guilty of encroaching on the fields of other retail businesses, pharmacists, encouraged by many of their editorial writers and association leaders, vocally and bitterly resent advances made by other retail outlets in adding to their stock in trade profitable items from the drug business that do not require too much professional knowledge for their distribution.

Pharmacists are encouraged by detail men and experts on store management to put even numerous pharmaceutical miscellany on a self service basis, their only professional contribution being the wrapping of the package and ringing the cash register. Then they go to the state capital and prate about their professional responsibility, in order to prevent another respectable retail outlet from doing the same thing. To many people it seems incomprehensible that a large part of the pharmaceutical curriculum is not devoted to training in methods of business administration. Actually the major training that a young pharmacist receives along these lines is obtained while he is serving his store apprenticeship. Hence, it is a trade-perpetuated custom, that has never intensively been made a part of the curriculum in pharmacy in many schools.

What are the real functions of pharmacy? From the time the apothecary first appears in history, his task has been the preparation of therapeutic agents in such manner that they are most acceptable and effective for the relief of illness. Literature, both Biblical and profane, classical and otherwise, refers to the "art" of the apothecary. Because the element of compounding has entered into the apothecary's daily duties from the beginning of time, it has been regarded as a "mystery" that developed into science, while other retail distributions have been only trades. The responsibilities of pharmacy therefore include all the services involved in the preparation of medicines, from the collection or manufacture of the crude raw material to the final compounding of the physician's prescription.

There are two major divisions into which science falls: pure and applied. Pharmacy very definitely belongs in the second group. Most scientists are today willing to admit that there is no sharp dividing line between the two classes, that no scientific conclusion is so abstract, so far away in the ethereal blue, that there is no possibility of it coming to a practical application; and none so practical that it does not win in some way substantiate a theoretical conclusion. While pharmacy falls into the second category because of its very practical applications in the maintenance or restoration of public health, it also belongs there because it represents the related practical applications of chemistry, physics, and the biological sciences.

Pharmacists have always taken great pride in pointing out how many of the earlier chemical discoveries were made by apothecaries. The discovery of chlorine by Scheele, of iodine by Courtois, and the alkaloidal discoveries of Derosne, Serturner, and Pelletier and Caventou are made much of, especially around Pharmacy Week. Likewise we note that Liebig's "Annalen," in which so much of the world's great chemical literature has appeared, was originally the "Annalen der Pharmazie." This, however, became the "Annalen der Pharmacie und Chemie," next the "Annalen der Chemie und Pharmazie," until finally it is today "Annalen der Chemie." This is said to symbolic of the growing apart of chemistry as a separate science, much to the credit of chemistry. It also indicates that many of the practitioners of pharmacy were becoming addicted to its commercial side, and that they were content to take such developments as were brought to them by those of other fields. Pharmacy, having become somewhat, pulled apart at the seams, is trying to pull itself together once more.

American pharmacy has passed through a series of periods in its development, whether one be thinking of the source of the drugs or of the style of professional practice. When a formal pharmaceutical practice began in America it was directed very much by the traditions and practices of the physicians and apothecaries who had come over from the old world. The mineral salts used were of course the same; among vegetable drugs were sought out the counterparts of those formerly used. Because large areas of the country were only sparsely settled, formal medicine became modified as to use of drugs by grandmotherly lore and also by gradually acquired contacts with the practices of Indian medicine men. The mechanics of pharmacy also adhered to tradition resulting in a continuation of the old world use of teas, tinctures and wines.

American pharmacy, however, from its beginning has not been held back for centuries by the very slow growth of science, nor by the fact that science was practically non-existent. Since many men of scientific attainment or manner of thinking were also likely to be original thinkers along other lines as well, they were frequently found among those colonists who crossed the ocean to escape the conservatism and oppression of Europe. Colonization began during the period of renaissance in arts and letters, and just when science was beginning to throw aside the monidy robe of the closet philosopher. Friends in America were in correspondence with friends back home, they heard of scientific advances as they appeared, and exchanged their own thoughts thereon. Thus, they were not held down to the crudest use of natural remedies, but at an early date began some chemical manufacturing. Efforts were made to systematize medical and pharmaceutical practice at the same time that our own governmental methods were being systematized. Witness the production of a pharmacopoeia for the use of the military hospital of the Continental Army at Lititz, Pennsylvania, in 1776, the publication of a pharmacopoeia by the Massachusetts Medical Society in 1808, based on the then current *Edinburgh Pharmacopoeia,* and one by the New York hospital in 1816. The originators of the *Massachusetts Pharmacopeia* had hoped to make it national in scope, but failed necessary cooperation. When the *New York Hospital Pharmacopeia* appeared, however, it became apparent that before long there would be serious confusion of authority, so Lyman Spalding four years later had little difficulty in persuading the medical societies and colleges to join with him in organizing the United States Pharmacopoeial Convention. American pharmacists, particularly their few colleges of pharmacy, had their scientific position so well consolidated that by 1840 they were rendering valuable assistance in pharmacopeial revision and in 1850 they were invited to become members of the Convention, fully activating that joint venture that today is regarded as the foremost work of its kind in the world.

While pharmacy and medicine were depending exclusively upon natural inorganic and organic drugs and their salts, botanical explorations were further extending the use of vegetable drugs and their derivatives. We may therefore speak of this as the botanical era of pharmacy, and consider that it was active until about 1880. The development of mechanization, when machines and larger manufacturing apparatus began to replace hand and laboratory scale operations, began about 1840 and grew most rapidly between 1880 and 1910. The demand for uniformity in strength of preparation, representing the inception of the period of scientific control, started when people began to migrate from one part of the country to another, and coincides interestingly with the rapid growth of steam transportation after 1860. The trend to biological products, introducing bacteriological and glandular drugs, leading up to such things as vitamins and hormones, was born about 1890, although Scheffer invented the salt process for isolating pepsin from gastric juice in 1872 and Fairchild produced scaled pepsin in 1879. The replacement of natural drugs with those of laboratory origin, involving, chemical reconstruction, parallels the progress of chemical science. But the actual use of the laboratory in this way comes so late in the last century that we may say that the era of chemical synthesis actually began about 1900.

Since we are considering the role of pharmaceutical education in industrial progress, I hope it is not presuming too much upon your patience to relate briefly the major developments in pharmaceutical industry in America. One of the oldest manufacturing lines in the field of pharmaceutical chemistry began in 1812 as Farr and Kunzi, later operating under the name of Powers and Weightman. The Rosengarten family began similar operations in 1829, and early in the present century effected a merger as Powers-Weighman-Rosengarten Company. In the late eighties the well known German firm of E. Merck established an American branch, which later came into control of the American branch of the family, and later, by absorption of the Powers-Weightrnan-Rosengarten Company became Merck and Company Incorporated. Two other American houses that have long taken a prominent part in the manufacture of pharmaceutical chemicals are Charles Pfizer and Sons and Mallinckrodt Chemical Works. And in naming these specifically we mean no disparagement to a number of other chemical manufacturers of pharmaceutical importance who have contributed largely to professional development.

Mechanical operations for processing drugs were slow to develop, it being near the middle of the past century when drugs were powdered in other than a mortar. One of the first examples of large-scale milling was the use of a stone paint mill by Charles Hagner of Philadelphia to powder cream of tartar. The French used percolators in 1813 for clarifying sugar solutions with bone-black, and in 1815 Count Real used a percolator for drug extractions, but European and American pharmacists generally preferred to make their tinctures by maceration. The first serious studies on percolation were made by William Proctor and Dr. Squibb. But a lack of refinement of what we now call chemical engineering caused many to fear the destruction of active principles by heat while percolates were being concentrated. During the 70s, for example, Parke, Davis and Co. advertised "we neither percolate nor use heat in any form," although shortly afterwards they were among the first to adopt large scale percolation and vacuum evaporation. Today, as every pharmacist knows, hand operations of any sort are required for only the most extemporaneous of preparation, and mechanization has been a triumph of American pharmaceutical manufacturing. In addition, new mechanizations are continually being developed for the production of new drugs or for the preparation of their dosage forms.

Science has advanced with engineering in pharmaceutical operations, the research laboratories providing new drugs to challenge the skill of the pharmaceutical engineers in their manufacture, and the control laboratories testifying to the precision of the manufacturing operations. Standardization has been one of the great contributions of scientific and industrial pharmacy during the past century. The majority of manufacturing operations were initiated, supervised and carried out by pharmacists, and done in accordance with the art of the apothecary. Standardization of procedure preceded that of the product. Standardization first established a ratio of quantity of preparation to quantity of drug for convenience in dosing, then turned its attention to the maintenance of potency.

We can all take pride in the fact that the use of laboratory control of manufacturing operations in pharmacy was both seriously considered and practiced by pharmaceutical industry when the larger part of American industry thought it either an expensive luxury or a silly fad, when Andrew Carnegie was viewed with suspicion by his fellow iron masters for saying that a chemist in the laboratory could better determine the quality of iron than the eye of the blast furnace foreman.

With the advance in knowledge of chemical methods of drug control, it became more and more apparent that chemical control could not satisfy the entire needs of the profession. It was then impossible chemically to characterize the active principles of some drugs, and others showed chemical characteristics that did not agree with their therapeutic behavior. As physiologists devised methods for measuring physiological reactions, it became possible to determine the strength of drugs that did not respond to chemical test. Probably the first biologically assayed preparation on the market was an extract of ergot introduced in 1894, the same drug that introduced the chemically standardized line fifteen years earlier. It was not long thereafter that the bio assay of digitalis was begun. Over fifty years of experience with these particular drugs has not brought knowledge to a state where there is no acrimonious discussion when pharmacologists get together, but bioassays have made safe and effective the use of some of our most valuable drugs.

Fifty years ago in the United States a scientific education, outside of the public health profession of medicine and the engineering fields, was looked upon primarily as a preparation for those who intended to enter the teaching profession, or as a qualification for research in academic circles. Business men, and particularly industrialists, were self-made in a large measure. Industrial leaders were often men who had risen from the bench because of their native ability. They prided themselves upon being practical men, and as practical men had no love, or at most only tolerated those persons who dealt in scientific and technical theory. Chemists might be tolerated in control laboratories, but their judgment was outweighed by the men of practical experience in the operating department of an industry. There were industrial research laboratories in some industries outside of pharmacy, and some distinguished names, but the relatively small number of graduates from the scientific schools and the membership of the scientific societies, outside of the teaching profession, testified to the little thought given to the value of scientific guidance in industry.

Robert Kennedy Duncan, who devised the system of industrial fellowships that was to eventuate as Mellon Institute, pointed out to his American readers that the technical preeminence of Germany in chemical industries was due to the fact that the leaders of German industry and finance alone had the vision of the worth of the knowledge in the reservoirs of their universities. He called attention to the partnerships that actually existed, that German scientists could go for support to manufacturers and bankers, and that the latter, having technical problems too deep for their own solution, could go to those same scientists for the leadership and relief that science could give. His teaching, and that of a few other publicists for science, together with the examples of the way in which those who had decided to take science into their confidence had profited thereby, emboldened others to take the same steps, with results that rapidly became apparent.

Industrial research laboratories today serve every conceivable field of manufacturing. The number of personnel employed ranges from one into the hundreds or several thousands, if all of the research and development activities of some of the large corporations be considered as a unit. The principal criterion that determines whether a laboratory group is entitled to be called a research laboratory is whether it is engaged in looking toward the future. It is most important that an industry look forward always to what it may be doing in ten to twenty years. In order to picture this it must give thought to what its competitors in the same line of products may be doing. Such a look into the future is always considered by some executives a figment of the imagination. But whatever prediction is made, it must not be discounted if it is based upon an accurate appraisal of the present state of knowledge, with particular attention to the trends which theoretical investigations seem to be taking, coupled with a careful look at present sources of raw materials or what seem to be becoming buyers' tastes.

I have never been able to agree with many research directors and still more business executives that effective research related to industry can only be carried out by those highly skilled in the art of that particular industry. Let me use the homely illustration of the village half-wit who recovered the strayed horse after the village had searched for hours without success. His explanation was as follows: "I just thought... if I was a horse where would I go?... and there he was." This fellow tried to project himself into the thinking of a horse, the supposedly normal citizens had confined their thinking to where the horses had been found in the past. The specialists of an industry are usually the most valuable men for a task of "trouble shooting." Their intimate knowledge of the relationship of operations in a sequence tells them almost automatically when something is out of step.

When it comes to venturing for a new process or product, many specialists in the line to be improved are actually handicapped by their experience. The fact that a thing has always been done a certain way is an almost irresistible push away from a new path. Not many years ago methanol and acetone were entirely primary and secondary products of the destructive distillation of wood. The processes were simple and the quantities of wood available for distillation were entirely adequate. The wood distillers were certain that nothing could challenge their supremacy, and therefore did nothing to determine whether there might be cheaper sources. Ammonia, likewise, was a by product from coking of coal. Today there is some requirement for charcoal, and a large demand for coke. However, the quantities of methanol, acetone, and ammonia, 90 obtained fall short of actual requirements: Methanol and ammonia today are made by catalytic synthesis in the vapor phase, and many other important chemicals likewise are produced by reactions in which air, natural gas, or the gaseous by products of petroleum refining furnish the raw materials. The assumption was made by the Japanese that silk could never be replaced, but synthetic fibers are made in such variety that silk today is but one of the quality textile fibers.

When it comes to this type of looking into the future the person most successful is, first of all, the one who has the soundest fundamental training in the basic sciences involved. Therefore a person trained in the methods of investigation, firmly grounded in the fundamental principles of chemistry, is more likely to be a successful long-range prognosticator than the person who knows the tricks of the trade but is not too firmly grounded in the means by which these were established. Every so often we hear it said that a certain person undertook a problem because he did not know it could not be resolved, and thereupon solved it.

Another reason for the necessity of sound fundamental training to be fortified by experience in the methods of the investigator is that, due to economic changes the need for further research in a particular field may suddenly cease. Under such circumstances the over-specialized research worker may suffer.

The broad applications to industry of chemistry are difficult for the less experienced students to appreciate. While teaching, I was also responsible for arranging the annual plant inspection trips of our upperclassmen. One day, while visiting a large chemical manufacturer in the Chicago district, the students were constantly asking to see the laboratory. Finally, in response to such a question, our guide pointed out a small building in the distance, and said, "That's it." With evident disappointment this student then asked, "But how many chemists have you?" To which the answer was, "About four hundred." "Well, where are they?" To this our guide answered, "I'm a chemist." "And what do you do?" "Oh, I am superintendent of the sulfuric acid plant." The fifteen students in that group then and there had their eyes opened to the importance of chemistry in industry. This same sort of thing had been pointed out to me nearly twenty years before in one of our large pharmaceutical houses, when my attention was directed to the compounding operations that must be carried out under the supervision of registered pharmacists.

As there are many things that pharmacists are called upon to do, it is desirable that the collegiate preparation of the pharmacist enable him to do these various things. Some of those things are daily duties, some are only possibilities. Formal courses of instruction in preparation for each of these possible duties are out of the question because they cannot be fitted into the curriculum. There is little utility in giving much formalized instruction to all students for duties they are seldom if ever called upon to perform. The subject matter of the curriculum should rather be calculated to enable the student, applying his professional knowledge, to accomplish those special things.

The pharmaceutical curriculum is a curriculum in applied physical and biological sciences. Fundamentally, it is a chemical curriculum, since pharmacy is, basically, the application of chemical knowledge and chemical procedures to the preparation of remedial agents. The operations in the pharmaceutical laboratory are, in general, basic chemical engineering operations, in which application is made of the general principles of chemistry and physics. Since the products of pharmaceutical operations are employed to influence life processes, pharmacy is also an applied biological science. Functionally, pharmacy refines natural products, or prepares products obtained by chemical or biological reactions, for the treatment of disease in accordance with the diagnosis and prescription of a physician. The function of pharmacy therefore is on a professional level with the function of medicine, the one being unable to accomplish its desired end without the professional cooperation of the other. Neither is subordinate to the other. Pharmacy is essentially applied natural science, medicine, applied biological science. The two, together, hold public health in their hands.

In every type of profession there is a large volume of routine work of a daily character that attracts no attention whatever, but is essential in the profession. One experienced structural engineer may conceive the plan for a huge bridge or a gigantic skyscraper. It requires uncounted hours on the part of other engineers in the drafting room to produce the working drawings for which all stresses and details have been calculated and by which procurement and construction are ordered. Public attention is directed to the attorney who conducts examination of witnesses and addresses ajury, or who argues an important case before a supreme court

The vast volume of work of the legal profession occurs in the drawing of documents and the assembly of references to statutes and decisions. These back office occupations never reach the public eye. The completion of a professional education is only one stage of a professional apprenticeship. Successive apprenticeships carry on office routine, and gradually emerge into junior executive positions from which advancement still continues. In every profession there are a series of levels, each successive one of increasing responsibility being of somewhat lesser area. These smaller areas of increasing responsibility are matched by the smaller number of persons of increasing ability and experience who can fill them. The old adage that there is always room at the top is usually true because of the many qualifications required of the man at the top. There is, however, a level at which each professional worker may find his place.

Whether or not a man is a member of a profession is not altogether a question of his occupation. A person may perform a scientific operation routinely, precisely observing all required steps, and still be only a workman, for he can at best pass only arbitrary judgment on what has occurred. On the other hand, he may approach each task as a new experience, presenting some new conditions for his consideration. The state of mind, the approach to a project, and one's manner of conducting that project determine whether one's occupation is professional, and not the surroundings or adjuncts among which the task is performed. The purpose of the sixty-five accredited colleges of pharmacy, the nine national associations, the many state, county and local associations, and the thirty-six pharmaceutical periodicals of the country, is to train and aid pharmacists in attaining and maintaining that state of mind.

Having talked all around the profession of pharmacy, and scientific and industrial research, I should like as my final point to discuss the relationship of research to our colleges of pharmacy. First, let us ask if research is only something attractive to brighten up the college, in the manner of a few good pictures? If it turns the college to better things, the answer is "Yes." It is also a necessary thing, of the structure rather than the ornamentation. A keen teacher is an inquiring teacher, his mental process stimulated, causing him to bring new inspiration with his teaching. A college of pharmacy is primarily an undergraduate college, therefore nothing must interfere with the quality of teaching. But pharmaceutical laboratory directors frequently express regret that the pharmaceutical industry has not absorbed more pharmaceutical scientists. They explain, however, that so many pharmaceutical students, in spite of the scientific background of their training, have never developed a scientific manner of thinking. This lack, I fear, can far too often be laid at the doors of those who are supposed to train students in their habits of thought.

Research training really begins at the graduate level, but under-graduate students must be inspired to reach that level. There is another need for rapid growth at the graduate level in addition to that for supplying industrial needs, and that is to develop a sufficient number of faculty replacements, and to make available more properly trained teachers to serve pharmaceutical education. The shortness of supply of top level teachers for the pharmacy curriculum is today the matter of most serious concern to the accrediting agencies. We would like to keep pharmaceutical education and pharmaceutical science just as far as possible in the hands of pharmaceutically trained personnel, and our investigative ability must be turned to study of the educational method as well as the pharmaceutical product.

In spite of criticisms that I have uttered or implied, I, nevertheless, insist that American pharmacy is a well balanced organization. It began during pioneer life as a self-contained and self-sufficient profession. It took from the best of old world science and added a new materia medica from a country of great botanical richness. It pioneered in applying and adapting engineering methods to its manufacturing industries, leading the world in developing novel specialized automatic machinery. It established a nation-wide system of professional education. It not only cooperated in securing, but actually initiated, needful regulatory legislation. It has very largely made its own standards of conduct both for men and merchandise. It has successfully combined scientific and commercial interests in one profession.

But pharmacy today requires skilled specialists. Such needful persons must be hired where they can be found, and it will be the fault of pharmaceutical education if its graduates do not flow into these positions. Pharmacy students who intend to embark upon truly scientific pursuits will find the avenue open, for in every research laboratory we have many assistants. There is more handwork than brain work in the research laboratory, and the lack of adequate assistance hampers the functioning of a brilliant brain. Students of pharmacy receive one of the best of manipulative trainings. They are among the best of raw material for apprenticeship to this scientific and industrial age. If our faculties are not strong enough to develop these apprentices, we must strengthen our faculties. If we raise our educational sights to encompass the research needs of pharmacy we also benefit pharmacy professionally. Pharmaceutical education and pharmaceutical practice of tomorrow are being determined in the teaching of students today. You are indeed being called to greater things. Answer the call, and you justify the contention that you are a profession. Fail, and you are tradesmen. ■

1942 Remington Medalist

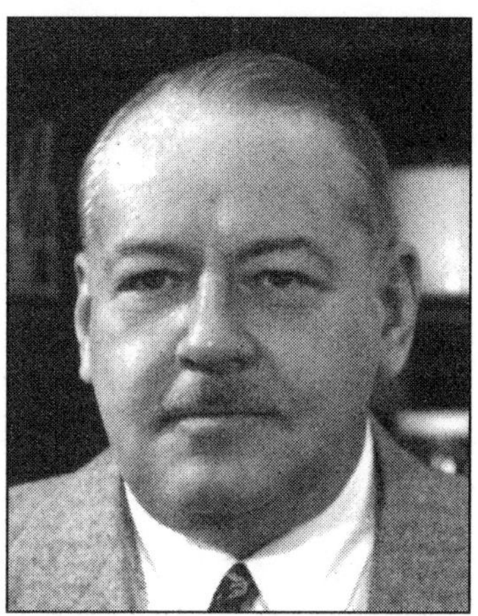

JOSIAH KIRBY LILLY, SR.

(1861-1948)

Josiah Kirby Lilly, Sr., born in Greencastle, Indiana, the son of Colonel Eli Lilly, founder of Eli Lilly and Company, received his initial pharmacy training in his father's establishment. Following graduation from the Philadelphia College of Pharmacy in 1882, he became superintendant of the Lilly Laboratories in Indianapolis. Upon the death of his father in 1898, he succeeded to the presidency of Eli Lilly and Company, continuing in this office until 1932 when he became Chairman of the Board. Lilly was a founding member of the National Association of Manufacturers of Medicinal Products, which, after a change of name, was merged in 1958 with another trade association to form the Pharmaceutical Manufacturers Association.

Under his direction, Eli Lilly and Company developed the first commercially available insulin in the U.S. and pioneered in the production of vitamins, ephedrine products, liver extact, and improved barbituric acid derivatives. His civic pursuits included service as president of the Indianapolis Y.M.C.A. and chairman of the Indianapolis Foundation. His cultural pursuits are best remembered for his collection of over 10,000 items associated with the life and music of Stephen Collins Foster and reprinting of first editions of Foster musical compositions, which did much to popularize this great American composer. Lilly served as APhA honorary president 1934-1935, and eight universities conferred on him honorary degrees. In selecting Josiah K. Lilly as the 1942 Remington Honor Medal recipient, he was cited for the "support of pharmaceutical research not only in the laboratories of his own company, but in APhA's Laboratory and in educational institutions throughout the country."

Life Is Like a Glass of Good Wine

Josiah Kirby Lilly, Sr.

The 1942 Remington Honor Medal Lecture was presented December 9, 1942, at the Hotel Pennsylvania, New York City. Since the text of the original Remington lecture has never been found either in the Eli Lilly Corporate Archives nor in the APhA Archives, the following excerpts of addresses and letters of Josiah K. Lilly, Sr., provide an insight into the life of the 1942 Remington medalist. They were selected from the Lilly Corporate Archives by Gene E. McCormick, corporate historian, Eli Lilly and Company, and published in an article entitled "Josiah Kirby Lilly, Sr., the Man (1861-1948)," appearing in *Pharmacy in History,* volume 12, pages 57-67, 1970.

Most gratefully does the boy treasure the personal contact with the great men of Pharmacy [Maisch, Remington, and Sadtler]. They not only taught their lines but inculcated into the students a high regard for true scientific pharmacy, impressed the fundamental need of the strictest integrity in all matters connected with dispensing medicines for the sick." (1940 manuscript entitled "Remembrances" by J. K. Lilly in the Lilly Archives.) In his address to the 1888 Philadelphia College of Pharmacy graduating class, J. K. Lilly, Sr. called upon the graduates to "make pharmacy a recognized profession and to maintain it on an equal footing with medicine because the pharmacist has a distinct service to render in promoting health care to mankind." He also urged the pharmacist to "avoid carrying credit with the wholesaler and purchase only what his resources would allow, for here there is a basic difference between the methods by which the pharmacist and wholesaler serve the common good." It was upon the conviction that the wholesaler, pharmacist, and physician each has a specific function in making medicines available to the sick that Eli Lilly and Company adopted a policy of distribution solely through the wholesaler. (Copy of *J.K. Lilly, Sr.'s address to the graduating class at the Philadelphia College of Pharmacy, March 16, 1888.)*

"That success may attend [our] efforts, a highly trained personnel is essential. It must consist of devoted men and women consecrated to the search for truth and must be free from commercial influence or control ...It should be recognized also that it must be a prosperous and reasonably profitable concern that essays to support, financially, extensive research. In short, it must supply its own endowment. Hence no apologies are necessary on the score of commercialism, but it is secondary and must never control." *(Address entitled "Research in Manufacturing Pharmacy" delivered lyj K Lilly, Sr. at the opening of the company's new research facility on October 11, 1935.)*

"It is a real accomplishment for any family to go on, generation after generation, in an honorable and creditable manner, especially if anchored to some field of endeavor that is useful to society at large. Of course, we all take out hats off to the Schieffelin family as the oldest in the field. No doubt our ancestors experienced great difficulties, just as we do today, but somehow, to be deeply anchored into a wholesome past is a tremendous help in time of need. So it seems that in these parlous days we should be of good cheer, keep on quietly in the channel of our ways day by day, building and building and building, for better and better things." *(Letter from J.K. Lilly, Sr. to WJ Schieffelin,Jr., president of Schieffelin & Company, June 20, 1946, in the Lilly Archives.)*

"Life is somewhat like unto a glass of good wine that one may drink hurridly, in great gulps, and have done with it; or it may be sipped slowly, deliberately, with good cheer and a smile, thus bringing us by easy and comfortable stages to the bottom of the glass, well satisfied that in the fullness of time we are permitted to make our exit hurridly, quietly and well content." *(Manuscript by J.K. Lilly, Sr. dated August 19, 1930, in the Lilly Archives.)* ■

1943 Remington Medalist

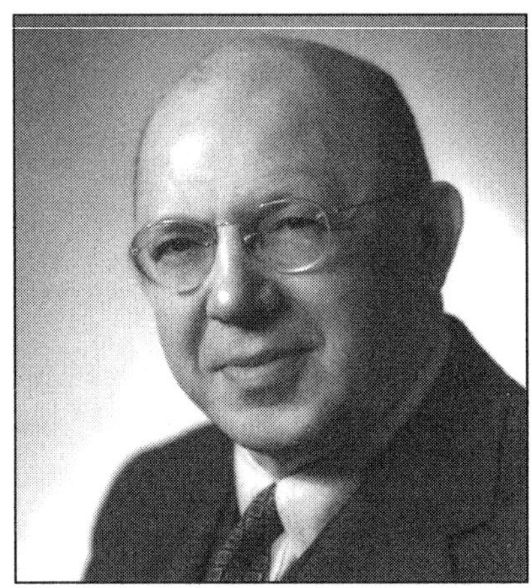

Robert Phillip Fischelis
(1891-1981)

Robert Phillip Fischelis was born in Philadelphia, Pennsylvania, and graduated from the Medico-Chirurgical College department of pharmacy in 1911. He joined the faculty of his *alma mater* until it merged with the Philadelphia College of Pharmacy; he then became dean of the New Jersey College of Pharmacy serving 1921-1925. He variously served as *Druggists Circular* assistant editor 1914-1916; H.K. Mulford scientific staff 1916-1918; Pennsylvania Pharmaceutical Association secretary 1916-1919 and president 1919-1920; *Pennsylvania Pharmacist* founding editor; *Industrial and Engineering Chemistry News Edition* managing editor 1922-1927; New Jersey Pharmaceutical Association secretary 1926-1929; *New Jersey Journal of Pharmacy* founding editor *1928-1935; and* New Jersey Board of Pharmacy executive secretary and chief chemist *1926-1944.* One of his most durable ventures into investigative reporting was *The Costs of Medicines* (1932) co-authored with C. Rufus Rorem. Military service included the U.S. Army Chemical Warfare Service during World War I and director, Division of Chemicals, Drugs, and Health Supplies, War Production Board, during World War II.

Fischelis joined APhA in 1912, serving as a member of the APhA Council 1923-1926 and 1933-1959; APhA vice president 1933-1934, APhA president 1934-1935; APhA Council chairman 1941-1945; and APhA secretary and general manager 1945-1959. He concluded his professional career as dean of Ohio Northern University College of Pharmacy 1962-1965. Several months before his death, he and his wife established the "Fischelis Fund," the largest single gift ever received by the American Institute of the History of Pharmacy.

Higher Professional Standards

Robert Phillip Fischelis

The 1943 Remington Honor Medal Lecture was presented December 7, 1943, at the Hotel McAlpin in New York City. Fischelis's address was published in its entirety in the *Journal of the American Pharmaceutical Association, Practical Pharmacy Edition*, volume 4, pages 379-382, 1943; and in the *American Journal of Pharmaceutical Education,* volume 8, pages 26-34,January, 1944. Abbreviated versions of the Remington lecture were published in *American Druggist* volume 109, pages 52, 110, 114, January 1944; and in *Wisconsin Druggist* pages 9, 24-25, January 1944.

While the Remington Medal Award confers a great honor upon the recipient, its purpose is also to commemorate the labors of a man whose leadership in the profession of pharmacy was the most outstanding of his time. Joseph P. Remington was a man of many talents. Charles H. LaWall, his pupil, assistant, coworker and successor, described him as "genial and eloquent, a keen student of human nature, a lover of the beautiful in art, music and literature, possessed of a fund of scientific knowledge of unusually broad scope, and with it all a consciousness of power that made him an acknowledged leader among men-these are some of the qualities that were combined in him to make a great teacher, a capable executive and a Christian gentleman, cleanminded and cleanhearted."

The twenty-five years that have passed since Remington was called to rest have been filled with stirring events which have left their mark upon American pharmacy. The period ahead of us looms as one of tremendous progress in the further conquest of disease. At this very moment we are in the midst of revolutionary changes in the treatment of diseases which have hitherto baffled those who have devoted their lives to the development of the healing arts. Apparently this global war is not to be without its compensations in the form of improved methods of fighting and preventing disease.

It is necessary for American pharmacy to gear itself to these revolutionary changes and to ask itself frankly and incisively whether it is prepared to play the part it should be expected to play in the general scheme of making these advances in medical science available adequately to all the people.

Neither pharmacy nor medicine can isolate itself from world affairs. Their services are part and parcel of the more abundant life for which nations all over the world are struggling and for which men are today making the supreme sacrifice in distant places.

The lofty idealism of the professions engaged in providing medical care must be translated into the practical performance of making the fruits of modem medical science available to the sick, the halt and the lame in all stations of life at a cost which they can afford to bear and under a system of distribution which will preserve their self-respect.

This is not a problem which the professions can solve alone. It is a problem for the people to solve through their chosen representatives in cooperation with the professions engaged in providing medical care. Members of the health professions must approach this problem in their dual capacity as citizens and as experts in this sphere of activity. As citizens they have every right to express opinions on the methods by which medical care should be made fully available and advocate the methods of distribution which to them seem best.

As professional men and women, skilled in one or more of the sciences or arts which constitute the practice of medicine in its broadest aspects, it is their duty to watch over the quality of medical care dispensed, regardless of the system of distribution which may be developed, and to achieve by moral persuasion and good example that excellence of accomplishment which cannot be secured by legislative fiat or regimented compulsion.

I am not one of those who subscribes to the oft-repeated statement that any change in the method of distributing and paying for medical care will lower its quality. I am aware of the indifference which job security and regimentation breed in some individuals who are not overly ambitious. But I am also aware of many complaints of careless practice, incompetence and cold disregard of the human being seeking relief from mental or physical ills under the present system of private practice. I also know that for many years the medical profession has exercised a firm control over admission to that profession and it has had a very large number of young men and women with high qualifications to choose from. Whether the aptitude and intelligence tests employed have served to select the combination of intellectual capacity, technical aptitude, character and social conscience required to make the kind of a doctor we like to read about, is still an open question. Certainly the right kind of doctor will give the best he has in him at all times and under all conditions and the same thing holds true for other professions in the health field.

After all, it is the men and women who enter these professions rather than the machinery set up for the discharge of their professional functions which determine the quality of medical care made available for the American people.

Pharmacy, like medicine, must exercise due care in the selection of its future manpower. The reduction in professional personnel caused by the war with its consequent elimination of some drug stores is not without its compensations. From all over the country comes the information that pharmacists are so busy practicing pharmacy in the drug stores of America that they have less and less time available for the extraneous merchandising activities resorted to in order to keep their shops going on a profitable basis, and they like it. This is a sign that in spite of the jokesmiths, pharmacists do place first things first, and the first duty of the pharmacist is to supply medicines.

In Remington's apprenticeship days pharmacists carried on considerable drug manufacturing in their own establishments, but in his lifetime he witnessed the gradual cessation of production of medicinal compounds in the average retail pharmacy and the increasing emphasis upon the distribution of ready-made standardized and tested products.

Like many others he did not welcome this transfer of functions to the large laboratory but realized that a change of function called for a readjustment of ideas and ideals to make them fit new conditions.

It soon became evident that the readjustment in pharmacy, like the readjustment in medicine, called for more and not less education of the pharmacist. Yet the educational program for pharmacists lagged behind that of medicine and dentistry and although rapid strides have been made in the past twenty years we have not had quite the courage of our sister professions in eliminating dead wood from the pharmaceutical curriculum, establishing pre-pharmaceutical education on a collegiate level and getting rid of unnecessary teaching institutions and incompetent, unprogressive or unproductive faculty members.

But all this is on the way and it is being hastened by war conditions. We ought to refrain from giving hypodermics to institutions and faculties which are not attuned to the demands of modern medical and pharmaceutical practice and concentrate upon the survival of those institutions which are willing to demand high standards of admission and support faculties whose outlook experience, ideals and abilities will stimulate students to look upon the practice of pharmacy as a public service as well as a method of earning a living.

Now is the time to seriously consider improvement of the future personnel of our profession by demanding pre-professional cultural training as is done in medicine and dentistry. We should hold the present minimum four-year course open for the returning war veterans who have partially completed the pharmacy course or who may wish to enter it upon completing their war service, but of all new students who have not had war service, pre-professional education on a college level should be required. This will put a stop to any effort to lower the present standard pharmacy course under the guise of doing something for the war veteran. The veteran will have the advantage of the present course, which like most other college courses will doubtless continue in a modified form of acceleration, while new students will be required to take the longer course. It is conceivable that under a partially accelerated program a pre-pharmacy college year plus the present standard four-year course could readily be completed in forty-eight months. The early inauguration of such a program will keep the number of new pharmacists down to a replacement level which will prevent the establishment of unnecessary numbers of new pharmacies. This in turn will keep the emphasis in our drug stores on professional activity and hold the remuneration of employed pharmacists at a level which is commensurate with the profession once more attractive to men and women who now seek other outlets for their abilities.

Had pharmaceutical education kept pace with medical and dental education and placed its pre-professional basic training on a separate basis rather than combining it with the professional training program, pharmacists would have received more equitable treatment by the Selective Service Administration and by the Military Services in the commissioning of personnel.

It has been difficult to convince these authorities that the college-trained pharmacist with a baccalaureate degree and some years of practical experience in prescription or manufacturing or hospital pharmacy, or in the wholesale drug and medical supply industry is a competent specialist who is in a much better position to render service as a medical supply officer, or as supervisor of pharmaceutical work in military hospitals than the medical doctors who are assigned to such duties. With the demand for medical doctors in the Armed Forces as great as it is and the civilian population being deprived more and more of the services of physicians, it seems only logical that medical officers in the armed services should be utilized for strictly medical duties and that supervision of pharmacies and supply activities should be assigned to capable commissioned pharmacists. It is time that any prejudice against the assumption of pharmaceutical duties by pharmacists should be laid aside in the public interest. The Congress of the United States has unanimously approved the creation of a Pharmacy Corps in the United States Army. What good reason can be advanced for failure to extend the organization of such a corps immediately to the Army of the United States? That is where commissioned pharmacists are needed today to relieve commissioned physicians of pharmaceutical and medical supply duties so that they may practice medicine either in the Army or be returned to civilian practice where they are sorely needed.

There is abroad in this whole great field of pharmaceutical endeavor an intense realization of the fact that pharmacy's responsibility for the preservation of health and life is on the same level of importance as that of medicine. It is a responsibility that must not be trifled with.

As science unfolds the causes of diseases, it also points the way to their prevention and cure. The day of mysticism and hocus pocus in medicine is rapidly disappearing. As it fades away we become conscious of a reduction in the number of medicaments, but the new single drug remedies are usually complex and difficult to produce. They are often as dangerous as they are beneficial. Their course from highly expensive laboratory curiosities to commercially available remedies is not only intricate but costly. To make such remedies universally available in quantities and at cost which are not prohibitive, there must always be available a combination of scientific knowledge, adequate finances and a keen insight into the economics of distribution. It is this phase of providing medical care adequately that many pharmacists find the most satisfying outlet for their abilities.

There will always be a demand for drugs and combinations of drugs required for the symptomatic treatment of the more common ailments and for diseases whose cause or specific treatment has not been discovered. The compounding of prescriptions for such use and the storing and distribution of specific remedies and making available full information on drug therapy in general will continue to occupy the hospital pharmacist, the prescription specialist and the neighborhood apothecary.

To distinguish these specialists from druggists who prefer to run variety shops with a bit of profitable pharmaceutical activity carried on as a side line, the time has come to emulate our medical specialists and establish Specialty Boards which will certify to the competence of such state licensed pharmacists as have met the higher qualifications which warrant their designation as Manufacturing Pharmacists, Hospital Pharmacists and Prescription Specialists.

The public will naturally gravitate to the well-informed and professionally competent pharmacist whether he makes his headquarters in a store on some prominent business corner or whether he chooses to operate his laboratory in an office building or as part of a group clinic or health center.

The first aid which the American public was accustomed to receive in a pharmacy in Remington's early days is no longer expected today. Hospital and clinic facilities are now more adequate and except for dire emergencies no medical attention is expected from the pharmacist. There is expected, however, considerable information as to availability of medical facilities and practitioners. The neighborhood pharmacist today must not and does not attempt to replace the doctor who has departed for military service, but it is his duty to keep informed of the availability of physicians and medical services so that he can direct inquirers to the places where they can obtain the necessary help. To this extent the pharmacist is the guardian of the health of his community and therefore his professional contacts must be broadened to include social welfare agencies as well as medical organizations and departments of health.

Prior to this date two years ago the American people were divided on the question of the extent of aid to be given to our present allies on this second World War. The events of December 7, 1941, galvanized our people into a united force with a single objective. We are all proud of the achievements of our military forces and of those who have produced and distributed the enormous supplies of fighting engines, ammunition and material which are now contributing so largely to the winning of this war for the allied nations.

Pharmacy and the drug industry have also worked with a unity of purpose during this period. Pharmacists in the War Production Board, in the Army and in the Navy have carried the responsibility for the production and supply of necessary drugs to the Services, to our Allies and to American civilians. So far they have met the essential requirements of all concerned by making necessary adjustments and by intelligent planning. In this they have had the voluntary cooperation of manufacturers, wholesalers and retail dispensers. If such team work is continued after the war ends, there should be little if any disruption of the distributive processes in the drug industry in the reconstruction period.

With its educational program adjusted to produce men and women who have a broad social and public health background as well as technical training; with a method of identifying specialists in manufacturing pharmacy and prescription pharmacy and with leadership that recognizes the limitations as well as the great potentialities for public good inherent in normal functions of pharmacy, the American public may expect from our profession in the future, as in the days of Remington, responsible, enlightened and effective service in its behalf. ■

1944 Remington Medalist

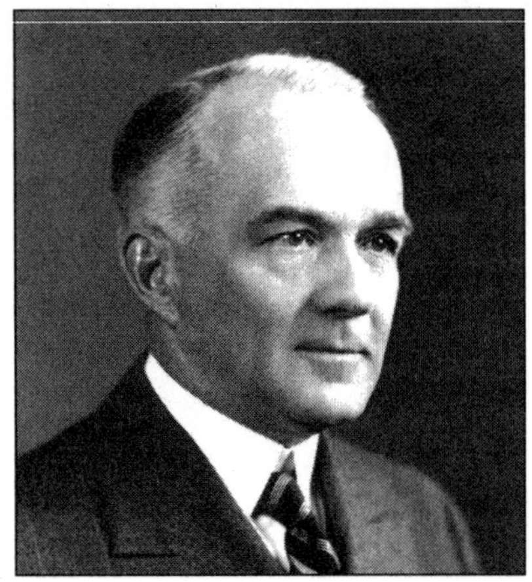

Harvey Evert Kendig

(1878-1950)

Harvey Evert Kendig was born in Newville, Pennsylvania, and graduated from the Medico-Chirurgical College department of pharmacy in 1901. He subsequently received an M.D. degree from the same college in 1905, and moved to Florida to practice medicine and to serve for one year as dean of the Florida College of Pharmacy. He returned to Philadelphia in 1907 to assume the chair in pharmacy at Temple University during which time he earned a Doctor of Pharmacy degree in 1910. He also held posts as associate professor of pharmacology at the Temple University School of Medicine 1914-1922, professor of pharmacology and toxicology at the Women's Medical College of Pennsylvania 1922-1926, and became dean of Temple University School of Pharmacy in 1932, a position he held until his death. He served as American Association of Colleges of Pharmacy president 1940-1941, and was one of the founders of the American Foundation for Pharmaceutical Education.

Kendig served as president of the Philadelphia APhA Branch; as a member of APhA's Committee on the USP 1934-1943; and for nine years as chairman of the joint Committee on the Status of Pharmacists in Government Service whose activity culminated in the commissioning of pharmacists in the Medical Administrative Corps and the subsequent creation of the U.S. Army Pharmacy Corps in 1943 by the U.S. Congress.

Pharmacy and the National Welfare

Harvey Evert Kendig

The 1944 Remington Honor Medal Lecture was presented in December 1944, at the Hotel Pennsylvania in New York City. Kendig's address was summarized in the *Journal of the American Pharmaceutical Association, Practical Pharmacy Edition*, volume 6, pages 57-58, 1945; and published in its entirety in the *American Journal of Pharmaceutical Education,* volume 9, pages 185-198, 1945.

I appreciate deeply the honor which you have conferred on me tonight; I am fully aware of the distinction which accompanies the Remington Medal. No one so honored can contemplate the life and work of the former recipients without being highly complimented that his services to pharmacy have been deemed worthy of such recognition. That the Remington Medal Committee looked with favor upon my work makes me very happy indeed.

I recognize the kindly intent which prompted the speakers to use words which, while pleasing to vanity and pride, are all too flattering for scientific accuracy. Due regard to the verities requires some clarification of the record, and especially as it refers to my part in placing a Pharmacy Corps in the United States Army.

When our country started to arm for participation in the current conflict, the National Committee on the Status of Pharmacists in the Government Service, representing the American Pharmaceutical Association, American Association of Colleges of Pharmacy, National Association of Boards of Pharmacy and the National Association of Retail Druggists, was charged with the duty of arranging for pharmacy's full participation in the defense of the country. As chairman of this committee I was blessed with the help of unusually able personnel and with the full support of the four national associations we represented. We secured the cooperation of every state, county and municipal pharmaceutical society in the country, as well as public spirited lay associations such as the American Legion. The untiring efforts of these thousands of pharmacists and laymen brought about the affirmative vote for the Pharmacy Corps Bill.

Knowing the facts as I do, as far as the Pharmacy Corps effort contributed to my selection for this honor, I gratefully accept the Remington Medal but not just for myself; also, I receive it in behalf of the pharmacists of America whose devotion, cooperation and hard work resulted in the unanimous vote in both the House and the Senate, and the President's signature on a Pharmacy Corps Bill after 60 years of effort.

Those present who have followed the work of the Committee will recall that in its annual report submitted to the member associations in 1943, due acknowledgment was made of outstanding contributions to the effort by individuals and organizations. Time will not permit repetition tonight of that list of names and the specific labors performed, but I believe it appropriate to refer briefly again to two or three men whose work was particularly valuable. They were indispensable men.

Foremost among these was the late, beloved Dr. E.F. Kelly. He was my constant advisor and together we worked out the strategy and planned the campaign. Happy indeed would I have been had his life been spared for still more achievements in behalf of pharmacy; happy indeed would I be had he lived to participate in this program.

Also, I want to pay tribute to Congressman Carl T. Durham and to Senator Robert R. Reynolds, both of whom rendered invaluable services in the Pharmacy Corps fight. Congressman Durham and Senator Reynolds were members of the House and Senate Committees on Military Affairs, respectively, and their knowledge of the routine to be observed was most helpful in obtaining Congressional approval of the Pharmacy Corps legislation. Pharmacy owes a great debt of gratitude to them, and I am privileged on this occasion to express the thanks of myself and the members of my committee for their help in this connection. Congressman Durham would have been present tonight and taken part in this program had it not been that he expected to join the Congressional group now studying war operations in England and on the Continent. I wish he were present that I might share your acclaim with him.

After paying due regard to the amenities, it is customary on these occasions for the honored guest to discuss his philosophy of life, or to explain his ideas of why the universe ticks. The character of these acceptance speeches stems from the age of the individual who is being honored; if he has reached the time of the sear and yellow leaf, he will essay the role of historian and the address will be weighted with the backward look. On the other hand, if the speaker is still ascending the sunny slopes of life's mountain, he will have the forward look and attempt to peer into the future.

Chronologically I qualify as a historian; biologically I still have certain priorities on things to come. Therefore, in conformity to the traditional expectation, I shall talk about two subjects which appear to be fitting for the occasion-the Pharmacy Corps effort of the past, and pharmacy's obligations under the premises in the future.

For the historical aspect I shall say a few words about the conditions existing when we decided to ask Congress to place a Pharmacy Corps in the Army. This action was not taken until it became evident that we could not expect the Medical Department of the Army to so organize the pharmaceutical service that it would protect the soldier in the use of medicines with the same safeguards enjoyed by him as a civilian under the protection of the pharmacy and drug laws of the forty-eight states.

The American Pharmaceutical Association had tried faithfully to bring about the desired changes in the Army procedure but without success. Former Congressional efforts had failed; our bills had never reached the floor of the House or Senate. They peacefully died in the files of committees. Notwithstanding these discouraging precedents, we were encouraged by our studies which showed that a number of forces operative during the earlier years had produced cumulative effects which converged and focused to our advantage with the beginning of the present national emergency.

Dr. Swain has stated that it was in 1885 that the American Pharmaceutical Association first sought to have a Pharmacy Corps established in the United States Army, and that successive committees, under successive chairmen, labored in vain to accomplish this end.

While I usually find myself in agreement with my good friend Dr. Swain, I cannot accept his version that the preceding committees or the preceding chairmen labored without results. It is true that the Pharmacy Corps objective was realized only in 1943, but there was a tremendous amount of constructive work done in the preceding years. These earlier efforts contributed much to a victorious conclusion, and fortuitous circumstances brought about a culmination of effort during my administration.

Also, during the nine years I served as chairman, I became more and more aware that the great improvement in pharmaceutical education weighed heavily in our favor.

During much of the preceding period our

educational program was in the process of evolution, and in fact, had only obtained recognition in academic circles a year or two before I became the chairman of the Committee. The most convincing argument presented by the Army in opposition to the Pharmacy Corps bills introduced in previous Congresses, was that the course in pharmacy did not meet the educational requirements established for the officer personnel of the Regular Army.

In 1936 the Surgeon General acceded to our importunities and approved our bill to commission 16 pharmacists for service in the Medical Administrative Corps. This was the first concrete evidence that we had overcome the objections to our educational program. The bill was passed by Congress at the request of the War Department, and while the officers were assigned to the Medical Administrative Corps, it was the first time in the history of the Regular Army that pharmacists were admitted to commissioned status because they were pharmacists. These officers were transferred to the Pharmacy Corps last year.

So, you see, in all of my negotiations with the Surgeon General and with the Congress, I had the advantage, not enjoyed by former chairmen and committees, of knowing that the pharmaceutical curriculum had been raised to standard collegiate levels, and that it was, therefore, no longer within the power of our opponents to look askance at pharmaceutical education.

Not only was the present excellence of pharmaceutical education a determining factor in bringing the Pharmacy Corps effort to a victorious conclusion, but I am convinced that we must look to pharmaceutical education as both the firmest foundation of pharmaceutical practice, and as the surest guarantee of pharmaceutical betterment in all respects. Superior education, too, will be the open sesame to participation in the broader social and political activities necessary on the part of all who believe in a democratic form of government if this nation is to continue to function under the constitution; indeed, I believe a crusading interest and participation will be necessary if the nation shall endure as a political entity having any resemblance to that form of government under which it has become the most powerful nation and the most beneficent nation the world has ever known.

The opposition of the Medical Department of the Army to any change was not supported by convincing or even reasonable argument. In refusing to place the drug function in the hands of pharmacists it proceeded contrary to the recognized system governing the employment of drugs in the cure of disease firmly established by one hundred years of precedent and practice. This procedure is for the physician to diagnose and prescribe and for the pharmacist to compound or provide the remedy. Furthermore, the opposition in general, was arbitrary and uncompromising. This type of opposition, as is always the case, further nurtured the desire and developed the capacity of pharmacy to render a service so peculiarly its own.

This is a time of unrest and change. So many of our old institutions and methods are being discarded and replaced by new mechanisms of service that the request for a Pharmacy Corps in the Army did not startle Congress as on previous occasions. The many measures designed to effect profound changes in this country's social, political and economic life, receiving legislative consideration, or innovations imposed by executive order, had so conditioned Congress to change that our measure was received by many as a matter of course. It did not provoke the antagonism and opposition engendered by earlier legislative efforts by your committee.

Furthermore, a general mental attitude, fostered by the well-defined movement toward a leveling process in the country's social life and economic structure, was a favorable influence. This leveling process carries with it the implication that too great power has been exerted by some who, possibly by tradition, have been placed in positions of control, to the detriment of those not so fortunately situated.

The condition of the pharmaceutical

service, to a considerable degree, grew out of the smallness of the Army in its early decades, as well as from pharmacy's lethargy and absence of an aggressive or even no policy at all. Pharmacy lacked vision during the first hundred years of the country's history.

I said the first permanent armed forces of the Republic were small. In 1784, Congress reduced the Army to one battery of fifty-five men and a detachment of twent-five infantry soldiers. Influenced by the fear of standing armies, the government under the Articles of Confederation established a small army of seven hundred troops for one year's service; the same number was continued until after the adoption of the Constitution. Some of us remember the small standing army of 25,000 of our boyhood days.

In those years when an emergency arose, the physicians and surgeons assumed the duties in the Army which properly belonged to pharmacists. Vigorous, effective protest from the drug men was not forthcoming. Gradually the pharmaceutical service came completely under the control of the members of the medical profession. When pharmacy grew in importance in keeping with the general progress in the medical sciences and turned to the armed forces, it was found that the medical men were in full charge of the drug function and had extended their control far beyond just limits.

The medical school curriculum has never trained its graduates for the manufacture or purchase, standardization, storage, compounding and dispensing of drugs, nor should it. Those are the functions of the pharmacist. The medical man majors in diagnosis and treatment; his drug knowledge is that of physiological action and its application. He may be skillful in the fields of pediatrics, obstetrics, ophthalmology or any other of the great divisions in his profession, but these branches of learning do not qualify him to replace the pharmacist in the ever widening area of drug knowledge and control. In fact, a knowledge of these sciences and arts precludes him from doing so. He cannot be a master of the one profession and have a practicing knowledge of the other also.

Bacon said, "Tempests in the State are commonly greatest when things grow to equality, as natural tempests are greatest about the equinoctia." Pharmacy had grown to equality in the field peculiarly its own, and the controversy we have just concluded was inevitable; the outcome was just as inevitable. The decision about who shall serve in a disputed province in a democracy is always resolved in favor of those best qualified by education, training and experience and who, therefore, are justly entitled to the opportunity. The opposite of this, the granting of positions or emoluments on the basis of favor or force is a characteristic of the totalitarian state and is the very thing we are fighting in Europe and Asia today.

History records the prominent part pharmacy has taken in the social and political advances achieved by this country during the past 100 years. During that period the education of the pharmacist was superior to that of the average or to that of most citizens, and clearer thinking and better planning and execution by him were to be expected. The profound influence exerted by pharmacists in every community, rural and urban, had as its base this better education of the members of the profession. They had more facts at their command, and superior reasoning and directing power due to disciplinary study.

As I have said earlier in my talk, it is unfortunate that pharmacy did not keep in line with medicine when that profession adopted the progressive educational program of 1918 which introduced, among other higher standards, a requirement of general cultural education on the college level as a prerequisite for admittance to an accredited school of medicine.

Medicine took this advanced step at about the time there was a resurgence of interest in higher education, an interest stimulated by private and public universities offering opportunities for advanced education to any young man or woman regardless of their economic situation. The enrollments in colleges and universities went up in leaps and bounds.

It was this broadened interest in the humanities and their significance in the developing sociologic pattern which brought about new concepts of our duty to the socalled submerged tenth, and which resulted in much of the more recent progressive legislation.

Rational social and sound economic progress in the future will stem from better and broader education. The problems with which this country will be confronted will be solved only by a clearer vision of the interrelation of life's component parts and this can be brought about only by increased knowledge and its scientific application or utilization.

President Conant of Harvard University, in an address on the occasion of receiving the Priestley Medal, said: "If we in the United States in the post-war years are to live up to our responsibilities, we must foster all learning-accumulative knowledge, philosophy and poetry. To this end we must see to it that as far as humanly possible all the potential talent of the country in all these manifold activities is recognized at an early age and given adequate educational opportunity. Stepping out of my role as a chemist for a moment and speaking as an educator, this means a vastly increased support of public educatio-federal funds administered through the states and a much fairer distribution of educational opportunities at the college level."

The strategic situation of the pharmacist and the peculiar nature of the service he renders the public, give him an extraordinary opportunity to mould public opinion and guide his contemporaries in sound thinking and constructive action.

However, if this profession is to exert an influence in public affairs comparable to that witnessed in former decades, it must offer or require of its practitioners a superiority in education comparable to the superiority enjoyed during those years.

Fifty years ago the two years of college training gave the pharmacist intellectual superiority over 99 percent of the people who addressed him from the other side of the prescription counter. That was the time when the number of college graduates in any small or limited area could have been counted on the fingers of one hand.

Today, in that same community, it is scarcely possible to cross the threshold of any even moderately well-to-do family without being greeted by at least one university graduate. The number of pharmacists has remained the same but the number of college graduates has multiplied many times since 1900. In the not far distant future, the chances are that the customer on the other side of the counter will have a standard four year college education. The pharmacist with his four-year degree will have equality but no longer will he enjoy the superiority he must possess to command the respect accorded him in former years.

The time has come for us to recognize the fundamental changes which have and are taking place in the theory and practice of this profession. Some of these changes result from increased scientific knowledge; some are caused by changes in drug economy incident to the industry adjusting its methods to the modern technology which has invaded the drug business and crowded out antiquated methods; and still other breaks in the established order are in conformity with the requirements of basic modifications of the procedure in the practice of medicine.

By way of illustration, our present information about the physiological activity of many substances and their specific actions in definite quantities makes assay and standardization necessary- a business and legal as well as a moral obligation.

Regarding the second point I made, it is scarcely necessary to mention the economic waste if in each of the 58,000 pharmacies in the United States was made the relatively small quantity of each of the commonly used potent preparations and then assayed and standardized. In many instances the quantity desired would not be more than the volume required for assay. One manufacturer can and does make at one time enough of one of these preparations to satisfy the requirements of several thousand retail pharmacists. He, the manufacturer, performs one assay and makes one dose adjustment instead of the several thousand necessary under the individualized production.

We must stop thinking of pharmacy as referring only to the retail drug business; we must enlarge our vision and widen our horizon to include every procedure connected with the production and distribution of remedies and corrective agents. Included must be every function from obtaining the crude materials, their refinement and use in manufacturing medicinal products; then distribution to the wholesaler and on to the retail pharmacist, the hospital and the coming medical centre, and finally compounding and dispensing to the individual consumer. This sequence represents American pharmacy today. We must adopt this all embracing conception of pharmacy to promote the unity of action required for the common good.

So many changes have taken place in the methods employed by the physician to cure and prevent disease that corresponding changes must take place in pharmacy. The advances in preventive medicine have canceled out many prescriptions and sick-room supplies which a generation ago required much of the time of the pharmacist. The prevention of malaria and typhoid fever by sanitary engineering removed a source of practice which will never return.

Diphtheria antitoxin and scarlet fever immunization and smallpox vaccination have transferred to the large biological laboratories the preparation of the substances now used to control these diseases. More recently the sulfa drugs and penicillin have removed from the list many diseases which hospitalized, or confined to the sick-room for long periods of time, those who were so unfortunate as to be stricken by these heretofore yielders of large volumes of pharmaceutical practice.

The declines in the death rate during the current century have been notable in pneumonia, malaria, typhoid fever, scarlet fever, whooping cough, diphtheria, tuberculosis, dysentery and influenza. This decline is due largely to preventive medicine and the methods employed call for little service by the retail pharmacist. Diminished death rates, the result of other than preventive measures, are due to the employment of the modern chemical instead of the many complex prescriptions formerly relied upon or used empirically in the search for effective remedies. The development of modern rational, scientific treatments, with substances such as the sulfa drugs, penicillin and other chemo-therapeutic agents, has revolutionized the practice of pharmacy and of medicine alike.

Pharmaceutical education is too narrowly conceived to meet the requirements of present day conditions. A curriculum which produces a scientist well-trained for practicing what is commonly referred to as retail pharmacy, would not prepare the graduate for service generally in the broader field which I said must be recognized as the present and future field of practice.

I think in considering the requirements of ordinary practice today we might well ask ourselves whether an educational pattern somewhat hastily put together in 1932, is adequate or even adaptable to conditions existing in 1944. For my own part, I think the time has come for a constructive factfinding survey of the pharmaceutical curriculum. As I have pointed out, there have been vast changes in medical practice, and it may well be that these should have been met by a more responsive attitude upon the part of our schools of pharmacy.

I think a good many questions might profitably be asked with respect to our current courses of instruction. Time does not permit me to enumerate on them, but broadly, could we defend the thesis that the pharmacy curriculum meets the current public health needs and provides for the fullest and most helpful cooperation between pharmacy and medicine and the other public health professions.

I think constructive, searching inquiry

will early indicate that the present curriculum includes much outmoded and needless material. In many respects the course content, especially in the professional subjects, has not changed much in the last several decades.

We are holding on to certain subject details whose claim to survival is largely historic. Much time is wasted on things of no practical value under present day conditions. They have sentimental value only.

If this task of elimination were done after a factual drug store survey, I believe the time and space would be found for building a modem curriculum expressive of modern needs.

Suggestive of my personal views, let me say that colleges of pharmacy need to greatly expand their work in the biological fields. Biology is assuming an ever increasing importance in medical practice, and it is entitled to a greater place in pharmaceutical education.

Well-equipped laboratories for the teaching of bio-chemistry, pharmacology, bio-assaying, and such other related subjects as may be necessary to a proper understanding of the drugs and medicines now coming from our research laboratories are urgently needed.

The mere fact that medical practice is becoming more and more dependent upon the research scientist leaves pharmacy no choice, if it is to survive as a professional pursuit and take its rightful place among the public health professions, except to put its educational house in order.

I am convinced, too, that one of our immediate needs is for more graduate work in pharmaceutical subjects. Under normal conditions, we have been turning out not more than 12 or 15 doctors of philosophy a year, and even this number has been sharply curtailed during the war.

Our new educational program must enable pharmacy to recapture the positions lost to the recipients of higher degrees from the old line universities and the colleges of liberal arts and sciences. An anamalous and embarrassing situation will exist just so long as schools of pharmacy do not supply the staffs for research, control, assay, standardization, and for pharmaceutical, biological and chemical drug manufacture in all of its ramifications.

It seems inevitable that there will be an enlarged demand both upon the part of colleges of pharmacy and the drug industry for men with high graduate degrees, if pharmaceutical education and the drug industry are to meet their responsibilities. Many of our colleges of pharmacy were operating with minimum teaching personnel before the war, and will be faced with the necessity of building up their teaching staffs to acceptable levels, once the war is over.

The same situation obtains in the manufacturing drug industry. The demand for men who have completed graduate work in their fields is bound to be acute, and under existing facilities this demand cannot be met. But, these men must be made available if pharmaceutical education is not to deteriorate and the drug industry become seriously hampered in its research development phases.

I should like to suggest that a joint committee of the drug industry and of pharmaceutical education be appointed to study the graduate personnel requirements of pharmaceutical education for the next several years, and the graduate personnel requirements of the drug industry; and to further study the facilities available in our colleges of pharmacy and to plan for their necessary expansion and improvement. If such studies could be made, graduate work could be developed in response to actual needs.

This study would enable us to maintain a proper balance between the requirements of both the retail and industrial branches of the profession. During recent years there has been a tendency on the part of the high scholarship graduates to accept employment with the manufacturers. A planned program would provide for industry without depleting the supply of superior graduates needed in retail practice.

I have been acutely aware of this need for a better graduate program for a long time; in fact, I have recommended to the President of the Board of Trustees of Temple University that a graduate school of pharmacy be added to the university ensemble. My plans call for complete divorcement of graduate work from the undergraduate school and faculty. The graduate school would be separately housed, have its own faculty and be presided over by its own dean.

I have refrained from talking about pre-college work for entry to a school of pharmacy. In the annual address as president of the American Association of Colleges of Pharmacy in 1941, I recommended that plans be made for this increase in entrance requirements to become effective at the earliest practicable time. I believe that the practicable date will come when the schools of pharmacy have replaced by graduation the practitioners lost by pharmacy because of the war effort and its interference with the enrollment of students, and with the educational process.

In conclusion, may I thank all who have had a part in this program. When Benjamin Franklin represented the colonies in France during the Revolutionary War, he wrote a letter to General Washington from which I quote:

"Should peace arrive after another campaign or two, and afford us a little leisure, I should be happy to see your Excellency in Europe. You would, on this side of the sea enjoy the great reputation you have acquired. Here you would know, and enjoy, what posterity will say of Washington. For a thousand leagues have nearly the same effect with a thousand years."

Philadelphians and New Yorkers are in agreement that in many respects, Philadelphia is a thousand leagues from New York. Therefore, I am sure my deep sincerity will be evident in my thanks to the New York Branch of the American Pharmaceutical Association for arranging this dinner, and for making possible the pleasant and delightful illusion of what posterity will say after a thousand years. ■

1945 Remington Medalist

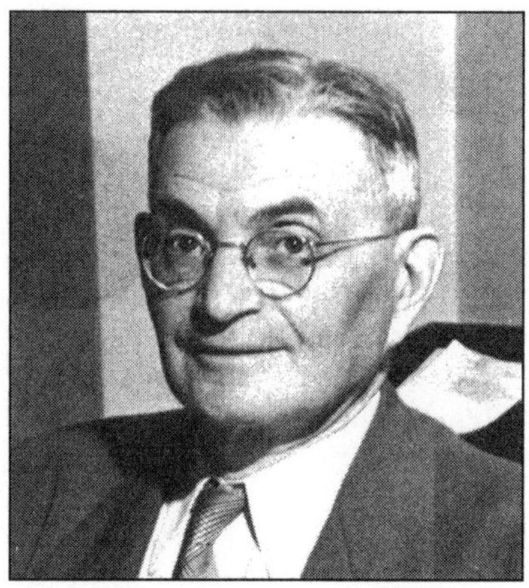

JOSEPH ROSIN
(1880-1969)

Joseph Rosin was born in Russia but came to the U.S.A. in his youth, earning a B.S. degree in chemistry from the University of Pennsylvania in 1909. He joined Powers-Weightman-Rosengarten Company in 1909 where he served as chief chemist from 1913 to 1927. When Powers-Weightman-Rosengarten merged with Merck and Company in 1927, Rosin became vice president and chemical director of Merck, serving 1927-1945. As foremost American authority on chemical reagents, he was a member of the American Chemical Society committee on analytical reagents 1922-1945, and served the USP revision committee 1910-1945 where he contributed more than any single individual to the development of official standards for the sulfonamides and the vitamins. His community service included first vice president of the Plainfield, NewJersey, Jewish Community Center and president of the Plainfield Temple.

Rosin joined the American Pharmaceutical Association in 1916, and served as a trustee of the Philadelphia College of Pharmacy 1937-1946. He authored the textbook *Reagent Chemicals and Standards,* served as chemical editor of *Remington's Practice of Pharmacy* (Ninth Edition), and as editor-in-chief of the *Merck Index* (1940 Fifth Edition).

My True Science Ever Becomes Extinct

Joseph Rosin

The 1945 Remington Honor Medal Lecture was presented on December 11, 1945, at the Hotel Pennsylvania in New York City. Rosin's Remington address was published in the *American Journal of Pharmaceutical Education,* volume 10, pages 202-207, April 1946.

Life is as strange as it is real. It is strange, and sometimes wonderful what a part accident, chance, or fate play in our lives and shape our destinies.

A few weeks after graduating, in response to my application, the late Dr. George D. Rosengarten called me in for an interview. After the usual interrogation, rather onesided, including a few embarrassing questions in chemistry, and when I thought the ordeal was over, imagine my mortification when he lifted a book from a nearby shelf, showed it to me and asked me the name of it and whether I knew of this book. I stuttered and stammered, but could not pronounce the name. It was the *Pharmacopoeia.*

Who could imagine then that this very book, whose name I could not even pronounce, would play such a role in my life, in my career, that it will make for me most cherished and inestimable friendships and would launch me on the road to this great honor.

From this you will readily see how little I knew of pharmacy, and was not even aware of the existence of the *Pharmacopoeia.*

Fortunately it was not long before fate threw me into contact with the pharmacy luminaries of that time and of all time. First and foremost was Professor Remington himself. I need not speak of his attainments in pharmacy and pharmaceutical education. His name speaks for it. He was also a very humane character. During many of the *USP* conferences held in his home library, he would relieve the strain of the deliberations by telling a suitable anecdote, or story, and he had a story for every occasion and nearly every drug. Well do I remember the last time I visited him. He was ill and when I came in he asked me to sit on his bed. After a while the conversation turned to iodides and he said, "Joseph, Syrup of Iron Iodide bothers me. (This preparation was then still at the zenith of its therapeutic reputation.) There is too much sugar in it, and in cold weather it crystallizes. Yet, if the quantity of the sugar is reduced, the syrup is unstable." Then, after a few moments of thinking, he said, "I think you and I should be able to do something about it." In a short time after he died.

George M. Beringer, a pharmacist of the city of Camden, New Jersey, was then a member of the USP Revision Committee, as well as of the succeeding committee. He was editor of a pharmaceutical journal, and one of the first Remington medalists (1924). He was also the toxicologist for the city. His learning in pharmaceutic sciences was amazingly wide and profound. To him every blade of grass was an open book, and the chemistry of drugs, no mystery.

Among the great it was my privilege to know and to associate with in the early days of my connection with the *Pharmacopoeia* was Harvey W. Wiley, then chief of the bureau of chemistry, Department of Agriculture, Washington, and who also was at that time a member of the *Pharmacopoeia* Revision Committee. Dr. Wiley was a physician who became a leading chemist of his time. To him the nation is forever indebted for the first Federal Food and Drug Act, achieved after years of hard labor and struggle. Through him the *Pharmacopoeia* and the *National Formulary* were for the first time given recognition by Congress as the law of the land for standards of quality and purity of drugs. It was an inspiration to sit with him in conference and listen to his discussion. His devotion to the cause of purity and truthfulness in foods and drugs kept him in single blessedness to his late sixties. He then married, had two splendid boys, and lived "by reason of strength" to the ripe old age of four score and five.

From them, and others of like statute, among whom is Professor E. Fullerton Cook, chairman of the *Pharmacopoeia* Revision Committee since 1920, I learned what pharmacy is, its high ideals and aspirations.

Pharmacy is frequently referred to as an art. Good pharmaceutic practice to be sure, does require art and elegance, but basically, pharmacy is a science, encompassing in its scope several branches of human knowledge and experience. From pharmacy was born lusty, aggressive and fast-marching chemistry. The youngest of her offspring, pharmacology, has already won a seat of equality with the older members of the body, scientific. Measured by Emerson's dictum that no science is a science unless it benefits mankind, pharmacy ranks high among the benefactors of humanity.

There are some who would have us believe that because the pharmacist no longer makes himself his extracts, tinctures, and so-forth, the sun of pharmacy is setting. This is inadmissible. No true science wanes or becomes extinct. Astrology, a pseudoscience, is gone and extinct, but not astronomy. A true science may take on new forms, it hews paths in new directions, but never ceases to blossom and bear fruit. It is ever fertile, ever multiplying and expanding. A single and simple discovery of a scientific fact ushers in many more in its wake, and opens up new avenues for human endeavor and aspiration.

Alexander Fleming's scientific eye spotted a tiny clear patch on a bacteriologic slide. It gave the world the wonder drug penicillin. Following penicillin came streptomycin, a remedial agent of great promise perhaps equal, if not greater, than penicillin. Streptomycin is one of the few substances that are active against gram-negative pathologic bacteria and, so far, the most powerful without pronounced toxic properties. The little clear spot observed by Fleming opened to the hope of mankind the new territory of antibiotics, a territory that may harbor great possibilities for the healing and relief of the ill and suffering.

Can we desist from speculating about the untold potentialities for a better world the atomic bomb holds, if we but temper its power with the engineering of the human heart?

Scientists are discontented individuals. They are not content with what "is" with the status quo of things with what they know and have achieved, and that is what makes them scientists. A group of mycologists, alias "mold hunters" were dissatisfied with the performance of the mold that produces penicillin, so they set out to study and learn more of the intimate life and habits of this mold, and behold! By means of X-ray mutants and other skills they developed a strain that, in the same unit of time, produces many times as much penicillin as before. Think what would happen if human workers should now increase their output to the same degree. Would it be a blessing? I wonder.

There no longer are acres of diamonds to be had for the picking, no wells bursting with oil. Our natural resources of materials are definitely diminishing, but when we recall the many times that scientists have been able to duplicate and even improve upon nature's work, we have no cause to be alarmed. The day may not be distant when knowledge will achieve for us almost complete independence of natural resources. Science creates. It creates both materials and work for thousands and tens of thousands. The younger generation may see the time when a nation's wealth will be measured not by the extent of her natural resources, but by the number of her scientists and research laboratories.

The future of mankind rests with science. Recent events have proven it. The military, too, see it. General of the Army Marshall puts scientific research as one of the first and most important points for future defense.

From the crucibles and test tubes of the laboratories, there will come redemption from many of the nightmares and ills that beset and pursue the human race. In them will be created new materials for man's greater comfort and happiness. From the laboratories of science may come the answer, if man but wills it, to the prayer of mankind for Peace Everlasting, the fulfillment of the prophet's vision, "When swords will be beaten into plowshares," and "no nation will lift up sword against nation, nor learn war any more."

Science, it may well be, is the power which the poet envisioned in the beautiful verse:

"All things by immortal power
Near and far, Hiddenly,
To each other linked are.
Thou canst not stir a flower,
Without troubling of a star."

Pharmacy too, will meet the challenge. Now that peace has returned it will resume its place among the progressive and advancing ranks of science. In the changing scenes of the world the field for scientific pharmacy is rapidly expanding. The program for pharmaceutic education and training should be broadened to meet the new conditions. There is a persistent call for pharmaceutic learning which may properly be called pure scientific pharmacy. Pharmaceutical manufacturing the practice of pharmacy on a large scale requires pharmaceutic engineers. Schools of pharmacy should act promptly. For in the words of Auchter, "In a world making such full use of science, you have to run fast to stay where you are. If you want to move ahead, you have to run still faster."

The *Pharmacopoeia* has been called the "bible" of the pharmacist. Like the Bible which from a small beginning has spread far and wide and became the possession of the world, the pharmacists can no longer claim sole rights to the *Pharmacopoeia*. Its scope has become much greater. It is also the bible of the pharmaceutical manufacturer a vigorous and responsible offspring of the practice of pharmacy, and of state and federal enforcement agencies. It is also becoming more and more a "materia medica" for the physician, and a book of reference for meclicinals of recognized merit.

When the *Pharmacopoeia* was first declared by Congress as the standard bearer for drugs, the action was not favored in some quarters. I venture to say that if the authority of the *Pharmacopoeia* were withdrawn, these very opponents would be the first to petition Congress to reestablish its authority. One can hardly imagine the chaos that would result in the quality and purity of drugs and in pharmaceutical trade if the responsibility of the *Pharmacopoeia* were cancelled.

It was not so long ago that pharmaceutical manufacturers were unwilling to have their new medicinal products in the Pharmacopoeia. Now most of the manufacturers are glad to have them in the book, because acceptance of a product by the Pharmacopoeia is a mark of recognition of its merit.

Pharmacy and the Pharmacopoeia are indissolubly linked. Together they progress to forward the welfare of the nation. ■

1947 Remington Medalist

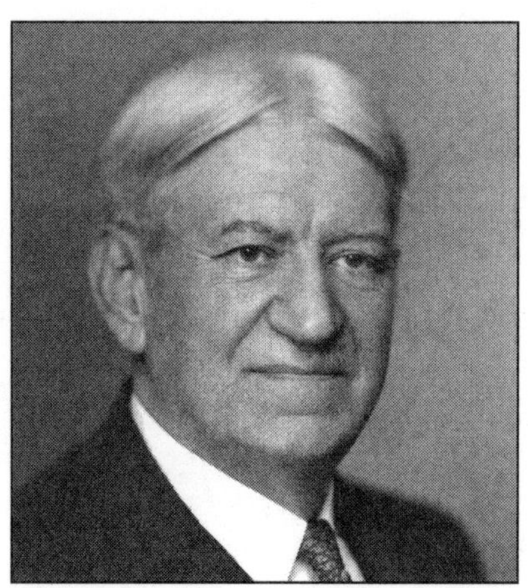

Rufus Ashley Lyman
(1875-1957)

Rufus Ashley Lyman was born in Table Rock, Nebraska, and graduated with an M.D. degree from the University of Nebraska in 1903. He practiced medicine for a time in Omaha before appointment to the faculty of his *alma mater* as instructor in pharmacology 1904-1908. He organized the University of Nebraska School of Pharmacy in 1908 where he served as director until 1915 when the College of Pharmacy was created by act of the state legislature. He was named dean of the new college serving in this capacity until 1946. He was then called to the University of Arizona at Tucson to establish a School of Pharmacy in 1947 where he served as dean until his retirement in 1950.

Early in the career of his adopted profession, Lyman became active in the American Association of Colleges of Pharmacy, serving as vice president 1915-1916, president 1916-1917, and chairman of the executive committee 1920-1923. He served as vice chairman of the American Council on Education 1929-1930, was founding editor of the *American Journal of Pharmaceutical Education* 1937-1955, and vice president of the American Institute of the History of Pharmacy 1941. In 1942, he was appointed editor-in-chief for a series of textbooks published by J.B. Lippincott Company, and he served as American Pharmaceutical Association honorary president 1952-1953.

Don't Confuse Training with Education

Rufus Ashly Lyman

The 1947 Remington Honor Medal Lecture was presented on December 3, 1947, at the Hotel Pennsylvania in New York City. Lyman's abridged address was published in the *Journal of the American Pharmaceutical Association, Practical Pharmacy Edition,* volume 9, pages 91-92, 118, 120, 125-128, 1948; and in the *American Journal of Pharmaceutical Education,* volume 12, pages 67-89, 1948. The following is an unabridged version of Lyman's lecture reproduced from his original manuscript.

It was still the era of the pioneer. Spring had come in the country of the Great Plains. The winds of March had spent their force. The April showers had refreshed the sod. The warm May sunshine had caused the Nebraska prairies to be clothed as far as the eye could see, with a mantle of green. Upon the crest of a hill overlooking a valley stood the Bunker Hill School House, one of those one room institutions of poetic fame. On the afternoon of the day of which I write a contest was to be staged for a Demorest Silver Medal. Seven small boys had been induced to compete. I was No. 7. The objective of all speeches was to dethrone King Alcohol. In my speech the King was personified as a serpent and his destruction had dramatic possibilities. I got some ideas from an evangelist at a Methodist camp meeting. I saw him kill sin, personified as the devil. And the Presbyterian minister in the church of my boyhood had some gestures which seemed to me both graceful and effective. I drew heavily on these sources in the preparation of the handling of that snake, only I went the evangelist one better by sinking some tacks into the heel of my boot. When I got those nails astride of that snake's head I performed a whirling deverish act and ground the snake's head into the floor. And as he lay there squirming in the agony of death I assumed the post of a Roman gladiator after he had broad sworded his victim and placed his heel upon his victim's neck. The applause of my school mates was deafening, and as I took my seat I could all but feel that shining medal against my chest. I was all the more confident because a great uncle of mine was one of the judges. But it was not to be. When the judges' report came, not the medal but place No. 7 was mine. As I passed my great uncle he glared at me and said "Just see how you marred the platform. I am going to tell your father, and if he don't give you a sound trouncing I know who will." The disappointment and humiliation of that hour was crushing. On that day medals passed out of my life, but my zeal to kill the serpent increased as the years rolled by.

More than three score years had passed. Again it was the month of May. I opened a letter and certain words stood out on the page. They seemed to jump at me. *"Lyman-Remington Medalist-1947-Hugo Schaefer."* I read it again, and then again. I thought of the snake of the olden day. I said it cannot be. The next day came a telegram from Dr. R.L. Swain. Then from Evert Kendig. Then I knew it must be so. Presbyterians are too Scotch to pay for telegrams that have no meaning. Then came letters from every corner of the nation-by the tens and hundreds all telling me it was so. All summer long they came, and they are still coming.

I like Arizona. I like its people. I agree with Westbrook Pegler who says, "When he retires he wants to go to Arizona and get a sports job on the Tucson *Citizen* or the *Republic* at Phoenix or the Brewery Gulch *Gazette* down in Bisbee, in a real country league, the Arizona-Texas, where they play the kind of ball the Yankees used to play and where they remember that to err is human, and never try to pretend they ain't." Arizonians do not claim to be anything they are not. I like that kind of people and I want to be that kind. I appreciated being awarded the Remington Medal, but I hesitated at accepting it because of my unworthiness. I had a similar experience on another occasion, many years ago, when I was ordained an Elder in the Presbyterian Church, when I knew, and God knew too, of my unworthiness.

In the due course of time the June 23rd issue of *Drug Topics* came. I turned to "Your Pharmacy and Mine" as I always do for a bit of inspiration or instruction, or both. What should stare at me from the page but "Lyman, Remington Medalist." I read the editorial and with fatherly pride I passed it to my younger son. He read it, much to my disappointment, without any sign of emotion. After a moment he said, "I thought you said Dr. Swain was the smartest man in American pharmacy." I acknowledged having so spoken. He said, "Well, I don't think so." Then after a thoughtful moment had elapsed, I said, "I'll take it back, but I can truthfully say he is the most generous Presbyterian I have ever known." And to that the son assented.

Then I scanned the list of Remington Medalists-twenty-four in all, from James H. Beal to Joseph Rosin. I knew them everyone. I matched my accomplishments with theirs and always to their advantage. The name of the beloved Eugene G. Eberle reminded me of an incident that occurred soon after the great Remington had passed. Dr. Eberle said to me" Remington's accomplishments in the field of pharmacy were many, but his outstanding characteristic was his ability to bring opposing forces together and direct them toward the common good." I realized the truth of that statement as I recalled the many occasions in our meetings when progress was blocked and adjournment seemed inevitable, and in a few cases secession was even suggested, that Remington rose to his feet, said a few words; the atmosphere cleared and cooperation was effected. At producing cooperation, Remington was a master.

The last day of June had come. I drew from a stack of letters one addressed in a familiar hand. It read: "Dear Lyman: The news certainly makes me happy (the reference is to Dr. Swain's editorial). For once I agree with Dr. Swain. Congratulations. Affectionately, Rudd." It took Rudd to tell me why I was a Remington Medalist. In one respect I had measured up to the great master himself. The most comforting thing that has come to me in more than forty years of endeavor is the unaminity of opinion that has been infiltrating our ranks through the years, which has at last, enabled pharmacy to present an undivided front in the effort to obtain its objectives as a profession of service.

The Milwaukee meetings were at hand. I had got no farther than the lobby of the Hotel Schroeder when I was confronted face to face with Hugo Schaefer, and with a directness that is commendable in a treasurer of the American Pharmaceutical Association he got right down to business. He said the matter of program for the Remington dinner must be settled at once, and that means right now. Then he continued "There will be several speakers who are well qualified to tell of your efforts, and then you will make a speech in which you will deny all the previous speakers have said." He made some suggestions as to who these speakers might be. I insisted as my right that Andrew DuMez come last because when he got through there would be less for me to deny. This is because Dean DuMez has become cold blooded by years of experience in evaluating men and schools of pharmacy, although in reality he has the tenderness of a mother cuddling her first baby. But Dean Schaefer was not through with giving instructions about my conduct at this dinner. He continued, "Furthermore, you should remember that this is your Swan Song. When you are through with this you are through. Then you will be on a basis comparable with the ex-presidents of the American Pharmaceutical Association, but without portfolio and without vote. You should remember also that you will not be talking to a group of school teachers alone, but in the audience there will be men of wealth, men who have made their wealth in pharmaceutical industry and collectively they represent an investment of and I'll not repeat the figure he used because I cannot comprehend its vastness. The figure was a monstrosity like many other monstrosities to which the New Deal gave birth.

I asked Dr. Swain what I should say to this group of men because he has become acclimated by hobnobbing with men on that level. He looked away off in the distance and said, "It doesn't make any difference what you say just so it is all Lyman." And then he left me to ponder over the meaning of that. Bob Hardt was helpful. He said, "If you want to win the everlasting gratitude of this group of men say just as little as you can, in just as few words as you can, and in just as short a time as is possible." Joe Noh dodged the real question, but he reminded me that I would be expected to appear in a dinner jacket, but if my hair was not Western, Nebraskans of the yesteryears would disown me. Rudd was not there, but I know what he would have said had he so been. It would have sounded like this: "Lyman, if you can't say something that would display a higher degree of intelligence than you have ever shown before you will render a pharmacy a real service by simply making a bow and saying nothing." Through many years of colleagueship and comradeship I have learned to respect Rudd's judgement. Bearing in mind the admonitions of these friends of mine, I now approach my subject.

It is difficult for one who has been engaged in pharmaceutical activities for four decades to bring anything new or challenging to his colleagues or to the practicing pharmacist or even the pharmaceutical industrialist, for our associations have been sufficiently close so that we all have a pretty clear understanding what the problems are. Some time ago I was asked to write an article which would convey to the retail druggists some "sound, hard hitting ideas for the betterment of pharmacy." That request struck a responsive cord in me, for through an active life of forty years I had been seeking such ideas, not to pass on to the pharmacist but for my own guidance, in order that I might carry out the task to which I had been assigned. So far as the retail druggist is concerned I had long ago discovered the thoughtful one was quite as much concerned about the betterment of this profession as a practitioner as I am as a so-called educator.

I do think it is worthwhile, however well we are familiar with pharmaceutical developments and attainments since the turn of the century, to pause for a few moments and retravel the road and see where we were at the turn of the century, how far have we come, where we are now, and what the prospects of the future are. Out of that way we may find some guide posts for the future conduct and, what is even more important, some inspiration for attacking the tasks that lie ahead.

Ordinarily I do not go back of the days when pharmaceutical education became my personal problem. That was the year 1908. It was the era of Remington and Caspari, of Edward Kremers, Henry Kraemer and James H. Beal, of Rusby and Searby and Hynson, of Hallberg and Oldberg, and Schneider, of Sayre and Stevens, and Arny, of Bradley and Scoville and Whelpley and Eberle and a host of others who have passed on. I think of them as Giants in the Earth in those days.

But I shall go back of that era for a moment to mention an event, which to me, is the most significant one in the whole history of American Pharmacy, namely the establishing of pharmaceutical instruction upon the campus of the University of

Michigan. That occurred in 1867. The man who was responsible for it was not a pharmacist. Albert B. Prescott was a physician and a chemist. This act brought to pharmaceutical education the moral and financial support of a great state supported institution and precipitated pharmacy into our system of state education. Not only did it do that, but it gave pharmaceutical education a stability it could not have acquired except by becoming a part of the educational system of the state and the responsibility of the taxpayer, and created a public consciousness of the importance of educating pharmacists. The significance of this act becomes all the more impressive when we recall that long before Charles W. Elliott retired from the presidency of Harvard University he was asked to name the ten men who he considered had influenced most of the thought of the world in the last two hundred years. In that list only two Americans were included. One was Ralph W. Emerson; the other was Horace Mann, a country lawyer who moved to Boston and in the course of time he became the secretary of the Board of Education and in that position he formulated a plan of education which became the foundation of America's educational system, the greatest system for universal education that the world has ever known. Prescott introduced pharmacy into that system.

We can rest assured that pharmaceutical instruction was undertaken by the University of Michigan not without opposition. It did meet with opposition, and that opposition came very largely from pharmacists themselves. The sentiment of the times is indicated by an action in 1871 at the St. Louis meeting of the American Pharmaceutical Association, and by the Association, when the (School of Pharmacy of the) University of Michigan was denied the recognition of being a college of pharmacy "within the proper meaning of our (the Association's) constitution and bylaws, it being neither an organization controlled by pharmacists, nor an institution of learning which by the rules and requirements insures to its graduates of the several colleges of pharmacy represented in this Association."

A few years ago I asked Dr. Edward Kraus of the University of Michigan whether the University undertook the task of pharmaceutical instruction out of a concern over the type of pharmaceutical instruction of that day or was it done out of its regard of and for Albert B. Prescott. His reply was, "I am afraid it was done out of regard for Prescott." After all, the why's and how's and where's are immaterial. It was done. It marked the beginning of a new era in pharmaceutical education, but out of a sense of justice credit should be given where credit is due.

It has long been an acknowledged fact that the greatest and most rapid progress in professional education has been made in those fields that first formulated and then most assiduously improved the educational program. Medical men were quick to grasp the truth of this fact and apply the principle to their own field, and that is why medicine today occupies an enviable position in the professional sphere and in the mind of the public as well. Medical men have pretty well set the pattern for progress in the field of the health sciences.

Another epoch-making event in the history of the pharmaceutical education took place in Richmond, Virginia in 1900, by the creation of the American Conference of Pharmaceutical Faculties which later, without any changes in its organization or its objectives, became the American Association of Colleges of Pharmacy. The objective of the Association was to improve pharmaceutical education and research. Albert B. Prescott was its first president, Joseph P. Remington its second, and Edward Kremers its third, and through its forty-seven years of existence its activities have been directed by the most constructive minds in American pharmacy. It is hardly necessary for me to say that this organization has been a potent factor in formulating the present educational program and has been a leading factor in promoting the legislation which has determined the standards for pharmaceutical practice.

It is not necessary to go into the details of this program or the results it has accomplished, but I do want to sketch a brief picture of the changes that have taken place within the realm of my own personal experience and observation.

In my time I have seen the requirements for the study of pharmacy increased from one year of high school (in some states the eighth grade) to four. I have seen the minimal college requirement increased from two years to four. I have seen the requirements for the practice of pharmacy increased from no academic requirements to the present four-year requirement including the bachelor's degree, and today there is sweeping through our nation the recognition of the necessity of going to prepharmacy training as well as the developing of graduate instruction.

I have seen pharmacy emerge from an obscure, and in many instances a degraded, position on our university campuses to an equality with other professional schools. I have seen the scholastic attainments of pharmacy students measure up to those of other professional groups. I have seen the time come when a large proportion of pharmacy students are given recognition by the honorary scientific society of its own.

I have seen pharmacy emerge from being a nonentity in national scientific and educational work to become active in the work of such organizations as the American Association for the Advancement of Science and the American Council on Education. I have seen pharmacy establish the *American Journal of Pharmaceutical Education,* the only journal in the world dealing exclusively with the problems of pharmaceutical education. I have seen it become a unit in the Medical Service Corps of the Army and of the Navy. I have seen it create its own standardizing agency.

I have seen it do for itself what some of the great foundations did for the other professions. I have seen the Commonwealth Fund spend $64,000 to make a functional study of the pharmacist to determine the value of his service and improve the educational program. I have seen the American Foundation for Pharmaceutical Education created to foster pharmaceutical education and research, and in these latter days I am seeing the Foundation back a nation-wide survey of pharmacy costing that organization around $170,000, conducted under the auspices of the American Council on Education and directed by the most experienced and brilliant minds in the educational and professional fields for the express purpose of discovering the needs of pharmaceutical education and practice in order that pharmacy may better fulfill its mission.

I have seen the American Institute of the History of Pharmacy become a reality, and because of that I have seen the first chair of the history of pharmacy ever to be established in a great American university, or for that matter, in the world, namely, at the University of Wisconsin. And most satisfying of all, and as a result of it all, is the increase of morale and the regard which the retail pharmacist has for the dignity of his own service and the increase in respect for his own profession.

This is but a brief resumé of the progress that pharmacy has made since the century's turn. There is no more amazing, yet unheralded, accomplishment in the history of professional education than the progress pharmaceutical education has made in the twentieth century. As we face the middle of the century with such a record of accomplishment well may we ask what are the problems that are in store for us ahead, and well may we think briefly about them one with another.

One thing is certain: For a profession to become static in its educational program is to go backward. If we wish to commit professional suicide that is the course to take.

For many years the American Association of Colleges of Pharmacy has had a standing committee, known as the Committee on Problems and Plans. The Association defined its functions as follows:

"It shall be the duty of this committee to define problems that pertain to pharmaceutical education and the welfare of the Association and to institute a study of such problems and suggest plans of attack upon them." This committee's membership is composed of thirty of our highly educated young men who have demonstrated their ability to do constructive thinking and have a willingness to do constructive committee work.

One of the major problems that the committee has given its attention to for the past two years was a product of our war experience. We were asked to study the problem as to what should be done to make pharmacy qualify for more effective service in the health field. Even before the days of the war Walter F. Meads, secretary of the Board of Pharmacy examiners of Iowa, had made the general statement that, "The pharmacist should get this point fixed firmly in his mind, that it will never be possible to promote successfully any legislation in the interest of the profession of pharmacy that is not backed by the sound policy of public health and welfare."

As a result of the committee's study there cam the following conclusions, unanimously:

1. In the future, as in the past, the usefulness of the profession of pharmacy in the health field will be determined by the character of its educational program.

2. In strengthening the educational program the first step is to place greater emphasis upon the basic sciences.

3. The undergraduate program should be revamped so as to make undergraduate instruction more effective.

4. We should confine our educational activities to things pharmaceutical.

5. Foster research in the pharmaceutical sciences, having in mind the production of inspiring teachers and research workers which will also be conducive to the production of high-grade pharmaceutical literature, including textbooks in greater abundance.

6. Finally, the declaration of a long-range program from the pre-pharmacy to and through the graduate level that will place pharmacy upon a sound educational basis comparable to that of the other health professions.

If these conclusions of the committee are sound, and I believe they are, the problem that confronts us is how are these suggestions to be implemented and our objectives attained?

And that brings us to consider briefly the Pharmaceutical Syllabus, which has been our guiding instrument through almost half a century of endeavor. Without intending to do so, and without any desire to do so, we made a monstrosity out of the Pharmaceutical Syllabus.

There is a railroad out in my country that is famous for making a schedule that it cannot maintain. They can't cover the distance in the time allotted. That's exactly what we did to the Syllabus. I had my finger in it almost from the beginning, and I am as guilty as anyone for what was done. Nevertheless, the Syllabus served a useful purpose. It was a sincere attempt to organize the pharmaceutical curriculum and bring order out of chaos. And it did. Further it made possible for the boards of pharmacy to organize state board examinations and make them more uniform, which in turn made possible the reciprocity arrangements so much to be desired. But we didn't have wisdom enough to know when to stop rolling the snowball, and so the Syllabus content grew and grew until it outgrew its usefulness. As Dean Ernest Little has often said, it left no room even for experimentation and when we reached that point, curriculum building became static.

When the American Council on Pharmaceutical Education abandoned the Syllabus as a measuring rod for the accreditation of colleges the organizations that had sponsored it through the years gave the act approval. Nevertheless, the Syllabus represented the best thought of American Pharmacists through four decades, and should be and will be used as a basis in this era of reconstruction of the curriculum which we are now approaching. And in doing so it will be well to bear in mind the words of wisdom of the late beloved Dr. Lotus D. Coffman, president of the University of Minnesota.

Speaking before the American Council on Education in the Hotel Mayflower in Washington a few years ago he pleaded for educators, both general and professional, to hold to the basic principles of education that have been tried through the years. He also pleaded for change, but not without applying the principles of scientific experimentation which would prove the value of such changes. And then in words which still thrill my very being, he said: "I agree fully with the English Association for Education in Citizenship which declares that "If democracy is to survive and develop as a living force, our educational system must produce men and women loving freedom, desiring to serve their community, and equipped with the necessary knowledge and possess powers of clear thinking to enable them to become effective citizens." It is because I believe in necessary knowledge that I make a special plea for education that puts lime into the bone, iron into the blood, and organized knowledge into the minds of the youth of this generation."

Dr. Coffman made no claim to being a scientist. He was an educator. But he believed in applying the methods and principles of science to the problems of education on all of its levels in all types. In the case of pharmacy, the Pharmaceutical Syllabus represents the principles of education that have been tried through the years. Our problem is to modify it or reconstruct it, using the scientific method in doing so.

The first step we must take is to quite trying to fool ourselves and the other professions and the public into thinking we have a four-year professional pharmaceutical curriculum. We have not and you can't make it one by constant repetition of the falsehood, any more than Coué could cure cancer by repeating the formula "every day, in every way, I am feeling better and better." We didn't fool the War Manpower Commission in the last war, and if we wish to fare any better in the next one we'd better correct this condition before the shooting begins.

If the first step is to stress the basic sciences, let's take general physics, the general chemistries, and the general biological sciences out of the four-year curriculum and give them pre-pharmacy status where they belong. The College of Liberal Arts can do a better job at stressing them then we can. That is their specialty. English does not belong in the professional curriculum. One should be able to speak and write well before he reaches the professional years. Neither does eighth grade arithmetic. And we don't fool the College of Liberal Arts either by giving it a more euphonious name like pharmaceutical mathematics or pharmaceutical calculations. Changing the name of an eighth grade subject doesn't elevate it to the college level any more than calling a horse a mule makes him a hybrid. We must quite doing those things that make us ridiculous in the eyes of educated men and women. Furthermore, we don't make our professional curriculum any more professional by introducing into it college algebra or trigonometry or the calculus. They again are basic science and belong in the pre-pharmacy level.

When all these basic courses are placed where they belong then, and not until then, are we in a position to build the professional pharmaceutical curriculum in such a way so that it will prepare the student for the practice of pharmacy and lay the foundation for specialized work on the graduate level. As the course now stands, there is not one student in a hundred that completes it that is qualified to pursue graduate work in any highly specialized field without taking a year or two in basic and broadening courses to prepare him for his work.

Until we correct this condition, the pharmaceutical industry will have to continue to seek men for the research and control laboratories and manufacturing plants from men who have had a more comprehensive training in physics, chemistry, and the biological sciences although any manufacturer will admit that if pharmacists had had more basic training in those subjects, their pharmaceutical training would be a tremendous asset in industry.

I shall mention only in passing that oft-repeated warning of the distinguished secretary and creator of the American Council on Pharmaceutical Education, Andrew G. DuMez, that we would make the greatest gain by confining our activities to things pharmaceutical and not attempt to make our pharmacy colleges preparatory schools to medicine, dentistry, business or engineering. I would not have been surprised if some pharmacy school had established a preparatory course for entrance to Princeton Seminary. It might be more to the point to ask Princeton Seminary to bring some ethics to our pharmacy schools.

When we stop to think it over, how foolish it seems for us to attemp to scatter our energies when we have so much to accomplish in our own field of endeavor and so little in the way of equipment and men with which to do it. I have never known any one to approve of this type of wastefulness except deans. Deans are a peculiar variety of the human species-they are not understandable. They are incomprehensible. The things they should do, they do not do, and the things they should not do, they do-and as a member of the craft I myself have done that very thing. That is why, many years ago, when I recognized this weakness in deans, I created the slogan: 'What pharmacy most needs is the funerals of a lot of deans." The truth of that statement has not yet become obsolete.

And finally we come to the graduate level. The objective of graduate work should be to stimulate and develop the creative instinct in man. If we are to have inspiring teachers and creative workers in all fields of pharmaceutical endeavor, suitable individuals must be discovered and their education must be one of our primary concerns. Education on the graduate level is not the function of the undergraduate college but of the graduate school. But the seeking out of those who have special talents for independent action and the inspiring of them by the warmth of a personality to work in the specific field of their choice and, usually, the directing of their work, fall to the lot of the instructors in the undergraduate college.

Unfortunately, on the campuses of many of our universities we find an indifference, if not an open hostility, toward graduate work in pharmacy. This is due in part to the fact that pharmacy is looked upon as an applied science. Yet in the same institutions graduate work in medicine is encouraged and well supported. This directly opposite attitude toward pharmacy and medicine is, of course, an untenable inconsistency, since all the health sciences are applied sciences in the commonly understood and accepted meaning of that term.

When the attention of the members of the graduate faculty is called to this inconsistency, and I speak from experience, they of course have no answer. We must credit them with basic honesty. Then they turn to the real answer, namely: graduates of the present four year course in pharmacy have not had as broad a background training as the students of medicine or those who have majored in the physical, chemical or biological sciences. And to that *we* have no answer, for we also are basically honest. This, however, is not a condition for which the graduate school is responsible. Only *we* are responsible for this and only we can correct this condition. It is the weakest link in the whole scheme of pharmaceutical education, and the quicker we correct it the more quickly we can take our place on a level with all other fields of professional education.

After having said all this I cannot refrain from making the statement that any of us can pick out any number of individuals, who have the doctorate in the major fields, that are lamentably weak in their background training. Bigotry is its outstanding symptom. These are the individuals a scholarly friend of mine brands as "PhD duds" or "blank cartridges." We have some of them teaching and administering in our schools of pharmacy. This, of course, is beside the point, but I feel better for having said it.

It is refreshing to know there are deans of graduate schools that have a broader conception of graduate work and the responsibility of graduate schools to professional education. One such is Dean Alpheus W. Smith of the Graduate School of Ohio State University, and it is with great satisfaction that I quote from an address at the 1943 meeting of that Association in Chicago. The address was published exclusively in a 1944 number of the *American Journal of Pharmaceutical Education* under the title, "To What Extent Should Graduate Education Become Functional as Directed to Meeting the Demands in Various *(Often New)* Occupations?"

"The responsibility of graduate schools for professional education may be illustrated by reference to medicine, dentistry, pharmacy and veterinary medicine. It is evident that the graduate schools have little to do with the formal training of dentists, physicians, pharmacists and veterinarians. That type of education is the responsibility of the faculties of the appropriate colleges. There remain, however, the training of teachers and research workers in medicine, dentistry, pharmacy, and veterinary medicine. It is one thing to organize existing knowledge and current practices. It is quite a different thing to provide leaders who will blaze new trails and create new understandings. Here the graduate schools have the same responsibilities as they have for research and education in fundamental fields like chemistry, biology and economics.

"Consequently the graduate schools should maintain graduate programs in medicine, dentistry, pharmacy and veterinary medicine with the same interest and enthusiasm they show for other fields of scholarship, but these programs like other graduate programs should be organized about research activities. They should not become extensions of undergraduate programs nor prolongations of training for practitioners. They should be designed to prepare for the creative work which will develop and recreate the profession...adhering to the principle that it is not the purpose of graduate schools 'to produce neither learned pedants or simple artisans', we arrive at the conclusion that they have great responsibility for the development of existing professions and creation of new ones in case these professions and occupations require the application of creative intellectual forces and form a social class of progressive guides and leaders." That is a masterly conception of the functions and the objectives of the graduate school as related to professional education, and if it could become the universal policy of such schools the present lamentable scarcity of qualified teachers would soon be corrected.

In this connection I want to express my concern over a matter that has been a source of irritation to pharmaceutical educators for many years, namely, the apparent lack of recognition on the part of pharmaceutical industry of any responsibility to pharmaceutical education; and, furthermore, I cannot believe that pharmaceutical industry has realized what it has been doing to pharmaceutical education. I am not criticizing. I am making a statement of fact which can be documented. In my day there have been many men who died multimillionaires, having made their wealth in the pharmaceutical industry. By their wills they left millions of dollars to great universities, to medical schools, to hospitals, and for other purposes that are beneficial to human welfare, but to this date I cannot find a single instance where more than a mere pittance was left for the betterment of pharmaceutical teaching institutions, which certainly had some part in the creation of their wealth.

And what adds to that irritation is the fact that industry has through the years robbed our institutions of many of our best men, cutting off their own supply, and has done nothing to aid these institutions to continue to be the source of supply of able men. I am not a business man. I am a school teacher, but it does seem to me that this constant impoverishment of the goose that lays the golden eggs is not good business. I do not object to pharmaceutical industry contributing to everything that in the end improves human welfare. In fact, I am proud of the industry for doing it. But not to give a just share to improve our own institutions is certainly in the language of the labor unions unfair. The creation of the American Foundation for Pharmaceutical Education is an indication that pharmaceutical industry is realizing its dependence upon the educative process, and in that realization there is new hope cast into the educational arena.

The greatest fear is the fear of fear. Fear was another monstrosity born of the New Deal. Fear of too little food drove us to plant more corn-raise more pigs. Before either was ready for the market the fear of too much food drove us to plow the corn under, and to massacre most of the pigs and to dump them into the river when people were still hungry. At that time Governor Bryan of Nebraska went down to Chicago, according to his own statement, to plan a course in birth control for the pigs that were permitted to survive. We still have a hangover of this use of fear in The Meatless Tuesdays and the Poultryless Thursdays. But the next day brilliant Washington declared that to be a mistake-so they opened up Thursday to the chickens, and then they saw that was a mistake and so they started the "Eat-a-Hen-a-Day-Club." Fear has been used more than any other weapon to drive Americans into regimentation and toward a totalitarian state.

Fear has become an infectious and contagious disease in our government and national life. It has reached the ranks of pharmacy, so that one month we are jittery because we have too few students, and the next month we have too many. We not only have too many students, but we have too many schools of pharmacy. And so we meet in annual conclave and condemn everybody and everything because of this situation, and we all declare something must be done to remedy the situation, and then we go home and do nothing about it.

It reminds me of what Dr. Swain once said. He was neither condemning prohibition nor defending it. He simply made a statement of fact when he said, prohibition went down the river because Senators said one thing on the floor of the Senate, and did another thing in the coat room. Now to paraphrase that to make it fit pharmacy, we might say we have enough pharmacists because deans said one thing in the conclave but didn't do anything about it at the registration desk. Perhaps that is the Creator's way of maintaining a sufficient supply of pharmacists. He knows that such a thing as an ever-normal granary of pharmacists is not possible.

Many years before the war Dean Evert Kendig began to call our attention to a decline in the number of pharmacists. The war exaggerated that condition, but there were other factors, including the advance in educational requirements and the standards for pharmaceutical practice, that caused a slowing up of production. It was a good thing for pharmacy in general.

I have stood practically alone in this country in believing there are not too many colleges of pharmacy. I grant there is an unfortunate distribution. There are too many in some areas, but the very areas where the complaints come from are the areas where those who could and should do something about it, do nothing.

The establishment of several new schools on the backbone of the continent has been criticized, but the criticism has not come from the people who live there. Take Arizona for example. There are few people living east of the Mississippi River that know that there are only four states in the union having a territory larger than Arizona, and that all of New England could be set down within its borders. They don't know that eleven states, including the Dakotas, have a smaller population. They don't know that millions of acre feet of water are locked up in its canyons, that in its valleys citrus fruit and date palms flourish. They don't know that its mountains are filled with copper, and silver, and gold, and other precious metals, and that cattle and sheep by the hundreds of thousands graze on the high mesas, and on the desert, and in the mountains. They don't know the grandest scenery on the continent is here and a climate that is therapeutically the envy of the world. They don't know its university has a registration of more than 6000 students, and there are other institutions in the state with a combined registration of almost that many more. And they don't know the determination of a people that insists on developing institutions of their own on a scale that will satisfy the needs of a state whose resources are still in the early adolescent stage.

It should also be remembered that a school of pharmacy has other functions than the education of students. It should be an intellectual, professional and spiritual center for the profession within the state. It should be an institution in which they can take pride, that they can work for and cherish. As such it becomes a creator of professional morale, and an asset to the state as a public health institution.

In editing a journal I am constantly on the alert for ideas that will be helpful to those of us who work in the pharmaceutical field. One source where I seek information is in the addresses of scholarly men. In my search this year the most helpful idea I have gleaned was from the commencement address of President Carter Davidson of Schenectady's Union College. Speaking at the University of Buffalo, he in substance said, "We Americans need to be warned against words and ideas that look much alike but have different effects. For example, we confuse size with importance, speed with progress, money with wealth, authority with wisdom, religion with theology, excitement with pleasure. We have confused training with education. Training is a process by which a pupil is taught to perform an act by imitating

"Education should acquaint a student with ways of analyzing problems he has never before seen."

Then I realized that throughout all the years of my service we have been training students rather than educating them. The time is opportune, now that we are in the business of reconstructing the curriculum; we will do well to bear in mind that from the pre-pharmacy to the graduate level our objective should be not training, but educating And if we educate instead of train, no man in this room will live to see the day when there will be an over-supply of pharmacists, for the areas of service and the avenues that lead to them will have become worldwide. ■

1948 Remington Medalist

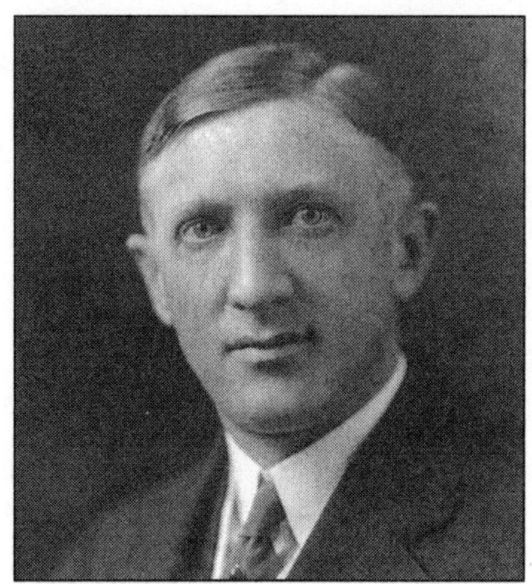

ANDREW GROVER DUMEZ
(1885-1948)

Andrew Grover DuMez was born in Horloon, Wisconsin, and graduated with a Ph.G. degree 1904, a B.S. in Pharmacy 1907, and Ph.D. 1917, all from the University of Wisconsin. He served as professor of chemistry at Pacific University in Oregon 1910-1911, and at Oklahoma A&M 1911-1912, and as director of the University of the Philippines School of Pharmacy 1912-1916, during which time he served as vice governor of the Philippines to investigate its colleges of pharmacy. He then served as pharmacologist for the U.S. Public Health Service's Hygienic Laboratory 1917-1918, and secretary of the Treasury Department's special committee to investigate the traffic of narcotics 1918-1925. He became dean of the University of Maryland School of Pharmacy in 1926, serving until his death. He also served as president of the American Association of Colleges of Pharmacy 1929-1930, vice chairman of the USP revision committee 1930-1940, secretary-treasurer of the American Council on Pharmaceutical Education 1932-1948, and consultant to both the War Manpower Commission and the Surgeon General of the U.S. Army during World War II. He was editor of *Digest of Comments on the Pharmacopeia* and the *National Formulary* 1916-1922, and co-author of *Quantitative Pharmaceutical Chemistry* (1931).

A life member of the American Pharmaceutical Association, DuMez served as chairman of the APhA Scientific Section 1920-1921, editor of the *APhA Year Book* 1921-1935, editor of APhA's *Pharmaceutical Abstracts* 1935-1940, editor of the *Journal of the American Pharmaceutical Association, Scientific Edition* 1940-1941, a member 1920-1941 and secretary 1920-1923 of the APhA Council, and APhA president 1939-1940.

The 1948 Remington Medal was presented posthumously at a joint meeting of the Baltimore and New York Branches of the American Pharmaceutical Association held on November 18, 1948, at the University of Maryland School of Law in Baltimore, Maryland. The selection of Andrew Grover DuMez as the 1948 Remington medalist was announced on June 28, 1948, but Dr. DuMez died on September 27, 1948.

1949 Remington Medalist

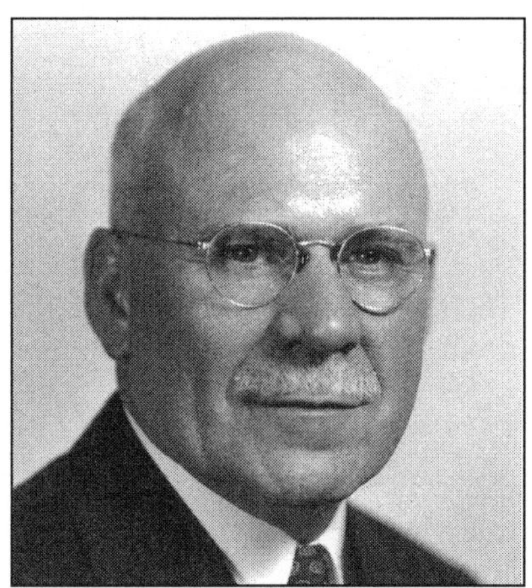

ERNEST LITTLE
(1888-1973)

Ernest Little was born in Johnstown, New York, and received a B.S. degree in chemistry from the University of Rochester in 1911, and a Ph.D. degree in chemistry from Columbia University in 1924. After serving as an instructor in chemistry at the University of Rochester 1911-1914 and at Pratt Institute 1942-1943, he joined the Rutgers University faculty attaining full professorship in chemistry in 1924. Two years later, he was named dean of the New Jersey College of Pharmacy, which later became the Rutgers College of Pharmacy. Little served as dean until 1946, and remained as professor of chemistry until his complete retirement in 1953. He served as treasurer of the New York sections of the American Chemical Society; president of the Newark, New Jersey, Rotary Club; president of the New Jersey Pharmaceutical Association and the Northern New Jersey APhA Branch; president 1934-1935 and executive committee chairman 1936-1941 of the American Association of Colleges of Pharmacy; and a member of the USP committee of revision 1930-1960.

As chairman of the National Drug Trade Conference committee on endowment, Little proposed the creation of the American Foundation for Pharmaceutical Education and served as its founding president, director 1943-1950, and acting secretary in 1950. He served as APhA president 1948-1949.

The Wide Walls of Pharmacy

Ernest Little

The 1949 Remington Honor Medal Lecture was presented on December 6, 1949, at the Hotel New Yorker in New York City. Little's abridged address was published in the *Journal of the American Pharmaceutical Association, Practical Pharmacy Edition*, volume 11, pages 27-29, 1950.

As I look back over thirty-one years, which is the length of time I have been associated with pharmacy, I find much which should act as a source of encouragement, as we face the problems of tomorrow.

In the field of pharmaceutical education progress has been rapid and profound. Three decades ago our colleges of pharmacy had, generally speaking, no entrance requirements and very low educational standards. Applicants with but two years of high school training, or even less, were admitted to our colleges in large numbers.

The curricula offered constituted, by and large, part-time two year courses. There were far too many part-time teachers on our teaching staffs. Laboratory work was sadly deficient. Indeed our whole educational program was in need of broadening and strengthening.

You know how splendidly such improvements have been made. We went to the minimum three year course in 1925 and the four year course in 1932. The so-called degree of Ph.G. (Pharmacy Graduate) has been abolished and the university degree of Bachelor of Science substituted.

Entrance requirements have been increased until today, they compare favorably with the entrance requirements of other university colleges.

Both the American Association of Colleges of Pharmacy and the American Council on Pharmaceutical Education are actively studying and seriously considering a six year program. We may rest assured that pharmaceutical education will not remain static but will continue to grow and develop as the needs of the profession dictate.

College prerequisite requirements are now in effect in all of the states of the union except one. Would that the citizens of that neighboring state could recapture some of the imagination and pioneering spirit of their ancestors.

Another encouraging circumstance in the field of pharmaceutical education is our rapidly developing graduate programs. Pharmaceutical industry and our colleges of pharmacy have need for many more Ph.D.s, who have done their undergraduate work in pharmacy, than are now available.

One of the many fine contributions which the American Foundation for Pharmaceutical Education is making to our profession is its support and encouragement of graduate work in colleges of pharmacy which are prepared to carry on graduate programs of high quality. The Foundation is spending in excess of $100,000 a year on graduate fellowships alone at this time.

It would seem that if the Foundation did no more than it is now doing in the field of graduate work, its continued existence would be fully justified. I sincerely hope that all of us, in all branches of the profession, will become increasingly interested in the American Foundation for Pharmaceutical Education and that increased financial support will be forthcoming from year to year. It represents one of the most fundamental and important developments within the framework of our profession during the past decade.

Twenty years ago we had no regularly organized accrediting agency operating in the field of pharmaceutical education. It is true that the American Association of Colleges of Pharmacy had performed such functions since the turn of the century in a most admirable manner, but the AACP was never intended to be and never considered itself primarily an accrediting agency.

Today we have the American Council on Pharmaceutical Education, made up of representatives of the American Pharmaceutical Association, the National Association of Boards of Pharmacy, the American Association of Colleges of pharmacy and the American Council on Education, operating in an efficient and considerate manner. This agency merits and should have our sympathetic understanding as it continues its good work in behalf of pharmacy.

We have recently witnessed the completion of a survey of American Pharmacy in all of its various ramifications. This survey was sponsored by the American Council on Education and directed by an unusually capable leader, Dr. Edward C. Elliott.

The Findings and Recommendations of this group should by now be known to all of us. I sincerely hope that we shall continue to give them general study, and exceedingly detailed study as they apply to the particular branch of pharmacy in which we are engaged.

This survey work has proven expensive. It has cost the American Foundation for Pharmaceutical Education in the neighborhood of $200,000. The expenditure of even such a sizable sum can be justified many times over if we will all play our full parts in helping to make its recommendations-realities.

It is up to us. Dr. Elliott can do little more. He is now diligently working with the American Council on Pharmaceutical Education helping to implement the recommendations of the Survey as they pertain to the important work on accreditation.

We must take up the work from here on. Dr. Elliott is available for consultation and advice but, as is so frequently the case, he can help only those who help themselves. It occurs to me that a similar comment has been made about an even greater personality than Dr. Elliott.

It would seem, from the above presentation of some of our more recent accomplishments, that pharmacy is about to go forward with a program more comprehensive and constructive than ever before.

Such should be the case. The necessary agencies are organized and in operation manned by capable staffs. Our recent survey has very clearly indicated the paths we should follows.

What then stands in the way of progress? Nothing, I should say nothing, unless it be a lack of unity, a lack of solidarity, a lack of singleminded determination, which are prerequisites to success in any field of endeavor. It is in these respects that we still have much progress to make. It is to this thought that I wish to direct my remarks for the next few minutes.

It is always dangerous to engage in superlatives, but for the sake of emphasis I shall say that in my judgment pharmacy's greatest need today is that we, its practitioners, should be freed from petty prejudices which keep us apart one from the other, weaken the very foundation of our profession and prevent us from making the over-all progress which should be ours.

Although I have tried to be generally active in the field of pharmacy, I am primarily an AACP man and it is there that my deepest interests lie. We are justifiably proud of the fine progress which has been made in the training and education of the practitioners of pharmacy during the past quarter of a century. Still, I would be false if I did not confess that we educators have been as narrow and possibly more provincial than the representatives of any other branch of our profession. We at times display unjustifiable suspicion of the motives and good intent of our co-workers in the manufacturing field, in the field of wholesale distribution and, to a lesser extent, in retail pharmacy as well. Our actions at times might even indicate that we are inclined to feel that we have more or less of a corner on virtue, one of the most dangerous attitudes which can threaten any man.

To those of you who feel that I may have been a little too severe with us educators, may I add that it seems appropriate, even when engaging in strictly constructive criticism, to start with self analysis.

We educators sometimes assume a 'holier than thou" attitude which is quite unjustified and certainly not conducive to progress in our profession. I hope that in the days ahead we shall strive, without the sacrifice of a single principle, to see the other fellow's point of view and to work more cooperatively with him.

Well, having antagonized my own colleagues in the field of pharmaceutical education, may I spend a few minutes alienating the affection of my friends in the fields of pharmaceutical manufacturing and wholesale distribution. For no logical reason except to save time, I shall consider them jointly.

We are all proud of the progress which has been made in the field of pharmaceutical manufacturing. We need to think only of the vitamins, more recently B12, the sulfa drugs, the whole field of antibiotics, antihistamine drugs and more recently cortisone, which may become the wonder of them all. A mere glimpse of these and many other equally profound accomplishments should cause us to stand in awe of the really profound achievements of our coworkers in the manufacturing field.

Yet these men do not always show an awareness of the need of cooperation in the pharmaceutical family which we would like to see. It is true that pharmaceutical industry has contributed several million dollars to the American Foundation for Pharmaceutical Education. This is something for us educators to be deeply appreciative of, but not something for pharmaceutical manufacturers to be unduly proud of.

As we review the potentialities of help from the manufacturing field for an agency as worthy and as obviously needed as the AFPE, we are appalled by the inadequacy of the contribution so far received. This may be due in part to the fact that the Foundation has not been sold to prospective donors as it should have been. I wonder, however, if at least to some extent, it does not also reflect an inadequate appreciation of the essential need of better cooperation and mutual help within the ranks of our profession.

There has been a discouraging decrease in contributions to the Foundation during the past several years. It is hoped that individuals and corporations in a position to do so, will think in terms of greater, much greater contributions than ever before. Such action could be amply justified from strictly selfish and hard-headed business considerations. I have too much confidence in the vision and in the enlightened generosity of our men of wealth in the profession of pharmacy to make any such uncomplimentary appeal.

Well, how about our retail pharmacists? Retail pharmacists have, by and large, shown an encouraging desire to cooperate, as best they can, in the upbuilding of our profession. They would be among the first, however, to confess that they have not done all that might reasonably be expected of them.

Seldom, during the twenty years that I was Dean of the New Jersey College of Pharmacy, did I talk with a retail pharmacist who did not profess to know more about how the New Jersey College of Pharmacy should be run than did the men then responsible for its administration. Possibly they were correct, but I could have told them how their stores could be greatly improved, sometimes involving nothing more profound than a more frequent use of the floor brush and dusting cloth.

The point is, they were making the mistake which you, and I too, frequently make. They were being too critical of their colleagues while overlooking or even being unaware of their own shortcomings.

Therein lies one of the big weaknesses of our profession, and one of our greatest challenges. Let us be more critical of ourselves, a little more tolerant of the other fellow, and much more determined to cooperate with him. That is the thought which I leave with you tonight. Will you consider it well? No branch of our profession can be stronger than pharmacy's weakest link. May we keep the over-all picture, the overall needs of our profession constantly before us, and develop a feeling of mutual confidence, an "Esprit de Corps" never before achieved.

I appeal to my friends, in all branches of the profession represented here tonight, to be generous in the interpretation of my remarks and try to understand the spirit which prompted them. I have made no attempt to give a scholarly address. I have tried to be neither complimentary nor critical. I have tried only to be helpful. One cannot always do that without running the risk of being misunderstood. Knowing you as I do, I am quite willing to take that chance.

I would like to conclude with a somewhat homely verse, written anonymously. It may not qualify as classical literature, but it appeals to me as being both stimulating and worthwhile. It is called "Wide Walls" and is as follows:

Give me wide walls to build my house of life

The north shall be of love, against the winds of fate,

The south of tolerance, that I may outreach hate,

The east of faith that rises clear and new each day,

The west of hope, that then dies a glorious way.

The threshold 'neath my feet shall be humility;

The roof the very sky itself infinity.

Give me wide walls to build my house of life.

May the walls of our house of pharmacy be built wide and strong. Wide enough to include all that is best from all sectors of our diversified profession, strong enough to resist undermining influences which beset it. From such a structure may we go forward together with a determination and a singleness of purpose which will result in accomplishments greater than ever before achieved, and which will make pharmacy's future worthy of its past. ■

1950 Remington Medalist

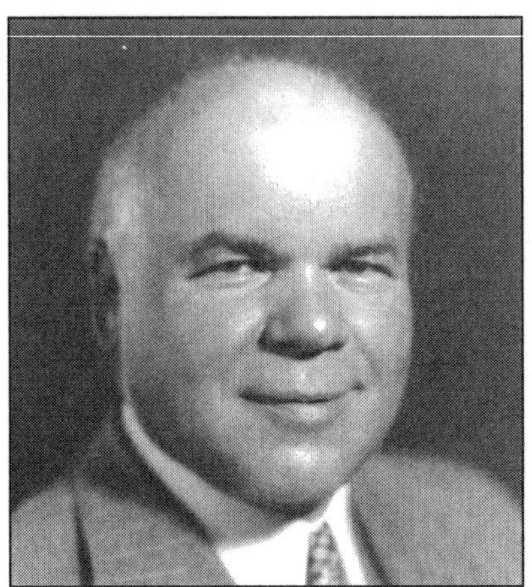

EDWIN LEIGH NEWCOMB
(1882-1950)

Edwin Leigh Newcomb was born in Vineland, New Jersey, and graduated with a Pharm.D. degree from the Philadelphia College of Pharmacy in 1905. Having specialized in bacteriology, he served as consulting engineer for the Vineland (New Jersey) Sewage Disposal plant 1905-1910, while teaching at his *alma mater.* He then joined the faculty of the University of Minnesota department of pharmacy 1910-1926, where he established a medicinal garden during World War I, and was instrumental in the cultivation and standardization of digitalis. During this period, he also served as secretary of the Minnesota Pharmaceutical Association, editor of *Northwestern Druggist,* secretary of the eight-state Northwest Pharmaceutical Bureau, and director of a five year study on pharmacy economics at the Minnesota University Business School 1920-1925. He was then elected as secretary 1926-1932 and executive vice president 1933-1950 of the National Wholesale Druggists' Association, and also served as a founding member and executive secretary of the American Foundation for Pharmaceutical Education 1942-1950, as well as chairman of the National Council of Wholesale Associations, secretary of NARD's Druggists' Research Bureau, and chairman of the Health Information Foundation finance committee.

Joining the American Pharmaceutical Association in 1906, Newcomb worked actively with H.A.B. Dunning in the fund-raising campaign for the American Institute of Pharmacy, headquarters building of APhA. In honor of the 1950 Remington medalist, NWDA established the "Edwin Leigh Newcomb Memorial Fund" to be managed by the American Foundation for Pharmaceutical Education.

The 1950 Remington Medal was presented posthumously at a ceremony held on December 4, 1950, in the Harkness Theatre of Columbia University in New York City, with eulogies presented by John W. Dargavel, Ivor Griffith, Ernest Little, and Theodore G. Kiump. The selection of Edwin Leigh Newcomb as the 1950 Remington medalist was announced on April 11, 1950, but Dr. Newcomb died on September 2, 1950.

1951 Remington Medalist

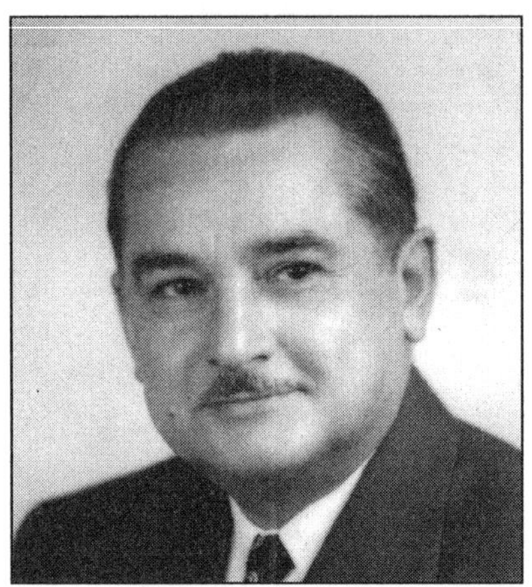

HUGO HERMAN SCHAEFER
(1891-1967)

Hugo Herman Schaefer was born in Brooklyn, New York, and graduated as a pharmacist from the Columbia University in 1913. He served as an analytical chemist for the New York Quinine and Chemical Works until 1916 when he joined the faculty of his alma mater as an instructor in chemistry. In 1923, he took a two-year leave of absence for graduate study at the University of Berne, Switzerland, where he received a Ph.D. in pharmacognosy in 1925. He was named dean of the Brooklyn College of Pharmacy in 1937, a position he held until his retirement in 1956.

Schaefer served as APhA third vice president 1921-1922, chairman of the APhA House of Delegates 1940-1941, and APhA treasurer for 26 years (1941-1967). He served as local secretary for the APhA annual meetings held in New York City in 1919 and 1937. As secretary of the New York APhA Chapter, Schaefer proposed establishing the Remington Medal and served as secretary of the committee on awards until his death. Service to his profession in New York included secretary of both the Bronx County Pharmaceutical Society and the Pharmaceutical Council of Greater New York, chairman of the executive committee of the New York State Pharmaceutical Association, chemist for the New York Board of Pharmacy, and president of the New York Academy of Pharmacy. On the national level, Schaefer was elected president of the American Association of Colleges of Pharmacy, the National Drug Trade Conference, and the American Institute of History of Pharmacy (subsequently as honorary president); treasurer of the American Foundation for Pharmaceutical Education; secretary of the USP revision committee; and director of the American Druggists Insurance Company. As a lasting memorial, APhA created the Hugo H. Schaefer Medal in 1964 to recognize unique contributions to the profession of pharmacy.

Pharmaceutical Advances Create New Problems

Hugo Herman Schaefer

The 1951 Remington Honor Medal Lecture was presented December 11, 1951, at the Waldorf-Astoria Hotel in New York City. Schaefer's Remington address was published in the *Journal of the American Pharmaceutical Association, Practical Pharmacy Edition,* volume 13, pages 28-29, 50-52, January 1952.

I suppose that it is only human on an occasion such as this to review the passing years, to evaluate the progress which has been made and the changes which have occurred in our profession. I refuse to acknowledge that I am rapidly approaching the age which would make me a suitable test animal for geriatric experimentation and observation, but this I fear is a form of self delusion or a state of mind which for the present must be set aside in order that I may qualify as one who can delve into the past so as to justify my comments on the future.

Forty-three years have passed since I began my apprenticeship in pharmacy and thirty-nine years since I graduated from college and became a registered pharmacist. As I look back upon these years I find little cause for regret. If I had to live them over again, I would try to correct some of my many errors of omissions and commission, but I would most certainly again choose the field of pharmacy as the sphere of my activities and interests. I would do so because of a convincing realization that pharmacy has made great forward strides in all its economic as well as professional fronts and that it offers a most promising and satisfying field of activity for those who make it their career. My faith in pharmacy forty-five years ago has been justified by passing events. While I devoted most of my years to pharmaceutical education, yet, my thinking, my activities and my interests are primarily those of the professional retail pharmacist. I will never forget my period of apprenticeship in the drug store, that period in my formative years which made such a great impression upon me. Since then, I have had an insight into all segments of our industry and a rather close relationship to several of them aside from my many years of activity in the educational field. I have had the benefit of a broad view of all aspects of the production and distribution of drug store products and still retain the firm conviction that the retail pharmacy is the keystone of our entire industry.

We can all look with pride upon the progress made by retail pharmacy. I need not describe the drug store of forty years ago and compare it with the modern pharmacy of today nor discuss the economic advances which have been made. These changes have been observed by most of you and have been reviewed on many occasions for the benefit of those who are not old enough to have witnessed them.

One often hears disparaging comparisons made between the pharmacy of yesterday and of today because of the increase in the prescription dispensing of manufactured preparations and specialties and the decline in the number of products compounded in the pharmacy as well as waning importance of *USP* and *NF* products as compared to branded name preparations. I, too, deplore this trend, but a mental analysis of the situation brings me to the conclusion that my feelings are based largely on sentimentalism just as I also regret that we no longer observe the characteristic drug store odor of many years ago and that the pharmacist has discontinued giving gum-drops, licorice and slippery elm to children.

Fifty years ago my father bemoaned the fact that most pharmacists were no longer making their own pills, plasters, tinctures and fluid extracts. Today we realize that it would be a practical impossibility to provide space, time and manpower for such outmoded activities. The underlying reasons for these trends go, however, beyond mere economic questions. Only large scale manufacturing procedures with elaborate scientific equipment and personnel can provide the necessary production refinements and controls which are more essential today than before because of the very nature of our modern medicaments. Consider, for instance, our vast production and use of the antibiotics. These drugs and their dosage forms must be prepared under the most painstaking conditions to insure full potency, purity, sterility and keeping qualities, and, in fact, samples from every lot must be submitted to the Food and Drug Administration for their examination before being released for distribution. Each step in the production of these so-called "wonder drugs" must be rigidly controlled and a patient's life often depends upon their effectiveness. The pharmacist should realize that these products must come to him and be dispensed in finished form and that this in no manner lowers his professional dignity. He must know all about the nature, action and uses of the antibiotics and this requires a vastly increased background of scientific and professional knowledge.

The necessity for accepting finished prescription products from the manufacturer is, of course, not confined merely to the field of antibiotics. A similar need for exacting production and control procedures exists in the vitamin field because of the very nature of the medication involved. In mixed vitamin therapy for instance, some ingredients are used in only microgram quantities. Chemical incompatibilities often require that some of the ingredients be placed in the tablet coating or in an interior pellet. Without such precautions rapid deterioration would result. Such products can only be properly produced in large laboratories.

Many other illustrations could be given. The production of most dosage forms of hormones, glandular products, and injectable substances must of necessity be left to the manufacturer. They require extensive research, elaborate equipment and continuous chemical and biological controls to safeguard the effectiveness of the finished product.

The fact that the pharmacist no longer compounds as many prescriptions as he did in former years is not a cause for his losing faith in his profession. He is dispensing more potent, more effective, more useful preparations today than ever before. He is not a mere purveyor of package goods, but rather a person with an extensive knowledge of the nature of this prescription products, one who can discuss them intelligently with the physician and who has a thorough understanding of their action and uses. Thus his education and training must cover a vast scope of newer medicaments undreamed of in past years and he must remain constantly alert to the many new and important medicinal agents which are being developed at an ever increasing rate. He compounds fewer mixtures in his prescription department, but this merely means a reduction in the time devoted by him to purely manipulative activities and the fact remains that he is filling more prescriptions than ever before and is dealing with preparations which require a far greater professional knowledge and are incomparably more effective and potent than those of earlier days.

We must face realities. We cannot afford to assume that prescription practices and procedures which prevailed years ago must go on forever despite our changing materia medica. We must have faith in pharmacy not just blindly, but with a complete realization of it is increased importance and responsibilities.

The present much discussed question of restricting many drugs to prescription use is an indirect tribute on the part of the law makers of this country and of its enforcement agencies to the importance of pharmacy in the health professions. In all recent legislative proposals and enactments the pharmacist has received increased recognition by being consistently designated as the only person who can be safely entrusted with such duties and responsibilities. Years ago there was no need for such added restrictions since the drugs generally used were relatively harmless and correspondingly ineffective. Greater responsibilities have been placed upon pharmacy by a changing medical world and this should create faith in our profession and do away with our fears for the future.

This change in general prescription practice from mixtures which must be compounded by the pharmacist to manufactured preparations has, however, created one situation which I deplore. I have in mind the apparent needless duplication of identical or closely similar mixtures marketed by different manufacturers under different trade names. That this is not exactly a new development can be gathered from the presidential address of Joseph Price Remington delivered at the 41st meeting of the American Pharmaceutical Association in Chicago on August 14, 1893. President Remington had been discussing the rise of synthetic organic medicinals in the materia medica of his day. He then spoke as follows:

"The effect upon pharmacy and medicine of this extraordinary activity in the synthetical departments of chemical science has been profound; new chemical compounds and new classes of compounds have been flooding commerce like a deluge, the more valuable ones being protected by letters patent or by copyright names; competition among the large manufacturers is extremely fierce, and the result to the average pharmacist has been to produce confusion, uncertainty, and annoyance; the representatives of one manufacturer no sooner visit him and the neighboring physicians, before a competitor follows on his heels with another remedy, claiming even greater advantages and which does not possess the disadvantages of the one that has already been added to the stock."

While pharmacists of the present day may willingly accept the premise that many of our newer medicaments can be made best in large laboratories under careful control procedures, yet, they strongly resent the fact that to a great extent these items are merely duplications of products made by other producers. Many such products vary in name only and not in composition or formula, and add nothing to our materia medica or to improved medication.

Considering the fact that a large percentage of prescriptions today call for single drug remedies and that the basic ingredient of these single drug remedies emanates, as a rule, from a limited manufacturing source, there should be some method of avoiding the economic waste and confusion resulting from the urge to supply whatever may be new in a form which indicates proprietorship. Proprietary rights are granted for a limited period under our patent laws for new and useful discoveries. But when the discovery is marketed by somebody other than the discoverer and the alleged proprietary right results only from adding a flavor or devising a clever dosage form and coining a name, we witness a type of competition which fails to recognize the elements of fairness and the principles of medical and pharmaceutical ethics.

I realize that all of the violations of good ethics and commercial fair dealing are not on one side. There is a reprehensible practice of some retail dispensers of drugs to substitute unbranded replacements for branded products without consideration for the legal rights of those who own patents or trade marks. Merely to mention these practices is to call attention to the fact that we have some unwholesome situations growing out of the commerce in drugs rather than the desire to render a high quality of professional service.

Pharmaceutical manufacturers today are spending millions of dollars annually for research which occasionally leads to the discovery and development of some new and more effective medicinal agent, but more often merely adds to the sum total of knowledge of chemistry and pharmacology. These contributions to scientific progress are possible only through expenditures which are recouped from the sale of products which have been successfully launched as new remedies.

In our colleges of pharmacy the faculties are continually urging young people to recognize the professional aspects of their calling whether they expect to practice pharmacy in retail establishments, in hospitals, in manufacturing institutions, or elsewhere. But we have great difficulty in explaining to these young people how a retail dispenser can establish himself without a rather large and to a considerable extent unnecessary expenditure for stocks of so called specialties, which in many instances are simply duplications of existing standard products.

And we have even greater difficulty in explaining how they are to overcome the financial loss resulting from the fact that so many of the new prescription products launched with ambitious advertising and sales campaigns become shelf-warmers after one or two prescriptions call for them.

I know that many leaders in the drug industry, as well as in the profession have given this problem much thought and are alarmed over the ultimate consequences of the situation which is clearly not in the interests of the sick or of the professions involved in treating the sick. Recognition of the problem is the first step towards its solution, and even though I am reiterating complaints recorded nearly sixty years ago by Remington, I am hopeful that the industry and the profession will take necessary steps to meet this situation before it becomes worse.

So far I have confined myself to observations of the prescription dispensing trends in pharmacy. I repeat that aside from the potential dangers created by the marketing of large numbers of needless items the prescription practice of the pharmacist has gained in importance both as a source of income and of increased prestige. This, however, cannot be said of his other activities. The sale of potent and dangerous drugs has become more effectively confined to the pharmacy both by legislation and by general public acceptance but we are now witnessing a reverse trend as far as other drug store products are concerned. The current inroad into general drug store sales by super markets and other non-pharmacy outlets is one such factor. Another one is the recent court decision nullifying the effectiveness of our fair-trade laws thus adding further fuel to undesirable competition and in addition to all this we are now threatened with encroachment of our traditional rights by court actions intended to challenge the purpose and scope of our state pharmacy laws and regulations.

These trends cannot be allowed to go on unchallenged. They have as their objective increasing the number of outlets for drug store products and this would result in bringing the pharmacy to the level of the ordinary merchant. We are told by many that this deplorable situation can best be met by adopting more aggressive merchandising procedures but such a policy I fear would only result in still further stressing the purely commercial aspects of the pharmacy. The future of our profession of pharmacy lies in our emphasizing the professional character of our retail establishments, the added services which we render and our specialized knowledge and training which make such services possible.

This, however, cannot be done without the full cooperation and understanding on the part of the other branches of our industry. Our manufacturing and wholesaling friends should realize that they have little to gain and much to lose by vastly widening their area of retail outlets. They have grown and prospered in a specialized field of activity, but this field is only specialized because of the fact that their products did not enter into general distribution channels and were confined primarily to the retail pharmacy. A widening of the nature of retail outlets for drug store products will inevitable cause a breakdown of the barriers with now create this specialized field for the manufacturer and wholesaler and he, too, will have vastly increased competition from completely unrelated sources.

I cannot help but reach the conclusion that while the prescription services in the pharmacy have become more significant both from the professional and economic standpoint that nevertheless the other phases of drug store activity are in danger of underlying changes which are not in the best interest of pharmacy or of public welfare. It is foolish to try to rely merely on the enactment of legislation to correct these conditions. Many of them require a better understanding and a greater degree of cooperation with the industry itself.

There must be a complete realization of the fact that the interests of any one branch of our industry and profession are common to all and that none can afford to have a weak link in our rather complex chain of production and distribution.

I feel confident that there is a growing realization of the need of such mutual understanding. Eventually we must and will have it, but the great danger is that we may wait too long before it becomes completely effective and much harm can come in the meantime.

Remington in his presidential address of 1893 also referred to the problem of encroachment of non-pharmacists on the prerogatives of pharmacists, and like myself he had no immediate program to offer to correct the conditions of which he complained. He said, "It has not been deemed necessary, to bring forward at this time for your consideration a new plan for the control of the sale of various medicinal preparations, which have long been sold by druggists but which have either shaken their allegiance to the apothecary, or have been appropriated by merchants in other vocations, who have for years cast longing eyes upon the much talked of profits from their sale.

"It would seem to accord with the universal 'fitness of things' to assert that the proper man to sell medicines is the medicine man, and it is surely in the interest of the common weal to have their sale controlled by educated and specially trained dispensers of remedies, which remedies are often dangerous in the hands of the inexperienced."

I can think of no better reason than that given in the foregoing quotation from Remington to appeal at this time for an early appraisal and study of prevailing policies of the different segments of the drug industry and the profession of pharmacy with regard to the effect of these policies upon the welfare of pharmacy as a whole and upon "the common weal."

In 1893 considerations of health had not reached the significance in the lives of our people that they command today. Americans are a health conscious people today and our nation has made tremendous strides in lowering death rates and extending the individual span of life. Pharmacists have contributed and are daily contributing to the general progress in creating and maintaining better health through the development and judicious use of drugs. Considering the fact that we have been able as a profession to solve intricate problems of production, standardization, and dispensing of complex medicinal agents, it would seem that it should not be too difficult to also solve the economic and social problems which arise from the rapid development in our professional services. ■

1952 Remington Medalist

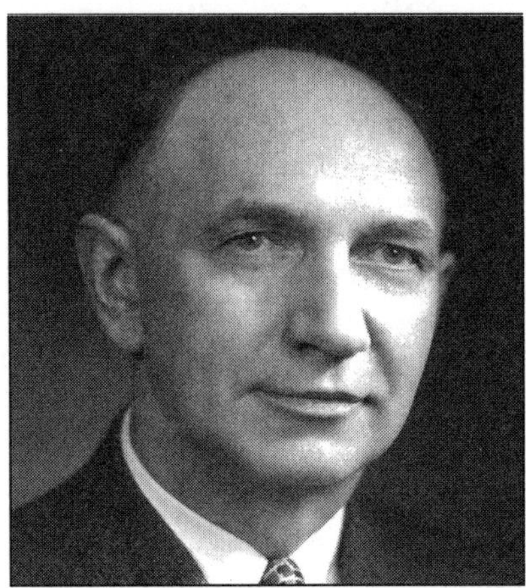

Patrick Henry Costello
(1897-1971)

Patrick Henry Costello was born in Sauk Center, Minnesota, and graduated from the North Dakota Agricultural College School of Pharmacy in 1917. He served as a pharmacist in the U.S. Army during World War I, returning to North Dakota in 1919 to open his own pharmacy in Cooperstown. He served as president 1924-1925 and treasurer 1927-1942 of the North Dakota Pharmaceutical Association, and secretary of the North Dakota Board of Pharmacy 1927-1942. Not neglecting his civic duty, he served as mayor of Cooperstown, North Dakota 1938-1942. For his work in the drug regulatory field, Costello was elected president 1939-1940 and secretary 1942-1962 of the National Association of Boards of Pharmacy during which time he gathered the first valid statistical data on pharmacists in the U.S., compiled the many varied elements of state pharmacy acts into the *NABP Survey of Pharmacy Law,* and developed a program of reciprocal licensure for pharmacists.

Costello served as chairman of the APhA House of Delegates 1933-1934, and as APhA president 1935-1936. He served as delegate to the U.S. Pharmacopeial Convention in 1940, 1950, and 1960, and was elected a member of the USP Board of Directors in 1945, 1950, and 1960. One of his most important contributions to the profession was his service to the American Council on Pharmaceutical Education serving as vice-president, president, and secretary-treasurer, helping to perfect and refine the Council's standards and requirements for accreditation which added immeasurably to the quality of pharmaceutical education.

LICENSURE AND RECIPROCITY

Patrick Henry Costello

The 1952 Remington Honor Medal Lecture was presented December 2, 1952, at the Hotel New Yorker in New York City. Costello's Remington address was published in the *Journal of the American Pharmaceutical Association, Practical Pharmacy Edition,* volume 13, pages 860863, December 1952.

Words cannot express how I feel about being the recipient of this honor and this medal. It is deeply appreciated. I should like to think that I am deserving of it. It is gratifying to know that others think so but the presence of so many on this occasion overwhelms me.

I feel greatly indebted to you, also to each of the speakers and to the New York Branch of the American Pharmaceutical Association, the sponsors of the award and of this occasion, and I most humbly and sincerely say "thank you all."

When the Remington Medal Award was first established in 1918, during the first World War, I was a newly licensed pharmacist serving in the Medical Corps of the Army of the United States. While in service I do not recall having ascertained any information about the establishment of this award or about anyone being the recipient of it but shortly thereafter I recall my reading an announcement to Mrs. Costello about Dr. James H. Beal being the recipient of the Remington Medal. Most everyone where we lived identified or associated the name Remington with arms and ammunition. Apparently Mrs. Costello also did because she immediately asked me if Dr. Beal was a sharpshooter as well as a pharmacist.

Now I am certain that she is fully as conscious as I am of the significance and the meaning of the award and shares the pleasure that comes with its presentation to me. We are delighted that our son, daughter-inlaw, nephew, niece and a sister are present this evening to share our happiness. I am sure it is a pleasant occasion to them, as it is to us, and the memory of it will always be cherished.

Publicity incident to the award which has been made to me refers to procedures which have been instituted for the purpose of evaluating and accrediting colleges of pharmacy and enabling practitioners in pharmacy in one state to acquire a license to practice in another state, both of which procedures are being utilized to great advantage and purpose.

The need for establishing some feasible provision which would enable State Boards of Pharmacy to grant licenses on a reciprocal basis was expressed at the first conference of representatives of such Boards which was held almost fifty years ago.

At that time formal education was not a required qualification for examination and licensure as a pharmacist in any state. Persons of legal age who had acquired the requisite amount and kind of apprenticeship training were required only to pass a licensure examination, prepared and given by the Board of Pharmacy, in order to obtain a license to practice. There was no uniformity in the scope or the method of examination or the manner in which the Boards of Pharmacy were performing other functions of the Pharmacy Laws of their respective states assigned to them.

Hence it was decided at that first conference to establish the National Association of Boards of Pharmacy as an interstate association to aid the Boards in improving standards for licensure and practice and to enable them to grant licenses reciprocally.

Since that time all but three states have made statutory provision for the issuance of licenses on a reciprocal basis. In accordance therewith a pharmacist who has acquired a license by examination to practice in one state may obtain a license to practice in any state in which he or she could have been deemed eligible at the time of original licensure by examination. Any pharmacist may ascertain his or her eligibility very quickly by completing and submitting a preliminary application form to the National Association of Boards of Pharmacy. Comparison is made of the data therein pertaining to the applicant's age and qualifications at the time of licensure and the statutory requirements which prevailed at that time in the state in which licensure is sought. Applicants who are deemed ineligible for the license applied for are so advised and given the reason. Applicants who are believed to be eligible are supplied with forms which must be completed by them, by the college which they attended and by the Board of Pharmacy that licensed them. The pharmacist who presents these forms, properly completed, to a State Board of Pharmacy may anticipate that he or she will be licensed by them.

Many of those familiar with problems of reciprocal licensure have expressed the belief that our procedure is an excellent one because of its simplicity and the fact that it disposes of all barriers except qualifications at time of licensure. It does not infringe upon the right of any state to determine who shall be licensed and how they shall be qualified. It takes cognizance of the right and privilege of any pharmacist who is properly qualified to practice his profession in the state of his choice and enables him to do so. Considerable more than one thousand pharmacists each year avail themselves of the opportunity and the privileges thus afforded them to remove from one state and secure a license to practice in another.

Four years prior to the time that the National Association of Boards of Pharmacy was founded the colleges of pharmacy had established the American Association of Colleges of Pharmacy to promote the interest of Pharmaceutical Education.

Both of these organizations have since held annual meetings in conjunction with the annual conventions of the American Pharmaceutical Associations and for several years a joint meeting of these organizations occurred at that time. For the past several years eight regional or district meetings have been held annually to enable all Boards and Colleges of Pharmacy in every section of this country to meet jointly for two days to consider subject matter that was relevant to pharmaceutical education, licensure and practice.

Attending all of such meetings were persons who believed it was the responsibility and should be the goal of each of the health professions, including that of pharmacy, to provide the best possible service to the public in their respective fields and said so; persons who believed that public health and welfare would benefit if the standards of pharmaceutical practice and the qualifications for licensure were elevated and said so; persons who foresaw the need for making educational requirements compulsory for licensure and said so; persons who believe that the prevailing programs of pharmaceutical education were inadequate and should be improved and persons who advocated other reforms in connection with the training and licensing of pharmacists.

The views thus expressed were almost never concurred in immediately. However, legislative enactments making formal education a prerequisite qualification for examination and licensure became effective in one state in 1905, in another in 1906, in another in 1910, in each of thirty-four more states at some time during the next two decades and in each of the remaining states at some time within the last two decades.

The imposition of educational qualifications as a requirement for licensure in the health professions is no longer looked upon as a barrier to entrance into the professions or to the free choice of a profession by an individual. Pharmaceutical education as now developed is universally accepted as the most appropriate training for the licentiate in pharmacy.

Significant credit should be accorded the American Association of Colleges of Pharmacy for their courageous endeavor to promulgate rules and regulations for their own security, but as is true with all organizations, it is seldom possible for the membership to provide unbiased judgment in matters of self-discipline. Thus we find that the leaders of this organization recognized that they could not establish their own privileges of educational freedom and at the same time police their own membership.

Wise indeed were the leaders of the Boards of Pharmacy who advocated that there must be some common ground upon which the practice of the profession could be established, even though the boundary lines of each state alienated the mandatory enforcement of the common principles enunciated in the rules and regulations which were established for reciprocal registration.

Laws which provided for the licensing of pharmacists specified that applicants must attain their educational requirements in colleges of pharmacy that were approved by the licensing Boards. The adoption of uniform standards to be used as a basis for the approval of colleges of pharmacy was advocated by the Boards of Pharmacy. It was therefore logical that the National Association of Boards of Pharmacy should give consideration to such a proposal and to ways and means of ascertaining which colleges should be approved.

The joint meeting of the Boards and Colleges previously referred to provided the medium through which a friendly exchange of opinion and a rationalization of differences between men and ideals were affected. Even after this step had been accomplished, there still remained the necessity of providing an unbiased judgment with respect to the evaluation of the divergent opinions expressed by the membership of the American Association of Colleges of Pharmacy and the membership of the National Association of Boards of Pharmacy.

By common consent and with the assistance of the leadership of men in the American Pharmaceutical Association, the American Council of Pharmaceutical Education came into being. Time does not permit a review of the incidents which preceded the formal constitution of the Council, nor an evaluation of the differences of opinion presented by each of the parent organizations.

The value of requirements for approval of educational programs depends upon the standards used and the ability of the approving agencies to measure accurately the compliance with the standards. Development of educational standards for and the inspection and accreditation of colleges of pharmacy by the Council may well become an important factor, if not the dominant factor, in determining the future contributions of pharmacy as a member of the health professions.

During this period of transition of delegated authority, or what might loosely be called "the police power," governing education, and in a sense licensure, many controversies have arisen. Yet, as a participant in these controversies, and as an observer of the results, I make bold to state that at no time have we turned backward from the ideals cherished by either the membership of the National Association of Boards of Pharmacy, or the American Association of Colleges of Pharmacy.

What I have delineated thus far is indicative that I think the Boards and Colleges of Pharmacy have played a significant role in the development of our professional practice as we know it today.

I would be remiss in my responsibility if I did not acknowledge the contributions made by the state and national pharmaceutical associations, the Charter's Survey, the American Council of Pharmaceutical Education, the more recent Pharmaceutical Survey, and last but not least, the American Foundation for Pharmaceutical Education. While no one of these agencies is entitled to full credit for the privileges which we now enjoy, yet it must be acknowledged that the men in each of these organizations were constantly inspired by a desire to provide a means by which men of sound judgment, unquestioned integrity and untiring efforts could not only justify their personal needs, but also remain ever-mindful of their responsibility to the members of our sister health professions and the welfare of the public.

Tribute for these contributions should be paid to men rather than to organizations. In fact, it is a matter of record that in many instances the persons who were responsible for the leadership of these organizations were bound together by their common allegiance to the principles established by the profession, which, whether written or unwritten, represents the sole security of the future practice of pharmacy which lies ahead.

The American Foundation of Pharmaceutical Education should receive a full measure of praise for its sympathetic understanding of our inadequacies and for its liberal financial support of the Pharmaceutical Survey, requested jointly by the National Association of Boards of Pharmacy, the Association of Colleges of Pharmacy, and the American Pharmaceutical Association. A survey of the strength and weaknesses of the profession could be a document ultimately to become lost in the files of pharmaceutical history. It is to the credit of the Foundation that it is preventing this from happening by providing the means of implementing several of the findings and recommendations of the Pharmaceutical Survey.

We have now reached manhood in terms of the establishment of mediums through which we may preserve all that is good within the present practice. Nevertheless, we shall stagnate unless we are willing to examine the challenges of the future with as much diligence and sincerity as did the men who are responsible for our present accomplishments.

Let us not, however, be guided too much by the element of tradition, for although tradition affords us a shrine of worship, it often precludes the possibility of our evaluating the challenges of the future. All around us men are engaged in the never-ending struggle of survival, and not infrequently we have committed ourselves, in desperation, to the destruction of those with whom we do not hold a common judgement. There are too few who are equally zealous in the utilization of their energy and wisdom in the betterment of a way of life or a professional practice. All too often we hear men say, "What is good enough for me is good enough for mine." Such an attitude closes the door of progress. It would therefore seem appropriate that we should approach with an open mind the recommendations of all men with respect to our needs of the next half century.

Much has been said with respect to the extension of the formal period of training required for degrees, and the raising of legal standards, by which a license may be secured. Such proposals should not alarm us, neither should they stimulate us to the organization of reactionary groups who would seek to undermine sound principles of education or legal standards of practice. Yet scarcely a year of my personal experience has passed without the threat of such formal challenge in the legislatures of this nation, and in some instances within the organization of our colleges of pharmacy. Perhaps there is some value to be derived from such a challenge simply because it forces us to re-examine more carefully the practices of the present. Experience has taught me that the simple establishment of legal statute, or of education requirement, does not fundamentally change the minds of men. Associations under titles are of no significance; it is the activities of the men who enjoy membership in organizations which determine progress.

My predecessor, the late Dr. H.C. Christensen, frequently stated that Boards of Pharmacy are very potent factors in determining the status of pharmacy in any state because the men appointed to serve on the Boards are men of influence. Likewise, members of college faculties and officers ofstate associations have, through their experience, developed qualities of leadership which have elevated them to the highest positions of responsibility in all of organized pharmacy.

Each, in his own way, and in accordance with his ability, has contributed to the common good of all. As a profession we have noted great improvement in the scope and quality of instruction. We have improved the methods of examining both the student and the candidate. We have supplied trained manpower to the industry, to the armed services, to Public Health agencies, and to the advancement of therapeutic practices in medicine.

These are accomplishments well known to ourselves. Yet withal, it cannot be denied that we have lost some of that public esteem which characterized the pharmacist of earlier generations. Some of this loss may be attributed to the natural forces of economic necessity, but I feel that a larger part of our loss has been sustained through our failure to proclaim adequate recognition for the professional services which we render, and for the indifferent attitude of those who do not volunteer to elect membership in the organizations which have for so long defended our frontiers against the attacks of the greedy and unscrupulous.

It has been argued by some that we are more of a merchant than men of professional dignity and stature. To those supporting this school of thought, I should like to point out that no profession known to man, law, medicine, or any of the healing art personnel, could survive without an economic remuneration. The only difference centers in the identity of the commodity or service for which compensation is demanded. In a professional sense, we are likewise dependent upon each other. A hospital could not exist without nurses, or pharmacists, or dietitians, as well as physicians. We should therefore strive to understand our responsibility to each other as members of the health professions, being ever mindful that our common objective is service to the patient.

In consideration of this important function of the pharmacist, I feel that our position would be materially strengthened if we were less critical of the minor encroachments in the marginal areas of professional practice or of the petty jealousies which might convey to the public that we may have lost concern for the personal welfare of the patient. This relates to a more wholesome respect gained through the medium of interprofessional activity, to the same degree as it relates to our willingness to consider our own inadequacies.

It is not enough that we should point with pride to our present accomplishments, as indicated by our present high standards of education, and to the excellence of the several practice acts which delineate the minimum standards by which the security of the profession as a legal entity exists. We must develop within our individual practitioners an awareness of the necessity of functioning at a level above and beyond such minimal standards as represented by the law.

Our constant purpose should therefore be directed toward the enlistment of all pharmacists in support of our cause, whether it be that of teacher, Board member, association official, or the practitioner in the humblest of surroundings. The needs of the patient do not vary with the particular geographic locality, since the ravages of disease or the frailties of body do not begin and end with the boundary lines of counties, states, or municipalities.

The mother of Abraham Lincoln once said to him, "Remember that no man will respect you more than you respect yourself." We have, therefore, an individual as well as a collective responsibility for protecting the professional status of the pharmacists by our personal willingness to stand up and be counted. If we sincerely believe in the principles which we have enunciated, then it is not only our privilege, but our duty to proclaim these qualities of professional practice which we render in daily service to those who are in need. ■

1953 Remington Medalist

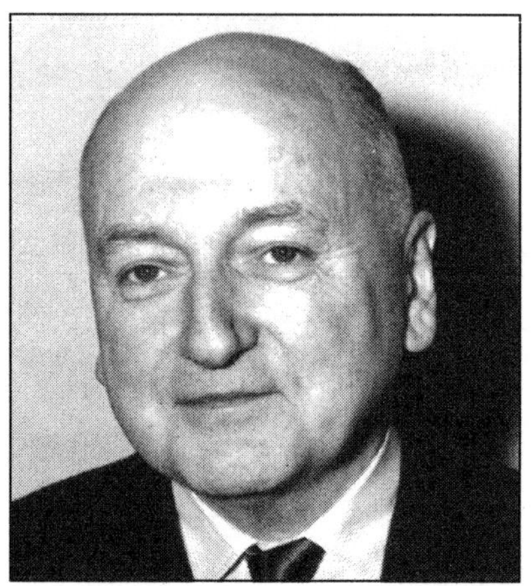

HUGH CORNELIUS MULDOON
(1898-1956)

Hugh Cornelius Muldoon was born in Truxton, New York, and he received a Ph.G. degree from Albany College of Pharmacy in 1912. He served as instructor in chemistry and Latin at the Massachusetts College of Pharmacy 1912-1918, professor of chemistry at Union University 1918-1920, and as dean at Valparaiso University School of Pharmacy 1920-1925. He was then called upon by the president of Duquesne University to establish a School of Pharmacy where he served as dean 1925-1955. He was a member of the USP revision committee 1930-1950, president of the American Association of Colleges of Pharmacy 1937-1938, and as an active member of the American Science Teachers Association; he also served as editor of *The Science Counselor.*

Muldoon joined the American Pharmaceutical Association in 1913 serving as chairman of the APhA House of Delegates 1946-1947, a member of the APhA mission to Japan in 1949, national chairman of the APhA committee on centennial celebration in 1952, and a member of the *National Formulary* revision committee. He served as editor of the American Pharmacy textbook series after authoring *Lessons in Pharmaceutical Latin* (1916), *Organic Chemistry for Students of the Medical Sciences* (1927), and *Laboratory Manual of Organic Chemistry* (1927).

The Strength of Pharmacy

Hugh Cornelius Muldoon

The 1953 Remington Honor Medal Lecture was presented December 7, 1953, at the Hotel New Yorker in New York City. Muldoon's Remington address was published in the *Journal of the American Pharmaceutical Association, Practical Pharmacy Edition*, volume 15, pages 25-27, 93-95, 116, 155-157, January-March 1954.

Praise can be pleasant. Criticism often hurts. Pharmacy and pharmacists have long been subject to praise and to criticism, both in liberal amounts. It is easy to find fault and to condemn. Pharmacy is not perfect-far from it. Pharmacists aren't paragons of virtue either. We don't find them pictured in stained glass windows, it is true. Neither do we find them in rogues' galleries.

Admittedly, pharmacy and pharmacists have weaknesses and faults, too many of them, both great and small. They distress us. We deplore them. But there is much about pharmacy that is right. If we look, we can find a multitude of things to commend, to rejoice in, to be grateful for.

Continued concentration on pharmacy's defects may blind us to its benefits. So, tonight, let's consider our profession, not in its commercial aspects, but pharmacy at its best, as an indispensable activity in the public health field. Let's examine its soundness, its merits, its excellences–not its demerits.

We have nothing startling or new to say, perhaps, but we may express our ideas a little differently. Our discussion will be one-sided and incomplete, deliberately so. Someday, someone else in another place may deal with pharmacy's defect and explain and apologize and defend. This evening, for a few minutes, let's consider some of the Strengths of Pharmacy.

Centuries ago, pharmacy was a clandestine art. It had to be. There were things to conceal. Today, there is nothing to hide. We have much to be proud of. Pharmacy is no longer a secret profession, but most people know far too little about it, about the pharmacist, his professional activities, his training, his competence, his ideas, his ideals.

With much of our profession the public has no contact. The casual observer is unaware of its extent and its diversity. Many think of the pharmacist only as a business man, not as the conscientious guardian of the health of the people he really is. It is time, I think, to turn the full beam of the spotlight of public attention on pharmacy. We should tell the public more about our profession and about ourselves. A one-day or a one-week program is not enough. It is a year-long task if people are to know well the men in whose hands every day they so confidently trust their lives.

Pharmacists are respected public servants. They should be. They labor competently and diligently to promote and to protect the nation's physical health. It is this valuable service and this service alone-thatjustifies the perpetuation, and the continued legal protection, of our profession.

Modern pharmacists perform a front-rank medical work, one that is essential to the well-being of society. They fulfill a great human need. Long centuries of dependable service, based on abundant competence, sound moral character, and demonstrated worth, have earned for pharmacists public trust, and confidence, and good will.

Pharmacy is not an ivory tower profession. It is now, and it always has been, close to those it serves. Patrons know their pharmacists personally. They rely upon them. They respect their counsel and advice. The pharmacist takes pride in his skill in human relationships. He serves with equal care and courtesy the eminent and the obscure, the aristocrat and the socially disinherited.

He is, of course, a proper source to the public of information on matters dealing with medicines and with general health and hygiene. His patrons consult him, too, on scientific and technical problems, and on personal matters far removed from pharmacy. As a personal, as well as a professional advisor, the pharmacist is a significant, but I am afraid, sometimes undervalued, social force in modern life.

He is an indispensable member of America's great medical service team. Joining with the physician, the surgeon, the dentist, the nurse, and other workers in the health field, he helps to provide an interlocking community service that is the envy of all the world. The members of the curative professions with whom he works most closely trust the pharmacist, and value his judgment, and appreciate the importance of the work he does.

The high regard of his associates in the related professions, and the richly deserved public confidence and good will he enjoys, constitute one of the greatest strengths of modern pharmacy.

American pharmacy is not native. It is derivative. It is derivative historically in that its roots lie embedded in the many foreign countries that contributed to Colonial pharmacy. For centuries, the pharmacy of the Old World was far in advance of that in America, and we drew upon it freely. As this country developed, our pharmaceutical self-reliance steadily increased. We needed less and less help from abroad. Eventually, we achieved complete independence. America became a drug supplier to the whole world. We are aware that we have not yet reached the apex of professional achievement, but we can, if we care to stand alone. We are beginning to realize increasingly, however, that for their benefit as well as for our own, we should establish and maintain close contacts with the pharmacists of all the free nations of the world.

America is now permanently involved in world affairs. Americans have become world-minded, and rightly so. Other nations look to us for the leadership we are glad to give.

We applaud pharmacy's steadily developing international outlook. We welcome to our schools foreign students and teachers. We interchange the results of our researches. For a number of years we have engaged in international agreements. Our *Pharmacopeia* is official in countries other than our own. We participated in the production of the *Pharmacopoea Internationalis* of the World Health Organization. Recently, groups of American pharmacists have journeyed to Europe and to Asia and South America, and to the other countries of our own continent. Last year, in Philadelphia, pharmacists from a score of foreign countries participated in the Centennial Celebration of the American Pharmaceutical Association.

The wheel is coming full turn. In 1753, we were recipients only. In 1953, it is our privilege to give as well as to receive. We gain strength in the giving.

Pharmacy, today, is highly developed. But we shall never know when or where or how pharmacy began. Its origin lies veiled in the mists of antiquity. Probably, in the beginning it was a home art. Later, it was practiced in the temple. Written records reveal that the art of the apothecary was surprisingly well developed in ancient Egypt and Assyria. Always linked to medicine, pharmacy advanced in Greece and Rome, and more rapidly during the Arabian period. By the Middle Centuries it had freed itself from a frustrating domination by medicine, and it was able to emerge and eventually to sustain itself as a separate calling.

Through the long centuries, pharmacy has continued to prosper despite the disruptions of war and the vicissitudes of peace. It has survived economic and political and social revolutions. Scientific and technological advances have assisted, rather than impeded, its progress. It continues to advance at a fast pace. Its long life and its sturdy endurance certify' to pharmacy's essentiality, and to its fundamental soundness.

When there was still a simple agrarian society, only plant drugs found any considerable acceptance. Chance or caprice often dictated their use. The rational scientific medicine of today was far in the future. Inorganic chemicals were first introduced, and then, at the turn of the present century, we began to use organic medicinals freely. As chemical medicines demonstrated their value, the use of berries and barks and leaves and roots, and preparations made from them, declined. Botanicals were subordinated but by no means obliterated. The trend away from plant medicines, however, continues.

A half century ago medicine changed its emphasis from cure to prevention. The search for specifics was intensified. During many years, great numbers of synthetic medicinals were tested. Later, we entered a biological era of serums and antitoxins and vaccines. More recently, came the introduction of the vitamins and hormones, the sulfa drugs, the antihistaminics, and the enzymes, and the antibiotics. The study of medicinal radioisotopes is now well under way. Our newest concern is geriatric medicine, the developing of methods and materials for treating the degenerative diseases of the aged.

All these changes and advances have been initiated, not by pharmacy, but by medicine. Medicine leads. It always must lead. Diagnosis must precede treatment. But we are proud of how well pharmacy has kept pace, step by step, with its sister profession in all its amazing progress.

New medicinal agents and new methods of treatment demanded of pharmacy new understandings, new adjustments, new procedures and new forms for administering medicines. Pharmacy responded well. We would expect it to, for one of the strengths of pharmacy is its willingness to face its problem as they arise.

Pharmacy made the new drugs pleasant and easy to take. It hurried to devise improved tablets and capsules and ampuls and other forms of medication. Just now, the needle is in fashion. More and more drugs are administered by injection, a practice that affects markedly the kind of work now being performed in the prescription room.

It is feasible to carry on only minor sterilizing procedures in the ordinary drug store. Necessarily, then, most injectibles are prepared by the large drug manufacturers. So are the thousands of pills and capsules and tablets, and other types of unit dose medication that America uses in such stupendous quantities. These require little preparation and handling by the pharmacist. As a result, increasingly he becomes more and more a distributor of medicines, and less and less a compounder. This is the 20th century's most revolutionary change in pharmaceutical practice.

The art of the pharmacist, while still important, becomes less used and less useful. Some of his once admired technical skills begin to show touches of rust. The manual labor of the prescription desk is lightened, but the pharmacist's responsibility in the handling of thousands of medicines, instead of hundreds, is greatly increased. He is now a head worker rather than a hand worker. The time he once employed in the preparation of medicines he now devotes to other professional duties.

Despite such changes and modifications, pharmacy is still the quadrate calling it long has been — art, science, business, and profession. Some 105,000 trained and licensed pharmacists practice their profession in 62,000 drug stores and pharmacies, hospitals, manufacturing plants, research institutes and colleges and universities. They dispense more than 400,000,000 prescriptions annually, and the number increases each year. Some 20,000,000 people a day visit the drug stores of America to seek the pharmacist's advice, to obtain medicines, and to purchase health supplies and the personal needs and conveniences that many pharmacists offer as a community service. The cash register rings up sales of four and three-quarters billions of dollars annually.

To satisfy a very real demand for non-pharmaceuticals, and to increase their incomes as well, many pharmacists have become a kind of hybrid pharmacist-merchant. In their stores business and profession meet. There need be no incompatibility between the two. There is no reason why a conscientious pharmacist shall not also be a competent business man. But the business of pharmacy can be, and sometimes is, overemphasized to the detriment of the professional.

In well conducted professional and semi-professional pharmacies, there is a proper fusion of business and profession, not a dichotomy. In localities where the demand for professional service is small, the commercial subsidizes the professional, and the public benefits. The many thousands of pharmacists who achieve a suitable balance between business and profession are the backbone of pharmacy. They give our profession great strength. We are proud of them. Pharmacy is willing to be judged by them as well as by other strictly professional pharmacists who approach more closely the ideal. Such pharmacists supply nothing but prescription service and sickroom needs. They give dignity and prestige to their calling. They increase steadily in numbers, importance and influence.

Specialists in hospital pharmacy form another group in which we take great pride. These men and women practice their profession in its purest form since in their service the profit motive does not enter.

At first, the pharmacists who resisted the transfer of medicine-making from the prescription room to the manufacturing plant, viewed the matter as wholly a personal and a pharmaceutical matter. But something more than that was involved. An industrial age, a mechanized civilization was developing. It soon became apparent that in no field could individuals compete effectively and economically against the large manufacturers' prodigal use of non-human energy, their automatic machines, their research organizations, and their specialized labor.

Pharmaceutical manufacturers appeared to have inexhaustible financial resources. They took advantage of every modern medium of communication and transportation to provide good service and rapid delivery. The elegance of the mass-produced medicines, and their economy, could not be denied. The products were of high quality. Pharmacists had to admit that extraordinary care was taken in their manufacture. There could be but one end. Individual and group opposition to the manufacturers abated. Pharmacists adjusted to the new situation.

Any expanding technology tends to depersonalize. Even in selling, machines may displace men. But there can be no robot pharmacies. In the true pharmacy, the professional advice, the professional service, and the professional responsibility of the skilled pharmacist can never be eliminated. The human touch will always be needed. The pharmacist's technical knowledge informs and protects the patient and the physician. The physician needs information concerning the new medicines he prescribes, not only factual information but evaluations and comparisons of the 8000 prescription products that are now available.

Whether or not he prepares them personally, the pharmacist is responsible for all the products he dispenses. He must have, and he does have, faith in those who make them. So well have the manufacturers served the pharmacist and the physician, and through them the public, that today no one would even consider a return to the old conditions.

We are proud to list our great pharmaceutical manufacturing industry, vigorous, alert, progressive, as one of the most important strengths of modern pharmacy.

Industry does more than make medicines. Its interests are broad. It looks to the future. It is not surprising, then, that pharmaceutical education has become one of industry's chief concerns. They know that men are the profession's most important resource. The colleges supply new manpower to the profession each year. It is largely through these college-trained men and women that the manufacturers' products eventually reach the sick room. Now, more than ever, the prescriptionist must be well educated for his work. Industry seeks for itself broadly trained and liberally educated men and women. It needs executives, researchers, production men, and other skilled workers. In the future, more frequently than it has in the past, perhaps, industry will utilize the specially trained graduates of our colleges of pharmacy. There will be more of them. They will be better prepared.

The manufacturers assist education individually and directly, but more often in recent years they have operated through the enormously helpful American Foundation for Pharmaceutical Education. This Foundation is one of the newest and most significant strengths of pharmacy. Through this organization, manufacturers, wholesalers, and other interested persons and groups have financed projects of inestimable value. They supplied the funds for the recently completed and very costly Pharmaceutical Survey that sought to discover what is right about pharmacy, and what is wrong, and what should be done about it. They continue to subsidize *The American Journal of Pharmaceutical Education,* the American Council on Pharmaceutical Education, and the stimulating annual Conferences for Teachers.

Foundation fellowships and scholarships have made advanced study possible for hundreds of able students who otherwise could not have afforded it. Financial aid has been granted generously to needy undergraduates. Last year alone, the Foundation's scholarship and fellowship expenditures passed the $100,000.00 mark.

Those who conceived this forward-looking organization, and those who direct and support it deserve, and have, the gratitude and the deep appreciation of the students, the colleges, and of pharmacists everywhere.

Pharmacy is proud of its 74 accredited colleges, and rightly so. Our educational system is one of our greatest strengths. Even so, we are not satisfied with it. I hope we never will be.

Once, apprenticeship or internship played an important part in the training of the pharmacist. It no longer does. Pharmaceutical education is almost wholly delegated to the college. Just now, there is a keen and widespread, and I think rather wholesome dissatisfaction with our schools and their curriculums. The professional competence of our graduates is not questioned; but many educators and practicing pharmacists, and even disinterested observers, point out that the colleges fail to give their students the well-rounded education to which, as members of a profession, they are entitled. Our critics say we graduate men and women of circumscribed interests, narrow specialists prepared only for living in a compartmented world. We are counseled to broaden our training by including more of those branches of learning that are conducive to culture, specifically the humanities.

If our training is to be preparation for all aspects of living, social, economic, and esthetic, as well as professional, we are not doing our job well. We are aware that specialization in any field, begun too early, is ill-advised. We know that pharmaceutical education is now and always has been specialized and utilitarian. Pharmacists are realists. They demand functional education. They are not interested in learning what they consider to be largely decorative if the professional has to suffer. Their first concern always has been and always should be, the safety of the public.

We know that no one kind of education can serve all the needs of all the people, or even today, all the needs of all kinds of pharmacists. We believe that our schools in their four-year course are making competent pharmacists for the retail field as we find it today. Even so, few will deny, I think, that we should give more attention to the pharmacist's non-professional learning. His personal life, as well as his professional life, deserves consideration. In college he should complete a well-balanced course of instruction which will include scientific and professional and cultural subjects that will enrich all his living. Such programs have long been offered, but they have not been mandatory.

To liberalize our basic training, we are advised to synthesize the vocational and the intellectual, to fuse our scientific and professional knowledge with more of the social sciences and the older humanistic studies that are commonly administered by the college of arts. Everyone will agree to that, I think, at least in principle. Certainly, we want to graduate men and women of culture. But they must be able and safe pharmacists, too; they must be well grounded in the basic sciences; and they should have at least some knowledge of the fundamentals of business. We want them to be good men, and good women, and good citizens.

Beyond that, we should like them to have a knowledge of economics and sociology and psychology and philosophy and a modern language or two. We want them to know something of what happened in the world yesterday and how it affects today. Their taste in music and literature and art should be cultivated. Our graduates should be prepared professionally and intellectually and socially for the important work they are to do, and for the dignified position they are to fill in modern society. We want them to enjoy the full respect of the public and of the allied professions. We want them to look across to the doctor, and not up.

That is an ambitious program. By extending our course of study a single year, we can accomplish only a very small part of it. We are not sure we could achieve all our aims even with much more additional time at our disposal. We do admit, however, that we have carried specialization too far. We do need a broadened curriculum.

But we point out to those who may have a tendency to over-rate the value of an arts college training, that we doubt if even the complete four-year arts curriculum, as it is frequently administered, fits a man much better than does our curriculum for life today in a complex and competitive world that is shaped so largely by science and technology. We do not disparage the arts course. Far from it. We merely point out that the curriculum in pharmacy has unappreciated values.

No one has yet proved that any one group of disciplines is the single and only way of liberating the mind. It is disturbing that so many educators, pharmaceutical and otherwise, in advocating the inclusion of more of the humanistic studies seem to feel that the pharmaceutical curriculum, with its fascinating variety of subject matter, has little or no moral or ethical or cultural value. I recognize no such limitations. The contributions of our curriculum are not wholly physical. Every subject in it, when properly taught, has cultural value.

We learn of the great discoveries in sciences, of those who made them, and of their effect on society. We learn of the great chemists and physicists and biologists and pharmacists. We even know about Beowulf. We develop the powers of reasoning, as well as understanding and memory. Our students learn to distinguish between facts and judgment. We encourage pride of self and pride of profession, and the development of self-discipline and self-reliance. At the same time we teach cooperation, and personal and group responsibility.

We inculcate sound moral and spiritual and ethical values by discussion and illustration and example. We teach respect for law, and the dignity of work, and the necessity for sincerity and honor and truthfulness in our relations with others. We encourage honesty and industry and accuracy and patience and perseverance. We nourish curiosity and initiative, creative power in thinking, and intellectual courage. We endeavor to develop sound attitudes and insight as well as professional skills.

We are concerned not only with what the student learns, but also with the attitudes he develops as he learns. We try to inspire as well as to teach. In some scholars, at least, we kindle a love of learning.

We need not be too discouraged with the results of our current efforts to educate pharmacists. We know that our graduates still have much to learn. But their college training is only the first and formal part of their lifelong continuing education. We believe that our young pharmacists are better fitted than ever before for a satisfying life.

But that isn't saying that we are satisfied with our product. It can be improved. We will be among the first to affirm that additional formal instruction will increase the actual and potential value of the pharmacist to society.

Some academically adventurous colleges of pharmacy already have in operation minimum five-and six-year programs. The question of extending the basic training in all colleges from four to five years is now under active consideration. Judging by the strongly affirmative votes on the question by our great national associations at their 1953 conventions, it is safe to say, I think, that the step will be taken in the not distant future. Many practicing pharmacists favor the change. Many others do not. Both groups offer strong reasons in support of their positions. If we do add a year, pharmacists must not expect immediate and spectacular results. Education is a long and slow and sometimes tedious process. It lacks drama.

Extent of curriculum, of itself, means little. It is content that is important. Sometimes we seem to measure education only by length, rather than by quality or substance. Our present course of study has not been lengthened since 1932, but everyone interested knows that there have been many significant advances in its administration and in its content. The Charters' Report and the Pharmaceutical Survey stimulated improvement. For many years, the powerful American Association of Colleges of Pharmacy, and more recently, the American Council on Pharmaceutical Education, have had enormous influence in promoting the development of our colleges, physically, academically, and professionally. The establishment of the Council was a mile-stone in modern pharmaceutical education. University administrators and state boards of pharmacy rely upon its judgment and accept its decisions. The studies made by the Council in evaluating our colleges have benefited notably not only the individual college and its parent institution, but all pharmacy. And all pharmacy is grateful.

In recent years, we have become interested not only in what our teachers teach, but in how well they teach. The seminars for teachers, conducted annually by the American Association of Colleges of Pharmacy under the patronage of the American Foundation for Pharmaceutical Education, are bringing new life and new vigor to pharmaceutical education. Just as we need to reinforce and broaden our curriculum, we need to vitalize our teaching. The quality of our product is influenced by the quality of our student material, and by the competence of our instructors. They should be forceful and imaginative and enthusiastic teachers, creative thinkers, and men and women of high moral and ethical standards. They should know their subject material, and how to teach it. They should develop and maintain student interest and enthusiasm. They should be fully convinced of the value of the work they are doing, and skillful enough to do it well. Pharmacy has had great teachers in the past. Remington was one of them. We have notable and inspiring teachers now. We shall need more of them in the future. The seminars can help.

For practicing pharmacists, study should never end. Minds must be refreshed and refurnished. Educators realize more keenly than do pharmacists, I think, that pharmaceutical education must be continuous. Many colleges offer refresher courses and workshops and seminars to keep pharmacists in service in touch with the latest professional and scientific developments.

The pharmacist returns to the college briefly for instruction. Some schools and associations provide itinerant instructors and advisors and offer other valuable extension services. A few college faculties even leave their campuses and go to the pharmacist to make it easy for him to learn the new. Teachers need to keep in touch with reality. They should know what is actually going on in practice. Close contact with the prescription room is essential. Teachers who participate in continuation education soon discover that teaching a voluntary group of mature pharmacists who are determined to learn, is quite different from instructing the captive audience of the college classroom. In every case the teacher as well as the pharmacist is stimulated.

Not everyone realizes to what extent pharmacy has become a specialized profession. Retail pharmacy, the most important and most familiar specialty, attracts by far the greatest number of our graduates. The major objective of our minimum course must be, therefore, to prepare men well for the retail field. But students with other career interests must be considered. One graduate out of ten enters hospital pharmacy or engages in drug production or sales or promotion; or in wholesaling or organizational work or journalism or government service; or in education or research, or in some other specialty. No one college can be expected to provide instruction in all of pharmacy's branches. But regardless of their individual choices, we serve all our students well when we provide a flexible curriculum with emphasis on a breadth of education, that is in turn based on sound fundamentals.

Each profession is responsible for its own development. To direct pharmacy in the future we shall need well-informed, creative minds, as well as skilled hands. Professional progress comes through research. One of the most important functions of pharmaceutical education is to prepare men for advanced study and systematic investigation. Colleges have an obligation to produce knowledge as well as to transmit it.

More that 600 students are now enrolled in our graduate schools seeking M.S. and Ph.D. degrees. We need many more, for industry and education engage these highly trained workers while their diplomas are still in their hands. Among the 4500 Bachelors of Science in Pharmacy we graduate each year, are scholars of ability and initiative who would if properly trained be able as researchers to make significant contributions. Those who have the capacity and the desire and the will, should be encouraged to undertake advanced study. Under wise direction they will grow and develop and learn to adventure independently into the unknown, in whatever fields they may choose.

Eventually, the results of their researches will be published in the technical journals for all to see. Publication is a way of obtaining an unprejudiced evaluation of a man's work by other specialists in the area. Professional journals permit communication among the members of a group. In them, new ideas, new methods, new materials are announced. Often, they are the only means the man in the prescription room uses to supplement his professional knowledge. Pharmacy is fortunate, then, that its professional literature is one of its developing strengths.

We take pride in the two *Journal of the American Pharmaceutical Association,* the *Bulletin of the Society of Hospital Pharmacists,* the *American Journal of Pharmaceutical Education,* the *American Professional Pharmacist,* and the most venerable of all, *The American Journal of Pharmacy.* All these compare favorable with the journals of the other medical sciences.

There are dozens of other useful journals published by associations and manufacturers and schools. An even larger number of national and regional journals, such as *Drug* Topics, and *The American Druggist,* and the *Journal of the National Association of Retail Druggists,* are devoted more especially to the news and to the business of pharmacy.

Textbooks, as well as formularies and

dispensatories and other reference books, are improving in quality and increasing in number. Publications dealing with the history of pharmacy come from the distinguished American Institute of the History of Pharmacy. Pharmacists have long been active and influential in preparing the many revisions of the *United States Pharmacopoeia* and the *National Formulary.*

The National Formulary is wholly the work of the American Pharmaceutical Association, our oldest and most eminent, national, professional organization. This admired and respected association, together with other societies that subscribe to its ideals, from one of pharmacy's superlative strengths.

Active, vigorous, expanding, the APhA is an organization of which all pharmacists can boast. For over a century, it has consistently advanced the prestige of pharmacy and extended its usefulness, arousing, encouraging, and informing not only its own members, but all other pharmacists who would listen. Unselfishly, it mothered numbers of other national, regional, and state associations. More than half the students enrolled in our colleges today are members of its student branches.

The APhA sets standards of professional conduct and excellence. It represents pharmacy's collective conscience. It gave us our exemplary code of ethics. It deals with members by the thousands, but it is happy to serve personally even the most remote and inconspicuous individual pharmacist. Inclusive, rather than exclusive, the Association welcomes to its ranks all who have a legitimate interest in pharmacy. Under expert leadership its thousands of members pool their wisdoms and experiences and hopes and ideals to determine the Association's policies. Its officers are leaders in national planning and action. The Association speaks authoritatively for the profession when a stand must be taken on controversial questions. As very recent history plainly shows, when it chooses to exert it, the APhA has a powerful influence on national legislation that affects pharmacy. Capitol Hill respects the advice and counsel that come from the APhA headquarters, Washington's stately white-marble American Institute of Pharmacy. Capitol Hill listens to other associations, too, but the mother society can speak able for all divisions of pharmacy.

There are more than a dozen strong national associations concerned primarily with the economics of pharmacy, with wholesaling and manufacturing and with other special interests. There are even important smaller specialized groups, such as the American College of Apothecaries, among the pharmacists who serve the public directly. In Rho Chi, the Phi Beta Kappa of pharmacy, we have a large and active society that encourages high scholarship in our colleges. Pharmacy is better organized today than ever before, but we need still greater solidarity.

Pharmacists have a personal and a group responsibility to see that safe, dependable, up-to-date pharmaceutical service is available to all. The state makes of pharmacists a privileged and a protected group. It depends upon them to provide continuously a special kind of indispensable health service that cannot be furnished by others. It must be modern, reliable, accurate, precise. The careful legal regulations that surround and protect the pharmacist are the state's indirect acknowledgment of the importance of the pharmacist's work. They strengthen pharmacy.

The many national, state, and local laws and rules and regulations that protect and guide the pharmacist, ensure safe service to the people. Pharmacists have, as they should have, great respect for the law. To a considerable extent pharmacists, through other pharmacists, police their own profession. Offenses against pharmaceutical ethics are the province of the professional societies. But there are laws which must be obeyed. The State boards of pharmacy, composed of experienced pharmacists, influence and guide legislation. They regulate the practice of pharmacy.

They license pharmacists, administer internships, and authorize the operation of drug stores. Under their direction infractions of the pharmacy laws are detected and punished. The boards guard against inefficient prescription compounding and the unauthorized sale of forbidden or restricted drugs. They apply legitimate pressures for the improvement of pharmaceutical practice.

The state boards are linked through the National Association of Boards of Pharmacy, a strong organization that works quietly but effectively for the betterment of pharmacy and the unification of the laws which govern it. Through district and national meetings it fosters a close and friendly relationship with the colleges. This splendidly directed Association is an invaluable aid in maintaining and extending the influence of pharmacy, and in protecting the public and the pharmacist. It adds to pharmacy's strength and professional prestige.

The regulatory work of the boards and the leadership of our associations is sorely needed at this special time when the nation's faith in moral values appears to have weakened, and the restraints that have always governed society seem to have become impotent or inoperative. With less effective colleges and associations and boards, the path ahead would indeed be dark.

Men are always apprehensive of the future. Just now, more than ever, we have a feeling of insecurity. World affairs cause great unease. We know that ahead of us lie political and social and economic changes. They are inevitable. If they come, as we hope, through the discipline of the law, they will not be catastrophic. Whatever the changes may be, and whenever they come, as sensible Americans and as responsible professional workers, we shall adjust to them. In pharmacy, we may expect frustrations and disappointments and, sometimes, failures. But there will be successes, too. Strength comes through struggle. Pharmacy will continue to have dignity and character and direction and purpose.

In a recent convincing editorial Dr. Robert L. Swain tells us that today the drug store is economically secure, and professionally sound, and competitively strong. We believe it will continue to be secure and sound and strong. We expect it to gain strength through firmer organization of those who practice it, through advanced educational standards, and through the improved understanding that will result from an enlarged public relations program.

Convinced of the soundness and essentiality of their profession, pharmacists will develop new public appreciation and support by telling the story of pharmacy truthfully and enthusiastically and perserveringly to all who will listen. Interprofessional relationships will be clarified and strengthened. International friendships will flourish. Industry will continue to assist the colleges in opening new doors into the future. The pharmaceutical curriculum will be extended beyond the five-year plan now under consideration. Graduate offerings will be enlarged and expanded. As the specialties of pharmacy grow in importance and attractiveness, they will receive the greater individual attention they already deserve.

The graduates of our present and projected educational programs will be able to employ effectively the most modern physical and chemical and biological and radiological tools of their profession. They will cope successfully with all the hoped-for progress that scientific research will bring to medical treatment. We are confident, too, that we shall have trained them sufficiently well in general areas that they will be able to maintain a serene inner sense of direction in the midst of confusing social change.

We admit, regretfully, that there will always be men engaged in pharmacy who differ in their choice of values. Many, many thousands, the great majority, will aggressively support their profession, understanding its primary purpose, aware of its past accomplishments, and proud of their own professional activities that promote the common good.

There will be other profit-seeking traders who will flaunt their disloyalty to an ancient calling and scoff at the imperatives of professional ethics. The separateness of the two groups will increase. Since environment can gravely affect the quality of pharmaceutical service, eventually we hope, the privilege of practicing pharmacy in highly commercial surroundings will be withdrawn.

We foresee no changes in the American pattern of life that will negate the pharmacist as a social force. His gracious human qualities will endure. Psychologically as well as pharmaceutically, he will continue to minister to a great fundamental need, and offer wise counsel as well, to the disturbed in mind and to the ill in body, helping both to orient wisely their living.

Pharmacists will always be what the *American Druggist so* aptly termed them-neighborhood statesmen. As patriotic citizens they will continue to enter wholeheartedly into the life of the community, contributing their special skills and wisdom and experience and judgment in the public service. Unselfishly, they will held others to obtain what they themselves seek; health, and independence, and security, and personal freedom, arid the right to enjoy the American way of life.

The conscientious young pharmacists of today are rightly concerned about the future. They look ahead. Sturdily independent, they will, we believe, want no share in a paternalistic economy planned from above. They are not unrealistic idealists. They desire only what we are confident they will have an opportunity to earn in a fear-free democracy a modest living for themselves and their families, practicing worthily the profession for which they have been trained. They have faith in the future. They have faith in pharmacy. They may well have, for pharmacy is strong today. It will continue to be strong.

It will continue to be strong—Because of the character and motivation of its personnel; Because of public trust based on agelong, faithful and intelligent services; Because of its respect for education; Because of its awareness of its problems and its willingness to face them; Because of its deep concern for the future. ■

1955 Remington Medalist

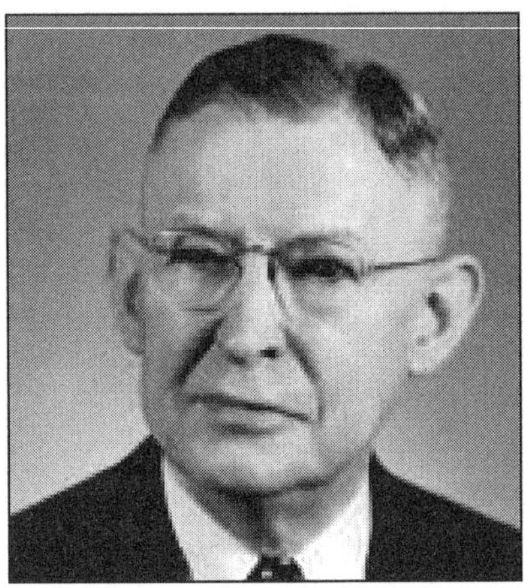

Roy Bird Cook
(1886-1961)

Roy Bird Cook was born in Roanoke, West Virginia, and while assisting his father in the publication of the *Weston Independent* newspaper, he apprenticed as a pharmacist with Minter B. Ralson of Weston. He took the state board examination in 1909 to become at 19 the youngest person ever registered as a pharmacist in West Virginia. He moved to Huntington in 1909 to form the Kelle-Cook Company, and ten years later he became treasurer of a chain of pharmacies in Charleston. Then in 1926, he formed the Older-Cook Drug Company, which became the Cook Drug Company in 1944. He served as president of the West Virginia Pharmaceutical Association 1918-1919, was appointed to the West Virginia Board of Pharmacy in 1926, and was elected secretary in 1932 serving until his death. He served as chairman of the APhA House of Delegates 1935-1939, and APhA president 1942-1943.

Unable to cleanse his hands of the printer's ink that he had acquired in his father's newspaper office, Cook served as associate editor of the *Weston Independent* and president of the Independent Publishing Company 1933-1941, president of the West Virginia Newspaper Council 1939-1940, editor of the *West Virginia History Magazine* 1939-1941, and author of a number of books on early West Virginia history. An authority on Stonewall Jackson, he collected one of the country's largest collections of Jackson memorabilia and gained national fame for his book *The Family and Early Life of Stonewall Jackson* (1924, 3rd edition 1948). A founding member of the American Instititue of the History of Pharmacy and author of *Annals of Pharmacy in West Virginia* (1946), Cook was elected AIHP honorary president in 1960.

Semi-Centennial

Roy Bird Cook

The 1955 Remington Honor Medal Lecture was presented on December 5, 1955, at the Sheraton Astor Hotel in New York City. Cook's address was never published, but his original manuscript has been preserved in the APhA Archives.

To the average, everyday man of this world there come few events which are of transcending importance. Being one of the most average men, I feel that I have been extremely fortunate in having had three monumental honors come to me during my lifetime. These have been even more gratifying since all were unsought, unexpected and certainly unhoped for.

The first of these great events came in 1938 when I was called before the assembly of graduates and friends at West Virginia University and had conferred upon me the honorary degree of Doctor of Laws. The second was the notification telegram telling me that I had been elected president of the American Pharmaceutical Association. Finally, in May, 1955, when I was at home, nursing one of the occupational ailments of a practicing pharmacist, I received word that I had been selected as the Remington Medalist for this year. Only those among you who have been so honored can know what my feelings were at that time!

Yes, I marvel as I stand before you, honored as I am tonight, that God and my fellowmen have been so gracious to me. And to friends here and elsewhere, from the hard working pharmacist to the leaders in all pharmaceutical field, I simply say, from the bottom of my heart, I thank you. For you know that any measure of success I have achieved, and honors which have come to me, have been made possible only through your confidence and help.

Some years ago a friend suggested that I might have taken for my life's motto that famous saying of "Teddy" Roosevelt: Aggressive Fighting For the Right is the Noblest Sport the World Affords. It is possible that this is true, but fifty years of work predicated upon such a thesis does not necessarily equip one to deliver a scholarly, scientific address on such an occasion as this. So, with your permission, I will remain in character, and reminisce for a brief time.

As if directed by some strange power, my selection as the 1955 Medalist came within a few days after I celebrated my fiftieth legal pharmaceutical birthday. In May 1905, after three days of trials and tribulations, I received a letter from the West Virginia Board of Pharmacy telling me that I had successfully passed the examinations for a registered pharmacist. Six years had just elapsed since I had graduated from my father's newspaper office, got the printers ink off my hands only have it replaced with gentian violet, iron and "opedeldoc."

What was this new world into which I had elected to spend my life? Let us take a looks at a typical pharmacy of 1905. Many here tonight can recall the days of their youth and the contacts they then had with the town pharmacy. It was headquarters for young and old alike. Usually it was in a good location, fairly well lighted with oil lights which had to be trimmed, or with gas lights which had porcelain tips or jets. Only a few had installed the new-fangled electric lights.

And what of the sign outside? Nearly all had a post on the curb with a mortar and pestle gracing the top. Also those who remember the cigar store Indian with its tomahawk raised in the air or the harness man's horse on wheels, will also remember the life-sized figure of a down-east fisherman, pointed and varnished in glowing colors, protected by an oil skin coat and hat, bearing on his back a cod fish that reached to the street. Each morning some pharmacist or his errand boy pulled this light but effective advertising of Scott's Emulsion out onto the sidewalk. Late in the evening, it was taken in again to protect it from the weather. Likely if used today it would be carried away and drowned in Central Park by some youthful citizen. Of course such items are in 1955 only of interest to antique collectors.

The front windows in winter were used to display *Frog In Your Throat* replicas or cardboard cutouts. In summer these were removed and seats for the fountain trade were inserted. Here society folk laid aside their parasols to partake of a claret ice or a drink of *Moxie.* It must be recalled that *Coca Cola* was not born until 1886 and that for twenty years thereafter people had to be offered special inducements to drink it. Along one wall was the soda fountain, probably made by Tufts of Boston, its design copied from some ancient temple. In its heart was a tank of carbonated water; many had a "Y" which dispensed either "soda" water or *Deep Rock,* depending upon which faucet was used. Here reposed patent medicines, now long forgotten, which cured everything, and some *Swans Down* face powder for any lady brave enough to buy it. The store owner who could afford a *Bang's* from Boston set of fixtures owned the show place of the town. Manufacturers vied with each other to see which could use the finest mahogany and plate glass in their fixtures.

No pharmacy worthy of the name was without a complete set of fine hand-made tincture and powder bottles which ran clear along one side of the store. Each carried a hand-painted label reading from *Hyd. Ox. Rub.* on the small bottles, on the top, to the fine herb section on the bottom shelf. In the finely labeled drawers one found a "great horn spoon", the real thing and not a plastic imitation; prepared chalk or "Tear Drops"which paved the way for miladies face powder-ground flaxseed and odoriferous foenugreek.

The pharmacist, who usually wore a black alpaca coat, presided over the general welfare. He was not above doing a little doctoring himself. He could recite stories of other days or repair a bruised toe. Irvin Cobb once observed that "nothing ever happens in a small town," then produced evidence to show that everything happens in just such places and especially in the town drug store.

Telephones in 1905 were still man-made and woman-operated. Three long and one short, plus some energy from a wet battery carried the voice quite a distance but drug stores were just beginning to install them.

In the rear of such stores in 1905 one found real pharmacies. Jars of glycerite of starch stood on the marble prescription cases, from which pills or soft mass capsules were compounded to heal the ailments of man. Big scales and little scales were on the counter and behind them stood *Remington's Practice of Pharmacy,* the *Dispensatory,* and often other books on drugs. Along the top shelves were boxes of the finest ground barks and herbs from the Baltimore market, which when packed into percolators, gave forth such color reactions as to drive the poor druggist frantic. Can any of remember the curious gourds of the aloes that had to be broken with a hammer and the effect they had even on the best of appetites? Or the arnica flowers to be bruised and packed in just the right menstruum, or finally the wonderful perfume of the vanilla beans which had to be cut up with scissors, pounded in the big mortar and made into choice extract. If you ever worked as a stock boy surely you remember the dozens of bottles which came packed in hay and straw.

This gives a fairly accurate picture of the store I started working in fifty years ago. Here prescriptions for the sick, written by the family physician, were filled by the gentle, loving hands of the family druggist. These prescriptions, many thousands of which are still filed away in basements, could tell many interesting facts concerning the history of various communities. In my own files, I have today such prescriptions for four and five generations of one family in my home town.

But what of the drugs which were dispensed from these pharmacies? This was the age of vegetable drugs. Dr. Henry Rusby and others were investigating botanicals and down Cincinnati way John Uri Lloyd and others were dispensing "specifics." Who is there to say that the quarter-pound jars of extract of taraxacum sold then was less effective than our modern day vitamins which didn't come upon the market until after 1912.

In 1903 a new drug with a long chemical name commonly known as *Acetozone* came on the market. It assailed typhoid fever and was a new venture in the field of pharmacy. Today one seldom hears of a case of typhoid fever but in 1905 it was not unusual for two percent of the population of a town to be stricken with this disease during a single summer. Anti-Diphtheric Serum had been discovered but was not yet in general use. There was no insulin, emetine, or adrenalin and arsphenamine had not be heard of. Xray, now sixty years old, was just coming into use, and, of course, radium was unknown. Think of what it meant to be druggists when they had to help administer to the sick without these helps.

To emphasize the lack of preventative medicines at the turn of the century remember that in the Spanish American War, the United States had 700 men killed in action while 5700 died of disease. It had just been discovered that typhoid and cholera came from unclean milk and water. Quinine was man's only weapon against malaria. It might not be out of place to say here that Walter Reed and William Gorgas likely did more for more people than any known military or political leader-unless it had to be George Washington.

It has been said that early Americans feared smallpox more than they did taxation without representation. This fear had not been completely dispelled in 1905. Even at that date many towns had their "pest houses" and the arguments over the merits and demerits of vaccination still went on. It was to take another twenty years to make vaccination mandatory thereby eradicating the disease which had claimed victims all over the world for many centuries.

The years from 1905 to 1930 were to bring about many changes, some of which should be mentioned, if only to emphasize their relative newness in the pharmaceutical field. The year 1906 was quite important. The Wright Brothers built a machine which would really fly, and the Pure Food and Drug Act was enacted. In 1912 an international meeting was held at The Hague, in The Netherlands, to consider ways and means of controlling the narcotic trade. Agreements were signed by many nations expressing the need for such controls, but the United States was the first country to pass laws legalizing its moral obligation. The Harrison Narcotic Act was passed in December, 1914. The speed with which our country acted in this matter was due to no small extend to the concerted efforts of druggists and certainly the phenomenal success of this law can be credited to the manner in which our profession has cooperated in enforcing it.

The younger ones here tonight well may wonder at the late date of enactment and also the need for such legislation, so let me say something about conditions that existed when I began the practice of pharmacy. At that time there was practically no restrictions on the sale of narcotics. Opium was sold openly over the counter, with no restrictions except that it be labeled poison. I own a catalogue which list "No. 10 bottles of laudanum at 75 cents a dozen." This could be in turn sold to anyone for 15 cents a bottle a very nice profit in those days. In some places, laudanum was known to have been sold in pints, with

Saturday night bringing in quite a few customers for that amount. In my home state, in Ohio, and other surrounding areas, 1/8 oz. bottles of morphine could be sold providing that the revenue stamp was not broken and the sale was recorded in the poison register. Some control had been established over cocaine by 1910 but I can remember when an ounce of it, mixed with a pound of flake acetanilid, was bootlegged via the back door of some disreputable stores in 25 cent packages. Heroin, known as "High Life," was much in vogue among industrial workers. Certainly it was due to the high moral standards of the majority of the druggists that narcotics were not more of a menace than they were at that time. This also tells you of the need for-and the importance of the Act passed in 1914.

The year of 1914 is also important to our profession also because it marked the beginning of a movement to enact fair trade laws. This year the Stephens Bill was introduced into Congress. It failed to pass, but it was a beginning toward a much needed control.

Now this year of 1914 seems to be of much interest to pharmacists in general, but to me it had special significance. That year the West Virginia Pharmaceutical Association held its annual meeting at Mountain Lake Park, a summer resort on the border line of our state and Maryland. In the early morning hours of June 24, a Baltimore and Ohio train arrived for the East, stopped and one of the principal speakers stepped off. He was wearing a sailor straw hat, which set off his genial face which was adorned by a typical nineteen hundred mustache. His face lit up when he met the President of our Association, Walter Dittmeyer, of Harpers Ferry, who was his former student. A few hours later the assembled druggists heard the slow, even voiced "Mr. Pharmacist of America," who was none other than Professor Joseph Price Remington, give the story of the evolution of the *U.S. Pharmacopeia* and heard him explain its growing importance and the new legal standard for drugs in the United States.

Professor Remington recounted many details of his work in the various fields of pharmacy. One of his observations was that, "physicians have abandoned the old time standards and many get their therapeutics from traveling salesmen." He continued, "There are enough medicines in the *Pharmacopeia* today (1914) for any doctor to practice successfully if he wants to use them." Later on he lamented, "the department of therapeutics in nearly all medical schools had lost the influence it once had." He made the prophecy that, "if things work out, we will put aspirin in the book."

Following his formal talk, a question and answer period continued for over an hour and one might imagine that the good professor could have used a bit of aspirin by then. But maybe he had already discovered the secret of licking his problems rather then let them lick him, which Dr. R. L. Swain has so recently recommended for all of us.

Professor Remington was born in 1847 and was therefor 14 years of age when his neighbors marched away in the Union Army. He died in 1918, during World War I. He graduated for the Philadelphia College of Pharmacy in 1866 and trained with and walked with men like Squibb, Parrish, and Procter. He was always close to the hearts of the practicing pharmacist for he was one of us, as he owned and ran a retail pharmacy. He served as dean of the Philadelphia College, he was one of the editors of the *U.S. Dispensatory,* president of the APhA, chairman of the U.S. Pharmacopeia Committee, and as early as 1885 he was bringing out his monumental *Practice of Pharmacy.* His activities and accomplishments would and do fill thousands of printed pages. Little wonder that West Virginia was honored by his presence at its Association meeting, photographs during his stay are yet prized possessions of many who were in attendance.

By some singular coincidence, there was read at this same meeting, following Professor Remington, a paper prepared by a young man who stands before you tonight, honored to be the recipient of the medal bearing his name. I might add that the title of my paper was *Lo, The Poor Druggist And Why! I* am not sure that the paper made any great impression at that time, and now in 1955 I am still looking for the Why.

Those here tonight who served in World War I remember 1914 for entirely different reasons. Those who remained at home and worked in stores remember the influenza epidemic of 1918, the frequent calls to the railroad stations to help care for the wounded who were passing through our cities. All of us remember that many wonderful pharmaceutical advancements came during and following this terrible war.

The completion of the research on insulin came to a successful close in 1921. What a blessing to mankind has been the work of Banting and Best. Alexander Fleming discovered penicillin in 1928 and started us on the antibiotic era. By 1935 the first combination containing Prontisil, a drug containing sulfanilimide, was announced in Europe. Soon it was found that this and its derivatives were a specific against a number of bacterial diseases.

Well I do remember by first contact with the "sulfa drug" age. In 1939 one of the most distinguished citizens of my home town was at the point of death with pneumonia. A well-known physician of Pittsburgh, who had done much research on this drug was called upon for help. He arrived in Charleston, by plane, and brought with him one ounce of this new chemical. He brought it to our pharmacy and there under his direction I weighed it out into powder doses. The patient recovered and is today, at the age of 88, still carrying on many of his usual industrial activities. Thus the "young man's enemy and the old man's friend" was practically conquered by pharmaceutical research. This drug also made obsolete the large stock of short-lived pneumococcus serums, types one to thirty three, which had been perfected only a few years before.

When World War 11 (1939-1945) came along the part played by drugs was quite a different story than that recorded in previous wars. This is indicated by the lower mortality rate, both among the wounded and those stricken by disease, or accidental injuries. All of us know how the pharmacists of American responded to the call for quinine. New drugs had taken the place of camphor, bromides, creosote carbonate, so much in demand during World War I. The contributions in the field by pharmacists was of the highest order. Many were misplaced or we might say misused, but from this came the creation of a Medical Service Corps in the Army by 1947. This did not remedy all of the just complaints of pharmacists but it was certainly a long step in the right direction.

Once again from a war came something good. The atomic bomb, tragic in its power to destroy, has brought for tracer elements to help the sick, and we have promise of even greater healing power to be discovered in this wonder of the century.

Besides the changes in the practice of pharmacy and medicine the past fifty years has seen remarkable changes in pharmaceutical education. In 1905 there were eighty institutions of learning listed as schools of pharmacy in the United States. However, of these only twenty-one were independent pharmacy schools, the remaining number being only departments of some medical college or university. Of this number many have been discontinued, although quite a few were then laying the foundations for some of our finest present day colleges of pharmacy. I cannot resist mentioning that in 1892 a school was opened in Louisville, Kentucky, known as the Louisville College of Pharmacy for Women. What became of this might make a nice story, but we all know that today our women students seek no separate institutions for their professional training.

Attendance at these schools was entirely voluntary. No state required college training for registration until New York passed such a law in 1905. Pennsylvania followed the next year, and from then on one-by-one other states established similar requirements until by 1921 seventeen required graduation from a college of pharmacy. But remember there was no uniformity in these college courses and an entrance examination had not been heard of. Most, if not all, offered two year courses. It was not until 1925 that three year courses were generally required and not until 1932 that the present four year course became mandatory in all states. Many here tonight played an active part in bringing about these higher standards. Now today we stand upon the threshold of the five year program.

During this same period has come a remarkable growth in professional organizations. Fifty years ago the National Association of Boards of Pharmacy was just getting started. Today we have reciprocity with and between all states except New York, Florida and California.

In 1905 your speaker had the opportunity of affiliating with either or both of the then existing pharmaceutical organizations-the APhA or the NARD. The APhA had been organized in 1852; the NARD) was only seven years old. Today I find myself a card-bearing member in eight organizations, all devoted to the advancement of some phase of pharmacy.

Yes, these have been fifty fabulous years in which to have lived and have worked in the field of pharmacy. The present generations of pharmacists have fought a good fight to bring about relief for suffering mankind. Many of the leaders must now pass the torch to younger hands. If I could make one wish it would be to have the power to look into the palms of these youngsters now entering the profession and to read there what they will accomplish by the end of this century. To this group I would pass on these words, copied from the base of the statue of Thomas Watson, which stands in the Capital grounds at Atlanta, Georgia:

"Democratic institutions exist by reason of their virtue. If ever they perish it will be when you have forgotten the past, become indifferent to the present and utterly reckless as to the future."

How many years remain for me to continue my life's work only God knows. Be they many or few I will continue working for the advancement of pharmacy, inspired by my realization of what has been done during my short lifetime, and stimulated and rededicated to my task because of this honor which you have so graciously bestowed upon me tonight. ■

1956 Remington Medalist

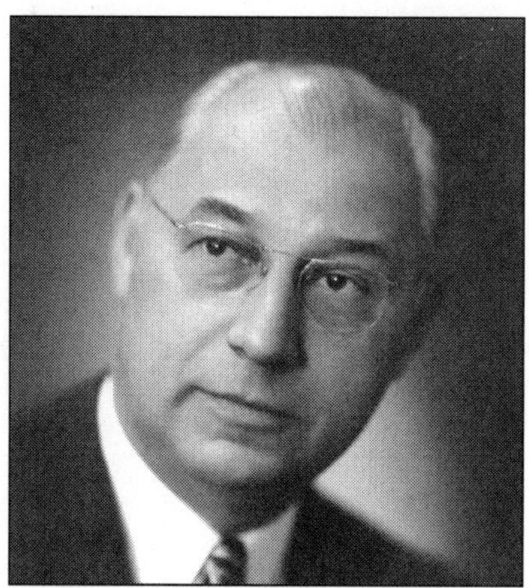

Frances William Moudry
(1895-1971)

Frances (Frank) William Moudry was born in Le Center, Minnesota, and graduated from the University of Minnesota College of Pharmacy in 1915. He was then employed by a pharmacy in Wauseca, Minnesota, in 1916 and later purchased a pharmacy in Waterville which he operated until 1930 when he founded the Moudry Apothecary Shop in St. Paul. He was elected president of the Minnesota State Pharmaceutical Association in 1928, and was appointed a member of the Minnesota State Board of Pharmacy in 1935, serving as secretary of the Board from 1940 until his retirement. During this period, he became a leading authority on pharmacy law enforcement.

Moudry served as the president of the National Association of Boards of Pharmacy 1947-1948, and the National Association of Retail Druggists 1949-1950, having first been elected as a member of the NARD executive committee in 1939, and as chairman of the Executive Committee in 1943. He was also a member of the Pharmaceutical Survey Committee and the American Council on Pharmaceutical Education. As the first chairman in 1952 of the NARD-American Medical Association Liaison Committee, he provided the leadership resulting in the creation with APhA in 1956 of the National Pharmacy Committee on Relations with the Medical Profession. Working with the Pharmacy Liaison Committee of the American Medical Association Board of Trustees, improved relations between medicine and pharmacy were obtained.

Improving Relations With the Medical Profession

Frances (Frank) W. Moudry

The 1956 Remington Honor Medal Lecture was presented on December 3, 1956, at the Hotel Roosevelt in New York City. Moudry's Remington address was published in the *Journal of the American Pharmaceutical Association, Practical Pharmacy Edition,* volume 17, pages 802-804, 1956; and in the *NARD Journal,* volume 78, pages 28, 38, 42, 44, December 17, 1956.

Over the past few years we have seen many great advances in our profession, both in the pharmaceutical field and in the area of merchandising. Many important scientific discoveries and the promise of greater ones in the future offer us hope for a wonderful tomorrow for pharmacy and better health for the nation. Hardly less amazing are the constant advances being made in our modern pharmacy, both in its appearance and its efficient merchandising techniques.

But modern merchandising is a mixed blessing because, among its many advantages for pharmacy, are some few trends which will in the long run do more harm than good for our profession. Some of these trends encourage non-pharmacists to enter the drug distribution field. Other trends tempt pharmacists to compromise the professional character of their pharmacies and drug stores and to identify themselves completely with extreme, unprofessional merchandising techniques.

We have to admit that, when others enter our field or when we pursue unprofessional merchandising goals, it is in both cases for the same reasons-greater profits. It comes down, then, to the problem of keeping the spirit of commercialism within the limits of professional operation. It has been the great objective of many pharmacists recently—and I am one of them—to preserve the professional spirit and at the same time to keep in step with the best modern trends of drug store merchandising. Today there are persons who lament that pharmacy as a profession is on the downswing; who forecast that because of modern merchandising competition all independent specialized retail outlets, including drug stores, will soon be absorbed as mere departments of the all-inclusive super-markets. Now that more and more retail outlets merchandise practically all drug products except prescriptions, the whole point of a drug store for the sale of drugs and medicines, say the pessimists, is lost.

That these are real problems, I do not deny. And they are serious because they affect our very existence as pharmacists and operators of retail pharmacies and drug stores. Yet I believe that the great American landmark, the retail drug store that blends professional health service with non-pharmaceutical merchandising, is not doomed. Our task is to see the dangers clearly, to think wisely about their solutions, and to inaugurate bravely the program that will preserve pharmacy as a profession and will safeguard the independent retail drug store as a major health center. To my mind this program, which is already under way, can be summed up in the following three objectives:

1. Renewal of professional ideals in pharmacy.
2. Modernization of pharmacy legislation.

3. Improvement of relations with the medical profession.

If we are going to preserve pharmacy as a profession, it is of fundamental importance that the term "profession" be more than just a word to us. A professional man is a man of idealism and pride and ethical conduct. He sees himself as a public servant, ministering to the health and well-being of his community. The drug store, despite the many merchandising services it provides, is essentially a health center, and the pharmacist is no ordinary citizen, and service should entitle him to the respect of the community.

Every day the pharmacist can rededicate his professional spirit by absolute integrity in the practice of pharmacy and by the professional health service he renders his customers. When we as pharmacists engage in unethical practices or condone such conduct in others, we not only undermine our own idealism but contribute serious harm to the prestige of the profession as well.

Perhaps there are cynics who would say that to talk of idealism and integrity and professional spirit in the present time of unscrupulous merchandising competition is to be naive and impractical. If the cynics are right and I am wrong, then it is time we face the truth and drop our masks and stop pretending to be something we are not.

It is especially in the area of merchandising that we need to apply our professional spirit. In our store operations, we should be modern in the best sense. As good businessmen we should adopt all the new, effective techniques that are in harmony with the professional dignity of a drug store.

To be specific, what about the trend of grocery stores and super-markets toward self-service operations? Should drug stores adopt this technique? Arguments in favor of it stress the reduction of overhead expenses and the value of open displays.

These advantages are undeniable. But the question remains: Does self-service harmonize with the professional goals of a drug store? I wonder. It seems to me that the sale of drugs and medicines under self-service does not provide sufficient protection to the public. It also eliminates the numerous intimate customer contacts by which the pharmacist could give valuable professional guidance and health information. Finally, are we not forgetting that the moment we place drugs and medicines in self-service we have admitted to the public that it is equally safe for grocery stores and super-markets to distribute them? Especially for these reasons, then, if we pharmacists sell drugs and medicines in the self-service operation, we fail to accept our professional responsibility to the safety and health of the public.

Some State Boards of Pharmacy have passed regulations prohibiting self-service of drugs and medicines, and we hope that all states will protect their citizenry by similar means.

Aside from the matter of integrity, there is great publicity value in the professional operations of a drug store. We all recognize the present need of improving public relations for pharmacy. While we wish great success to programs now underway, it is clear that no program can accomplish what an individual pharmacist can, in his own drug store.

For example, when a customer steps out of his local drug store, has he spoken to a professional man, or just to another businessman; has he been in a health center, or in just another retail variety outlet? In the final analysis, good public relations must originate in the local drug store. Before we can expect that legislatures, courts, and consumers look on us as professional men, we must first see ourselves in that light and display to the public a professionally operated drug store.

Another important area for the future of pharmacy is the matter of legislation. The individual pharmacist needs help in serving the health needs of the community. He alone cannot protect his neighbors for the dangers of unrestricted sale of medicines. Such protection is the purpose of pharmacy legislation, which should be as modem and effective as up-to-date merchandising.

Unfortunately, many states have outmoded pharmacy laws, with statutes long obsolete in terms of protection for the citizens of today.

When the profession of pharmacy works to revise and modernize these laws, it too often encounters misguided opposition. I have in mind at the moment the fight that pharmacy is waging in several states to restrict the sale of so-called proprietaries or packaged medicines.

Competent testimony is unanimous in its opposition to promiscuous distribution of packaged medicine. Nevertheless, many manufacturers and distributors right now are campaigning vigorously to make every kind of retail outlet a legalized supplier of packaged medicines. They oppose the enactment of legislation proposed by the profession of pharmacy which would safeguard the health of the public through statutory restrictions on the sale of socalled proprietaries to the drug store.

Why all this strenuous opposition? Perhaps we can better understand it from the comment of a spokesman for the organized food merchants of New York before a joint legislative committee at Cooperstown, N.Y. He declared that grocers should be allowed to sell packaged medicines because these products carry large gross margins and the profits from their sale would enable merchants to keep grocery prices down.

There in plain words is the motive that urges the majority of the grocers and the operators of supermarkets to favor promiscuous distribution of packaged medicines. To them, protection of public health is secondary to profits.

As we can see, the manufacturers of packaged medicines are strongly motivated, well organized, and alert to mobilize and all support for wide-open sales of their products. Grocers and peddlers and operators of super-markets have been induced to help oppose pharmacy legislation. This combined pressure amounts to a strong political influence which makes it very difficult to enact effective pharmacy laws for the protection of the public.

At the present time in my home state we are engaged in just such a struggle. The Minnesota Board of Pharmacy, under the provision of the Pharmacy Act, restricts the sales of drugs and medicines to licensed stores. There are now, in a district court, injunction lawsuits directed against a food chain and ajobber for refusal to stop selling packaged medicines in violation of the State Pharmacy Act.

The defendants have asked the district court to dismiss the lawsuits, on the ground that to grant an injunction against them would be contrary to legal procedure, since they are entitled to be prosecuted in a criminal action. All this legal terminology may seem confusing but the significance of this judicial wrangling is clear. The defendants intend to break down the authority of the Minnesota Board of Pharmacy. Where there is so much at stake for public health, we can only hope that the court will give a favorable decision to the Board of Pharmacy.

To modernize pharmacy legislation certainly requires idealism, watchfulness, and perseverance of us. This is a real challenge. But an even greater challenge-and our ultimate goal-is not to defeat those who disagree with us but to cooperate with them in finding common ground for conciliation and mutual solution of mutual problems. It is difficult enough to engage in legal battles. It is more difficult still to enter that field of arbitration and cooperation that will produce a solution satisfactory to both parties and will serve the public interest. I sincerely hope that we will find the peaceful settlement.

This final objective is the threefold program for the welfare of pharmacy could be the most vital to the economic survival of the American drug store.

The drug industry, we know, is booming today, and the future holds even greater promise. The profession of pharmacy is the public servant that makes these drugs available to the public. But our role is an intermediary one, between the physician who prescribes a medicine and the patient who buys it. In other words, we are a dependent profession. For the benefit of public health as well as for the economic prosperity of the pharmacist, it is important that the two professions-medicine and pharmacy-act ethically toward each other and cooperate on the most cordial terms.

To promote better professional relations between medicine and pharmacy we now have a joint committee known as the "National Pharmacy Committee on Relations with the Medical Profession." The membership consists of three members of the American Pharmaceutical Association and three members from the National Association of Retail Druggists. On January 5, 1956, this committee met with a similar committee, the Pharmacy Liaison Committee of the Board of Trustees of the American Medical Association, to consider matters of mutual interest.

In particular, these committees discussed the 1955 change in the Principles of Medical Ethics of the AMA, which would permit physicians to own and operate pharmacies. This was a reversal of their code of ethics, and has been very disturbing to the pharmacists of the country.

We have found that the leaders of the AMA are as eager as we are to promote friendly relations between the physician and the pharmacist in each community. They understand and are sympathetic with the danger of economic encroachment on pharmacy. However, the power of the officials is limited since they must abide by the decisions of the House of Delegates (the legislature of the AMA).

Since the joint committee meeting last January, the AMA at their convention in June 1956 again revised their Principles of Medical Ethics to provide that physicians should limit the income of medical practice to services rendered the patient. To be effective, this change has to approved by the House of Delegates.

I have said before on numerous occasions and I repeat again that the local medical society is the logical and most satisfactory place for the solution of the problem created by physicians entering the practice of pharmacy. Big stick tactics will not be successful. What is needed is tact, diplomacy, and a willingness to cooperateon both sides.

The problem of physician-owned pharmacies is an instance where we enlist the cooperations of the medical profession. But the relationship is mutual, and pharmacy is in a position to support medicine. The outstanding current example of this cooperation is the constant, vigorous support which pharmacy has provided in the medical profession's struggle to remain free from government domination. Medicine has always found her allied profession, pharmacy at her side in the fight against socialized medicine.

In my 41 years in the profession, I have come to know many of the persons connected with the drug industry. The foresight, determination, and integrity of these men are my personal hope for the future of pharmacy. I only wish I could divide the honor of the Remington Award and could give each of these professional friends the recognition they deserve. And if I could make such a division of honor, even that little credit that would be left for myself, I would receive with humility and treasure with gratitude. In this spirit, I thank the New York Branch of the American Pharmaceutical Association for this Remington Honor Medal and for all the arrangements that have made this evening one of the great moments of my life. ■

1957 Remington Medalist

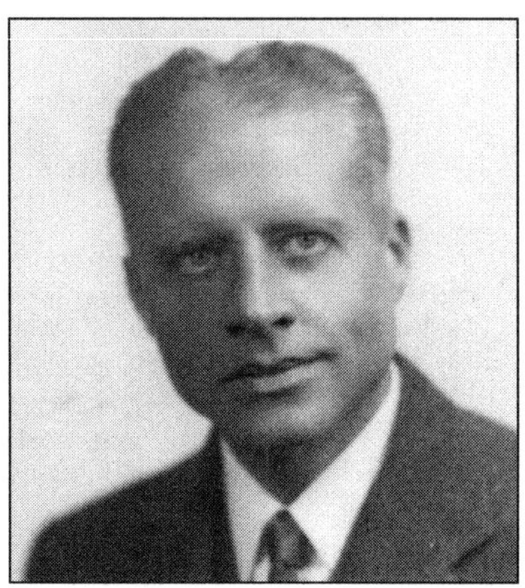

William Paul Briggs
(1903-1977)

William Paul Briggs was born in Washington, D.C., and received a B.S. degree in pharmacy from the George Washington University in 1928, and a Master of Science degree from the University of Maryland in 1930. He operated his own pharmacy in Washington, D.C., for two years before joining the faculty of George Washington University in 1927, where he served as dean of the School of Pharmacy from 1932 until 1947. During the last two years as dean, he inaugurated the "hometown pharmacy service" program for the Veterans Administration. He served variously as secretary of the District of Columbia Pharmaceutical Association 1934-1939, secretary of the National Drug Trade Conference 1936-1938, and treasurer of the *U.S. Pharmacopeia* Board of Trustees 1940-1970. He was a member of the Pharmaceutical Survey committee and author of *Systematic Prescription Pricing Digest* and co-author of the 1949 edition of *American Pharmacy.*

Briggs served in the U.S. Naval Reserves 1942-1945, advancing from the rank of lieutenant to commander. He returned to the U.S. Navy in 1948 as head of pharmacy service for the Medical Service Corps. He relinquished this post in 1951 to become secretary and executive director of the American Foundation for Pharmaceutical Education, a position he held until his retirement in 1974. For his 23 years of AFPE service in raising funds to support both undergraduate scholarships and graduate fellowship, he was elected posthumously as an honorary member of the American Foundation for Pharmaceutical Education, and the "W. Paul Briggs Memorial Fellowship" was created in his honor in 1978.

A Moratorium on Pharmacy Introspection

William Paul Briggs

The 1957 Remington Honor Medal Lecture was presented on December 2, 1957, at the Hotel Roosevelt in New York City. Briggs's Remington address was published in the *Journal of the American Pharmaceutical Association, Practical Pharmacy Edition,* volume 18, pages 726-728, 1957.

This is an historic occasion for me. It marks the culmination of a long series of personal good fortune and generous judgements by my colleagues

I am aware that this is not a purely personal honor. Rather, I am acting tonight as the representative of many pharmacists, educators, drug industry leaders, association officials, Government and naval associates, and a host of other cherished friends whose own work has reflected favorably upon me. In this role, I accept the coveted Remington Medal with humility and appreciation.

With all its inspiring traditions and heart warming glories, I am sure that even the Remington Medal cannot confer divine wisdom upon recipients. However, no metaphysical powers will be needed for my comments to you on marriage, manpower, and a moratorium.

The most perfect marriage in the drug world occurred when the American Foundation for Pharmaceutical Education was solemnized by the unanimous action of every segment of Pharmacy.

On its 15th anniversary, this year, the Foundation can look with loving pride upon its offspring. It has raised a large and flourishing family of 1,505 pharmacists who were aided in their education by AFPE Scholarships. This year 150 more top grade pharmacy students will receive AFPE undergraduate scholarships. The Foundation has provided 394 Graduate Fellowships and, during the current academic year, is supporting 70 outstanding scholars who are working toward their Doctor of Philosophy degree at 24 universities. One hundred seventy five Foundation Fellows are now teaching in 70 of the 76 U.S. Colleges of Pharmacy, with many others engaged in research and related professional services within the industry and in Government.

The Foundation, in 1946-49, financed The Pharmaceutical Survey, conducted by the American Council on Pharmaceutical Education. This was the most exhaustive study of Pharmacy ever attempted. It cost $186,000.00, and its findings provided the basis for many of the constructive programs now being carried on to insure a better Pharmacy tomorrow.

The Foundation provided $110,000 to the American Association of Colleges of Pharmacy in support of its current pharmacy student recruitment campaign, including production and distribution of two splendid movies. In addition, the Foundation has stimulated other pharmaceutical organizations and individual companies to use their own resources to aid in this work. This joint effort over the last few years has cost upwards of $300,000. Through booklets, movies, magazine and newspaper articles, TV and radio, the story of Pharmacy as a career has reached parents and prospective students in more than 50,000,000 homes.

The American Council on Pharmaceutical

Education has made a major contribution in the improvement of all Colleges of Pharmacy, and in the licensure work of State Boards of Pharmacy. The Council has been supported since 1946 largely by the Foundation.

AFPE also supports the *American Journal of Pharmaceutical Education.* Another important activity is its financing of the annual Teachers' Seminar. These week-long, intensive courses serve to refresh and stimulate pharmacy college teachers. The Seminars have been held each year since 1949 and are attended by staff members from all our colleges.

The Foundation provides Teaching Fellowships in Business Administration for pharmacy college faculty members. This program is producing competent teachers of business subjects, so that tomorrow's pharmacist will be a good business man as well as good professional man.

The Foundation administrators Memorial Awards and Fellowships in the names of Edwin L. Newcomb, S. Barksdale Penick, Gustavus A. Pfeiffer, E. Mead Johnson, Charles R. Walgreen, H. A. B. Dunning, and J. K. Lilly. It carries on still other fundamental activities that are designed to strengthen education in Pharmacy.

The Foundation has already "invested" in pharmaceutical education nearly $3,000,000, received from the leading manufacturing drug, surgical dressing, prescription accessory, container, and related industries; the wholesale drug trade; chain drug stores; individuals; the medical and pharmaceutical press; advertising and associated industries; and the producers of commodities usually supplied through the pharmacies of the U.S.

We have barely begun our planned work. With the continued support of the business of pharmacy, The Foundation hopes to bring new vitality to pharmaceutical education, research, and the practice of Pharmacy in America.

The Foundation Board of Directors representing industry, practice, trade, and education, meets in united strength to pool minds and money for the common good of Pharmacy. Here individual objectives are quietly submerged in devoted efforts to benefit Pharmacy. We hope and believe that the happy, wholesome family life of the American Foundation for Pharmaceutical Education will, by example and accomplishment, bring new resources to the profession. I think it is quite appropriate to characterize the American Foundation for Pharmaceutical Education as the true "love child" of the happiest marriage in Pharmacy.

It is impossible to condense an account of the monumental achievements of the Foundation, but I shall hope this brief reference will soften the hearts, and especially the treasuries, of our friends in the business world of Pharmacy.

The second of my three topics-manpower-is the one most urgent and basic problem facing Pharmacy today. Pharmacy simply cannot survive without adequate numbers of competent pharmacists to carry on our essential function as a member of the health team. And the American people cannot survive without Pharmacy.

Pharmacy is not alone in losing students to the lure of quick earnings in occupations that may be entered directly from high school. Nor is it alone in losing talent to currently glamorous fields, such as engineering, that do require college training. And it shares with all professions the shameful annual losses of brilliant students lacking the means to pay for their eduction. A recent study supported by the National Science Foundation stated that last year "some 150,000 high ability students... would have gone to college had adequate financial support been offered them."

It is quite simple to give away money and not overly difficult to find takers for tuition loans. Yet Julius Rosenwald, who gave away his vast fortune during his own lifetime, said he found it "nearly always easier to make one million dollars honestly than to dispose of it wisely."

Career bribery, through scholarships, is not a lasting substitute for genuine career interest. We need Pharmacy-motivated young men and women, not "gift shoppers" or "drafted volunteers." How can we insure the adequacy of pharmaceutical manpower? I have no broad-spectrum specific to offer.

But I am sure of the absolute necessity of starting with ability and motivation, instead of just dollars. Of course, we need scholarships and tuition loan funds, but money alone will not solve Pharmacy's manpower problem.

The search for pharmacists of the future cannot be conducted in a vacuum. It must be related to our educational system and the environment of the practice of Pharmacy. Education, in any field, must be geared to the academic background of the student; the intended utilization of new knowledge; and the moral obligation of teachers to provide preparation for living, as well as preparation for working.

We must aggressively seek to enlist for our team every superior science-minded high school and junior college graduate we can find. We must give them the best possible scientific eduction, and we must try to stimulate these young people to undertake graduate study. We can place all the men and women we can get with this kind of training, as teachers and industry scientists. I never expect to see a surplus of top flight, graduate-trained pharmaceutical scientists. But not everyone wants to be a teacher, or researcher. This is fortunate.

With equal vigor, we must seek for our colleges profession-minded students and provide for them stimulating professional and technical training. We can absorb, in satisfying and rewarding positions, many more pharmacists with such preparation than we have any likelihood of getting in the immediate future. Hospital pharmacy, professional pharmacy services, and many Government, trade and industry openings await superior young pharmacists with talent and motivation toward these growing activities. But not everyone wants to work in Government, or industry, or a hospital, or a professional pharmacy. And this is fortunate.

In our search for total manpower we should also look for desirable high school graduates and Junior College students who are instinctively impelled toward the modern practice of Pharmacy with all its challenging professional, retailing, and management aspects.

The drug store is going to be here a long, long time. It will continue to render an essential professional service, but it will also continue to meet the wants and demands of the people for a variety of non-pharmaceutical services and supplies. Many thousands of drug stores, in county seats and great cities, must be staffed with pharmacists, by law and in the public interest.

As we find these "practice-minded" students, there may be some who did not follow the technical program in high school or Junior College, and thus may be apprehensive of their ability to master the imposing scientific courses that make up so large a portion of the typical Pharmacy College curriculum.

I am still talking about sound education and superior students. A student can be superior to other students without being strongly motivated toward science. A Pharmacy College program can be educationally sound without being overwhelmingly scientific. Superior students are to be found in all shapes, sexes, and sizes, with interests in every discipline from agronomy to zoology including the science, the profession, and the business of Pharmacy.

Many young men and women in pharmacy will not want to be teachers, or researchers, or serve in professional pharmacies, or hospitals. But they will want to own or operate retail pharmacies, enter the wholesale trade, or engage in other services. And this, too, is most fortunate for Pharmacy.

I hope all our future graduates will be equipped to live, and love living, in their world of tomorrow. I want them to be trained for contentment and comfort in the area of Pharmacy where their natural abilities and motivations direct them. For some this may require a program of basic liberal art courses, but with concentration on scientific disciplines, in preparation for teaching and research; for others, perhaps greater emphasis upon technical and professional courses; and for still others-indeed the far larger number -a well-balanced program in general education subjects with entirely adequate, but not superfluous, scientific and professional courses.

Clarence B. Randall, former Board Chairman of Inland Steel Company, pointed up the comparative importance of liberal, versus scientific, education when he said, "Most of the problems (of management) would be just the same had the atom never been split. They require, not knowledge of the nature of matter, but a clear mind, the power of logical analysis, wisdom born of experience, and a talent for communication." Here is ajudgement to ponder.

It seems probable that flexible training programs, with the individual rather than a rigid curriculum as the teaching guide, would attract, in both quality and quantity, the essential manpower for Pharmacy.

If college admission requirements should provide for acceptance of professional and business, as well as science-minded students, and elective programs of pharmaceutical education are thus indicated, then I think these are luxuries we cannot afford to forego. Education should provide preparation for life -let us not allow it to become of idealistic carving of round pegs to fit square holes. Dynamic pharmacy needs many kinds, not just one kind, of pharmacist, and education should serve, as well as shape, the career choices of students.

My final comment is concerned with our need for a moratorium on the dispensing of pharmaceutical defeatism. To be sure, the practice of pharmacy is changing-but who says the public does not love Pharmacy?

A great deal of sheer nonsense has been written about steps that should be taken to "save" or "change" or "restore" the practice of Pharmacy to its former pristine glory. While I am ashamed of some drug stores, I am not convinced there is much that is fundamentally wrong with the practice of Pharmacy today, or that it without its proper share of glory in the discerning eyes of the people.

Eloquent and sincere persuaders have suggested that by making every drug store a professional pharmacy; or by enrolling every pharmacist in one or another of our various organizations; or by adopting a longer college course; or by enacting certain legislation; or by subscribing to a new code of ethics; or even some form of magic, we can overnight create a new and better pharmacy. I do not condemn such proposals as being without merit. But I do consider it ridiculous to start out with the assumption that pharmacy is less vital today than it was 25 or 100 years ago, or that it is in imminent danger of passing from the American scene. I do not concede that the public is dissatisfied with pharmacy. On the contrary, I believe most drug stores enjoy a warm affection with the American public. Furthermore, in my view, there is convincing evidence that pharmacy is merely hypersensitive to professional claustrophobia and normal public indifference. Pharmacy lives and thinks too much within itself and indulges in imaginary fears of public disapproval. The public does not disapprove of pharmacy; it simply takes it for granted.

Like many faithful husbands, the American people just do not take time to proclaim their love for pharmacy every day. We may yearn for some display of affection, but we should find comfort in the fact that the American public keeps coming home to pharmacy day after day after day. This is the real test, and we score a high grade. I have not detected any mass movement toward a pharmaceutical Reno.

I submit that pharmacy can achieve its own psychological emancipation from fear and frustration by living in the sunshine of its values, rather than dwelling in the darkness of its difficulties. Praise is free-use it generously.

I am a Pollyanna, and I do not believe I am about pharmacy. I am aware of the faults of pharmacy and of the many problems of our practitioners. But I am just plain tired of hearing, in microscopic detail, of every defect in pharmacy with rarely a reference to its advantages to pharmacists, and its very real value to the public.

If the honor I received tonight gave me the necessary power, I would declare a one-year moratorium on pharmaceutical introspection, sadistic self-depreciation, and unrealistic comparisons that make pharmacists-but not the public-question the importance of pharmacy on the health team and its useful community service.

I urge each of you to list the obvious values of pharmacy and to use this catalogue as a preamble to every utterance, public and private, during the next 12 months. After doing this, it will not matter how vividly you describe our problems or how vigorously you fight for a better environment for pharmacy.

And I predict that every undertaking will come closer to accomplishment because it then will start from strength rather than weakness. Won't you join me in a pharmaceutical jubilee year of rejoicing for our assets, even as we continue to press for a better pharmacy tomorrow?

I am grateful to the New York Branch of the American Pharmaceutical Association and to all who have paid me the honor of attending this diner. I will try to justify my selection by the past presidents of the American Pharmaceutical Association, and I will undertake to earn the right to sit with the illustrious past recipients of the Remington Honor Medal. ■

1958 Remington Medalist

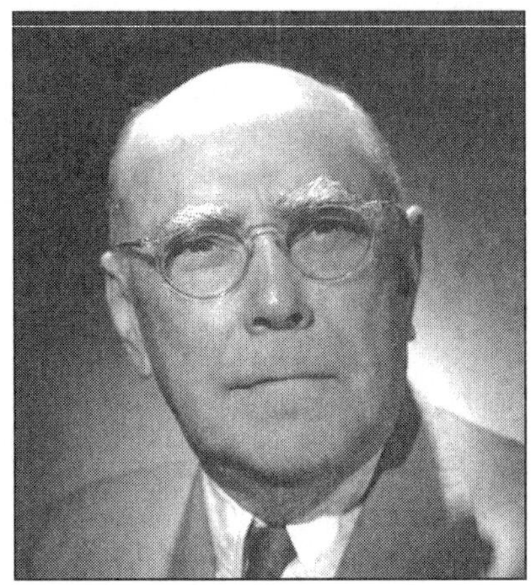

Eli Lilly
(1885-1977)

Eli Lilly was born in Indianapolis, Indiana, and received a Ph.C. degree in 1907 from the Philadelphia College of Pharmacy. He then joined the company founded in 1876 by his grandfather, Colonel Eli Lilly, and became superintendent of the manufacturing division in 1909. He then served as Eli Lilly and Company general superintendent 1915-1920, vice president 1920-1932, and president 1932-1948. Following the death of his father, Josiah K. Lilly, he became chairman of the Board of Directors serving 1948-1961 and again 1966-1969, and then as president of the Lilly Endowment, which he helped establish in 1937. He served as president of the Indiana Historical Society 1933-1946, president of the Indiana Academy of Science 1938, chairman of the Historic Landmarks Foundation of Indiana, and he helped to organize the Indianapolis United Fund in 1957, serving as its honorary chairman.

A member of the American Pharmaceutical Association, he served as APhA honorary president 1953-1954, and as a director of the American Foundation for Pharmaceutical Education. He was noted for his extensive collection of Indian relics and prehistoric artifacts of the Mound Builders, which is now preserved at Indiana University, and he authored *Prehistoric Antiquities of Indiana* (1937); *The Little Church on the Circle* (a history of Indianapolis Christ Church, 1957); and *Early Wawasee Days* (1960, second edition 1965). The governor of Indiana proclaimed April 1, 1969, as "Eli Lilly Day" as a tribute to his contributions to the state and its citizens.

A Period of Remarkable Progress

Eli Lilly

The 1958 Remington Medal was presented December 10, 1958, at the Roosevelt Hotel in New York City. Lilly's Remington address was not published, but a copy of the manuscript was obtained from Anita Martin, archivist, Eli Lilly and Company, Indianapolis, Indiana.

The shades of Demosthenes, Cicero, Edmund Burke, and Daniel Webster have been singularly unresponsive to my desperate appeals for words, phrases, and ideas which would properly express my deep appreciation and thanks to those generous persons who have honored me with the Remington Medal of 1958. It is accepted with joy, humility, and thanksgiving and with the certainly that, for the most part, the great credit of the honor belongs to the many wonderful people with whom I have come in contact in pharmacy, medicine, and business. Without their examples and assistance, I might have existed in a state of mild inadequacy.

The New York Branch of the American Pharmaceutical Association and the Committee of Award have taken a grave risk in presenting this year's Remington Honor Medal. My father repeatedly said that it was always dangerous to honor a living man, for there was no telling how big a fool he would make of himself before his life's end.

Then again, it might work to the undoing of the recipient. A very dear business associate said that several men who had served as Rex in the Mardi Gras, at New Orleans, acquired delusions of grandeur which persisted forever after. It must be said, however, that there seems to have been no tendency of this kind connected with the Remington Medal. Let us hope that good record may continue.

Related statements by two famous men fit exactly my prevailing thoughts. Dr. Oliver Wendell Holmes once observed, "Everyone is an omnibus in which his ancestors ride," and Dr. Albert Einstein said, "Many times a day I realize how much of my own outer and inner life is built upon the labors of my fellow man, both living and dead."

All of us are interdependent and are largely influenced and formed by our myriad of personal relationships. The pollen of ideas carries capability from mind to mind. I wish it were possible to name all the persons who have cast their lights upon my way, that they might be given credit for their share of this Remington Medal. Since this is not practical, permission is requested for an oldtimer to reminisce briefly and in so doing to drop the names of just a few of the many people who have been influential in his life.

Ours has been the privilege of participating in pharmacy during a period of truly remarkable growth and progress. My grandfather used to say there were only two drugs that would cure disease: quinine was specific for malaria and sulphur for the itch. Imagine how astounded he would be today at the life-saving drugs on prescription department shelves, exciting evidence of the successful blending of the scientific knowledge and professional skills of many dedicated people.

It is appropriate at this time to "Praise famous men, and our fathers who begat us," and to remember the twenty dedicated men who, on their own initiative, founded the American Pharmaceutical Association some one hundred years ago. The glorious accomplishments of this society, in working tirelessly in the best interest of human health, has had marked effect upon the lives of the whole nation. No less do we owe to those who have guided this Association and its branches throughout the years and to those now in the saddle, of whom Dr. Hugo H. Schaefer and Dr. Robert P. Fischelis are shining examples.

A young related organization now ably assisting is the American Foundation for Pharmaceutical Education, headed by such tireless workers as Charles S. Beardsley, George Doerr, W. Paul Briggs, and many other able men.

In thinking back on the influences that have shaped my life, I recall fond memories of devoted men in the field of education.

On the charming personality, ability, and deep understanding of his subject and of human nature possessed by Professor Joseph P. Remington, I need not dwell tonight. I shall simply say, stealing and changing a statement of Emerson, "He had precious goods on his shelves and brilliant show windows." The honor medal could not bear a more exalted name. Both my father and I absorbed his lectures and influence with joy and pride.

The quiet dignity and effectiveness of Professor Sadtler, who lectured with mildly apostolic fervor, the enthusiasm of Professor Henry Kraemer, and the able backing of these older men by Professors LaWall, Stroup, Newcomb, Moerk, and Cook are ever remembered with deep appreciation. Of all the staff of the Philadelphia College of Pharmacy in 1907, only Dr. E. Fullerton Cook has survived, continuing to serve the public and pharmacy with outstanding ability.

As just demonstrated by our dear friend president Ivor Griffith, the high voltage of the staff of the old college has been maintained. I should imagine that whenever he is scheduled to speak, students come "like feeding time at the zoo."

I suspect that a psychiatrist would classify me as being normal in thinking frequently about the past. An item regarding Dr. Elliott P. Joslin, of Boston, in a recent issue of *Time* recalled long-ago experiences connected with the development of insulin; they were intensely fascinating.

My relations with Doctors Banting, Best, Collip, and MacLeod were of the highest order, and contacts with the canny Scots among the Toronto University trustees were indeed a sizzling course in negotiation.

The item in *Time* Magazine mentioned that Dr. Joslin, at age 91, was still examining patients six days a week. A decade ago he attended a celebration at Toronto, afterward leaving on the night train for Buffalo. Dr. Clowes, then our research director, and I were aboard the same train. We decided that since Dr. Joslin's day had been quite strenuous and he was getting along in years, we would not disturb him. No sooner had we determined this than the good doctor popped into our compartment with his benign smile and discussed things diabetic until the small hours. His sincere interest and love for his patients are proverbial; and if he had lived in the days of Abou Ben Adhem, the latter would have had to play second fiddle.

One of the pleasures and privileges of being in this field has been my association with scientists from all over the world. Several years ago, Mrs. Lilly and I were privileged to have a dinner for Sir Alexander Fleming of antibiotic fame. He surprised us greatly by saying it was the first time he had been invited into a private home since his arrival in America. He was a charming, quiet, effective person who clearly belied the old pun that "Daniel was the only man who wasn't spoilt by lionizing."

Many times a day, as Dr. Einstein said, I realize how much of my life has been built on the labors of my fellow man. My "coaches" from within the drug distribution field have been numerous. How I would love to name them all.

One I will mention; dear old Uncle Paul Schuh, wholesale druggist of Cairo, Illinois. It was he who in the company's earliest days gave our first salesman, Uncle James

E. Lilly, such a whopping order that he was called off his territory to help make the goods.

When my father first started to really push our sales in 1899, one of the first trips he made was to Kansas City. Having always served in the factory, he was at first noticeably nervous and uncertain in the field. The elder Mr. Faxon, Henry's father, sensed the situation and so encouraged the young man that a very warm place in our hearts has forever been held by the Faxon family.

Then there was the attractive and gentlemanly Charles A. West, who had just the right amount of the proper Bostonian. My father and mother once visited in the home of Mr. and Mrs. West and at breakfast heartily praised the fragrance and flavor of the baked beans. Mrs. West had a can sent in from the kitchen, and behold it was from the Van Camp Packing Company of Indianapolis.

I would love to tell you stories about many, many more; Augustus Kiefer, for one, who encouraged my grandfather to enter manufacturing pharmacy; also the Murrays, Van Gorders; the Mooneys, Muellers, Moxleys, and Leichs in Indiana; the Doerrs, Davises, Meyers; the Hutchinses, McPike, and Ellises. And the Schieffelins — Dr. William Jay Schieffelin spoke so kindly at an occasion like this when my father was honored with the Remington Medal sixteen years ago.

I would like to say much about a far-sighted leader in pharmacy, John Dargavel. His shoulders are broad and he always has the interests of his brethren at heart.

It is extremely fortunate, too, that our "university of experience" faculty in charge of publicity and public relations has been so blessed with strong, forceful, and discriminating men like Robert L. Swain, Fullerton Cook, William S. Auchincloss, Irving Rubin, and Wallace Werble whom I have personally known.

Early in these remarks I mentioned Oliver Wendell Holmes' statement that everyone is an omnibus in which his ancestors ride. My own chief claim to some of the glory of this Remington Medal rests in the possibility of having unconsciously influenced the stork to land me in a certain family in Indianapolis.

That I might serve as the omnibus to carry at least some of the genes of grandfather Colonel Eli Lilly and of father J.K., Sr., has been a ruling passion. Modesty dictates that their proper praise be not indulged in, but those of you who knew them will understand in part what is meant. My own affection and admiration for them has an unknown depth.

It is also very fortunate that I have had my brother, J.K., Jr., and that we see so many thinks alike. Wally Werble once said, "It is well known in the trade that the Lilly brothers work very close together." Nothing in public print has ever pleased me so much.

It would be a serious oversight not to pay tribute to my immediate family, for no outsiders could ever have had the influence that an understanding wife and a fine, talented daughter provided. Best friends say that Mrs. Lilly made a different man of me. That was a very desirable accomplishment.

Death has recently called two revered associates-Charles J. Lynn and Dr. G.H.A. Clowes. Mr. Lynn's lifelong and effective service to the drug trade will long be remembered. As a citizen he contributed his time, judgement, ability, and financial strength to every good cause. His heart was not just a pump. He was often and justly called Mr. Indiana.

Dr. Clowes was one of the pioneers in the field of cancer research, and also cooperated with the University of Toronto in developing the first, large-scale pre-marketing clinical testing program. This was for insulin in the early 1920s. Dr. Clowes was also a leader in art and musical circles in Indiana, for the sandblast of science had not worn off his deep interest in the humanities.

As for other associates in our organization, past and present, whose examples have motivated me, their names are legend. To think of them, from bottle washer to president, revives basic faith in human nature. They are a cross section of the best in America, and it is impossible to praise and thank them too much. I realize how much of my life is built upon them.

As we retire from active life and have more time to value first things first, the soundness of certain teachings becomes more and more clear. These turn out to be almost copybook maxims, but their significance is cause for enumerating them:

There can be no substitutes for quality and integrity.

We should strive constantly to improve in all fields of our endeavor and especially to capture and keep the human touch, remembering that miracles can be wrought when people work together for the good of all.

We should obey the unenforceable laws of kindness, compassion, and unselfishness.

And finally, all things come to him who does not wait.

What Oliver Wendell Holmes said about the individual being an omnibus in which his ancestors ride applies quite as well, I think, to a profession or an industry. Pharmacy today is an omnibus which reflects the ideals and the integrity and the conscientious work of many able men and women who have labored over the years to bring better medicines to the people of the world. Their accomplishments eloquently speak for themselves. Moreover, there is every reason to be confident that the great traditions of the profession of pharmacy will be carried on with distinction by our present and oncoming leaders. Let us be every hopeful that the combined efforts of all will continue to demonstrate, beyond all socialistic propaganda to the contrary, that free enterprise in all areas of the health field will best insure the quality of medical care that the citizens of this great country have come to expect as their natural right.

Since I wish to avoid the dangers of old age, prolixity and gout, I will end with this note of confidence before both my friends and the grave begin to yawn, and before you follow the example of the ancient Scythians who ate their grandfathers as they became old and troublesome and began to tell long stories.

My dear friends, my heartfelt thanks and appreciation are yours forever. ■

1959 Remington Medalist

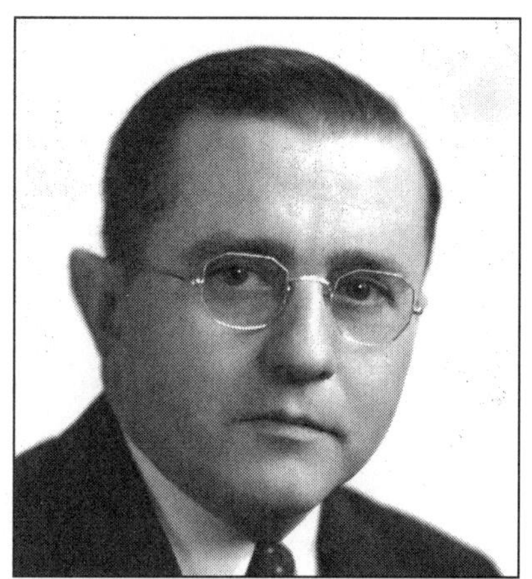

Justin Lawrence Powers
(1895-1981)

Justin Lawrence Powers was born in Tokonsha, Michigan, and after service as a sergeant in the U.S. Army Medical Department during World War I, he graduated from the University of Michigan with a Ph.C. degree in 1919, a B.S. in pharmacy in 1924, and an M.S. degree in 1927. In 1935, he received a Ph.D. degree from the University of Wisconsin for research in plant chemistry. During this period, he variously served as an instructor in pharmacy at Washington State College of Pharmacy 1919-1923, pharmacist at the University of Michigan Health Service 1919-1923, assistant professor of pharmacy at Oregon State College School of Pharmacy 1924-1926, and as a professor at the University of Michigan College of Pharmacy 1926-1940.

Powers joined the American Pharmaceutical Association headquarters staff in 1940 serving variously as director of the APhA Laboratory 1940-1947, editor of the *Journal of the American Pharmaceutical Association, Scientific Edition* 1941-1959, and as director for an unprecedented five revisions of the *National Formulary* 1940-1959. He also served on the USP revision committee and as chairman of the National Research Council's Committee on Purity of Chemical Products. He headed the U.S. delegation to the first Pan American Congress of Pharmacy in Havana, Cuba, in 1948, and served as a member of the expert advisory panel of the *International Pharmacopeia* 1952-1957. Following his retirement from the APhA staff, the APhA Foundation named a Research Achievement Award in his honor in 1961, and he served as director of the National Academy of Sciences *Food Chemicals Codex* 1960-1966. He was elected APhA honorary president 1975-1976.

Two Pharmaceutical Heritages

Justin Lawrence Powers

The 1959 Remington Honor Medal Lecture was presented on December 9, 1959, at the Roosevelt Hotel in New York City. Powers's Remington address was published in the *Journal of the American Pharmaceutical Association, Practical Pharmacy Edition,* volume 21, pages 30-32, 1960.

The Remington Medal is referred to as the highest award of pharmacy, and I so consider it. In the citation and in the presentation, reference was quite properly made to the *National Formulary* with which I have been identified for nearly 20 years. It must be emphasized that the present status of the *National Formulary* has not been achieved through the efforts of one man or even a small number. The production of five editions during a 20-year period is the result of the combined efforts of hundreds of individuals who have had an appreciation of the importance to the public of the *USP* and the *NF.*

I feel I was chosen to receive this year's award as a symbol of what the *NF* has accomplished, and as a representative of all who have contributed to its success. With this understanding, I am most happy to accept the Remington Honor Medal. I cannot begin to express adequately my deep feeling of appreciation and pleasure for having been selected to receive this outstanding honor.

Cooperation in creating new editions of the *USP* and *NF* comes not only from the pharmaceutical industry, but from other sources. These include pharmacists, educators, staff members of the Food and Drug Administration, other government agencies, independent institutional laboratories and many individuals in other categories. Without the co-operation of the pharmaceutical industry, the *National Formulary* and the *USP* would be severely handicapped in carrying on their revision programs. It might be possible to devise suitable official standards of quality for drugs without any help from this source, but in the United States it is neither practical nor desirable and, fortunately, is not necessary.

In many countries the close working relationship between pharmacopeial commissions, pharmaceutical manufacturers, and law enforcement agencies, as we know it here, does not exist. For example, in certain countries it is sometimes necessary for pharmacopeial commissions to obtain a sample of a basic drug, needed for the establishment of standards, by extracting it from a dosage form, and then to proceed with no knowledge of the quality control methods used by the manufacturer. The final quality specifications obtained in this way may be satisfactory, but the method certainly is not efficient.

The *USP* and the *NF* are two pharmaceutical heritages which are now taken for granted. Their importance often is not appreciated and their significance, under present conditions of pharmaceutical practice, is often forgotten and sometimes questioned.

Much time and effort are expended on pharmaceutical interprofessional and public relations programs. As an illustration, National Pharmacy Week is a public relations program designed to emphasize the professional aspects of pharmacy. In the promotion of this program, the USP and *NF* are seldom mentioned. More extensive reference to them as professional pharmaceutical contributions might serve a twofold purpose (1) acquainting the public with their significance and at the same time (2) reminding pharmacists of their obligation to the official compendia and the benefits they derive therefrom. I should like to review briefly the present positions of the official compendia and to discuss their significance and some of their future needs as I see them.

Some of the legal requirements relating to the manufacture and distribution of drugs in the United States are unique, and nothing comparable to them will be found in any other country. The *United States Pharmacopeia* and the *National Formulary* provide standards for drugs, established by organized groups of private citizens, which are enforceable by the terms of state and federal laws. The details of providing these standards are delegated to committees, by democratic processes, but the responsibility for the *NF* resides in the American Pharmaceutical Association and that for the *USP* in the U.S. Pharmacopeial Convention. Both of these organizations have always functioned in the public interest. If they had not, the official compendia could never have attained the positions they now occupy.

Their present status stems from the authority derived from the Federal Food, Drug and Cosmetic Act. One section of this law requires that drugs in the USP and the *NF* must conform to the standards prescribed therein. Minor variations are permitted when certain labeling requirements are met.

The same section, authorizes the administrator of the act to prescribe tests where none has been provided or where those designated are considered to be insufficient. Before this provision can be invoked, the official compendium concerned must be given a reasonable opportunity to correct the deficiency. It has never been necessary to resort to this safeguarding provision of the law. This seems to be a significant indication of the good character of these two books.

It has been said that the provision of the new drug section of the Food, Drug and Cosmetic Act decreases the significance of the official compendia, but this is not valid. There is no reason to believe that this section was designed to supersede the *USP* and the *NF* Information required in a new drug application is privileged and none of it, including quality control methods employed by the applicant, is available to the public. On the other hand, the official compendia offer an authoritative process for setting up open, objective, practical, and generally applicable standards for the quality of drugs. Control methods described in a new drug application do not comply with all of these criteria. They apply only to the products of the applicant, whereas, official specifications, particularly for dosage forms, should be suitable for products of all manufacturers. Usually drugs are removed from the new drug class when they become official. The *USP* and the *NF* have performed useful functions during the 22 years that the new drug section of the Act has been effective and they will continue to do so.

On March 29 and 30, 1960, a decennial meeting of the U. S. Pharmacopeial Convention will be held in Washington. This is of great importance to all phases of pharmacy. The convention will elect new officers, a board of trustees, and a committee of revision. To the 60 committee members will fall the work of producing two new revisions during the next ten years.

The *National Formulary is* a responsibility of the American Pharmaceutical Association, but the Council of this Association functions in a manner comparable to that of the board of trustees of the *USP*. The Council elects a director of revision, an executive committee of ten members and 50 participating members to constitute an Advisory Panel, from which subcommittees may be formed as required. Thus, the formal working bodies of the *USP* and the *NF* are substantially the same. The work of both committees is supplemented by several joint and individual special advisory committees.

The scope of the *USP* and of the *NF* differs to some extent. The content of the USP is determined by a subcommittee on scope, composed of 20 physicians and five pharmacists. The first *Pharmacopeia* was designed to serve as a therapeutic guide to the medical profession and its scope was restricted to drugs believed to possess the greatest merit. Therapeutic essentiality and the avoidance of extensive duplication of drugs in the same pharmacological categories have continued to be the principal criteria for admission of drugs to the *USP*.

The *National Formulary* also bases admission of drugs upon therapeutic merit as determined by an advisory committee on admissions, composed of physicians and pharmacists. Care is taken to avoid any conflict of interest with the *USP* and no drug ever appears in both books in the same form, but closely similar forms may appear.

Synthetic medicinal chemicals in the same categories are often quite closely related structurally and the narrow shades of differences in their efficacy are often difficult to determine. As a result there are many drugs, for this and other reasons, which are not admitted to the *Pharmacopeia*. In part, it is for such drugs that the *National Formulary* provides official standards. Thus, the appearance of drugs in the *NF* does not mean that they are inferior to those of the *USP*. Most items deleted from the *USP* during the course of a revision period are routinely admitted to the next edition of the *National Formulary*. In this way, official standards for many well-established drugs are maintained.

The revision and publication programs of the *USP* and *NF* run concurrently. The directors of revision of the two books work in close co-operation and maintain a free exchange of information. For example, the sections covering general tests and general notices are kept as nearly identical as possible. In addition, use is made of joint *USP* and *NF* advisory committees established to assist in the development of specialized procedures required in both books. It is hoped that in the future this co-operation can be expanded in joint efforts aimed at placing the two official compendia on a truly continuous revision basis.

In the preliminary planning for specifications, both the *USP* and *NF* depend upon several sources for background information. The principal sources of basic chemical information for most drugs are the pharmaceutical manufacturers who developed them. Commissioner George Larrick recently said, "Today's responsible firms exercise a degree of control that assures the American consumer of the finest drug supply ever produced in the world's history." With this I think we would all agree. Specifications for dosage forms obtained from these sources, while adequate for internal control, are not necessarily satisfactory as official standards because they apply only to one formulation. To adapt such methods so that they are generally applicable to all possible formulations, regardless of the nature of added inert substances, such as bulking agents in tablets, often requires an inordinate amount of time and effort. Moreover, no specification for a drug should ever be adopted as official before an independent determination has demonstrated its validity. This necessitates study in laboratories staffed by qualified chemists who have an appreciation of the needs of the official compendia.

For laboratory service the *USP* has depended largely upon members of the revision committee who are connected with academic, institutional, or industry laboratories. The *National Formulary*, however, has relied to quite an extent upon the staff of the American Pharmaceutical Association laboratory to supplement assistance from other sources. The results by both approaches have been equally satisfactory.

Until recently, considerable help has come from the specifications developed, with industry's co-operation, by the American Medical Association chemical laboratory. This laboratory operation has been discontinued recently and facilities to replace it are needed. Service from academic sources is becoming increasingly difficult to obtain, and the necessity of an independent laboratory specializing in the development of specifications for drugs to meet the needs of the *USP* and *NF* is apparent. There exists within the headquarters building of the American Pharmaceutical Association, the physical facilities, but not the personnel, for such laboratory assistance. It is hoped that means can be found to staff this laboratory so that its services will be available to both the *USP* and the *NF.* Plans are being formulated to accomplish this purpose.

There is one striking dissimilarity between the organizations sponsoring the USP and the *NF.* The United States Pharmacopoeial Convention is composed of representatives of organizations. Its sole function is to provide for the periodic revision and publication of the *Pharmacopeia.* It operates under a constitution and bylaws that define clearly the function of the *USP*, the duties and responsibilities of the board of trustees and the director of revision and the procedures to be followed by the revision committee.

The *National Formulary* on the other hand, is sponsored and published by the American Pharmaceutical Association, which is engaged in many activities in addition to those relating to the *NF.* In the Constitution of the Association, its first objective reads:

This Association shall exist...

1. To improve and promote the public health by aiding in the establishment of satisfactory standards for drugs, and to aid in the detection and prevention of adulteration and misbranding of drugs and medicines, and to take such steps ... as will assure the production and distribution of drugs and medicines of the highest quality.

The *National Formulary* is not mentioned in the Constitution, but is referred to in two sections of the bylaws, one outlining the duties of the officers and the Council and the other relating to standing and special committees. In view of the many and varied interests of the American Pharmaceutical Association, it might be well for it to consider defining the *National Formulary,* and referring to it in the Constitution as one of the means by which the organization's first objective is being accomplished.

Because of the important position to which the *NF* has risen over the years, and because it is a traditional fundamental activity of AMA, it would also seem desirable to provide a special chapter for it in the bylaws. This added chapter could clearly define the attitude of the Association toward the *NF* and indicate, in a general way, the duties and responsibilities of all who are directly concerned with its compilation and publication. Such changes would increase the prestige and recognition of the *National Formulary* and place it in a stronger position.

The official compendia render a service to pharmacists and pharmaceutical manufacturers by providing specifications for the procurement of drugs used in dispensing, prescription compounding, and manufacturing. Their greatest significance is the fact that standards developed by organized pharmacy as a public service, through recognition by law, protect the consumer against the distribution of inferior drugs. This recognition of the professional integrity of pharmacy possesses an inherent, but intangible value, which is all too often forgotten.

It is hoped that the positions now held by the *USP* and the *NF* will never be lost through default by those who have responsibility for supporting their revision programs. ■

1960 Remington Medalist

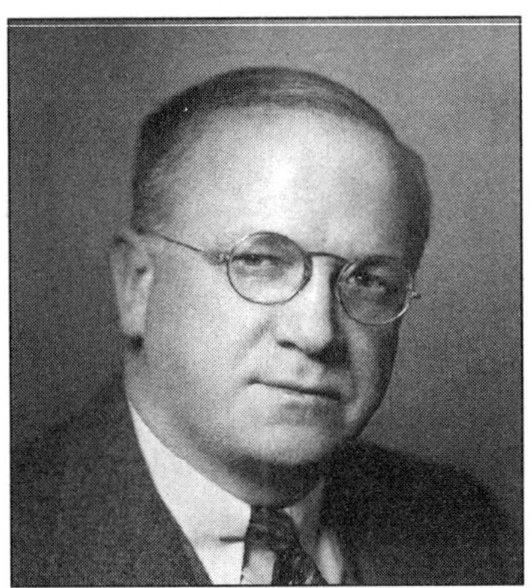

IVOR GRIFFITH
(1891-1961)

Ivor Griffith was born in Rhiwlas, North Wales, and came to the U.S.A. in 1907 where he obtained a Doctor of Pharmacy degree from the Philadelphia College of Pharmacy in 1912. He practiced pharmacy at the Stetson Hospital in Philadelphia 1913-1915, after which he joined the faculty of his *alma mater* serving as instructor 1916-1922, associate professor 1922-1936, professor 1936-1940, dean 1936-1959, and president 1941-1961. He also served as director of research for the John B. Stetson Company, professor of organic chemistry at the Wagner Institute of Science in Philadelphia, president of both the Welsh Society and the St. David's Society of Philadelphia, a member of the National Research Council committee on pharmacy 1943-1946, and is credited as the founder of the National Quinine Pool of the War Production Board in the early days of World War II.

Joining the American Pharmaceutical Association in 1916, Griffith served as secretary and president of the APhA Philadelphia Branch, chairman of the APhA Section on Practical Pharmacy and Dispensing 1920-1922, and APhA president 1943-1944. His numerous contributions to the literature include editor of *American Journal of Pharmacy* 1921-1941, "Notes and Queries" editor of *American Druggist,* editor of the 1926 edition of the *United States Dispensatory,* editor of 12 volumes of *Science Talks,* and as author of *Recent Remedies,* a scientific miscellany called *Lobscows,* and a book of poems and essays entitled To *the Lilacs.*

Creed of the Pedagogic Rebel

Ivor Griffith

The 1960 Remington Medal was presented December 7, 1960, at the Roosevelt Hotel in New York City. Griffith's Remington address was not published, but a copy of the manuscript was obtained from the archives of the Philadelphia College of Pharmacy and Science.

It goes without saying that I relish with much heart-warmth this fine award which commemorates the great dean, Joseph Remington, of Philadelphia. Man among men, teacher among teachers, author among authors, statesman and spokesman for Pharmacy his whole life through and whose influence still persists. Although he lived when the light of Pharmacy shone much more dimly than it does today, he gave a full life of devotion to its progress. As a teacher he taught his charges how to think for themselves and not just how to remember. He knew how to press his factual points into his pupil's mind with the adhesive lubricant of a bit of good humor. I take the liberty of reciting a bit of verse which I wrote some time ago in my salad days when I was green in judgment and I called it the *Creed of the Pedagogic Rebel,* but it was really a reminiscence of Remington.

I teach–try to teach–
To my ultimate objective, not with formulas collective–
Not with methods pedagogic, nor with regimented logic.
I detest mundane statistics, and those lecture hall ballistics.
Let the Czars of Education
Take their concrete transportation,
I'll take those enchanting by-ways,
Far removed from plotted highways;
Paths of beauty through the valleys–
Paths of duty through the alleys–
I shall learn as well as teach,
I shall pray as well as preach.
And I'll make a happy landing
Sooner far than those outstanding
Exhibitionists of "Teach."
For my lads, grown men, will say
"He taught us how to watch and pray,
And live rejoicing every day."
Happy Day–O! Happy Day
When teachers all shall teach that way!

Such a teacher was Remington for he knew that the capacity to live rejoicing every day is the hallmark of a truly educated man. And now may I hope for your pardon if I refer to some intimate introspections and retrospections. Firstly let me tell you how and why it pleases me to be a Welshman who wilfully and properly became an American; why I am proud to lay my microscopic accomplishments at the altar of such a Welsh ancestry. The Welshman, you must know, has evolved from a background quite complex. His racial ancestry, though fundamentally Celtic, is as complicated as the pattern of a crazy quilt. In him is a little Pictish - Scotch-Iberian-Hebrew -Roman -Norman. And you might expect from so composite a pattern-an eccentric sort of a creature. And the Welshman is a creature of many moods and as changeable as a modern teenager's face. He can be as stubborn as a Kentucky mule (ask the wife of any Welshman), yet with proper smoothing he is as pliant as a willow wand in June. He is always

Godfearing, yet often Godforgetting.

Happy as a picanniny in the morning, he may come home at night with a face as long as a canal boat, and expect his wife instantly to overlook his moods, but never his pipe and slippers. His sense of humor is as gentle as the morning dew and he does more inside laughing than anyone I know.

In short his is a most contradictory personality. To be the wife of a Welshman is therefore not only a great privilege but a tremendous responsibility for when a woman marries a Welshman she marries a dozen different men and her polyandric adventure entails a hazard high, wide and handsome.

His hymns with their plaintive, crying cadence, are the most glorious Godly, simple music of all time. He sings them to his God and to his sweetheart, at church and at the picnic, at the graveside and the banquet. Yet, indeed, you may even hear him sing them, not hum them, when Barleycorn is in his brain, and his head chuck-full of vapor. Whether the Welshman rises to the eminences or falls to the deepest depressions, the unquenchable residues of Godly fire never leave his heart or mind.

From a gentle Welsh mother, far gentler than I, and from a good father, better than I can ever hope to be, each of them born and bred as I was, in those glorious heather hills, came this imponderable bequeathment, this intangible inheritance of clear faith, which is mine and shall be time without end.

To them I now humbly, but reverently, devoutly, turn my fond rememberings and high appreciation. God keep forever green their kindly memories.

Secondly, I rejoice in the character of the several institutions with which my life has been thus far fortunately and, I hope, fruitfully spent. All have been institutions founded upon high ideals. All have been institutions stabilized by the traditions of an honorable and lost past. There is something to such survival beyond the mere coincidence, and from such contacts comes a comfort that is communicable, and a content that is contagious.

I am proud of my long relations with the institutions that bear the honored name of Stetson, of McNeil, of Samuel Wagner and his institute of Science, institutions whose ethics, whose sense of service, and whose integrity are beyond reproach.

Particularly fine have been my associations with that venerable institution, The Philadelphia College of Pharmacy and Science, where first as a student, and then as a teacher, and now as president, I have largely lived and loved my work these past three decades. This is an institution of which Philadelphia and the world of Pharmacy may well be proud.

In it have I learnt and taught these many years. Here gained I the guidance and the great friendship of men like the beloved LaWall, Remington, Sadtler, Moerk, Wetherill, Stroup, Sturmer, Cook, and many others. Here in an institution dedicated to the never ending work of finding balm for human pains, and of training young men and women in the sciences serving public health, I have spent more than a half century of my active life.

Here I first met the great Remington. I was his last assistant. Here I was inoculated with a growing respect for the practice of pharmacy and it has been growing ever since.

Unfortunate it is for a young fellow to meet a man of great intellect, of fine attributes, of national renown, when his sun was near setting and his career nigh ended. In his time he had illumined with a great and good light practically every phase of Pharmacy, and his name commemorated in this Gold Medal Award is a fine tribute to his greatness. His two faithful followers, Drs. Cook and LaWall, gave proof over the decades that their Dean, their *Pharmacopoeial* guide and counsellor would be worthy of such a memorial and it is sweet to remember that both LaWall and Cook earned the Remington award. Both felt greatly glorified and may I publicly commend the New York APhA Branch upon their kind initiative in recognizing before quiet Philadelphia ever did, this grand token of respect to the Philadelphia

Remington. And I am proud, too, of the illustrious men with whom I served my apprenticeship in Pharmacy. Modern educators have found it difficult to endorse, and possibly for good and sufficient reasons, the old system of preceptorship. Yet I gained from my preceptors more honest respect for discipline and learned much more of human relationships that I ever did at college.

Pray tell me where is the Remington of today, the Henry Hurd Rusby, and Maisch, the Arny, Caspari, Anderson, LaWall, and many other kindred eminences in men. Men who taught Frank Ryan, Josiah and Eli Lilly, Silas Burroughs, Henry Wellcome, and many others.

These are not the wailirigs of one bewildered by the years but rather the yearnings of one who remembers that colleges of pharmacy in those days taught the enduring values. I am not too sure that our extended curricula are making their mark in extending discipline and character.

The fact is that however hard we try, we are not making the men in Pharmacy today that the teacher of old was wont to inspire in spirit and in truth.

And I seize this moment to make an observation which is in propriety and good order. Such an opportunity as is presented to me tonight to speak to so distinguished and representative an audience might easily tempt me to break out into a critical rash which would bring nothing to me but an itch and a discomfort and a feeling to my listeners that I had not preserved the esthetic unities.

So I will venture nothing on certain conditions obtaining in Pharmacy which may change its conduct on every level of practice. I shall even refrain from more than airy reference to the Tennessee mountaineer senator and his inquisition of the industry. He selected for his advisors ill-informed and fractious doodle heads who fiddled with figures while his reputation alledgedly grew great at the expense of the much greater.

But listen, I pay my diligent respect to the pharmaceutical representatives who trimmed his sails with an issue of dignity and truth.

Eugene Beesley, Harry Lloynd, Arthur Munn, Dr. Connor, Dr. Austin Smith, and others grew great in contrast with the pin-headed pygmies that gained the headlines in season, but only low lines in real performance.

I remember a strangely formative turn of my life when I lost, in a brief span of a year, my beloved parents, my brothers, my life companion, and the dear Dr. LaWall, who brought arrangement into my life.

In my saddening I gained a gladdening. I grew through a sorrow a sense of dedication, a sense of devotion that centered in our beloved College, and a fine association with my comrades, the busy John Kramer, Linwood Tice, Arthur Osol, Marin Dunn, Lou Gershenfeld, Robert Jones, George Rossi, and many others. But I don't mind telling you that ultimately I gained another life companion who has brought the glow of her afternoon sun to bless me and who has made my waning years luminous and livable.

And so in accepting this gold medal, this honorable award, I do so with a deep sense of reverence and appreciation and with a proper humility.

My deep appreciation goes to my beloved lifelong friend and counsellor, Colonel Wetherill, to Professor Gershenfeld for his well intentioned accolades, and to Eli Lilly, long my esteemed friend.

One long and persistent remembering remains with me always. Hilda and I had the great privilege of walking with Eli and Ruth early one morning when the Indiana blossoms, and particularly the Shooting Stars, were at their glowingest and where the old Indian archeological shards reached out to long ago, and I shall always remember what was quietly said that morning by Eli Lilly although he may not so recall. 'We should have more time for thinking and resting in places like this." And, indeed, that was not the first time that this was said.

Spring mornings have said it ever since the First Sheriff sent the shivery sinners from their Paradise in Eden to a sunless subterranean cave. The birds said it and every blade of grass that bends with jewelled dew at dawn of day. And the wind, soft on your face in the morning and bearing burgeoned balm from every wood and thicket said it. The longing stream that sometimes finds the sea and the trout that dailies in the eddies said it.

Hail the day when Mr. Lilly's wish becomes more universal. We should have more time for rest and contemplation, and in a world where peace shall reign forever.

May I now give as my parting salute a little Welsh verse translated into the much less lovely English

Happy are we met
Happy to remain
Happy shall we part
Till we meet again. ■

1962 Remington Medalist

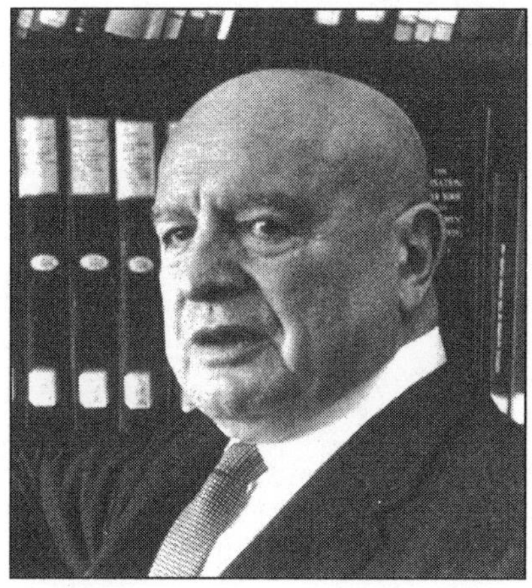

HARRY JACOB ANSLINGER
(1892-1975)

Harry Jacob Anslinger was born in Altoona, Pennsylvania, and studied at Pennsylvania State University and Washington College of Law where he received an LL.B. degree in 1913. He joined the U.S. State Department serving on the staff of the American Legation in The Hague 1918-1921, as vice consul in Hamburg, Germany 1921-1923, as consul in La Guaira, Venezuela 1923-1935, and as consul in Nassau, Bahamas 1926. He then joined the Treasury Department serving as chief of the division of foreign control 1926-1929, and as assistant commissioner of prohibition 1929-1930. In 1930, he was appointed to the newly established position as U.S. Commissioner of Narcotics, a post he held under five presidents until his retirement in 1962. During this period he served as chairman of the American Bar Association's Advisory Committee on International Cooperation in Criminal Law, as a member of the board of governors of the Diplomatic and Consular Officers Retired, as a member of the National Research Council's Committee on Drug Addiction, and as co-author of several books including *The Murderers and The Protectors.*

Anslinger represented the U.S. on many international commissions including delegate to the Conference on Suppression of Smuggling in London 1926, the Conference of Limitation of the Manufacture of Narcotic Drugs in Geneva 1931, the Conference for Suppression of Illicit Traffic in Narcotic Drugs in Geneva 1936, and a member of the League of Nations Opium Advisory Committee 1931-1939. He subsequently served as U.S. representative to the United Nations Commission on Narcotic Drugs 1946-1962.

Four Roadblocks To Truth

Harry Jacob Anslinger

The 1962 Remington Honor Medal Lecture was presented on December 4, 1962, at the Roosevelt Hotel in New York City. Anslinger's Remington address was published in the *Journal of the American Pharmaceutical Association,* volume NS3, pages 86-87, 95, 1963.

This is one of the few times during my slide down the banister of my career that splinters have pointed in the right direction.

The shortest acceptance speech by a Remington medalist was by Paul Briggs, who took sixteen minutes. The longest was by a medalist who took two and a quarter hours. I intend to break one of these records, and I have selected Paul Briggs. I was toastmaster at a dinner in Washington at which Paul spent exactly two minutes lauding the honored guest. I commented that college professors like him are too long-winded.

Secretary Reed is in charge of a multiplicity of agencies, Bureau of Customs, Alcohol & Tobacco Tax Division, Secret Service, Intelligence Unit, Bureau of Narcotics, Coast Guard, and a number of other agencies. He is like the fellow in my village who received a letter from a pharmaceutical house asking him to collect $60 from the local drug store and, failing to do so within 60 days, to give the case to a lawyer. The reply was "I own the drug store and am president of the bank, so my credit is good. I am the only lawyer in town and if it weren't for the fact that I am also the Methodist minister, I would tell you to go to hell."

The bureau rarely issued an order or regulation which applied to pharmacists without first consulting the duly accredited representatives of the pharmaceutical associations. We worked out our differences before the regulations or orders were issued. Accordingly, there ws no need for long, expensive and tiresome hearings. We have confidence in the pharmacists' policing themselves.

Since 1909 the United States has been the leader in bringing about nine treaties and protocols to suppress the abuse of narcotic drugs thoughout the world. In the United States during a fifty-year period as a result of international control, implemented by Federal and State laws, drug addiction has declined from one in 400 to one in 4,000, or a 90% reduction. The pharmacists were of invaluable assistance in bringing this about.

During the current wave of addiction, I have always been extremely happy to tell Congressional and State committees that no one can lay a finger on the pharmacists as being in any way responsible for one case among the 46,000 non-medical addicts known to the authorities.

As an example of the wonderful cooperation afforded the Bureau of Narcotics, when they saw a legible prescription for narcotics, or when they saw a doctor's signature was not identical and decided it was forged, they called in our agents, who quickly made the arrest. The pharmacists accounted for uncovering more forged prescriptions than Federal, State, and City authorities combined. I hope the doctors will continue to write illegible narcotic prescriptions, which only the pharmacists can understand.

Pharmacists are responsible for handling a greater volume of narcotic drugs than any other group of persons. The profession has always graciously accepted that responsibility in its very close cooperation with the Bureau of Narcotics throughout the history of the Bureau.

On many occasions I have been privileged to point with justifiable pride to the well-nigh spotless record of the pharmacists in maintaining the most effective control of these drugs that are so important to the well-being of mankind. No one is in a better position to understand so well as the pharmacist the consequences of loosening the reins of control over the production and dispensing of narcotic drugs.

The pharmacist undoubtedly experiences his full share of frustration and annoyance in continuously carrying out all the necessary precautions and details involved in safeguarding and accounting for every vestige of his narcotic stocks in the course of his day-to-day routine. He must throughout his professional life be thoroughly conversant with the requirements of both Federal and State laws and regulations that provide the very necessary control of all narcotic substances which he daily dispenses.

This traditional adherence of pharmacists to the spirit and intent of the Federal and State laws and regulations governing narcotic drugs convinced us that it would be both possible and feasible to relax the Federal law covering certain narcotic preparations having little addiction liability so that pharmacists could accept oral prescriptions for them, and could sell entirely without prescription those having no addiction potential. Thus we placed the entire responsibility for dispensing these substances at the discretion of the pharmacist. The splendid spirit of dedication and continuous vigilance that has pervaded the pharmacy profession has always merited the greatest respect of the Bureau of Narcotics. No words of commendation can adequately express the profound appreciation of the Bureau for the excellent professional relations and genuine friendliness that have flourished through the years.

During the recent meeting of the United Nations Narcotic Commission, the French delegate complained about the large number of new drugs coming on the market and used a term *FARMOCOMANIA*, stating this was a serious problem which confronted pharmacists. He said eight new products were on the market. In the United States there were 78, which is another proof of the industry and resourcefulness of the American pharmacist as compared wit his opposite numbers in other advanced countries. The American pharmacist is the envy of the world.

At the last session of the United Nations Narcotic Commission, an attempt was made to place barbiturates under international control. This would have put these useful drugs under the same strict control as narcotic drugs, including estimates, import and export certificates, a requirement to license all dealers, keep separate records, and a multitude of other duties. The United States, with the help of other nations, was able to defeat this proposal. It would have entailed administrative burdens on the government, the drug industry, and the professions. There is no need for such control, as there has been no international illicit traffic. A resolution was adopted urging all countries to place manufacture and distribution under control.

The nine treaties and protocols controlling the international narcotic traffic include limitation of production, limitation of manufacture, control of distribution, and regulation of the trade. All nations participate in this cooperative effort except two. You must have universality for complete control. When these bullies who strut across the international stage, ready to draw the sword if they are not obeyed, are a thing of the past, then we will have universality. We can then join the Indian philosopher who said, "If I be dust, then the whole world is my country, and everybody in it is my kin."

Former Secretary of State Cordell Hull stated, "In no field of international relations has there been greater cooperation than in the field of narcotic drugs." And here is a similar analogy on our national scene. In no field of relations between government and industry has there been greater cooperation than between the pharmacists of the United States and the Federal Bureau of Narcotics.

There are four roadblocks to truth which I have encountered:

The influence of fragile and unworthy authority; Custom; The imperfection of undisciplined senses; And most important - Concealment of ignorance by ostentation of seeming wisdom.

These the pharmacist must keep in mind in his important profession. ■

1963 Remington Medalist

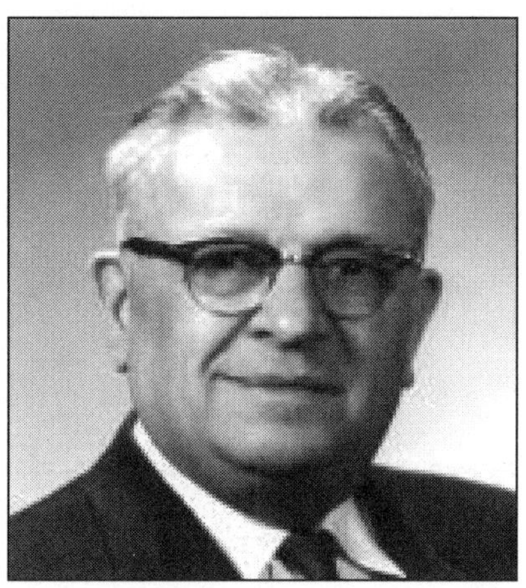

Glenn Llewellyn Jenkins
(1898-1979)

Glenn Llewellyn Jenkins was born in Sparta, Wisconsin, and after service in the Student Army Training Corps during World War I, graduated from the University of Wisconsin receiving B.S. (1922), M.S. (1923), and Ph.D. (1926) degrees. He served variously as instructor in pharmacy at the University of Wisconsin 1926-1927, and professor of pharmaceutical chemistry at both the University of Maryland 1927-1936 and the University of Minnesota 1936-1941. He was named dean at the Purdue University School of Pharmacy in 1941, a position he held until his retirement in 1965. He served as chairman of the Indiana Interprofessional Health Council 1941-1956; chairman of the Indiana State Board of Health 1958-1960; national president of Rho Chi 1930-1934; president of the American Association of Colleges of Pharmacy 1944-1946; and a member of both the USP revision committee 1940-1960, and the American Council on Pharmaceutical Education 1948-1952.

Jenkins joined the American Pharmaceutical Association in 1927, receiving the APhA Ebert Prize for medicinal chemistry research in 1936, and the APhA Foundation's Achievement Award for the Stimulation of Research in 1962. He served variously as chairman of the APhA Section on Education and Legislation 1929-1930; chairman of the APhA Scientific Section 1936-1937; APhA second vice president 1937-1938; vice chairman 1938-1940 and chairman 1940-1941 of the APhA Council; chairman of the APhA House of Delegates 1943-1944; and APhA president 1949-1950. In 1949, he chaired the APhA Mission to Japan to advise General MacArthur's staff on pharmacy education and practice.

The Most Courageous Thing I Ever Did

Glenn Llewellyn Jenkins

The 1963 Remington Honor Medal Lecture was presented on December 3, 1963, at the Astor Hotel in New York City. Jenkins's Remington address was published in the *NARD.Journal* volume 86, pages 14-15, 39, January 20, 1964.

My profound appreciation to all of you. It is with great pleasure and pride that I accept the Remington medal, particularly in recognition of my work in the area of advanced education. The first place ranking (Walter Crosby, "Leading American Graduate Schools," *The Association of American Colleges Bulletin* volume 43, No. 4, December 1957) of the school which I head for graduate work in the pharmacal sciences could only be developed on the foundation of a strong and sound undergraduate program. Of course, I recognize that at this moment I am basking in the reflected achievements of almost three hundred former graduate students. Not a single one of those with whom I have been associated in this advanced study and research has proven a liability to our profession, to science, or to me. This shows that a sound four year baccalaureate followed by well designed advanced study is the true road to progress. I am pleased, too, that the medal is given for work in education, for it is my opinion that education holds the key to the future advancement of our profession. As the recipient of the Remington medal I am only the representative of many colleagues at Purdue and elsewhere who labor for the greatest and noblest of all the professions, the development of the minds of men.

This seems to be the year when medals are given for saying "no." I am not happy to be placed in company with the recipient of a political gold medal. I suspect that I'm not being given the Remington medal for my opposition to the minimum five-year course in pharmacy. But I should have been because it was probably the most courageous thing I ever did in my professional public life, and I stood almost alone. And I was right, for the extended program can lead only to mediocrity or chaotic conditions. This statement deserves some elaboration.

Economists now recognize that the live dynamic forces introduced into the economy by education and research may well spell the difference between economic stagnation and faster rate of growth. This statement summarizes the efforts being made in most nations of the world to meet the crisis in education precipitated by the impact of science on human society. Science and human capital in the form of superior scientists who develop it are now the real basis for wealth of any nation, industry, or profession. Science through the dynamic factor in the advancement of technology and the scientific method is the prime manner by which a profession can fulfill its function in society.

Science has altered the conditions of human life in this world more radically in the last 100 years than anything that has happened in past history, and the rate at which it is expanding its control over and power to alter our existence is beyond our imagination.

Modern science concerns itself with the understanding of all nature including our physical environment, all living things, and especially man himself. It is a part of our health, food, transport, defense, and economic well-being as well as our social and political life. It has become a major element in our way of life. It is growing and creating a high and expanding demand for able personnel with advanced training. Pharmacy needs quantity and quality of manpower both for professional practice and for scientific and technological work. The competition for able superior students to enter the sciences such as biology, chemistry, engineering, and physics is intense. In this competition a program extended beyond four years for the baccalaureate is at a great disadvantage; it is incompatible with graduate education. The factors of time and median level instruction repel rather than attract the science oriented students to our professional schools. The experience requirement adds just one more barrier to the attraction of intelligent youth.

We have now had enough experience with the extended curriculum to know that we cannot secure our fair share of the superior and exceptional students motivated toward a career in science under our programs. There is an increasing opinion that the educational program, for example in chemistry, biology, and physics where the upper strata of students completing the undergraduate program are selected for graduate work are superior to extended programs in professional education. In fact, the four-year baccalaureate is the American way of entry into the study of science. Consequently, some of our schools of pharmacy seek to recruit the four-year graduates with majors in chemistry, biology, and other sciences. When these finish their graduate work and enter teaching they may be quite competent but they will not have the allegiance and the *esprit de corps* desired in a profession. Some schools have established and others are establishing four-year non-professional degrees in the basic pharmacal sciences, e.g., medicinal chemistry, pharmacology, bionucleonics, and physical pharmacy. These programs are necessary if pharmacy is to salvage even a low level chance to participate in the present scientific age. They will cause some confusion and chaos in the profession, but our great universities will not be denied fulfilling their chartered obligations.

There is a logical alternative. I recommend a restructuring of the plan for education in pharmacy and the pharmacal sciences. The elements of the new plan which I believe to be sound are as follows: A four-year program leading to the B.S. degree. This might be an integrated program with all four years in the pharmacy college or a pre-pharmacy year or years followed by professional and scientific instruction. This B.S. degree should form the base for additional education leading to various specialties, e.g. professional practice in community pharmacy or hospital pharmacy. It should also form the base for graduate work for those who can qualify for admission to graduate schools. The length and content of the specialized education could be changed to meet changing conditions. The basic B.S. degree would permit cross over from one area of specialization to another such as from hospital pharmacy to community pharmacy with a minimum of lost time and expense as barriers become erected in the various specialties. It would be flexible and would permit those who wish to enter such areas as research, production, control, education, professional service representation, or industrial management to specialize in advanced courses with graduate credit toward an advanced degree when qualified. If they wished to gain professional licensure they could fulfill the requirements for professional practice.

This plan would provide economy of time and money better than the present program, and it would enable the B.S. graduate to select the career of his choice after he had reached a mature level. It would upgrade the quality of instruction in our schools of pharmacy. It would insure the flow of superior students into advanced fields of study to provide the qualified manpower necessary to extend the frontiers of pharmacy through scholarly effort and research. It would give each school autonomy to emphasize areas of specialization where superior staff and facilities can be provided.

I also recommend that the apprenticeship system as we have known it be abolished as a legal requirement for licensure. Voluntary apprenticeship would always be available. The old art and processes of collecting, grinding, preparing, extracting, and mixing drugs were almost ideally adapted to the concept of a preceptor and a neophyte working together and the transfer of knowledge from master to beginner. The art of pharmacy has been largely replaced by science. The tempo of modern business does not lend itself to leisurely personal preceptorship. It is an obsolete system characterized by the exploitation of youth, maintained largely by greed and selfishness, and is a prime cause for the breakdown of the idealism and ethics in the youth who enter the profession. Licensure should follow completion of the basic and professional education with a "diplomate" or other rank for those who qualify in a specialty.

The thoughts I have expressed are brief and unsupported by lengthy argument, but I believe that the conclusions are obvious.

Finer language might have been used, which reminds me of the story of an American speaker who used the expression, "That ain't hay." He was followed by a gentlemen from Britain who, using clipped Shakespearian actor's enunciation, said,

"That is not the clipping from yon meadow." I am quite sure that what I have said is understandable. It is interesting to note that mature individuals who ascend to leadership forget what they were like when they were young. I am sure that our mature leaders have forgotten the careful analysis and comparative evaluation which they employed. Talented young men and women did not and do not fumble and bumble their way into a scientific career.

Had pharmacy education in my student days borne the same relationship to all other fields of education that it bears today, I would not be the Remington medalist now. Likewise, I have learned from inquiry that a substantial majority of the Ph.D.'s who are leaders in pharmacal science would be in other career fields. Is further argument necessary?

I thank you for the honor you have bestowed upon me. For pharmacy through our professional education, I wish a new era characterized by excellence in professional practice, teaching, research, and all our proper efforts. Through unselfish service I'm sure we can make pharmacy a great and vital force in this age of science. ■

1964 Remington Medalist

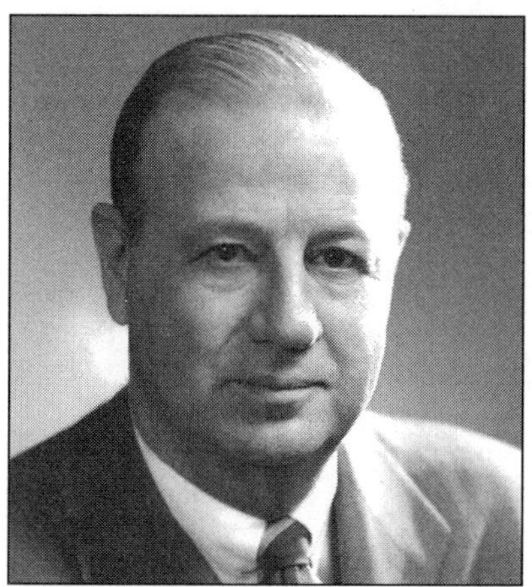

ROBERT ANDREW HARDT
(1901-1978)

Robert Andrew Hardt was born in Friend, Nebraska, and after military service during World War I, graduated from the University of Nebraska College of Pharmacy with a Ph.G. degree in 1922. He commenced practice in his father's pharmacy in Hastings, Nebraska, arid was appointed secretary of the Nebraska Board of Pharmacy in 1923, the youngest person in the country to have served in such a capacity. He joined E.R. Squibb and Sons in 1926 advancing to the position of vice president in 1946 when he moved to Hoffmann-La Roche as vice president 1948-1957, and to Armour Pharmaceutical Laboratories as president 1958-1963. He subsequently served as a consultant to various firms until his retirement to Delray Beach, Florida. He authored *The Pharmaceutical Industry* (1946) and co-authored *Drug Research and Development.*

As president of the American Pharmaceutical Manufacturers Association 1954-1955, Hardt organized at Rensselaer (New York) Polytechnic Institute a three-day program at which more than 1,000 social science teachers learned how pharmacists serve the nation. He served as president of National Pharmaceutical Council 1956-1957, and as president of the Fourth Pan American Congress of Pharmacy held in Washington, D.C. 1957 for which he was honored as the 1957 *American Druggist* "Man of the Year." Hardt joined the American Pharmaceutical Association in 1938, serving as a member of the APhA international relations committee 1959-1961, and a member of the APhA Council 1962-1965.

Responsibilities of Pharmacy's Leadership

Robert Andrew Hardt

The 1964 Remington Honor Medal Lecture was presented on December 9, 1964, at the Roosevelt Hotel in New York City. Hardt's Remington address was never published but is preserved as an original manuscript in the APhA Archives.

To merely say that I am grateful for the honor you are bestowing upon me this evening would be an anemic declaration; in other words, a cliche, if I did not make my gratitude clear to you in some other way.

Perhaps I have done so already by my selection of the two fine young speakers who have preceded me at this lectern. Perhaps, I can do more to show my deep appreciation before this meeting is adjourned. One way would be to conclude this speech within the span of human attention which I understand is a maximum of 20 minutes.

When the secretary of the Remington Award Committee, Dr. Hugo Schaefer, notified me that I had been nominated for the medal, he made what, I hope, was a facetious remark in his letter requesting biographical data. As I recall the letter, he wrote: "Now just because you have been nominated doesn't mean you have been chosen, so don't rush out and buy a new tuxedo. Others have also been nominated and the APhA past presidents must vote and they are not stupid."

Such candor is quite characteristic of Dr. Schaefer and the statement was quite proper, if not prophetic.

In paying my tribute to Dr. Joseph P. Remington in whose honor this cherished award was named, I am glad to say that the Remington Professor of Pharmacy at the Philadelphia College of Pharmacy and Science, Dean Linwood Tice, is in this audience and I consider this a special honor.

I am indebted to Dean Tice for biographical data concerning Professor Remington which I explored with avid interest.

For a period of at least 25 years, Professor Joseph P. Remington was the foremost figure in American pharmacy. Genial and eloquent, a keen student of human nature, a lover of the beautiful in art, music and literature, he possessed a fund of scientific knowledge of unusually broad scope. These are some of the qualities which were combined in him to make a great teacher, a capable executive and Christian gentlemen.

Inasmuch as I never knew Professor Remington, I researched his career for some common ground; some few things which would enable me to become even remotely identified with him. At last I found them. We were both once associated with E. R. Squibb & Sons and my wife is probably distantly related to his mother.

As some of you know, I normally have a well stuffed satchel of punch lines, many of which have been filched from others. However, tonight I find my self constrained to deliver a message rather than entertain with jokes and wise cracks. Nevertheless, should I find that you are not concentrating on my material, I promise a quick shift to the less serious.

Tonight I have chosen to say something about the responsibilities of pharmacy's leadership. In doing so, I do not flatter myself that I am a part of that leadership because I am quite certain this is not the case. I do feel, however, that I have had a small part in the indoctrination of some of the new leaders and for this experience, I shall always be grateful.

As you well know, the profession of pharmacy has problems. Some are not easily solved. If I were to stand here and give easy answers for their solution, they would be no answers at all.

Our new generation of pharmacists have developed a style and grace which is not only admirable, but reassuring to the older generations.These new leaders, in my opinion, have the dedication, the selflessness, and the intelligence to solve our problems. For this we should consider ourselves fortunate.

As many of us have learned by long experience, a person can accomplish much he doesn't care who gets the credit.

In organizations, in governments, in industry, and even in families, personal, ambitions frequently transcend the real objectives of a program. Human nature being what it is, this problem will always be with us. Indeed, it is one of the basic reasons for the failure of nations to live with each other in harmony and peace. Discouraging and frustrating as this obstacle may be, progress can come from strife.

Fortunately, however, there are always a few people who rise above bickering and jealousies and who can see the worthwhile goal for all.

In speeches made to pharmacists and to industry during the past two decades, I have frequently made predictions and I propose to do so again tonight. Some of these predictions have not materialized, others were wrong as to timing, but a good percentage were fulfilled and this encourages me to try again. I am no prophet and I have no crystal ball, so let me preface these predictions with some philosophy which may cause you to have more confidence in them.

Sir Arthur Conan Doyle once said that from a drop of water, a logician could infer the possibility of an ocean or a Niagara Falls without having seen or heard of one or the other.

People who really know and think about their subject are seldom surprised by the course of events. The reason is that events have a logic and rhythm of their own. If we master one and become attuned to the other, it is quite possible to predict with an accuracy that might look like black magic to the uninitiated.

By a logic of their own, developments in Venus arising from the waves and skipping the normal processes of gestation.

Keeping this philosophy in mind, I venture to make the following predictions relating to the profession of pharmacy.

Prediction #1

The profession of pharmacy in the U.S., as represented by its various organizations, will assume even a greater role in world leadership. More and more U.S. pharmacists will travel abroad and make their influence felt in many ways. In a recent visit to 12 countries in the Middle and Far East, I saw evidence of this. There were numerous copies of U.S. journals in college and pharmaceutical industry libraries. One Australian pharmacy dean said, "I almost feel I know Dr. Apple from his writings." Others told me of numerous people in U.S. pharmacy whom they greatly admired for thcir dedication to the profession.

All are watching our progress with the greatest interest because they have similar problems.

Prediction #2

We shall soon see more pharmacies convert to pharmaceutical service centers of the type innovated by Eugene B. White of Berryville, Virginia. I suggest that all pharmacists watch this development with interest. It can create new interest among young men and women who are seeking a professional career... and it can solve some of our recruitment problems.

The shortage of pharmacists will become even a more serious problem. Demographers warn us that we shall have another doubling of our population before the end of this century... a mere 35 years. When we realize that the first doubling of our population from year 1 A.D. required 1600 years, we are shocked into realization of what is now occurring. This new public of 6,000 million instead of our present 3,000 million must be more health conscious to even survive.

Prediction #3
More and more of our pharmacists will be employed in hospitals, by government, by medical centers, by co-ops and insurance groups, by industry, and by new bureaus whose functions and existence will be influenced by social trends. This does not mean that the community pharmacists, as we know them today, will disappear. Quantitatively, they may be diminished, but qualitatively they will be strengthened.

Prediction #4
Pharmacy organizations local, state and national will grow in membership and in services and thus in power to the point where they can really make their voices heard in government and in society in general. This may come about as an essential element of progress and even survival in a changing world. To me it seems quite clear that in those countries where pharmacy has been nationalized or socialized, pharmacists manage best when they are well organized.

Prediction #5
Therapy, complex as it is today, will become even more complex as more and more pharmaceutical discoveries are made. We have reached an age where not only new agents are being discovered, but also an age when drugs are being administered to people who are perfectly well. For the first time in the history of mankind, several million persons are taking a drug to alter physiological functions. I refer, of course to estrogen progestin combinations which are now being taken by healthy women for 20 days each cycle to prevent or postpone ovulation.

Other such breakthroughs may be anticipated in the future. Let us hope that one of these will be for the prevention of cancer, or coronary disease, or both.

Prediction #6
I predict that in the future all organizations in pharmacy will work together for the common good of the profession. This is what the membership of various organizations is hoping for and even demanding. The new leaders of the profession know this and they also know the value of such cooperation. There are problems involved; problems of human relationships, problems of semantics and socio-economic problems. Nevertheless the will to accomplish this is emerging and there is reason for optimism.

Prediction #7
Those pharmacists who wish to do so, will play an increasingly important role as therapeutic consultants to the medical profession. I say those who wish to do so advisedly because not all pharmacists are enthusiastic about practicing their profession to the extent of serving as drug consultants to practicing physicians. Yet, they can do so if they gradually make it apparent that they can serve as an intelligent, objective source of information about the most dynamic and complex side of the practice of medicine drug therapy.

Prediction #8
We shall have reclassification of drugs in one way or another because the need is becoming increasingly clear.

This reclassification will include the following categories of drugs: 1. Those to be dispensed at the request of a medical practitioner and renewable at the prescribers discretion. 2. Those to be dispensed at the request of a medical practitioner and renewable for a reasonable period at the pharmacists discretion. 3. Those to be dispensed personally by a pharmacist at his professional discretion at the request of the patient. 4. Those to be sold to the public without supervision or control.

The question has been raised by some thoughtful people, “would reclassification be a burden or a betterment”? It would, in my opinion, be both. The burden of increased responsibility and the betterment of pharmaceutical service and thus the public health.

When we became pharmacists, we accepted the privileges and responsibility of our professional license. The new generation of pharmacists are willing to accept increased responsibilities without waiting to have them forced upon them.

Prediction #9

Pharmacists everywhere will take giant forward strides in eliminating the feeling of insecurity which is probably caused by being halfway a professional and halfway a merchant. Thus according to psychologists, the pharmacist, has misgivings about his selfimage and social prestige.

For a more searching self-analysis, I refer you to Dr. Dichter's new book *Handbook of Consumer Motivations. I* don't think we should permit psychologists to "bug us" nor make us feel even more insecure in our role. However there is much to be learned about ourselves and what makes us think and act the way we do.

Prediction #10

Medicare, in some form, seems inevitable. This could mean the by-passing of the community pharmacist and also the whole saler unless organizations representing them are alert and vigilant.

Everything possible should be done to avoid destruction of the traditional relationship between community pharmacists and patients whether covered by medicare or not.

There is a rhyme attributed to Sir William Osler, the distinguished physician, who in an era when retirement was earlier because the life span was shorter, wrote: "Brothers, I am sixty-one, now my work on earth is done, calm should follow after storm, hand me down the chloroform."

My approach is to be somewhat different and will be: "Brothers, I am sixty-five, now's the time to be alive, if I should run out of steam, please pass me some Benzedrine."

The world around us is changing. We cannot ignore these changes as they affect the nature of the practice of pharmacy.

Our profession was not built by men who were striving to be common. It was built by men and women who were trying to distinguish themselves.

Our organizations were fashioned to move with our times as well as the future. They were fashioned to meet the changing needs of the profession and the public. They will, in my opinion, do so on an accelerated basis under organized pharmacy's contemporary and future leadership. ■

1965 Remington Medalist

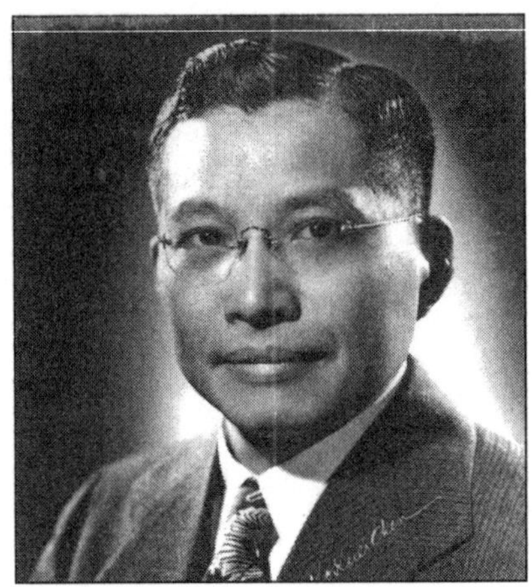

Ko Kuei Chen

(1898-1988)

Ko Kuel Chen was born in Shanghai, China. After graduation from Tsing Hua College in Bejing in 1918, he came to the United States where he graduated from the University of Wisconsin with a B.S. degree in 1920 and a Ph.D. degree in pharmacology in 1923. He returned to China for two years (1923-1925) to care for his ailing mother, during which time he conducted research at the Union Medical College in Bejing on the ancient Chinese drug *ma huang* from which he isolated ephedrine in 1924, and co-authored with Carl F. Schmidt a textbook *Ephedrine and Related Substances* (1930). He returned to the United States in 1925 to become an associate in pharmacology at Johns Hopkins University School of Medicine where he received an M.D. degree in 1927.

Chen joined Eli Lilly and Company in 1929 as director of pharmacological research, a position he held until his retirement in 1963. During this period, he served as president of the American Society of Experimental Pharmacology and Therapy 1952-1953, as chairman of the executive committee of the American Societies for Experimental Biology 1953-1954, and as U.S. delegate to the first general assembly of the International Union of Physiological Sciences 1956. Upon his retirement from Lilly, Chen was appointed chairman of the pharmacology panel of the U.S. Office of Science and Technology in 1964, and served as professor of pharmacology at Indiana University School of Medicine until his final retirement.

In Pursuit of Science

Ko Kuei Chen

The 1965 Remington Honor Medal Lecture was presented on December 1, 1965, at the Roosevelt Hotel in New York City. Chen's Remington address was published in the Journal *of the American Pharmaceutical Association,* volume NS6, pages 27-28, 1966.

I want to lose no time in thanking the past presidents and the New York Chapter of the American Pharmaceutical Association for the award of the Remington Honor Medal conferred on me. I am simply overwhelmed. Dr. George Armstrong and Dr. George Hager have tried their utmost to justify the action taken by the officers of APhA. To all medical officers of the army and to all Chinese physicians, Dr. Armstrong is the general and the authority of the medical sciences at all times-in peace and in war. Dean Hager has been my colleague for a long time and we now meet more often at the same study sections and training grants committee of the National Institutes of Health. I am very grateful for the generous remarks of these men and naturally proud of their approval.

Some of you may be interested in knowing how I happened to come to this country to study pharmacy. In China sick people were treated with preparations of native herbs on an empirical basis. When I was graduated from a junior college in Peking in 1918, I made up my mind to analyze these interesting herbs reputed to have healing properties. My teachers in China advised me to matriculate at the University of Wisconsin and wrote letters of recommendation. When I arrived at Madison, the registrar of the University did not know where to put me so referred me to Professor Edward Kremers, the tenth Remington medalist. Professor Kremers mapped out my program with great emphasis on chemistry, including his own course on phytochemistry. My initial expenditure was on the sixth edition of *Remington's Practice of Pharmacy* and the *US. Pharmacopeia, IX Revision,* which was completed under the chairmanship of Remington. I learned how to use the U.S. *Dispensatory, 20th Edition,* by Remington and Wood. I did not dream that one day I would be eligible to receive the precious medal named after Remington.

After I obtained my bachelor's degree in pharmacy, Professor Kremers assigned to me a research problem on the essential oil of Chinese cinnamon leaves and twigs which he imported from China through the courtesy of the American embassy at Peking. The results were published in the December 1923 issue of the *Journal of the American Pharmaceutical Association.* While Professor Kremers urged me to concentrate my mind on scientific pharmacy, I figured that I should know something about the profession of pharmacy. I got myself a part-time job in a drugstore. For the first few weeks my preceptor asked me to work at the prescription counter. Being satisfied with my work, he let me wait at the soda fountain.

As my research on *Cinnamonium cassia* was in progress, I noted that there was a gap between pharmacy on one hand and physiology and pharmacology on the other. The scientists of the latter category had their own problems and would not be interested in investigating any pure substances I might isolate from the Chinese herbs. I gave this matter a great deal of thought and I transferred from the pharmacy school to physiology and pharmacology while still at Wisconsin.

Professors Bradley, Meek and Loevenhart advised me to register in the medical school because the prerequisites were identical. In 1923 the university awarded me a PhD degree in physiology and pharmacology.

At that time I was obliged to return to China because my mother was seriously sick. I took her to a modern hospital and within a short period of treatment she regained her health and lived 13 happy years thereafter.

Before I left Wisconsin in 1923 I was successful in arranging for a teaching position at Peking Union Medical College. There I had the first opportunity to apply my knowledge of pharmacy to medical research. My uncle, an herbalist, told me that a very toxic drug, called *ma huang,* when used properly, would reduce fever and stimulate circulation. By sheer luck I isolated an alkaloid ephedrine without prior knowledge but it actually was already known in 1887. My superior, Professor Carl F. Schmidt, collaborated with me and we concentrated our efforts on its pharmacological action and then on its clinical applications. Since then many more sympathomimetic drugs have been introduced into medicine and ephedrine has been totally synthesized by a novel process.

In 1925 I came back to the United States and continued my medical studies at Johns Hopkins University. It was my good fortune that Professor John J. Abel, the father of American pharmacology, took me on his staff. His laboratory was not only full of scientific atmosphere but was also adapted to conversations of daily life at the lunch table.

While it was a privilege to work in Professor Abel's laboratory, my ambition was to go back to China if a university or a medical school with research facilities would offer me a position so that I could utilize my education in pharmacy, chemistry, pharmacology and medicine. My work had been cut out to prove the scientific value of numerous Chinese herbs, especially because my studies on ephedrine could serve as a model.

Meanwhile the management of Eli Lilly and Company sent for me and asked me to set up a pharmacological laboratory entirely for research. In the depression year of 1929 I was fearful of taking responsibilities in industry. I told J.K. Lilly, also a Remington medalist, "I do not know the drug business."

He immediately replied, "We will run the business but you do what you have been doing in the university." This started my 34 years of pleasant work at the Lilly Research Laboratories.

Like all of you, I witnessed great advances and revolutions in pharmacy and medicine. My associates and I investigated 18 crude drugs imported from the Orient but after pharmacological evaluation and preclinical trials, a majority of the pure substances could not be justifiably introduced into medicine. Nevertheless I did not lose faith in empirical medicine and drugs of natural origin because ergonovine, digitoxin, reserpine, dicoumarol, antibiotics, vinblastine and vincristine all arrived during my lifetime. Vitamins belong to the same class. Beriberi, scurvy, rickets, pellagra and xerophthalmia have become rare diseases.

As *USP* and *NF* continue revisions, we cannot help noticing the disappearance of galenical preparations and their replacement by synthetic organic chemicals. The short-acting barbiturates not only give patients sleep without hangover but some also qualify as anesthetics in place of ether. The whole gamut of autonomic drugs has been studied by pharmacologists for more than one-half century. New chemotherapy has brought the morbidity and mortality of major infections to a minimum-I refer to pneumonia, tuberculosis, gonorrhea, malaria, syphilis, trachoma, poliomyelitis and measles. Effective antidotes are available against poisoning by cyanides and heavy metals. Hormones and steroids correct endocrine disorders and even regulate our population growth. Non-addicting analgesics have become a reality.

These amazing developments are made possible by human efforts. The faculties and students of pharmacy and medical schools today have higher standards of education and are therefore more capable of carrying out pharmaceutical, chemical and biomedical research. The support given by the government, industry and private foundations has relieved the handicap of space and equipment. How can one help not finding things new in biological and pharmaceutical research? More and more industry is making original and important contributions.

Pharmacists, community practitioners, hospital pharmacists, wholesalers and pharmacists in industry and physicians of every specialty work hand in hand for the patient care and public health. They communicate with one another to render the best service to the sick. The learned and professional societies offer continuing education at annual meetings and through their scientific and professional journals. I am particularly glad to see the formation of the APhA Academy of Pharmaceutical Sciences. It is important to point out that in the health field, a profession must be founded on a solid scientific base, otherwise it will lost its ground and may eventually deteriorate. Pharmacists everywhere are indebted to the American Pharmaceutical Association for never having lost sight of this fact and I am sure that much of the growth of our national professional society and its prestige is a direct result of its pursuing this fundamental philosophy. Our shrine is in Washington, but our influence is felt all over the world.

Since I spent almost one-half of my life at Eli Lilly and Company, I would like to give you a few observations. Our management generously allowed me to conduct both academic and applied research with full freedom. There was a staff of competent scientists and each problem was solved by a group of employees. Ultimate decisions of marketing products were based on scientific merits. I have no claim for the rapid growth of this organization because my contributions are trivial but I have certainly enjoyed my long association with the Lilly Company.

I do want to take this opportunity to acknowledge my heartfelt gratitude to the United States as a whole. I mentioned the junior college that was Tsing Hua College established by the Boxer Indemnity Fund. I was there from 1916-18. I was in China from 1923 to 1925 but my connection was with Peking Union Medical College of the Rockefeller Foundation. The rest of my adult life has been spent in this country.

I wish specifically to thank the University of Wisconsin, Johns Hopkins University, Eli Lilly and Company, through the good offices of Eugene Beesley, and Indiana University. I also wish to thank Dean William S. Middleton, Professors Harold C. Bradley and Carl F. Schmidt and the late Professors Edward Kremers, Walter J. Meek, Arthur S. Loevenhart and John J. Abel. I will continue to teach and do my research as long as I am able so that I may deserve my selection for this significant recognition. ■

1967 Remington Medalist

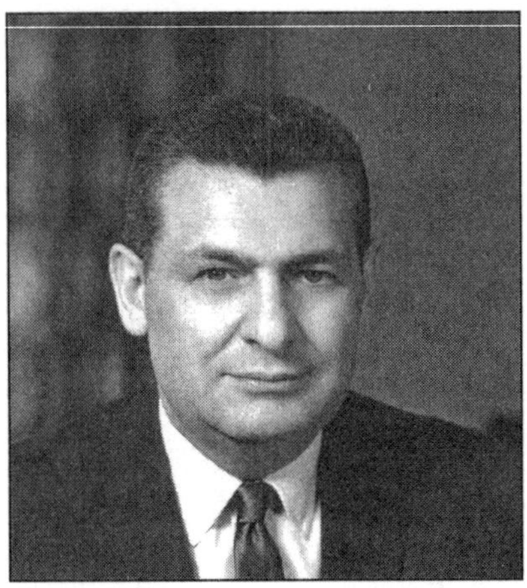

William Shoulden Apple
(1918-1983)

William Shoulden Apple was born in Spokane, Washington, and reared in Duluth, Minnesota. He enlisted as a private in the U.S. Army and rose to the rank of major after graduation in 1944 from the Command and General Staff School in Fort Leavenworth, Kansas, serving in the Pacific Theater during World War II. After attendance at Wayne State University 1945-1946, he received a B.S. in pharmacy in 1949 from the University of Wisconsin and practiced pharmacy for a time in Phillips, Wisconsin. He returned to the University of Wisconsin to obtain an M.S. in business administration in 1951, and a Ph.D. in 1954. He joined the faculty of his *alma mater* serving as pharmacy instructor 1951-1953, assistant professor 1953-1956 and as the first head of the department of pharmacy administration 1956-1958. He served as president of the Wisconsin Pharmaceutical Association 1956-1957 and was elected executive secretary of the state association early in 1958. But before he assumed that position, he was elected secretary-nominate of the American Pharmaceutical Association 1958-1959 becoming APhA chief executive officer in 1959. During the ensuing 25 years as APhA chief executive officer, Apple pioneered such concepts as the "professional fee" and "drug product selection," and doubled the membership of APhA.

Apple served variously as vice president of the National Health Council 1961-1968; president of the American Council on Pharmaceutical Education 1964-1968; president of the National Drug Trade Conference 1970; and charter member of the Committee of 100 for National Health Insurance. He received worldwide recognition as vice president of the International Pharmaceutical Federation 1974-1979.

Declaration of Independence

William Shoulden Apple

The 1967 Remington Honor Medal Lecture was presented on November 29, 1967, at the Statler Hilton Hotel in New York City. Apple's Remington address was published in the *Journal of the American Pharmaceutical Association,* volume NS8, pages 8-9, 51, 1968.

The man who suggested that the profession perpetuate in a fitting manner the memory of Professor Joseph Price Remington was Hugo H. Schaefer. If this evening only afforded me the opportunity of expressing my respect for Hugo Schaefer and honoring his memory, I would have all the recognition I need.

The man who had the distinction of being the first Remington medalist was an educator, scientist, writer, diplomat, legislator and dynamic leader of the American Pharmaceutical Association during one of the most controversial periods in American pharmacy. When James Hartley Beal received his medal, he paid the following tribute to Remington:

"When I first became a member of the Association many years ago, Professor Remington was one of the first to extend the hand of professional fellowship and from the day of that first acquaintance until the last his sympathetic advice and encouragement were unfailing."

As many of you know, Dr. Schaefer was my Professor Remington.

Pharmacy like other professions is a jealous mistress and pharmacists expect their official spokesman to express their viewpoints publicly. Only on such a rare occasion as this would I claim the privilege of speaking for myself.

The historian Henry Adams once said, "A teacher affects eternity; he can never tell where his influence stops." I have had the good fortune of being exposed to many wise and stimulating teachers, both inside and outside of the classroom. They taught me that nothing is so perfect that it can't be improved. They taught me that men who attempt to preserve the status quo march to battle on a treadmill. They taught me that hard work can be fun. They taught me that the majority is never right until it does right. And, they taught me that every man is an unpredictable combination of strengths and weaknesses. To all my teachers, wherever they are, I say-thank you.

As you have been told, I was a college professor for a brief period. My colleagues at Wisconsin could tell you that I spent as much time on the affairs of the profession as I did on my teaching responsibilities. As I think back, I recognize that I was just as interested in what pharmacy graduates would be doing with their education as I was with helping to give them that education. This was the period in which the Elliott Pharmaceutical Survey was reported and widely discussed. Most of my classmates were veterans of World War II and many of my students were veterans of the Korean conflict. The experience of fighting for country and ideals is not easily dismissed. As good as things were in pharmacy, the young turks thought the profession could and should be improved.

Many consider World War II as the end of the "what you do" period in pharmacy and the beginning of the "what you know" period. It marked the end of the philosophy that pharmacy was not pharmacy unless it involved the individual practitioner's compounding and dispensing the medication. It marked the end of the period in which the majority of the profession concentrated on manipulative functions. It marked the beginning of the period in which pharmacists concentrated on the scientific knowledge of drug therapy. It marked the beginning of the period in which our graduate studies in pharmacy rapidly expanded to meet the insatiable demand of industry for pharmaceutical research and production scientists.

Today, pharmacists in industry who contribute to the discovery and improvement of drugs, or who are engaged in their production and distribution, are held in esteem by that part of our profession which directly serves the public. Most of the pharmacists I know who went on for graduate degrees and found their niches in the pharmaceutical industry have not lost their empathy for the pharmacist in general practice. They recognize that he too must find professional independence and psychic reward.

A decade ago, my colleagues and students were talking about the need for pharmacy to draft and declare its own contemporary declaration of independence. At that time, foremost in their minds was the economic separation of pharmacy from medicine. Pharmacists always have been willing to recognize that the demand for their professional services is partially a derived demand. But, so it is too with the anesthesiologist who must wait until the surgeon operates. Pharmacists want to be treated as professional colleagues, not as captive professionals.

The battle for the economic separation of the pharmaceutical from the medical profession still continues. It is indeed unfortunate that organized medicine forced the battleground to be shifted from the private conference table to the public arena. Recent actions of Congress reflect the public's support for pharmacy's position.

More recently, pharmacists have added to their declaration of independence, the economic separation of the profession and industry. I think we explained in detail the feelings of the profession on this subject when we appeared recently before Congress. Again, the profession has been forced to fight in the public arena.

The profession wants a strong, independent, prosperous pharmaceutical industry. The profession has said time and time again that it does not want to see the industry made a public utility. The profession wants the elimination of price discrimination and other injurious practices. For example, the profession can't understand or accept the idea of a physician's getting a drug for a fraction of the cost a pharmacist pays. This industry practice only encourages physicians to take time to dispense drugs when our citizens desperately need their diagnostic services.

The other day I saw an advertisement in a trade publication for a prescription drug which the manufacturer suggested the pharmacist should sell for $19.50. The manufacturer's suggested price to pharmacists was $11.70. I don't think any pharmacist in good conscience would ask a patient for a $7.80 fee for dispensing 100 tablets of that or any other drug. The members of the profession want to determine for themselves the value of their professional services, just as the manufacturers want to determine the value of their products.

It has been little more than a decade since Abrams, Apple, Evanson, Fuller, and McEvilla started explaining to pharmacy students, pharmacists and anyone who would listen that prescription drugs are not ordinary consumer goods and that pharmacists deserve to be reimbursed for their professional services on a fee basis. For a while, it was only possible to evaluate the merits of this principle by observing who opposed it.

Now that the idea that pharmacists should be reimbursed on a fee basis has received private and public endorsement, pharmacists must be prepared to justify the fees they ask and we welcome the opportunity.

Medicine, pharmacy, and the pharmaceutical industry are inseparably joined in the common challenge of serving sick people. Each has its own special contribution to make. Each must act according to its own conscience. Pharmacy always stands ready to cooperate with medicine and industry but the profession must speak for itself.

As I think back to my experiences in pharmacy before I came to Washington, I would have to describe it as a period during which I listened to others proclaim our aspiration for pharmacists to become full-time health professionals. Since 1958, I have sought to champion this cause nationally.

A few decades ago, management of the drug chains looked at the professionally minded pharmacist with suspicion. Pharmacists were assigned many nonprofessional duties because the activities of most chain prescription departments could not justify their professional salaries.

How things have changed! After World War II, chain management realized that a liability could be converted into a handsome asset and, just as industry developed a demand for pharmaceutical scientists, chains now have an insatiable demand for pharmacists who want to practice pharmacy.

If the independent, private practitioner is to remain independent and private, he must employ to the maximum the one asset he possesses which competition cannot devaluate his professional knowledge and competency. A pharmacist who spends only a small fraction of his time practicing has to spend as much time and effort maintaining his professional acumen as does the pharmacist who devotes all of his energy to providing professional service. If he does, his return on that invested time is considerably less. If he doesn't spend that time, he is not in a position to give the public the quality of service it deserves.

For the past several years, the profession has been able to demonstrate that its recent practitioners have been trained to practice as therapeutic specialists. In a few years, some of the pilot educational projects which bring pharmacy students into direct bedside contact with patients, physicians and the latest diagnostic and treatment procedures will be part of the pharmacy curriculum and internship. Perhaps, in a decade, the profession will be able to demonstrate that its current graduates are qualified to participate directly in the prescribing function.

A few years ago, pharmacy students politely asked now they demand to know what opportunities the profession offers for them to use and expand their knowledge. Consciously or otherwise, pharmaceutical education is moving pharmacists in a direction which will require them to be fulltime health practitioners.

Certainly, there is no question in which direction our country is moving with regard to improving the distribution and quality of health care. We need only refer to the work of the National Commission on Community Health Services, the National Conference on Medical Costs, and the recent report of the National Advisory Commission on Health Manpower. There are signposts all around us, pointing the direction in which the country is moving in health affairs. Pharmacists, like all others concerned with providing health services, have the choice of putting on blinders and winding up on a dead end road or of observing all of the signs and taking the roads which are marked "opportunity to serve mankind."

As all of you know from the press, the recent report of the health manpower commission includes a recommendation that physicians and other health professionals be relicensed periodically "...on the basis of acceptable performance in programs of continuing education, or on the basis of challenge examinations for those who choose not to participate formally in continuing education."

The fact that I have mentioned this subject might tempt some editor to use the headline "Apple Demands Annual Pharmacist Exam."

I don't mean to imply that I would be intentionally misquoted but I do recognize that it is becoming exceedingly more difficult for all of us to communicate in our hurried existence. What I am suggesting is that pharmacy not remain a bystander while other health professionals discuss the commission's recommendation. It is not too early for pharmacy to study the application of this relicensing procedure to our profession.

As some of you know, in the last 100 days we testified before three Congressional committees. We reported that pharmacists were not unhappy to see the "brand name percentage markup" era come to a close. I understand that a few people have taken exception to our observation. If they interpret the "brand-markup" system as the criterion for quality, then I can understand their irritation. Apparently they do not understand our premise that quality must be built into a product; it isn't derived from the name on the label. The American Pharmaceutical Association, since its inception in 1852, has promoted zealously the principle that sick people deserve to be treated with safe and effective drugs.

I don't see why Abbott, Bristol, Burroughs Wellcome, Ciba, Geigy, Hoffmann-LaRoche, Lederle, Lilly, Merck Sharp & Dohme, Parke-Davis, Pfizer, Robins, Rorer, Schering, Searle, Smith Kline & French, Squibb, Upjohn, Warner-Chilcott, Winthrop, Wyeth, and the many others which have contributed so much to the war against disease, pain and even death would want to masquerade their proud corporate names behind brand gimmickry and promotional fads. Some of these company names are well known to generations of physicians and pharmacists and I suspect that all of these firms would like to be known for generations to come. It would seem to me that the name of the manufacturer is the most important hallmark of quality that could be featured on any label.

Pharmacy has been generous to me. It not only has provided me with a useful life and purpose, but it has brought me into contact with health leaders around the world. I am especially pleased that some of the voluntary health association executives are here tonight. Usually, testimonials about the quality of a product are not very reliable, but I am sure you will understand my willingness to accept and treasure the testimonials from which Betty Schaefer read. While the people who wrote those testimonials haven't always agreed with me, they have contributed much to my education, progress, and life.

At this time, I would like to thank the past presidents of the Association for having selected me for this honor. I also would like to thank the thousands of pharmacists who, over the years, have given me their encouragement, support, and advice. I am proud of the men and women in our profession and of their unselfish and devoted efforts to serve society. Those of you who have come in contact with the Association in recent years understand and share my appreciation for the dedication and competency of the men and women who work with me at 2215 Constitution Avenue. Their efforts form the mold out of which this year's Remington medal was cast.

In announcing my selection as the 1967 Remington medalist, Dr. Schaefer said many nice things about my work. But I have not forgotten his admonition:

"Dr. Apple is an extremely fitting recipient of this medal because of what... he will do... for American pharmacy and APhA itself."

Dr. Schaefer knew me well enough to expect that when I accepted this medal, I would also accept this challenge. ■

1969 Remington Medalist

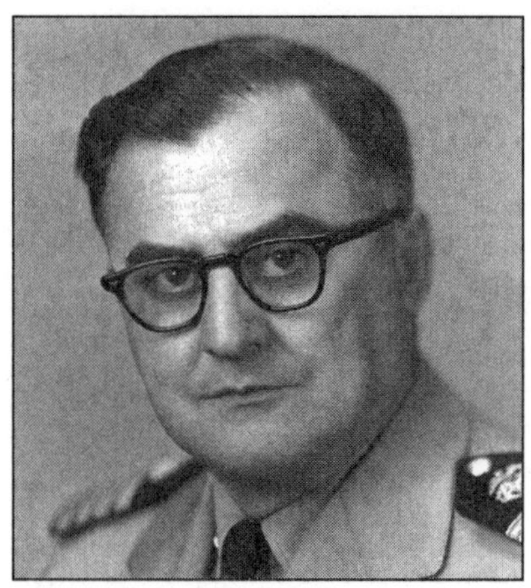

George Francis Achambault
(1909-2001)

George Francis Archambault was born in Springfield, Massachusetts, on April 29, 1909, and after graduating with Ph.G. in 1931 and a Ph.C. in 1933 from the Massachusetts College of Pharmacy, he served as lecturer on the faculty of his *alma mater* until 1943. He received an LL.B. degree from the Northeastern University School of Law in 1941, was admitted to the state bar in 1942, practiced law for a time in Massachusetts, and was admitted to the U.S. Supreme Court Bar in 1976. He served with the U.S. Public Health Service as chief of pharmacy service at the Boston Marine Hospital 1943-1945, and as director of professional relations for the Liggett Drug Company in New England 1945-1947. He was commissioned as a pharmacy officer in the U.S. Public Health Service in 1947 serving as chief of the pharmacy branch, division of hospitals 1947-1965, as pharmacy liaison officer to the Surgeon General 1959-1967, and as pharmacy consultant to the USPHS division of medical care administration 1965-1967. He then served one year as dean of the University of Florida College of Pharmacy and as a consultant to the United Mine Workers Health and Retirement Funds 1970-1976.

Archambault joined the American Pharmaceutical Association in 1931, serving as secretary APhA Section on Pharmaceutical Economics 1946-1947, president APhA Washington Chapter 1950-1951, APhA Council chairman 1959-1960, and APhA president 1962-1963. He also served as a member of the *USP* revision committee 1950-1960 and a *USP* trustee 1960-1975; as president of the American Society of Hospital Pharmacists 1954-1955; as vice president of the American Association for the Advancement of Science 1958-1959; as *Hospital Formulary Journal* editor 1967-1978; and as *Drug Intelligence* and *Clinical Pharmacy* Washington editor 1979-1983. He died January 1, 2001.

UNFINISHED AND NEW BUSINESS

George Francis Archambault

The 1969 Remington Honor Medal Lecture was presented on December 2, 1969, at the Hotel Roosevelt in New York City. Archambault's Remington address was not published, but an actual copy of the presentation was provided by the recipient.

I am told that it is customary for the recipient of the Remington medal to present his views on American pharmacy-past, present, or future, or to discuss some particular phases of pharmacy of special interest or concern to him.

Probably the most comprehensive presentation made by a Remington medalist was delivered by Hugh Muldoon in 1953. His "Strengths of Pharmacy" Remington address traced American pharmacy's professional relationships from its colonial origin to 1953. In his concluding remarks, remarks as valid today as they were in 1953, Dean Muldoon stated, "Men are always apprehensive of the future. Just now, more than ever, we have a feeling of insecurity. World affairs cause great unease. We know that ahead of us lie political and social and economic changes. They are inevitable. If they come, they will not be catastrophic. Whatever the changes may be and whenever they come, we shall adjust to them. In pharmacy, we may expect frustrations and disappointments and sometime failures. Strength comes through struggle. Pharmacy will continue to have dignity and character and direction of purpose."

I am sure that all agree with me that pharmacy is indeed showing dignity, character and direction of purpose in 1969, as it attacks the many political, social and economic changes now enveloping pharmacy and other health professions. I refer to such matters as third party payers for medications including Medicare, Medicaid and Champus, unionism, continuing education, professional fee approach to medication costing, the use of technicians, unit dose packaging, the changing roles of health professionals, biological availability of medications, and the current strength of the profession as witnessed by its new rules for membership in state, county, city and local associations.

In reviewing the current literature of American pharmacy and in noting the topics under discussion by specialty associations and the APhA, I found most topics of national concern well covered. Not only are the associations doing a goodjob, but our national and regionaljournals are reporting the issues.

There are however three topics that have not been noted to any great extent by pharmacy that deserve our attention: 1. The new strength of American pharmacy. 2. The changing roles of health professionals, and 3. The legal implications involved in this change-over period as to professional duties and responsibilities and the use of aids or technicians.

It is indeed heartening to witness state, county and city pharmaceutical associations opening their membership to other than pharmacy owners.

The recognition of "employee" pharmacists (employees of hospitals, government, chains, and 'independents") is indeed a healthy one.

Today "employee" pharmacists outnumber the "self-employed" or independents." They seek a platform where they may debate local and national matters of health affecting pharmacy. State and local associations meet this need.

Pharmacy's strength becomes stronger because of this new policy. Already one notes these associations making use of this new talent by election of new members to executive committees and other leadership posts. This is indeed a new strength for the profession, one moving pharmacy closer to a "united front from local levels on through to the national level.

Due to the growing shortage of physicians with little possibility of increasing the output in the immediate years ahead, medicine now seeks means to conserve its medical manpower. The removal of certain routine functions from the physician and the placing of these responsibilities on others is under active study. Hospital corpsmen returning from the Services, individuals with two years of special medical training, and specially trained nurses are being trained to serve as "medical assistants."

Dentistry and nursing, recognizing their manpower shortages, have reviewed in detail the nature of their responsibilities and duties As a result we note an increase of dental hygienists, licensed practical nurses, and the gradual phasing out of training schools for registered nurses.

Pharmacy has not been untouched by this problem of health manpower. While it would appear that there is a sufficient supply of pharmacists, if properly placed for professional services, we know full well that economically relocations are impossible. Many of the nation's pharmacists must continue to provide pharmaceutical service in rural and other areas where their total time is not consumed in pharmacy compounding and dispensing. To bridge this gap we note that pharmacy is being surveyed by itself and others, as to how best utilize its manpower in the delivery of pharmaceutical services.

Already pharmacy associations and practitioners have started to debate the issue of pharmacy technicians. Universities and junior colleges, some with and some without the advice of pharmacy, are considering the training of such individuals in two year programs. As of the moment, hospitals are looking into this subject of pharmacy technicians as a possible means of solving their manpower problem.

We need to take note that pharmacy helpers have long been a part of the hospital personnel structure, with job descriptions calling for "the immediate and direct supervision" of these individuals by pharmacists. Since these "helpers" are trained on the job, without approved professional courses, such positions are "dead end." However, with junior college or other formal courses of two years, might this not be a "ladder" health career whereby one might obtain credit for some of the courses and at a later date, switch over to a recognized pharmacist curriculum? Some have proposed this.

The rearranging of work loads to stretch present health manpower appears to be moving in this fashion. Physicians will, in their offices and in hospitals, make use of specially trained medical assistants who will relieve them of the more routine duties, thus conserving medical manpower for the more important diagnosis and treatment roles.

Nurses, already in short supply, will along with the other two sources of manpower (Service Health Corps and specially trained medical assistants), move into this "medical assistant" category. Nursing, now already overburdened, will divest itself of its responsibilities in medication administration, thus releasing considerable time for patient bedside care.

Pharmacy will move into drug administration in institutions, and also recognize the technician position in as much as pharmacists will be serving in two new roles that of "drug administration" and as medication consultant in a more formal manner than at present.

While such technicians are intended for hospital pharmacy service, it is quite likely that chain and independent pharmacies, in their search for manpower, will also show considerable interest in this matter.

At present, hospital pharmacy uses this type of sub-professional personnel under the "direct and immediate supervision" of pharmacists. Such individuals are normally referred to as "pharmacy helpers." The proposed "Pharmacy Technician," will operate not under the direct and immediate supervision of a pharmacist but under indirect supervision and his duties will include "counting and pouring" activities.

This brings up the legal implications in using personnel for acts currently reserved by state law to specific health practitioners. As this relates to pharmacy, let us look to the pharmacist's new duties in drug administration and his utilization of pharmacy technicians.

In recent years we have seen the education of a pharmacist change from one of product orientation to patient orientation. Educational pharmacy today, through such courses as Clinical Pharmacy and Clinical Pharmacology is deeply involved in developing these aspects of modern day pharmacy service. The goals, however, vary from college to college; some are of the opinion that the goal should be one of developing "medication experts" or "drug therapy consultants." Others are of the opinion that we need go further and include the nurses' role of drug administration, i.e., the actual giving of the medication to the patient.

Recently, national nursing and hospital pharmacy associations met to discuss the matter. All appeared to agree that nurses are better qualified in the techniques of drug administration because of their training in the rapid recognition of changes in the vital health signs. Also all seemed to agree that the pharmacist is better prepared to serve as the drug consultant.

Discussing the subject with staff nurses and older pharmacists, one senses that many will be resistant to change. However, it is my opinion, one shared by others, these changes in pharmacy are coming. In fact, some teaching research hospitals are already with us to some degree.

In this change over of responsibilities, one being brought about by a need to utilize to the greatest extent possible, the training and experience of the health professionals, one notes with concern violations of the health practice acts of the individual states. This matter currently needs study by pharmacy and the other health professions involved.

The question is raised, can pharmacists in institutional practice legally serve in the administration of medications (a nursing function) and may pharmacy technicians in hospitals, and possibly in chain and independent pharmacies, legally perform basic pharmacy duties such as "counting, pouring and labeling" without direct and immediate supervision of a pharmacist?

In capsule form, the situation at present is as follows: The use, as pharmacists, of nurses, pharmacy aides, and helpers is one of the more disturbing legal issues in hospital pharmacy practice today. Should chains and independents seek to use similar trained helpers, they too will be concerned with the problem.

The health practice acts were placed "on the books" in the early 1900s for the protection of the public health and patient safety and regulations in connection with the acts have been made piecemeal through the years.

In 1969 the health professions are confronted with this dilemma. In attempting to conserve highly trained manpower now in short supply, the utilization of non-licensed but trained sub-professionals in basic roles designated by state statutes and regulations to named professionals is under active consideration and appears to be in violation of the law.

We note from such reports as the HEW Task Force on Prescription Drugs, recommendations to the effect that the use of aides be considered for the "count and pour" and other activities currently confined by law to licensed pharmacists. The report also recommends that a "pharmacy aide curriculum" be considered by junior colleges and other schools (possibly in the health related professions schools at health-centered universities).

To repeat, as a nation we are moving in

the direction of utilizing lesser talents in certain areas that are today considered the sole province of medical, nursing, and pharmacy practitioners.

Until legislation catches up with this trend, pioneers (hospitals, administrators, and pharmacists) find themselves confronted with two real possibilities. (1) Criminal charges of violations of state practice acts, and (2) charges of tort administrative negligence in the event of injury. To date, to my knowledge, no one has been challenged directly on these issues where federal grant money is involved. However there are cases on record both on the criminal and tort side, holding parties liable for such violations in hospital and community practice.

A professor of preventative medicine recently indicated that current state practice acts do not permit the delegation of such tasks to non-licensed personnel, and he has suggested that model legislation be drafted for consideration of the individual states. He suggests that such considerations might well be patterned after the Federal Food and Drug Act and regulations as these pertain to investigational drugs. He indicates that "patient consent" might well be a requirement where such technicians and aides act in place of the customary licensee.

The subject of legalizing health manpower utilization studies and the use of other than customary licensees in certain basic duty areas is indeed one long overdue for study, debate and resolution. At present those involved in such studies or activities operate at their peril as to violations of the state practice acts and in the event of patient injury.

While it may seem at first glance this problem is of concern only to institutional practitioners, the increasing shortage of pharmacists, will bring these matters to the attention of those in independent and chain practice as well as state board members.

I have attempted in this presentation to call attention to (1) pharmacy's new and growing strength, that is the membership of employee pharmacists in local and state pharmaceutical associations; (2) the current thinking that is now prevailing as to the new roles for pharmacists as drug consultants in community and institutional practice and in the administration of medications; and (3) the legal implications involved in the use of pharmacy technicians who perform acts now restricted by law to licensed pharmacists. I hope I have remained within the allotted 20 minutes, and I wish to thank you all very much. ■

1970 Remington Medalist

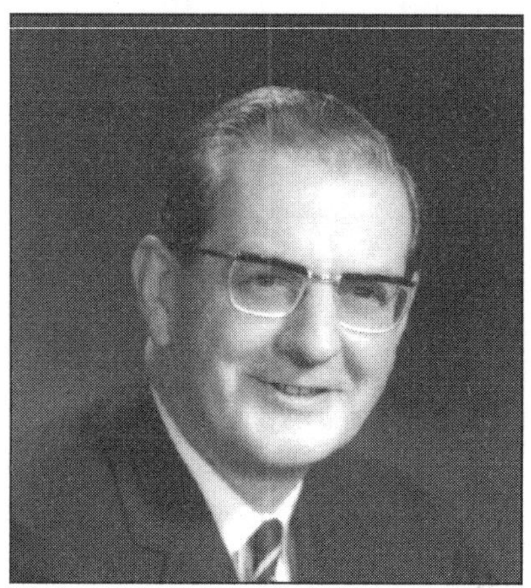

Don Eugene Francke
(1910-1978)

Don Eugene Francke was born in Athens, Pennsylvania, and received a B.S. degree in pharmacy in 1936 and an M.S. in 1948, both from the University of Michigan College of Pharmacy. He served as lecturer 1948-1951, assistant professor 1951-1962, and associate professor 1962-1963 at his *alma mater* during which time he also served as director of pharmacy services, University of Michigan Medical Center 1944-1963; director of the Michigan Academy of Pharmacy 1947-1957; member of the Michigan Board of Pharmacy 1950-1952; and associate editor of the *University of Michigan Medical Bulletin* 1950-1958. He then headed the department of hospital pharmacy, University of Cincinnati College of Pharmacy where he served as director of pharmacy service at the Cincinnati General Hospital 1967-1971. After a brief period as special assistant to the Veterans Administration chief medical director, he established his own publishing company serving as editor and publisher of *Drug Intelligence and Clinical Pharmacy* 1972-1978.

Francke served as a member of the American Pharmaceutical Association Council 1948-1956, and as APhA president 1951-1952. But he is best known for his service to the American Society of Hospital Pharmacy where he served three consecutive terms as ASHP president 1943-1946, as editor of *the American Journal of Hospital Pharmacy* 1944-1966, as director of the Audit of Pharmaceutical Services in Hospitals 1956-1959, as founding editor of both the *American Hospital Formulary Service* 1963-1966 and the *International Pharmaceutical Abstracts* 1964-1966, and as ASHP director of scientific services 1963-1966. He served as president of the International Pharmaceutical Federation (FIP) Press and Documentation Section 1964-1978, and FIP vice president 1958-1966. As a lasting tribute, ASHP established the Donald E. Francke Memorial Library.

Medicine, Medical Care, Manpower, and Mankind

Don Eugene Francke

The 1970 Remington Honor Medal Lecture was presented on December 1, 1970, at the Roosevelt Hotel in New York City. Francke's Remington address was published in *American Journal of Hospital Pharmacy,* volume 28, pages 410-421, 1971.

The stirring words of the American Declaration of Independence make it one of the most inspiring documents known to mankind. This document has done more to reshape the world than all the armies of mankind of all time. Over the years in many lands it has fomented rebellion, fostered revolution, led to social reforms and changes, corrected abuses and slowly but consistently led to improvement in the status of the individual as nations attempted to bring its message into reality.

Equally inspiring are the thoughts expressed in the Preamble to the Constitution of the World Health Organization, thoughts which are slowly creating a similar revolution in the delivery of health care in the United States, transforming it from the privilege of the few to the basic right for all regardless of economic status or other considerations.

"Health," it says, "is a state of complete physical, mental and social well-being and not merely the absence of disease or infirmity.

"The enjoyment of the highest attainable standard of health is one of the fundamental rights of every human being without distinction of race, religion, political belief, economic or social condition.

"Governments have a responsibility for the health of their peoples which can be fulfilled only by the provision of adequate health and social measures."

Dissatisfaction with our present system of the delivery of health care is moving the country rapidly toward an expansion of the availability of health insurance benefits and a strengthening of our national health programs. What the public demands is equal access to high-quality comprehensive health care on the basis of need rather than either the ability to pay or charity. We now have a comprehensive national health service for almost 30 million veterans. In Medicare, we have the beginnings of a comprehensive national health insurance program for about 20 million of the aged. It has been proposed that this be expanded to include the disabled and others. In Medicaid, we have a far less satisfactory beginning of a national health program for several million children. Medicaid, however, is too dependent upon the resources, interests and action of individual states to be a long-range answer to the health-care of children. In reality, it makes as much or more sense to develop a national health program for children as a program for the aged. If the health of a child is safeguarded the nation's future is guaranteed. Much of our need for health service is poverty-related and the constantly rising cost of medical care is rapidly creating medical indigents out of many more than the 40 million so-called disadvantaged in the nation since private insurance now pays for only about 30 to 40% of the total costs of health care.

More important, however, are the stirrings among the people who are demanding health care as a right. At the end of World War II, Great Britain created a National Health Service which Americans said we could not then afford. The British did it despite the tremendous devastation and destruction and great manpower shortages which the war brought to them. The Right Honorable Jennie Lee, British Minister of State Department of Education and Science and widow of Aneurin Bevin, the first Minister of the National Health Service, quotes a statement by some American friends: "We made a mistake after the Second World War. We came out of it in very comfortable economic circumstances not realizing that if you leave considerable numbers of your young under-educated, under-doctored, badly housed, you are going to have an explosion."

Today we are witnessing the results of this explosion in our society. And it is a chain reaction which will continue to erupt for decades until people obtain better health care, are better housed, are no longer hungry, and have an opportunity for education and jobs, according to the concept of health as expressed by WHO. People who are angry that the idea of health as a privilege has prevailed in this country for so long. They are beginning to realize that the United States is one of the few remaining industrialized countries in which the citizens must buy their health on the open market like any commodity. They are beginning to realize that the United States ranks behind every industrialized nation in the world in the two health statistics considered the most accurate indices of medical progress. In infant mortality the U.S. ranks 19th in the world; in mean life expectancy at birth it ranks 16th. They are beginning to understand that what they have been told about America's having the finest medical care in the world is not true for them or for their children or for their family or their neighbor. They are beginning to learn, for example, that in 1966, 16 governments were spending more than $20 per capita that the U.S. was spending for health and that 15 other nations have a higher ratio of hospital beds to population than we. They are beginning to learn that many other nations have forms of readily available comprehensive health services which puts ours to shame.

The pressure for reform is irresistible. Pushed by the people, politicians of both parties, liberal and conservative, are voicing the demands of society. Medicare and Medicaid were passed over the objections of most of the health professions. President Nixon has proposed a new health plan for the poor. Walter Reuther's Committee of One Hundred has called health care in the United States a "disorganized and disjointed, antiquated and obsolete nonsystem" and is actively working to bring about a new system of health care. Governor Nelson Rockefeller has proposed that the federal government assume all of the country's welfare costs, including those related to health. Representative Griffiths, Senators Javits, Kennedy and Percy and others have each introduced legislation to improve delivery of expanded national health insurance programs. The U.S. Surgeon General recently told an audience that he sees no possibility of finding all the resources to meet all the demands placed on the nation's health services. He added "the public" is not going to stand for the present confusion much longer.

The organization and distribution of health care in America is undergoing rapid changes. Neither the physician nor the American Medical Association is any longer in the driver's seat; nor is the pharmacist or the American Pharmaceutical Association. Society will decide our fate and, should we continue along present lines, will no longer finance the education and training of pharmacists to serve the public health in the manner they have been serving it in the recent past and at present.

The ferment existing today regarding national health insurance, considerations relative to the delivery of health care through the redesigning of the system, the great health manpower shortage and the resulting redefinition of the roles of all health team participants, give to pharmacy the opportunity to move into the mainstream as a public health profession. If pharmacy is to become a health-centered profession it must swallow a strong cathartic and purge itself of many of its present patterns. Among other things, it must develop means to (1) reorganize pharmacy schools and make them a part of a larger school of the health professions and redesign pharmaceutical education to make the pharmacist a more valuable member of the health team, (2) greatly accelerate research and projects through which community pharmacists may develop new health-care related roles, (3) find a way to make all who call themselves pharmacists really a part of the profession, (4) negotiate the prices that may be charged to the pharmacist and to the public for drug products, (5) provide a better means of monitoring the quality of drug products, and (6) find a way to separate pharmacies and drugstores.

Pharmacy could take a big step in the direction of becoming a health-oriented profession if its colleges were made part of a much larger school of health professions such as has been developed in some countries. This comprehensive interdisciplinary school would be responsible for the education of all health professionals including physicians, dentists, pharmacists, nurses, inhalation therapists, social workers, pharmacy technicians, other technicians and allied health workers of many varieties. Such a school would provide for both upward and outward mobility, permit all students to take at least some of their classes together, permit them to learn to appreciate the knowledge and abilities and special skills of the others and encourage greatly the development of the new public health roles for each group.

Within such an interdisciplinary setting the pharmacy student would be able to undergo the type of socialization which would produce in him the health role relevant psychosocial characteristics required of a health professional, as has been described for the medical student. But probably the most important benefit would be the opportunity for the pharmacist to develop new health-related roles which could very well include the prescribing of drugs for certain types of patients such as those requiring continuous drug therapy, as suggested by Dean Ebert of Harvard. However, little along this line can be developed until pharmacy is recognized as a health profession. The prevailing attitude of the public and of the allied health professions toward pharmacy is reflected in a multitude of ways. An example is in an article on "The Student Health Organizations" which appeared in the *New England Journal of Medicine.* This article describes the purposes, development and activities of a national coalition of health science students. Students of pharmacy are not even mentioned or included. This attitude of other health professions toward us must be changed.

In the near future, a school of pharmacy that does not establish close ties with a teaching health center should not be accredited, so essential is its role in the training of health-oriented pharmacists. Years ago I used to feel quite smug and superior when I learned that pharmacy and medical schools in foreign countries had a mixed faculty. Naively, I told my foreign colleagues, "American pharmacy schools are completely separate and independent," not appreciating at the time now much we had lost by this separation and independence. Francis Stewart discussed this point in 1920 when he said, "Pharmacy can never secure recognition as a profession until the practice of pharmacy is conducted in conformance with the professional ideals upon which the practice of medicine was originally founded." At that time Stewart was discussing the reorganization of the American Pharmaceutical Association and actually opposed the idea of a federation of all pharmaceutical organizations because he felt that the APhA would be dominated by druggists rather than by pharmacists.

Many pharmacy schools are moving in this direction by becoming part of the overall health or medical center of the university, and it is my personal opinion that this has greatly accelerated the development of clinical pharmacy in schools of pharmacy.

It is also for the first time giving pharmaceutical education a clinical component. Not long ago I heard of a dean of a college of pharmacy who was talking to his new administrative superior, the vice president of the university's medical center. "Tell me," asked the vice president, "why is it that your school is the only one among the health sciences that has no practitioners at the medical center?" Embarrassed by his inability to give a satisfactory reply to the question, the dean hurried to develop a clinical faculty as many others have done, I suspect, for similar reasons. However, at this point in time health education is not coordinated and developed as the interdisciplinary effort that it should be and one day will be. Incidentally, I understand that a national conference is to be called to define clinical pharmacy. Clinical pharmacy can be conceptualized and discussed but in my opinion, it would be unwise to constrict it by definition at this point. Not enough work has been done in the area of clinical pharmacy and much more experience has to be gained before we kill it by defining it. And when they succeed in defining a clinical pharmacist I predict that it will be anyone who has a patient oriented attitude toward pharmacy in other words, anyone who calls himself a clinical pharmacist. It seems to me that before we try to define clinical pharmacy we should first be able to define pharmacy itself. Attempts have been made to do this without much success.

Now that pharmaceutical education is beginning to adopt a clinical component to give the students a better understanding of the patient and to enhance his ability to communicate with the physician, it should turn its attention toward establishing community prescription pharmacies for the education and training of professional practitioners. I am not talking about a college operated student health service pharmacy, but rather, one that serves the population of a town or city and thus would be a pharmacy servicing a representative population. There must be a concerted, nationwide effort on the part of the colleges to train pharmacists in clinical practice under ideal conditions to an establishment operated, controlled and supervised by the college. The pharmacy should be designed and constructed for teaching and research purposes and should be operated by professional practitioners holding appointments on the faculty.

Such a pharmacy would reflect the best in pharmaceutical practice for students to emulate. It would establish patterns, explore new possibilities, conduct research, investigate unmet health needs and test new potential roles for pharmacists. It would be a living, viable, dynamic part of the college's instructional program with which the prospective community pharmacist could identify, in a manner similar to the way in which hospital pharmacists identify with the hospital in which they serve their residency. The pharmaceutical center could provide a model for all undergraduate students and would be an essential tool for the training of Doctor of Pharmacy candidates. I know the arguments against colleges engaging in activities of this type, but those in favor of it are so overwhelming that it could gain strong support from community pharmacists if properly explained. Community pharmacists who oppose the undertaking of such a project by the colleges for fear of losing prescription business are sowing the seeds of their own destruction.

While community pharmacists spend their energy in opposing the opening of one pharmacy by a college of pharmacy, a corporation may open ten or more units in the same city and pharmacists are powerless to do anything about it. In many cases, pressures from local and state pharmaceutical associations and pharmacy owners make it impossible for the college to move in this direction. In these cases, I suggest that it would be entirely appropriate for the clinical faculty of the college to establish a nonprofit corporation whose tripartite objectives would be patient service, education and research into new roles for the pharmacist in group practice situations. These proposals would be similar in nature to those group practices now established by the faculties of 38 schools of medicine.

They are extremely important to the future development of pharmacy as a public health profession. I understand that at least two colleges of pharmacy are now recruiting for a faculty member to operate a pharmaceutical center which will be used for the training of undergraduate and graduate students. Let us hope that others will develop rapidly. Because as Ulan has said, "Present pharmacy graduates are not prepared to work in a healthcare system."

As Brodie has so well pointed out, "the classical professional purpose for pharmacy as we have known it will not sustain us in the future." I agree with Brodie when he says that the most important single factor in the development of the drugstore since the 1930's "is the failure of pharmaceutical education to provide the leadership that would assure the profession of practitioners with the professional and scientific maturity to withstand the intrusion of non-professional interests." Too many pharmaceutical educators are pharmaceutical scientists who have abandoned the community practitioner. "Get the pharmacist out of the drugstore and into professional practice in a manner that will identify him as a pharmaceutical specialist by the public and by practitioners of other health professions," says Brodie. Too many educators today like the drugstore as it is or are the captives of other interests. How else can we explain the appalling lack of research into community practice when every need of society calls out loudly for it and when the great health manpower shortage demands it?

At this time I want to pay tribute to the excellent way in which hospital pharmacists are developing. The principle reason for this is that, in the main, they are health-care oriented professionals working in a healthcare oriented institution in close association with other professions involved in patient care. During the past couple of decades they have developed so many pharmacists with advanced professional degrees that, if continued, in a few years hospital pharmacy will have an additional 5,000 elite practitioners with specialized education who cannot help but greatly influence the future direction of the profession as a result of their research, professional practice and teaching.

In many countries pharmacy musters great strength because all pharmacists belong to their national professional society. Not so in the good old United States! Here a student can complete pharmacy school, pass his state board examination and thumb his nose at both his state and national professional societies for the rest of his life. And most of them do exactly this. When I was president of APhA, we had about 1 out of every 10 pharmacists as members; today we are doing much better, but not nearly well enough, with almost 30% of all pharmacists as members but with 70% as non-members. This makes the national professional society a ship without a rudder, a captain without a crew, unable to direct, powerless to persuade and, in essence, unable to lead because two or three times as many pharmacists on the team he is leading are going in several different directions at once. This may be pluralism at its best but it is not the way responsible members of a profession devoted to the public health conduct themselves.

The mission of pharmacists is to serve the public health needs of society-but most of us never stop to think about that. In the name of individual liberty we have substituted individual license to do as we please. The plan for a federation and unification of American pharmacy goes back at least to the beginning of this century and was outlined by APhA Presidents Wulling and Dohme at the end of the First World War. APhA Past-President Curt Nottingham again fostered the plan in the early 1960s and during the past several years the APhA has been able to gather in about 15 states as affiliates. Although I commend the APhA for what it has done and would not want it to abandon the plan before a better one is developed, it is not very comforting for pharmacy to have to project a waiting time to the second or third century of the third millennium for unification!

Many things can and will change before that time arrives. But times are changing. Herman and Anne Somers have pointed out that:

"In all countries regardless of differing economic or political systems, medical care is changing from a private relationship between two individuals into a medical social institution, or, more precisely, a great network of specialized institutions, which make it possible to provide better care to more people than ever before. The United States is no exception. This is the overriding fact of twentieth century medical care-as it is of education, industry and government."

Or as Bently Gilbert said of the evolution of national health service in Great Britain, "A system of public relief deliberately made hideous for its recipients could not long outlast the grant of universal franchise." If pharmacy service is an important part of health service to the public, society itself will find ways to establish and maintain its quality by encouraging pharmacists to become more professionally oriented. Uniform nationwide standards can be promulgated pursuant to legislation under any plan of national health insurance, and in my mind this would make it possible for the American people to have a type of pharmacy service that most of them have never experienced-a health-centered service rendered by health-oriented pharmacists. This could be done by establishing uniform, national requirements for pharmacists similar to those established for physicians in Senator Javit's bill to establish a National Health Insurance program. In almost every country of the world, the pharmacist is part of his profession and assumes certain obligations toward it and is subject to some type of national professional control. The sooner we develop a similar plan here the stronger our profession will be. I personally believe that a national plan for the unification of health-oriented pharmacists will be developed within the next decade. The pluralistic laissez-faire, permissive attitudes of the past are too costly to be sustained. One of the significant effects of current and impending social legislation is the greater degree of public control over the nation's hospitals. The enormous investment of public funds in hospital care will lead to increasing emphasis on controls relative to costs, promotion of efficiency and the planning of resources in general. Hospitals will be increasingly regarded and treated as an integrated public utility rather than an agglomerate of independent private institutions.

The American public has come to equate quality of pharmacy service almost solely with the price of the drug product. Many pharmacists have encouraged this. Others who want to give a more comprehensive public health service are discouraged by competition from offering it because their profit is too closely related to the cost of the drug. In addition, there has been for years justified or not a public clamor about the excessive cost of drugs to the public and the high profits of the pharmaceutical industry.

Many countries have solved this dilemma by arriving at prices to be charged to the public after negotiation between representatives of pharmacists and governmental authorities. In turn, the government has negotiated prices the pharmacist may be charged for the drug product by the producer. The Drug Tariff which results from negotiation between the Pharmaceutical Society of Great Britain and the Ministry of Health is an example of a document controlling the price of drugs to the public. For the control of cost of drugs to the pharmacist, the British Health Ministry has established a Voluntary Price Regulation Scheme with the pharmaceutical industry which permits the negotiation of a percentage profit which will vary with many different circumstances and considerations. The scheme is flexible and the pharmaceutical industry in Great Britain has flourished under it. Without becoming a public utility, the industry submits to voluntary price controls.

The greatest advantage of these price controlling plans is that the public is represented and, therefore, its interests are protected. At the same time a professional fee and other items of remuneration and reimbursement can be worked into the formula for compensating the pharmacist, based on the level of pharmaceutical service he gives. Perhaps a capitation fee for each person registered with a community pharmacy could be paid in addition to the fee for each prescription, as is done in The Netherlands. Since the government will soon be paying most of the bills for drugs and related professional service, it is inevitable that it, as a representative of society, will exercise some control over them.

A cooperative scheme to adjust the price of drugs to the public makes much more sense to me than current plans by many health agencies to control the price of drugs by putting a ceiling on the amount they will pay for certain drugs, often ignoring completely the reliability of the source of supply or the quality of the drug product.

The health of the public can be safeguarded only if the quality of drugs dispensed to them is assured. It was, in fact, the importation of adulterated and substandard drugs into our nation that served as the prime reason for the founding of the American Pharmaceutical Association. I base my belief that the quality of drugs in this country is not yet well-monitored principally on the published findings of the Defense Personnel Support Center. Stated briefly, it has found in surveys over the past five years that about 50% of its pre-award inspections of manufacturing plants resulted in their disqualification because of deficiencies in either control of housekeeping. More amazing is that about 50% of those that do pass the inspection fail to submit acceptable pre-award laboratory samples. If we apply these statistics to, for example, 20 producers of reserpine, 10 out of the 20 plants would be eliminated by poor quality control or housekeeping. Of the remaining 10, five more would be eliminated because their pre-award sample failed to meet specifications and standards. This is an extremely poor performance.

The recent USP Convention recognized the threats to public health and confidence in USP products brought about by the distribution of sub-quality drugs when it voted to recommend "establishment of a program designed to make known to pharmacists and physicians information that would be helpful in the assessment of the quality, strength, efficacy and safety of USP drug products available on the market."

This question of drug quality, it seems to me, is much more basic and fundamental than that of drug product equivalency which is, of course, also of great importance in its own right. The APhA Academy of Pharmaceutical Sciences has called attention to this in its statement on "Drug Product Quality."

In a study of illegal practices among pharmacists, those who violated the law regarding the compounding and dispensing of prescriptions, Quinney found that violations occur with the greatest frequency among the business-oriented pharmacists and least among pharmacists with a professional orientation. The pharmacists' orientation was measured by their responses to a series of questions including the following: "In terms of your pharmacy career, how important is each of the following?" There followed ten randomly placed questions. The professional role items were: (1) reading the professional literature, (2) being a part of the public health team, (3) using and encouraging the use of official drugs, (4) attending professional meetings, and (5) compounding and dispensing prescriptions.

The business role questions were: (1) maintaining a business establishment, (2) being a successful businessman, (3) arranging window and counter displays, (4) being a good salesman, and (5) handling a variety of sundry goods. Each respondent had two role orientation scores, professional and business, and each was given a low or high rating for each role. Those who did not orient toward either role were judged "indifferent pharmacists" while those about equally oriented toward both roles were placed in the category of "professional-business pharmacists."

It is interesting to note that in his sample, Quinney found only 16% of pharmacists had a profile by which they could be rated as professional. There were no law violators in the professional group. The business oriented pharmacists made up 20% of the sample and 75% of them were prescription violators. The professional-business oriented pharmacists made up 45% of the sample and 14% of them were violators. The indifferently-oriented pharmacist made up 19% of the sample and 20% of them were violators.

Thus prescription violation is related to the structure of pharmacy. Even if all of APhA's approximately 30% of pharmacists are professionally oriented, it does not seem to me in the interest of public health to remove all legal constraints against substitution from the business-oriented and indifferent pharmacists.

I find it very difficult to reconcile these facts with the proposal of the APhA to repeal all state anti-substitution laws and to thus remove all legal constraints from the nation's pharmacists. Especially do I find it difficult to reconcile when the APhA has no power of moral suasion over about 70% of the nation's pharmacists, and when it accepts no responsibility for the quality of drugs as done by the pharmaceutical societies of many countries such as Belgium, Scotland, Holland, Sweden and Finland.

Over the years, I have supported the concept of "conscious current consent," such as the medical staff of a hospital gives to the pharmacist to dispense alternative brands of the same basic drug with the pharmacist controlling the source of supply. The significant difference in this situation is that physicians daily visit their patients and can readily monitor the evidence of physiological and therapeutic effects of the drugs on their patients, and the pharmacist is readily at hand to receive any complaints relative to the ineffectiveness of the drug and can take appropriate action. Drugs dispensed to outpatients are produced by the same manufacturer as those medications given to inpatients and hence one serves as a control on the quality of the other.

Community pharmacists in dialogue with physicians have also been able to obtain their consent to dispense alternative brands of drug products.

I voted against the APhA proposal to repeal antisubstitution laws, however, because their repeal would remove the penalty from pharmacists who substitute another brand without the consent of the physician. Concerning this point, the APhA argued that "repeal of the antisubstitution laws would not disturb the existing prescriber pharmacist relationship or deprive the prescriber of the right to insist that a particular product be dispensed. Repeal of antisubstitution laws would simply act to remove the state as a decision-maker in the prescribing and dispensing of medication."

This argument seems particularly weak since the penalties for the act of substitution without the consent of the prescriber are removed and since the APhA has no program for the certification of the quality of drugs upon which the pharmacist can rely for his choice of products to dispense.

Another argument put forth by the APhA in support of the repeal of antisubstitution laws was that "the pharmacist's training and expertise qualify him as an expert on drugs and permit him to make judgments about the quality of the drug products." Two conditions are necessary to make this statement valid. One, the pharmacist must have available to him a wide variety of expensive, sophisticated analytical equipment and the competence to operate it and interpret the results. Second, he must have the cooperation of physicians who can monitor the effects of the drug products on patients. Even in hospitals, the presence of the first requirement is rare, and thus great dependence is placed on the latter.

This is the reason that "conscious current consent" is valid when the physician is a partner in the selection process, and becomes valid when he is removed. With the sophistication of today's analytical instrumentation and its unavailability to the vast majority of practicing pharmacists, it is absurd to say that the average pharmacist is able to judge the quality of drug products, particularly in view of the absence of a simplified analytical approach to drug quality as has been developed for the Danish pharmacists. He may be competent to do so but he lacks the necessary tools. I also agree that the physician's judgment of drug quality is principally empirical. But he is prescribing for the patient and he has a right to know the drug product his patient is taking. This, if nothing else, is a matter of courtesy.

The British, under their National Health Service permit "conscious current consent" to operate in their hospital system, but in pharmacies where physicians are not in close contact with pharmacists they insist that the pharmacist not change the physician's prescription without his knowledge. Rather than trying to control the price of drugs for the National Health Service through the use of mandatory formulary systems, they do it by negotiating prices with the manufacturer and issuing a drug tariff for use by the community pharmacist. To me, this seems like a much better way to achieve the same objective.

The United States has more than 50,000 retail establishments known as drugstores with which are included a few thousand pharmacies. This great heterogeneous mass makes it impossible for the public and the allied professions to clearly discern, to carefully distinguish or to recognize in any way the pharmacist practicing in them as a professional person. Drugstores in America so greatly outnumber pharmacies that when pharmacies are called drugstores and drugstores are called pharmacies, the terms pharmacist and pharmacy become meaningless to the public because they are equated with druggists and drugstore.

Far too many American drugstores, especially those of multiple unit operating corporations, can only be described as commercialized jungles which dull and tarnish and blunt the professional drive of pharmacists as they seek to practice their profession within their walls. The participation of pharmacists in an environment of diverse non-professional activities such as the selling of lunches, hardware, clothing, garden tools, radios, jewelry, sheep dung, motor oil and other general store items confuses the public as it does the pharmacist who practices in such a setting.

The drugstore, redefined and restructured, could be a respectable and acceptable institution. I bear no ill will against the drugstore, per se. I protest strongly, however, its identification with pharmacy. It is this identification which is destroying pharmacy as a profession in America.

The public can associate neither the drugstore nor the pharmacist in it as serving the health needs of society. It cannot esteem a man who works in such an environment; he may sell a health-related-product-but he is not accepted as a member of a health profession. One can find no fault with society's judgment of pharmacists when one reads the studies by the Professors Knapp and their colleagues. As a drug adviser to the physician, pharmacists in their sample failed five out of six questions; as an adviser on self medication, 83% of pharmacists sold patients they believed to be diabetic, products contraindicated in this condition; and several similar actions. The authors state:

"It is painfully and deadly obvious that the pharmacists in our sample utterly failed the tasks presented them-failed to the point of exposing their patients to the unnecessary risk of possible death in the third phase. Statistics are of little use in cases such as this, both because of the overwhelming nature of the incorrect responses and the severity of the consequences of the pharmacists' actions."

I believe that the interests, motivations and rewards of the community pharmacist are so greatly diluted and dispersed by all the other activities of his store that he cannot help but fail when tested as a professional practitioner concerned with public health. We must find some way to separate these two institutions because at present the relatively few pharmacies are engulfed, enmeshed, submerged and choked by the many drugstores. The public simply cannot and will not accept today's community pharmacist as a member of the health team. As Brodie has said, one of the first things we must do is to get the pharmacist out of the drugstore so that he can be identified readily as a pharmaceutical specialist by the public and by the practitioners and other health professions.

In another study, Knapp found that the pharmacist is placed closer to the concept of a technician than he is to the concept of professional by the public, by physicians and by other pharmacists.

The idea of making a separation of pharmacies and drugstores has been in the minds of a few of pharmacy's leaders since the founding of the American Pharmaceutical Association. For example, W.E. Stone in 1919 said, "There will not be much chance for elevating the standard of the profession as long as it continues to be a mere adjunct of a general department store business;" or to listen to Charles LaWall writing under the intriguing title of "Bolshevism in Pharmacy" who said, "That pharmacy is separating into two distinct classes no one will deny." Or to Albert Dewey who in 1915 said, "Commercial pharmacy practices a type of pharmacy wholly independent of the medical profession... whether or not professional pharmacy can even be separated from the hodgepodge we now call the drug business is a question." Or to James Hartley Beal who, in the first Remington address, said that the frequently deplored commercialism of pharmacy is a beginning of the separation of its merchandising features from its purely professional features and that this tendency is toward the same end as those who advocate legislation to create two classes of pharmacists.

Or come to the 1970s when we hear a physician, the vice president for health affairs at a major university say, "The public does not look on the pharmacist as a member of the health profession. He has been regarded as a dispenser of pre-compounded medications in various forms as ordered by the physician. Many consider him basically as a merchant selling medication and health items and also a great variety of non medical items including toys, hardware, gifts, and sporting goods."

One of pharmacy's leaders recently said, "In our economic and legal system, the multiple unit operating corporation has as much right to own a pharmacy as the individual practitioner." Perhaps it does have the economic and legal right but does it have the moral right to merchandise with such abandon and lack of constraint that it prostitutes and degrades the profession whose name it uses and abuses? Yes, anyone can own a drugstore but not everyone can practice pharmacy. If deans of pharmacy schools would be less willing to sell their profession and students to the multiple unit operating corporations, if the faculties would not give their support by silence or by saying, "We are only giving the public what it wants," perhaps the students could be given such pride in their profession that they would be loathe to work in such establishments. I look to today's young pharmacists and students to provide the leadership to carry us forward to the realm of a true public health profession. It is only in the English-speaking countries that the law allows pharmacies to be owned by other than pharmacists and then allows those owners to own more than one pharmacy. It is only in the English-speaking countries that the pharmacist is held in such low esteem by the public and by the allied health professions. Can you imagine what would happen to medicine or dentistry if physicians' and dentists' office practices were taken over by multiple unit operating corporations? In 1949, President Elliot of Pharmaceutical Survey fame referred to these stores as "jungles of commerce." Completing his survey after several years of study he said:

"... the outstanding factor determining the future of the profession of pharmacy is fundamentally moral in nature. The profession must contain a far greater proportion of members who are ever sharply jealous of the high reputation of the profession."

I pray we shall find a way to invoke the moral law and separate pharmacies and drugstores. In the first Remington address James H. Beal said:

"It may be too early to ask for legislation dividing pharmacies into different classes according to the character of the patronage they seek, but it ought not to be too early to encourage the progress of such a separation through voluntary action on the part of their proprietors."

There are numerous possible ways such separation could be brought about if enough of us put our minds to it. The profession should no longer permit its degradation by the continued combined existence of pharmacies and drugstores. Let us affirm our determination to return pharmacy to those professions practiced with dignity. History has demonstrated that great social changes and this is what we are talking about as we discuss new directions for our profession great social changes when they occur in a profession do not alter the attitudes and values of its members until a significant number of them assume new roles and perform successfully in them for two or three generations. A British colleague, after completing a study of pharmacy, wrote:

"This thesis has led me to the conclusion that it is time for the general practice of pharmacy to cease trying to run with the hare and hunt with the hounds at one and the same time. A choice must be made between the professional and commercial activities .... On the one hand, commercialism is becoming completely incompatible with a system of small scale pharmaceutical retailing as we know it today; on the other, legislation is dictating, and the health and social welfare services welcoming, the whole-hearted cooperating of pharmacy. It is to be hoped that the profession will choose to capitalize the standing achieved through its educational policies. If it elects to provide a professional service only, it can rightly expect both the government and the community to give it complete recognition both in status and by financial reward; it will simultaneously, regain its own professional satisfaction through the nature and practice of the work entailed."

"I like the dreams of the future better than the history of the past," said Thomas Jefferson. Yet, as Galsworthy wrote, "If you do not think about the future you cannot have one."

In closing, I would like to thank the past presidents of the APhA for having selected me to receive the Remington Medal for 1970. I also want to thank the officers and members of the New York Branch of the Association and especially the chairman of this Dinner Committee, my friend Frank Pokorny. And to you who honored me by your presence, I am especially grateful. Thank you. ■

1971 Remington Medalist

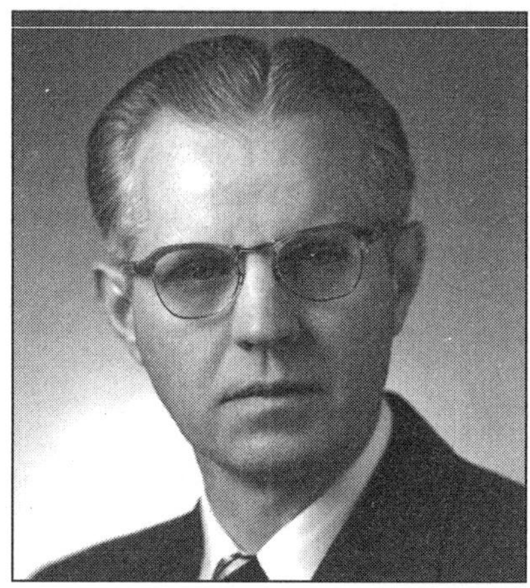

Linwood Franklin Tice
(1909-1996)

Linwood Franklin Tice was born in Salem, New Jersey, on February 17, 1909, and commenced working in a pharmacy at the age of twelve. After receiving a Ph.G. from the Philadelphia College of Pharmacy in 1929, he served on the faculty of Baylor University 1930-1931. Returning to his *alma mater,* he earned a B.S. in Pharmacy in 1933, an M.S. in Chemistry in 1935, and served as assistant professor 1938-1940, professor of pharmacy 1940-1975, assistant dean 1941-1956, associate dean 1956-1959, dean 1956-1975, and from 1975 until his death on August 18, 1996, as professor emeritus. During this period, he served on the *USP* revision committee 1940-1960 and as a *USP* trustee 1960-1975, on the American Foundation for Pharmaceutical Education board of directors 1954-1959, as vice president of the American Council on Pharmaceutical Education 1964-1966, and as president of the American Association of Colleges of Pharmacy 1955-1956. He was technical editor of *El Farmaceutico* 1941-1959 and *Pharmacy International* 1946-1959; associate editor of *Remington's Practice of Pharmacy* 1948-1963, and editor of *American Journal of Pharmacy* 1941-1977.

Tice joined the American Pharmaceutical Association in 1931, serving as president of the Philadelphia APhA Chapter 1944-1945, as a member of the APhA Council 1960-1968, as chairman of the APhA House of Delegates 1964-1965, and as APhA president 1966-1967. As chairman of the APhA Committee on Student Branches 1952-1955, he was instrumental in the creation of the APhA Student Section; and as chairman of the APhA Committee to Study the Qualifications for Membership 1959-1962, he was a strong supporter of limiting active APhA membership to pharmacists.

Values Based on Love and Respect

Linwood Franklin Tice

The 1971 Remington Honor Medal Lecture was presented on December 2, 1971, at the Statler Hilton Hotel in New York City Tice's Remington address was not published, but it is preserved on a tape recording in the APhA Archives that has been transcribed for this volume.

One cannot be selected as a Remington medalist without mixed emotions-happiness, but also humility. The legendary James Beal received the first Remington medal when I was only ten years old. Over the years, we have seen many other distinguished leaders of American pharmacy receive the Remington medal, and they all contributed much to our profession. It is therefore deeply satisfying for me to have achieved the distinction of becoming a Remington medalist.

Since Joseph Remington's successor Charles LaWall, and his successor Ivor Griffith, were my predecessors at the Philadelphia College of Pharmacy and Science, and since both LaWall and Griffith received the Remington medal, the chain remains unbroken down through the years. So too has the indelible mark left by Joseph Remington and his philosophy which surely must continue to be passed down to successive generations of our faculty and students.

I know that it is somewhat traditional for a Remington medalist to use such an occasion to give a blueprint for the future. I shall not do so! I have belabored audiences and my readers for years on this subject without any noticeable effect, and I shall spare you this exercise in endurance.

I have tried to analyze why I am being honored tonight. Quite frankly, I have never been convinced that any one of us deserve all the credit we receive for our achievements. We inherit certain genes, and we accept ourselves at an early age in an environment not of our choosing. Our destiny is shaped and molded by various influences, and it is the special influences in my own life that I wish to discuss.

My grandfather was a firm and resolute man whom I idolized. I worked for him on his farm, and in time I joined him in his commercial fishing venture. He taught me to endure hard work, and well I remember how on one windy night when I was at the oars straining with every once of energy I had, he turned and looked at me with his pipe clinched between his teeth and said, "son, it never does any good until it hurts." And my mother taught me determination, and set me on a course of Christian living.

I attribute my entrance into pharmacy to an old preceptor, Dr. James L. Tuohy. I was working at the age of twelve at a sidewalk fruit stand on Saturdays, and it was here on one cold day that Dr. Tuohy stopped by and asked me if I would like to work for him. I accepted, I now suspect, to get out of the cold. This began a friendship which lasted until I helped lay him to rest many years later. He took time to teach me many things in his pharmacy where I worked all through high school. He then encouraged me to enroll at the Philadelphia College of Pharmacy where he had graduated in 1903, and it was from him that I first learned about the great Joseph Remington who was one of Dr. Tuohy's teachers. I enrolled at the Philadelphia College of Pharmacy when I was seventeen, commuting each school day almost 100 miles while still working for Dr. Tuohy. As a student, I was scared to death of Dr. Louis Gershenfeld, but in later years he became my confidant and advisor. It would be difficult for me to give credit to all of my early teachers because each contributed much to shaping my career. My first degree was received in 1929, after which the late Dean Charles LaWall asked me to assist him in some research which he was conducting in cooperation with Dr. George Beal whom I got to know very well. These old friendships are important.

In 1930, I accepted a position at Baylor University. But I must have done something wrong because they closed the school the following year. So I returned to the Philadelphia College of Pharmacy and Science in 1931 to continue my studies. It was then that I met a young chemistry professor, Dr. Arthur Osol, who encouraged me in my work. We even co-authored some research papers which were published. Somewhat later, Dean LaWall invited me to join his department beginning my faculty service which has lasted to the present. This brought me even closer to a former professor whom I admired as a student. It was Dr. Ivor Griffith's encouragement during his long tenure as dean and then as president which led me to my rapid advancement at the College.

My *Pharmacopeial* service began when I was recommended by the late Edward Newcomb to fill an unexpired term on the revision committee during 1940-1950. I credit my early assignments with the American Pharmaceutical Association to Dr. Hugo Schaefer who over the years did as much for our national professional society as any other person. I first met Dr. William S. Apple when he was waiting to be interviewed as the successor to Dr. Robert Fischelis. I know that Bill Apple has been controversial. The British would have gladly shot George Washington for his part in the War of Independence, and Lincoln was shot for freeing the slaves. I have watched Bill Apple closely from many vantage points, and I am convinced that he has but one goal-to emancipate our profession. I pray he will succeed.

In summation, it has been the opportunities given me by others which made my career possible, and in almost every stance a Remington student, a Remington disciple, or a Remington medalist has been responsible. I must also recognize the great advantage which I have had by reason of my tenure at the Philadelphia College of Pharmacy and Science. It has long been our tradition to give great freedom of action to our staff and to encourage participation in professional, scientific, and community affairs. In many cases, I am sure that my frequent absence from the campus placed a burden on others, and at times my activities might well have been cause for dismissal in an institution not subscribing to complete freedom of expression and action.

Many others deserve great credit including my dear wife of 42 years, my administrative assistant who has worked with me side-by-side for over 20 years, my many colleagues at the College, and my students who have always been a source of deep satisfaction.

From these reflections of the past, each of us can learn a lesson. Whether intended or not, each of us in our daily life influences countless others for better or for worse. A seemingly insignificant word of encourage mentor praise, a letter of endorsement, or an expression of faith may turn out to be their turning point in life. If I were to break my promise and write a prescription for the future, it would be simple. Pharmacy must reverse the trend of depersonalization. Modern life with its total preoccupation with technology has dehumanized us all. People cry out in pain and desperation for the help of just one human being who really cares.

We have such opportunities every day in the practice of pharmacy. Nothing can ever take the place of sympathetic listening and living by values which are based on love and respect for one's fellow man. Those of us who have been blessed by loyal, helpful friends have an even greater obligation to extend a helping hand to others. I surely owe much, if not everything, to others. I thank you one and all, and may God bless you as he has blessed me throughout my life. ■

1972 Remington Medalist

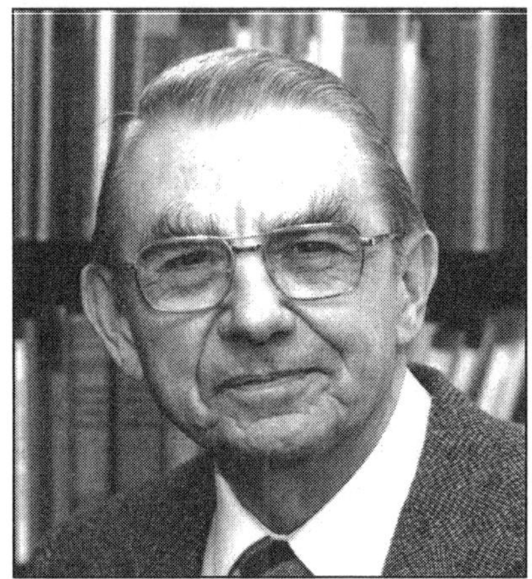

GLENN ALLEN SONNEDECKER

Glenn Allen Sonnedecker was born in Creston, Ohio, on December 11, 1917. He received a B.S. degree in pharmacy from Ohio State University and was licensed as a pharmacist in 1942. He joined Science Service in Washington, D.C. 1942-1943, and served as American Pharmaceutical Association staff member 1943-1948. He then entered graduate school at the University of Wisconsin earning an M.S. 1950 and a Ph.D. 1952 in the history of pharmacy, and subsequently served as assistant professor 1952-1956, associate professor 1956-1960, and professor 1960-1986. During this period he served as chairman of the AACP committee on pharmacy college libraries 1954-1955; as Rho Chi executive council member 1957-1959; as contributing editor of *American Professional Pharmacist* 1957-1960; and as editor-in-chief of *RPh* magazine 1978-1980. But he is best known for his service to the American Institute of the History of Pharmacy as secretary 1949-1957, executive director 1957-1973 and 1981-1985, founding editor of *Pharmacy in History* 1959-1963 and 1985-1986, and chairman of the AIHP Council 1988-1989. He served as president of the International Academy of the History of Pharmacy 1983-1991. Among the most notable of his many publications are 1963 and 1976 revisions of *Kremers and Urdang's History of Pharmacy*.

Sonnedecker served APhA variously as editor of the *Journal of the American Pharmaceutical Association, Practical Pharmacy Edition* 1943-1948; secretary of National Pharmacy Week 1946-1948; chairman of the APhA committee on terminology 1949-1952; chairman of the APhA Section on Historical Pharmacy 1951-1952; APhA research consultant 1964-1965; chairman of the 1969 task force on sub-professionals in pharmacy; chairman of the 1985 APhA-Academy of Pharmaceutical Sciences joint task force; and APhA honorary president 1985-1986.

American Pharmacy—A Retrospective Future

Glenn Allen Sonnedecker

The 1972 Remington Honor Medal Lecture was presented on December 12, 1972, at the Statler Hilton Hotel in New York City. Sonnedecker's Remington address was published in *Journal of the American Pharmaceutical Association,* volume NS13, pages 128-130, 146, 1973.

The values of history have never included prophecy. So it seems appropriate to take an historical perspective in assessing some circumstances of the American pharmacist from today's vantage point, in the year 2072. As Ambrosius of Palermo declared in 1287, "Pharmacy stands at the crossroads!" Each year since 1287, this has been reiterated by pharmacy's leaders. The question remains, do we know which crossroads we're at? We do know, of course, that the pharmacist would not want the road back to that half-civilized time of, say, the 1970's, with its underdeveloped profession and relatively primitive drug therapy. Nor were pharmacists then entirely united as a profession, or united in their views of what the profession should be, according to Professor Strompelthwaite's historical study. He found evidence that American pharmacy in that remote time had not recovered from a delayed impact of the Industrial Revolution, for which pharmacists seem to have been ill prepared. Already in the 19th century, however, the old unity of pharmacy's function-the collecting and processing of ingredients, the preparing of medicines, the assurance of quality, the dispensing itself as a single role had begun to fragment.

It appears from surviving records that by the 20th century pharmacists were spending a good bit of time telling each other that the loss of their centuries old central function, the making of drugs, was not really an important event. It had been merely manual labor. Pharmacists were warned about whistling in the dark, however, at the conclusion of the National Pharmaceutical Survey in 1950. The director, in his final report, observed that, "Mass manufacture of medicinals has caused the practicing pharmacist to serve more and more as a mere distributor... Whether pharmacy is to be able to have and to hold a real professional status, or whether it is to become stabilized, in the most of its practice, as one of the subordinate technological occupations of modern civilization, may be considered to be debatable questions—Vigorous offensive action is clearly indicated ...." At first, action seems to have been limited largely to debate about the dimensions of "pharmacy," and therefore about its future. The actual regeneration scarcely began before the late 20th century when-at a decisive moment in history-doors closed by tradition were sprung open by the impact of American medical care itself being restructured. Out of this regeneration was born to the 21st century the diversified, pharmacy-based careers that may strike us in 2072 as remarkable, at least in contrast with the 20th century, when pharmacy had been unified largely around a distributive function.

If the profession became more vigorous, it also became smaller. This can be attributed partly to an influx of pharmacy aides and other auxiliary personnel. Insecure about their own role, many pharmacists resisted the idea of welcoming a subordinate class until well after technical assistants were commonplace in the pharmacies of most other countries and in literally hundreds of newly structured semi-technical occupations in America. Many other complex functions traditional in society had been reduced to components designed for minimal education and a control system, if not actual automation.

The intensified need for quality rather than quantity can be attributed even more to a basic change in the workplace of the pharmacy practitioner-a subject even today, in 2072, still somewhat painful and perplexing. Perhaps no one here is old enough to be able to remember the 20th century, but some are old enough to recall a time when there were as many pharmacists working in public shops on street corners as are now employed in a strikingly different way in our health centers, group medical clinics and other types of institutions.

All but the younger pharmacists here may be aware that what we know as "druggists: sundry shops" evolved, only a couple of generations ago, out of pharmacies in the same locations. A few of the old "druggists" in these shops are former pharmacists who failed to pass the periodic relicensing examination, or even still hold a license to practice pharmacy; but most "druggists" (you may recall) have little formal training, often being pharmacy technicians who aspired to a higher income. Since these ubiquitous sundry shops may still be operated much in the old capitalist pattern, the income of the druggists often equals that of the pharmacist in a health center or clinic, even though the druggists are not permitted to mix or manipulate drug ingredients in any way or dispense drugs from broken packages. Thus, in ultra-modern guise, America seems to have resurrected an old functionary of European communities, the "druggist" of bygone times, whose shop had nothing to do with the profession of pharmacy.

Today American pharmacists do not feel either in conflict or in competition with the druggist, since the uniform law of the year 2013 removed prescription drugs from the druggist's sundry shop and stopped public advertising of even the rather innocuous range of medication they were still permitted to stock.

But to understand fully how the old conflict was resolved, and how the roles of the pharmacist and the druggist came to be separated, we must remind ourselves briefly of a remarkable turn of events in the organizational history of pharmacy.

Soon after the end of the 20th century, the imagination of young pharmacists was captured by a supposedly new slogan-"One voice for pharmacy!" Actually, these were antique and magical words that had been conjured up periodically over the preceding half century in an attempt to exorcise the controversy between the National Association of Retail Druggists and the American Pharmaceutical Association. That can be documented from yellowed journals of pharmacy still preserved, which at that time were still being printed in bound volumes much like the books that had transmitted information since the invention of printing.

What pharmacists now attained was a merger of the two organizations, renamed the "American Pharmacists' Association." It was more than a political ploy. Pharmacists wished to make clear that the organization represented pharmacists wherever they might serve, yet make explicit even in the name that the association did not represent all elements of the pharmaceutical field.

The stark difference between the dimension of pharmacy and of the pharmaceutical field, which seems obvious to us, for some reason seems to have been confused or obscured during much of the 20th century. In any event, older pharmacists here may recall the explosion that occurred from this incompatible mixture of the two organizations.

It is one of the ironies of history that many of these retail establishments, by the time of the schism, no longer found it worthwhile to maintain their qualifications to be designated as pharmacies. Thus it was the obsolete term "druggist" came to be resurrected, refining the flavor of an old tradition as well as accommodating to new conditions. To serve these druggists the National Association of Retail Druggists was resurrected, which research shows had existed during most of the 20th century as a business-oriented organization of drugstore owners. Truth indeed can be stranger than fiction!

The vigor and verve of today's compact profession stems in no small part from the challenging full-time demands placed upon the pharmacist by physicians, nurses and other health care professionals. Professor Ischkin, the historian of 20th century pharmacy, claims that an eloquent and daring spokesman for pharmacists named Arple was insisting already in the 1960's that making the average pharmacist a full-time practitioner was crucial to the future of the profession. Why this was considered a radical idea can no longer be discerned from surviving records, although it is obvious that Arple is a misprint for a leader named Apple... William Apple.

Even though these full-time roles are not all of a kind-as the multi-path curricula in our schools of pharmacy reflect and indeed guarantee-nevertheless, from our vantage point in 2072, we can see that there has been achieved a greater sense of common roots and shared aims despite the specialization.

The practitioner usually called "pharmacist" today finds his antecedent in the practitioner who was termed "clinical pharmacist" during about a half century prior to 2030. The intent had been to differentiate clinical pharmacists from those who were geared by training and experience to mainly a distributive function. This distinction became superfluous after the affectionately regarded "American drugstore" proved to be crucially handicapped in sustaining clinical pharmacy services within the new, more tightly integrated system of medical care. Thus, the pharmacies formerly existing as separate shops gradually withdrew from the structure of professional pharmacy or amalgamated with some type of institutional pharmacy.

Within the new professional hierarchy the so-called "clinical pharmacologists" have become somewhat of a self-defined elite, bringing a new source of friction in its wake.

Professor Pestlepusher concludes from his study of pharmacy during the early 21st century that this specialized segment of pharmacy became legitimatized mainly through two circumstances. First, the advanced standard of training that had been made available to selected pharmacists proved adequate, once they were declared eligible to take the board-diploma examination in applied clinical pharmacology. Second, the number of clinical pharmacologists holding an MD degree had remained totally inadequate for practical therapeutic needs since at least the mid-20th century, hence they no longer felt threatened by the candidates for qualification that arose with increasing frequency in the domain of pharmacy.

While it would be unbecoming for me to speculate about the future, it appears that the main thrust of pharmacy will continue to be in the health center, whose forerunner had been known in its pioneer days by the rather bureaucratic term "health maintenance organization." In recent decades of course, these often have been not only physically unified or interrelated but contiguous to traditional types of hospitals. This has simplified the sharing of facilities and resources, such as electronic information retrieval facilities and supersonic transport of emergency cases to specialized treatment facilities. If there's one feature of these operations I would urge changing, it is the flying pharmacies that serve the remaining rural areas and are manned only by a pharmacy technician and, sometimes, a physician's assistant. This type of service in a flying pharmacy merits a fully qualified pharmacist quite as much as a more sophisticated facility in a health center.

Probably we should comment more specifically on some of the services that we have come to expect of the public practitioner-as contrasted with pharmacists educated to specialize in industrial sales; in the legally required supervisory positions in manufacturing and wholesale pharmacy; in information storage, retrieval and evaluation; in applied pharmacology, and so on. At one time separate curricula were required to qualify fully in these branches, which are distinct and yet today are taken so much for granted as components of the same profession of pharmacy. Professors Winldestump and Pillendreher once came to blows over whether or not curricula in the schools had proliferated in response to public need or only in response to government capitation grants. In any event it had constructive results, even though more sporadic and often less formal means of advanced education have become popular, now that specialty board examinations are open in most of these fields to anyone with a basic pharmacy degree. However, it is the public practitioner of the health center, clinic or hospital whom Fred Thimblethwaite of Oshkosh, in his presidential address, termed the "backbone of medical care since time immemorial"although to be historically precise, I would say that the public pharmacist in this sense did not dominate the field of pharmacy until about 2030 or even later. What strikes us about this pharmacy practitioner is the long tradition and respect he holds as an expert in monitoring symptomatology and blood levels, and in controlling the drug depot implanted in a patient to achieve the physician's prescribed therapeutic objectives. Unfortunately, it is coming to seem old fashioned for a pharmacist to make house calls for this purpose, since most pharmacy departments now have an electronic console adequate to handle a normal patient load by remote control.

When stockpiles of artificial as well as natural limbs, organs and tissues-and electronic substitutes for the senses-began to be of practical importance several years ago, it appeared that providing surgeons with this range of resources would become an important new service of the pharmacist. There remains a strong argument for reuniting this responsibility with a related one the pharmacist already holds-I refer to formulating and monitoring the delicate regimen necessary to inhibit antibody reactions after surgeons have made the grafts onto defective bodies.

Perhaps most of us can scarcely imagine the practice of pharmacy without a computer-based operation. Yet, we need not reach back into history farther than the 20th century to understand that it was perfectly feasible for a chief pharmacist to function effectively without computerized inventory, without automatic ordering, without audioprint and computer input when designing a drug regimen, without centrally computerized medication profiles, without automated dispensing of drugs and typing of labels. Indeed there was a time-still within the limits of what we call the modern period-when there was not even a pharmacy aide to type labels, and this often was done by the pharmacist himself. To those who think pharmacy has become old-fashioned and tradition-bound in employing computer technology, I would remind you that it has been only a century since pharmacists were keeping hand-written medication records in their own pharmacies.

What we must keep in mind is that the pharmacist then did not have complex drug delivery mechanisms for which he was responsible in the medical-care team; did not have many drug entities with which to cope, and particularly had only a fraction of the preventive regimens that the pharmacist now routinely administers; and he did not have responsibility for information retrieval and evaluation in therapeutics from the massive resources made possible by national and international data processing, and by a cadre of auxiliary personnel in medical-computer technology. Indeed, much information was brought to the pharmacy on hundreds of printed pages monthly, usually travelling by gasoline and diesel-powered conveyances such as you have seen in museums.

In Dr. Pennyweight's penetrating little essay called "Reminiscences of American

Health Science Under Capitalism," he related that during the transitional system under health insurance, there were as many as 1.5 billion third-party claims per year. The present data-processing system thus can be seen as an artifact of this insurance method of compensating for pharmaceutical services; and the desired re-tooling has been inhibited by the enormous cost.

Moreover, a lack of complete compatibility among regional data banks and computer networks serving the health professions has been aggravated by the increased mobility of patients since the abolishment of customs and immigration barriers over nearly two-thirds of the earth's surface. Another problem of information storage and retrieval is more basic than system redesign. I refer to the hazards of placing utter reliance upon man's common language, globa-lingua, in such highly specialized areas as pharmaceutics and pharmacology. Moreover, deviations from the international system of pharmaceutical nomenclature in the reports from some parts of the world make it unfeasible to rely upon standard code numbers alone.

In the field of education we should be eternally grateful to the martyred deans who rejected federal grants they believed not to be in the best interests of the profession thereby committing academic suicide. This traumatic time yielded a somewhat smaller network of remaining schools, which meanwhile have expanded in size and influence within their respective medical-education centers.

Building upon a full development of the concept of clinical pharmacy toward the end of the 20th century, most faculties moved toward strengthened assurances that graduates of the core curriculum would be confident in their use of systems of drug administration, drug monitoring and drug reaction reporting; ingrained with the concepts and practices of control systems made mandatory by the number of different professionals and subprofessionals complexly involved in drug therapy; expert in health-data processing far beyond the level of their technicians, and masters in reading (if not speaking) globa-lingua. Perhaps more surprising has been the insistence of a majority of the faculties that students have a small amount of humanistic and social study of pharmacy to help prepare them for a place in the intellectual and professional community.

Moreover, at least a third of the schools instituted vigorous research programs to analyze historical trends as they affect pharmacy and to study pharmacy with social science tools as a major resource in expediting knowledgeable change. I think particularly of the demonstrated utility to the profession of some of the alternative models that have been project-tested under controlled field conditions concerning professional techniques, concerning patient relationships, concerning demographic factors, concerning measurable effects of guiding the mushrooming use of non-medicinal drugs and so on.

From the symbiotic effect of the technical and social studies we are getting young practitioners with both the content and cast of mind that makes them effective in patient care and enthusiastic colleagues. Looking back from the vantage point of 2072, we must admit not being so successful, however, in resisting a trend toward controls and programs that foster the enlargement and welfare of the state perhaps more than the enlargement and welfare of its citizens. Yet, the average pharmacist has maintained-even more than in pharmacy's so-called "golden age of the '80's"-his own conception of his duties and responsibilities toward the patient and toward the core concept of an unwavering professional judgment. The enlargement of these responsibilities under public mandate, during the 21st century, may be partly attributable to the pharmacist's involvement and outreach in all areas related to medicinal supply and therapeutics.

Perhaps above all, it links into pharmacists having made obvious the unique safeguard, and continuous and collective commitment, that only they so uniquely offer society toward safe and effective use of physiologically active substances.

As we look upon these developments in pharmacy we share the feeling of that master pharmacist of New York, Frederick Hoffmann, who said in 1902 before the APhA, "... The art of traditional pharmacy...has undergone a sweeping change in recent years and has suffered a displacement of its original essential functions, brought about by the prodigious advance in the kindred sciences and arts, by specialization in most domains of application, but more rational and restrictive methods of medication, and... abolishing the apothecaries' laboratory of old ...." Although the changes experienced in our time may not seem as dramatic as those faced by Frederick Hoffmann, as pharmacists entered the 20th century, the historical record suggests that we have progressed in redefining the roles of the several specialties of pharmacy as full-time occupations for the average practitioner; that we have progressed in making these roles an integral and compatible part of medical care.

If I have seemed to imply what the next century might bring, I have not meant to do so. A forgotten historian of pharmacy of the late 20th century, Glenn Sonnedecker, often expressed conviction that the value of history did not include prediction. Yet, he was not above the whimsy of looking at the future retrospectively. Probably he would not be surprised (if he could know) that things have turned out quite differently from what he imagined. ■

1973 Remington Medalist

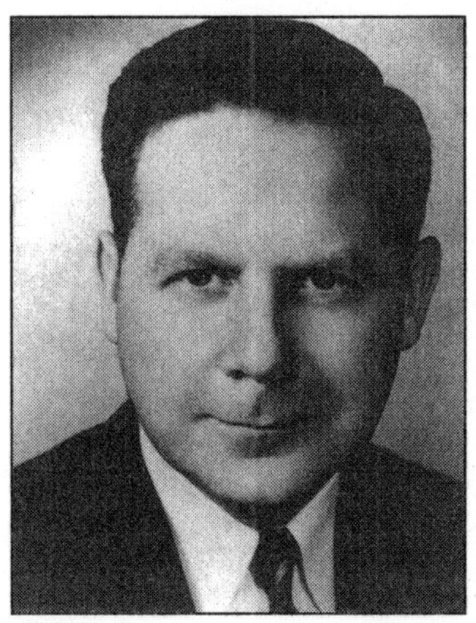

GROVER CLEVELAND BOWLES, JR.

Grover Cleveland Bowles, Jr. was born in Piedmont, Missouri, on February 15, 1920, and received a B.S. degree in pharmacy from the University of Tennessee in 1942. After service with the U.S. Navy Hospital Corps during World War II, he interned in a hospital pharmacy at the University of Michigan 1946-1947; he became chief pharmacist at Strong Memorial Hospital in Rochester, New York, and served on the faculty of the University of Rochester School of Medicine and Dentistry 1948-1955; as associate director of the Memorial Hospital Association of Kentucky 1955-1956; and as director of pharmacy service at the Baptist Memorial Hospital in Memphis, Tennessee 1956 until his retirement in 1984. He served on the faculty of the University of Tennessee College of Pharmacy 1958-1993, Memphis Retail Druggists Association president 1958, Tennessee Society of Hospital Pharmacists president 1948-1949, and American Society of Hospital Pharmacists president 1952-1953. He was a member of the *USP* revision committee 1960-1970, Tennessee Hospital Licensing Board 1962-1981, and American Council on Pharmaceutical Education president 1982-1986.

Bowles joined the American Pharmaceutical Association in 1943, and was first elected to the APhA Council in 1956. He subsequently served as APhA House of Delegates speaker 1960-1962, APhA Board of Trustees chairman 1963-1964, APhA president 1965-1966, APhA treasurer 1967-1979, and APhA Foundation vice president 1991-1993. He traveled to South Vietnam in 1969 under sponsorship of the U.S. Agency for International Development to survey pharmacy, and he served as contributing editor to both the *American Journal of Hospital Pharmacy* 1958-1968 and *The Modern Hospital* 1956-1967.

VIEWING THE FUTURE WITH OPTIMISM

Grover Cleveland Bowles, Jr.

The 1973 Remington Medal was presented August 6, 1974, at the Conrad Hilton Hotel in Chicago, Illinois, during the August 3-8, 1974, American Pharmaceutical Association annual meeting. Bowles's Remington address was published in the *Journal of the American Pharmaceutical Association,* volume NS14, pages 550-553, 564, 1974.

I am honored to be the 1973 Remington Medalist. I am grateful to my colleagues and friends who are here tonight and to all who have wished me well on this most important occasion in my life.

When I selected Dr. Apple and Dr. Latiolais to speak on my behalf, I did not attempt to offer either of them any advice about what they might say. It would have been bad manners and futile. Both of these leaders are always very frank in their observations, and I appreciate their candor tonight.

As citizens, all of us are concerned about the credibility crisis in our national government. Many of us still don't understand what happened, how it happened or why it happened. But all of us recognize there is a lesson to be learned and learned well if your republic is to survive. It needs to be learned by those who are governed just as much as it does by those who are entrusted to govern. While the current focus is on Washington, the issue is integrity of government to every level-precinct, city, county, state and national. All of us are involved, and none of us can deny our responsibility.

If you have heard or read any of the law school commencement speeches this year, you know the special emphasis on integrity and accountability. The public image of the legal profession has been badly tarnished, and its leaders recognize that it won't be wiped clean by the guilty pleas or convictions of a few dozen former government officials.

Dr. James Barber, chairman of the Department of Political Science at Duke University recently observed that:

"The reputation of nearly every national institution is drifting down: Professors, doctors, the press, even 'science' is in decline, with politicians leading the pack. The American people say in plain terms that they are disgusted with the way things are going and with the men in charge."

Dr. Barber also observed that V*ox populi* is no *vox Dei* and as sore as the present public is, there is strong evidence that they are American to the core, "... above all, watching and waiting for the leadership to express and effect their new sense of the country's commitment to community, humaneness and candor."

It is not my intention tonight to offer any appraisal of the current reputation of pharmacy or to suggest which way it is drifting. It should be obvious to every pharmacist that whether we are better or worse than doctors or lawyers is not relevant. Our concern should be-do we have what it takes to stop drifting and start paddling?

One cannot be involved in the political structure of pharmacy government for several decades without forming some impressions and opinions. Tonight, I would like to share a few of mine with you.

First, pharmacy is not a "captive" profession although many pharmacists still be have as serfs. Second, pharmacy education is maintaining pace with technology, but there has been little improvement in preparing pharmacy graduates for the humanistic responsibilities of professionalism. Third, pharmacy is organizationally weak because pharmacy leaders are provincial and lack selfdiscipline.

Now, I would like to expand on these observations.

Pharmacy is not a "captive" profession although many pharmacists still behave as serfs and are held in bondage by an inbred inferiority complex that is neither becoming of a profession or necessary at this point in time.

Schooled to a comfortable complacency, too many pharmacists are content to function in a subservient capacity and fail to see the crippling effect of their attitude on the profession. They are inclined to place greater credence on the views and advice of those outside the profession than that of our own leaders. It is this group of pharmacists who think that if the APhA would just stop rocking the boat everything would be alright. They're quite willing to face the future as they have the past knowing-"That's the way things are; that's the way things have always been; and that's the way things will always be." To them, acquiescence and don't rock the boat are the only options open to the profession in dealing with conflict and in charting our future.

Nowhere is the pharmacist's inferiority complex more visible than in his relationship with the physician.

Growing consumer sophistication, the coverage of prescribed medication by governmental and private third party programs with freedom of choice clauses and other changes during recent years have been helpful in freeing the pharmacist from the economic domination of the physician. As a result few pharmacists today provide physicians with imprinted prescription blanks, there are not as many direct telephone lines between doctor's offices and pharmacies as in previous times and I suspect that fewer pharmacists feel obligated to give gifts to physicians during the holiday season and on other occasions. However, physicians who own professional buildings or clinics have no difficulty in finding pharmacists in the community who are willing to enter into a percentage lease agreement for pharmacy space on the assumption their financial future will be secure.

Although much progress has been made in physician/pharmacist relations, the fact remains that few pharmacists are comfortable in discussing the drug therapy of a patient with the prescriber. Even when it is necessary to question a dose that appears to be too high or too low, or to bring a possible drug-drug interaction to the attention of the physician or to raise other questions involving the professional judgment of the prescriber, the pharmacist's inferiority complex begins to surface. While pharmacists may complain to each other about the difficulty in getting through to the doctor, the truth is that all too often, the pharmacist is more comfortable discussing problems with the office nurse than with the physician. When the pharmacist does discuss a problem with the physician he does so apologetically and with hesitation even when he knows that he is technically correct and is acting in the best interest of the patient.

In the area of product selection, I know more pharmacists who are afraid of offending the physician than I do who are concerned about their lack of competency to select drug products of acceptable quality. I know still fewer pharmacists who feel comfortable suggesting to a physician that the same benefits for the patient can be obtained at substantially less cost by using the drug product of another manufacturer rather than the one specified, when multiple sources are available.

Over years, pharmacists have generally followed the dictates and wishes of organized medicine and the pharmaceutical industry in supporting health-related legislative proposals, even to the detriment of the profession.

A good example of the failure of pharmacists to examine what they were being encouraged to support in the light of how the legislation, if passed, might affect the profession and pharmacists personally, was the support by pharmacists of organized medicine's opposition to the Medicare amendments to the Social Security Act. As pharmacy blindly pursued a course of loyal support of medicine's public opposition to Medicare, organized medicine's leaders were privately negotiating a sweetheart deal with the Administration. As a result, pharmacists were left out in the cold and out-of-hospital drugs are yet to be included as a Medicare benefit.

It is highly doubtful if the industry sponsored state anti-substitution laws could have been passed without the almost unanimous support of pharmacists, their state associations and their national professional society. It took pharmacy almost two decades to realize that these laws protect the brand name pharmaceutical industry, not the public or the profession.

The Durham-Humphrey amendment to the Federal Food, Drug, and Cosmetic Act, widely supported by pharmacists, has had the most devastating effect on the professional prerogatives of the pharmacist of any legislation enacted in my time. Had pharmacists of the late 1940s and early 1950s been politically alert they would have worked to either defeat this legislation or to expand it to include a third class of drugs to be dispensed personally by the pharmacist. Unfortunately, pharmacists of that era, like many today, simply did not want the responsibility for making professional decisions.

If pharmacy has a real function in society then we have the right to professional freedom. We must exercise this right by getting rid of the inferiority complex which has been passed from one generation of pharmacists to the next. This calls for reorientation and a changing of attitude for many pharmacists. We must convince ourselves that pharmacy is an independent profession and that we can stand on our two feet. If we are to avoid becoming a captive profession we cannot leave our future to be determined by others.

While we live in a time of rapid change, we don't experience our lives and the surrounding conditions changing so rapidly.

It is when we look back over two, three or more decades that we see the magnitude of the changes that have occurred. Public opinion is also constantly changing and these changes are reflected in a variety of ways, including the decisions handed down by our courts. The unanimous decision of the U.S. Supreme Court late last year in overturning the Liggett decision, followed more recently by the unanimous decision of the North Dakota Supreme Court upholding the state statute requiring pharmacy ownership control of pharmacies, reflects the change in public opinion that has taken place over the years. These decisions offer much encouragement and hope to pharmacists in their struggle to keep the profession free and independent.

Of equal or even greater significance to the profession was the decision handed down by the U.S. District Court upholding the APhA position in the methadone case. While this case is being appealed, it demonstrates the profession's ability to defend itself from the onslaught of governmental bureaucracy assuming we have the desire to do so.

Now I would like to move to my second observation.

Pharmacy education is maintaining pace with technology but there has been little improvement in preparing pharmacy graduates for the humanistic responsibilities of professionalism.

Most of us, perhaps all, will agree that pharmaceutical education is maintaining pace with technology. We point with pride to the many advances in the sophistication of the scientific courses in today's curriculum compared to that of 10, 20 or 30 years ago. The application of this new knowledge in clinical settings outside the classrooms and laboratories of the college of pharmacy is bringing students into direct contact with patients and other members of the health care team for the first time. These are major changes when we remember that the vast majority of pharmacists now in practice were educated in the day when the emphasis was on the preparation of dosage forms and on drug product knowledge with little time spent on the disease processes and no contact with patients.

The Dichter Study concluded that many of the pharmacist's problems can be traced to his failure to adequately communicate the value of his services to his patients. The same might also be said about our problems with the medical profession and governmental agencies. If pharmacists are to function effectively in clinical settings and if they are going to restore their rapport with people, pharmacy students must have more exposure to the behavioral sciences and to courses that sharpen their communication skills.

If you have participated in the sessions of the Academy of General Practice of Pharmacy or reviewed their excellent program for this annual meeting, you know the emphasis they are placing on the importance of improving communications and building a professional image. Yet one state having mandatory continuing education will not allow credit for the Monday morning session on "How to Build Your Professional Image" or the Thursday morning session on "Understanding Human Behavior" but will give credit for all sessions of the Academy of Pharmaceutical Sciences.

In the field of professional competency it is important that pharmacists face up to the fact that we are going to have to demonstrate our capacity to the public. I am convinced that the best way to do this is not to turn over responsibility to the state but to demonstrate that we can do it ourselves as a matter of professional pride and responsibility. Mandatory continuing education and mandatory patient drug profiles, it seems to me, again demonstrate the strong tendency we have to pass laws with compulsory aspects almost as a symptom of our psychotic feeling that we have to be forced or ordered to do things by someone above us.

There has been somewhat of a tendency over the years on the part of pharmaceutical educators to attempt to give the student the total package as if during his life cycle of practice the graduate is not going to have the opportunity to expand his knowledge. As a result many students leave school over prepared in technology but under-prepared as human beings and to function as professionals. This points up the important work of such groups as the Task Force on Specialties which recognized that there is much to be learned after graduation and that those who are willing to learn it and function in a special way deserve to be recognized for this accomplishment.

More than a quarter of a century ago, the Pharmaceutical Survey concluded that, "the outstanding factor in determining the future of the profession of pharmacy is fundamentally moral in nature." Our Code of Ethics was revised a few years ago and we are fortunate to have a judicial Board to aid in its interpretation and to give us advisory opinions. All too frequently when the Code of Ethics is discussed in the classroom it is in the abstract sense and by those who are more familiar with the printed words than the application of the Code in real life situations. There is little time for discussion among pharmacy students of moral and ethical values as they relate to professional practice.

Speaking about the development of the student as a professional person, Dr. Hugh C. Muldoon in his 1953 Remington Address said, "We inculate sound moral and spiritual and ethical values by discussion and illustration and example. We teach respect for the law, and the dignity of work, and the necessity for sincerity and honor and truthfulness in our relations with others. We encourage honesty and industry and accuracy and patience and perseverance. We nourish curiosity and initiative, creative power in thinking, and intellectual courage. We endeavor to develop sound attitudes and insight as well as professional skills. We are concerned not only with what the student learns, but also with the attitudes he develops as he learns. We try to inspire as well as to teach. In some scholars, at least, we kindle a love of learning."

This brings me to my third and final observation. Pharmacy is organizationally weak because pharmacy leaders are provincial and lack self-discipline.

If we make an honest appraisal of pharmacy's organizational strength, we will have to conclude that even the American Pharmaceutical Association which has the largest membership of any pharmacy organization in the United States still doesn't have a clear majority of the pharmacists belonging to it. But even more disturbing to me is that if we took all the resources of all the national pharmacy organizations and pooled them with the resulting efficiencies that might come about, we still couldn't claim to be organizationally strong and effective, considering all the obstacles and problems in the constructive activities that should be undertaken.

How then are we to adjust to changing circumstances, to new complexities and to new challenges? Is it not clear that the time has come for all elements of our profession to work together and speak with one voice?

APhA and NARD leadership demonstrated their sensitivity to this need in the formation of the Committee on Pharmacy Economic Security. COPES, now more than a year old, is no panacea nor is it going to solve all the problems of American pharmacy. No one recognizes this more than the leadership of APhA and NARD. However, leaders of both organizations have found that a result of discussing issues thoroughly and taking into consideration the effect that a certain position is going to have, not just on their own constituency, but on the total profession and the public, they have moved closer together.

I have supported the affiliation movement since its inception and during my year as APhA president, three states signed affiliation agreements. While I would be the first to admit that the affiliation movement has not progressed as rapidly as I would have hoped, I am gratified to see the ripple effect that it has had on pharmacy organizations at the state and national levels. Many states that have not yet affiliated have or are in the process of implementing the basic recommendations made by APhA during the early days of the affiliation movement. Here I refer to the adoption of a House of Delegates structure which provides broad-based representation and for the use of democratic procedures in the nomination and election of officers such as the mail ballot. Some state and national associations have carried implementation of these democratic safeguards to a high state of sophistication with the addition of reference committees which provide for open and frank discussion of committee reports and the opportunity for input from the membership on the vital issues of the day.

It has always been rather interesting to me that the leadership in a number of states strongly supports reciprocal membership agreements within the state boundaries but is vehemently opposed to reciprocal arrangements between the state and national associations. This is one aspect of provincialism that is difficult for me to understand.

Many pharmacy leaders, and I am referring specifically to those who hold elective offices and committee appointments at the local and state levels and to whom the membership looks for guidance, lack self-discipline. When these so-called leaders are unhappy with a situation the first thought that always comes to mind is to create another organization or to go out and tell the troops to withhold their support until they get what they demand.

When I say that pharmacy leaders are provincial and lack self-discipline I should also point out that many do not prepare for leadership roles and fail to recognize the responsibility of leadership. There are always some who are more concerned about the next office they may obtain than they are about accomplishing something in their present office by speaking their minds with candor.

Now in defense of the leaders, I hasten to add that there are times when they are not completely at fault. Sooner or later most leaders find it necessary to stand their ground on unpopular issues and it is not uncommon for the troops to find it hard to accept a realistic appraisal of the situation and turn on their leader for telling the facts of life. We often lose good leaders in pharmacy because we fail to back them up and they are unwilling to take the carping criticism which is the habitual pattern of reaction among pharmacists. They either wash their hands of organizational activity entirely or lend half-hearted support, preferring the pursuit of personal interests to the politics of pharmacy.

Pharmacists criticizing APhA are always quick to point out that what we need in pharmacy is an organization like AMA. The American Medical Association is an effective voice for organized medicine. Physicians may grumble about organizational problems but when the chips are down and medicine has battles to fight, there is no doubt in anyone's mind that AMA speaks for the physicians of the country.

Like AMA, the American Pharmaceutical Association may be far from perfect, far from what we should have in pharmacy-but remember one thing, APhA is the best we have and is deserving of the profession's support. I often ask myself, why should we in APhA be apologetic about what we have done? Has anyone, anywhere, anyplace done so much?

One of pharmacy's major problems is that we are hung up on the past and seem to be hell-bent on keeping it alive. There is nothing to be gained by thrashing old hay. It is time to put the past behind us and look to the future. It is time to count our blessings and good fortunes-to stop measuring progress against perfection.

In closing, I should like to say that as I view the future I see much cause for optimism. We are no longer running away from the issues. We are not trying to run away from the problems. We are not trying to run away from our weaknesses and our differences. I sense that we in pharmacy are ready to set our own goals and make our own commitments. All this augers well for the future.

And one thing is certain, there will be a future. The question as I see it is not so much do we have the foresight to understand the future, but rather do we have the courage to change it? As we ponder this hard question, I hope that we will be guided by Theodore Roosevelt's advice, "Far better is it to dare mighty things, to win glorious triumphs, even though checkered by failure, than to take rank with those poor spirits who neither enjoy much nor suffer much, because they live in the gray twilight that knows not victory nor defeat."

I thank each of you for making this most memorable occasion for me. ■

1974 Remington Medalist

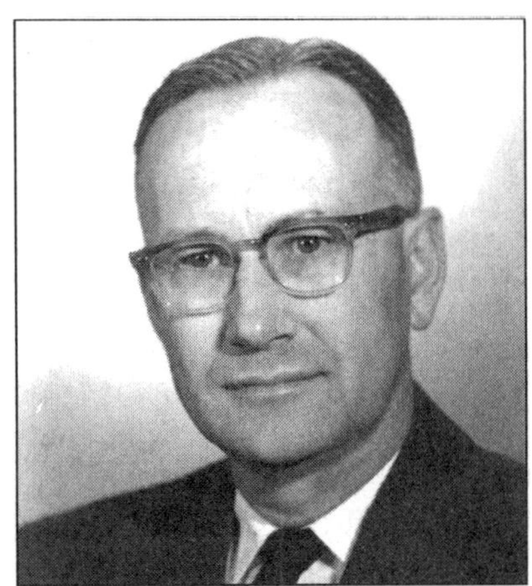

Lloyd McClain Parks

Lloyd McClain Parks was born in Scottsburg, Indiana, on March 21, 1912, and received a B.S. in 1933 and M.S. in 1936 from Purdue University School of Pharmacy, and a Ph.D. in 1938 from the University of Wisconsin. After working for a year as assistant manager of Myer Brothers Drug Company in Mishawaka, Indiana 1933-1934, and as graduate assistant at Purdue University 1934-1936, he joined the faculty of the University of Wisconsin serving as instructor 1938-1940, and associate professor 1942-1946 during which time he was on leave during World War II serving three years in the Mediterranean theater of operations as chemical officer for the 12th Air Force Service Command. He returned to the University of Wisconsin as professor of pharmaceutical chemistry from 1946 until 1956 when he became dean at Ohio State University College of Pharmacy, serving in this capacity until his retirement in 1977. During this period he variously served as a member of the *USP* revision committee 1950-1962, as president of the American Association of Colleges of Pharmacy 1961-1962, as president of Rho Chi 1961-1963, and as a member of the American Council on Pharmaceutical Education 1962-1968.

Parks joined the American Pharmaceutical Association in 1938, serving as chairman of the APhA Scientific Section 1951-1952 receiving the APhA Ebert Prize in 1952 and the APhA Foundation Research Achievement Award in 1966. He also served as APhA vice president 1970-1971, as chairman of the APhA Council 1967-1969, as APhA president 1971-1972, and as chairman of the APhA Task Force on Specialties in Pharmacy 1973-1974. Irene Comiskey Parks (1915-1979), wife of Lloyd Parks, served as president of the APhA Auxiliary 1964-1966, after which the Auxiliary Student Loan Fund was named in honor of Irene Parks.

Putting the Cart Before the Horse

Lloyd McClain Parks

The 1974 Remington Medal was presented April 22, 1975, at the St. Francis Hotel in San Francisco, California, during the April 20-24, 1975, American Pharmaceutical Association annual meeting. Parks's Remington address was published in the *Journal of the American Pharmaceutical Association,* volume NS15, pages 448-451, 457, 1975.

To be chosen as the 48th recipient of the Remington Medal is the highest honor in my professional life. When I look at the long list of previous recipients and contemplate their contributions to American pharmacy, I am humbled by the comparison. There are many among my contemporaries who are worthy of this honor but there is none who will cherish it more than I.

It would be impossible for me to acknowledge the many persons who, through their guidance, inspiration and support, have been important in my professional career but I would like to mention a few. Dr. Charles 0. Lee, long-time professor of pharmacy at Purdue University and my first teacher of pharmacy, encouraged me by his quiet but effective example and steered me to the University of Wisconsin for further graduate study under the late Edward Kremers, who was the Remington Medalist in 1930. Dr. Kremers attempted to teach me much more than I was able to learn but one of his precepts has always remained with me and that is that nothing can substitute for hard work and effort.

I spent many happy hours on the faculty at Wisconsin and, under the gentle but wise tutelage of Dean Arthur H. Uhl, served a sort of apprenticeship for my own later years as a dean. Among other things, I learned from him that a wise dean gets good men on his faculty and then stays out of their way so they can get the job done. It was there that I first came to know and appreciate Bill Apple, first as a student and later as a faculty colleague. Even as a student and faculty member, Bill was as impatient with the status quo as he is today; but I have learned much more from him in the years since than he learned from me as a student.

It was at Wisconsin also that I met Irene and asked her to become my wife. From that day forward she has been my biggest asset. Her devotion and love as wife and mother, her support and patience with my impatience, her understanding and unselfish suppression of her own interests, wishes and desires to the interest of my career and professional activities have been more than I ever can repay.

It has been my good fortune to have been associated, as student, faculty and dean, with three colleges of pharmacy that have been ranked by their peers as among the top seven in the United States, all three of them in the mid-west. This ranking confirms what I have long subscribed to and which I dare to say here in the Golden State-that the mid-west has been and is the heartland of pharmaceutical education in the United States. It is somewhat reassuring that Ohio State is regarded highly, in some quarters at least, for something besides its football team.

My special thanks are due Linwood Tice and Bill Apple for their much too generous remarks about me. I have been following such people as Linwood Tice and Bill Apple in American pharmacy for a long time and I hope some of their good qualities have rubbed off on me. But I would ask you, if you can, to appreciate the awesome spot in which such a build-up places the recipient. It is as though here were made an instant sage in pharmacy and that he must now deliver the final words of saving wisdom. I am reminded of the situation that President Gerald Ford found himself in when he delivered the commencement address last August at Ohio State University. He observed that, just a few months earlier, he had become the country's first instant vice president and just a few weeks earlier he had become the country's first instant president. Then he remarked, "The United States Marine Band is so confused that it doesn't know whether to play 'Hail to the Chief' or "You've Come a Long Way Baby."

Perhaps it would be more appropriate, and probably more appreciated by the audience, if the recipient, after basking in the glory generated by the testimonials, would follow the example of the late, beloved Walter Brennan of movie and television fame. He became famous for the shortest and most appreciated response when he received his first Oscar by saying, "Thank you." When he received the second he said, "Thank you very much;" and on the occasion of his third Oscar he gave his longest response, "Thank you very, very much."

But, frankly, I don't have the audacity to break with the tradition for the recipient to make an address on this occasion, so I shall make some remarks and leave it for a future recipient to break with precedent. Since my professional life has been devoted to pharmaceutical education, it should not be a surprise to you that my remarks will be largely confined to that area, since it is the one in which I feel most comfortable.

Those who have followed the development of pharmaceutical education in this country know that, in 1900, at the time of the formation of the organization now known as the American Association of Colleges of Pharmacies, two of the pressing problems were the lack of an adequate science foundation for the curriculum and the need to upgrade the faculty to provide that science foundation. We have succeeded so well in solving the second problem and, subsequently, the first that we now find ourselves with other problems as a result. The Carnegie Commission has said, "Professional knowledge usually consists of an underlying discipline, and applied science, and a component of skill frequently viewed as the art of professional practice. The professions differ in the degree to which these three elements come together in professional training."

Pharmaceutical education, as it has developed in the past few decades, is certainly not lacking in providing our students with the underlying disciplines. Our pharmaceutical science faculties, by and large, are of excellent quality and they are doing a commendable job in teaching their portion of the curriculum. There is not a clear distinction between what is a basic science and what is an applied science in our programs and the latter tends to blend into and become an extension of the former. If pharmacy is a clinical discipline, and I submit that it is and has been even before the appearance of the term "clinical pharmacy," then it is something more than the mere application of the basic sciences and the pharmaceutical sciences. This is where we get into philosophical and semantic difficulty in our curriculum planning.

Molecular pharmacology or medicinal chemistry may be basic to resolving the mechanism and site of action of adrenergic drugs, for example, but there is some question as to whether that is basic to, or even contributes to, what the pharmacy practitioner does or should do in his services to the patient who is being treated with such a drug. It seems to me that we must get some agreement among our faculties on the distinction between what is basic to the scientific advancement of a field and what is basic to the practice of a profession. In much of our thinking and curriculum planning we have confused these two objectives.

It is in the component of skill, or the art of professional practice, that we have found wanting in our educational programs. In our commendable zeal to overcome the deficiencies of the old apprenticeship-type of training we have manipulated the pendulum to the other extreme. With our curricula becoming filled with more and more science and with our faculties becoming dominated by science oriented teachers, we have largely come to disregard the part of professional practice and relegated that part of our students' education to the internship requirement that is administered by the state boards of pharmacy. Now we are confronted with the new accreditation standard of the American Council on Pharmaceutical Education that requires, as a part of the curriculum, a clinical component along with clerkships and externships and live practice settings that are of such caliber so as to serve in lieu of the internship requirement for licensure. Thus, there is being exerted a force to swing the pendulum back toward the middle.

The challenges that this new requirement represents to our colleges of pharmacy and our faculties are not to be taken lightly. Our pharmaceutical sciences faculties, to whose vested interests this represents a threat, must exhibit some real educational statesmanship in adjusting and accommodating themselves to it; in improving their communications with our clinical faculties, and in making more of an effort to make their own courses more relevant to the needs of their students in the practice environment. Our clinical faculties, who are viewed with apprehension by all of the others, must likewise improve their communications with the science faculties; must explain the objectives of their efforts and aspirations with such convincing clarity that they will be accepted, and must make more effort to bridge the gap between theory and practice in their teaching. Finally, our colleagues as a whole face the challenge of insuring that the clinical courses, clerkships and externships will measure up to the same academic standards that have been set and accepted for other courses in the curriculum.

It is not enough to place our students in the clinic or professional practice environment for the purpose of observation only. Nor is it sufficient only to lecture to them on what the pharmacist does or should do in such an environment. They must be involved in doing, under proper supervision, those things that the pharmacist does, including that the pharmacist does, the physician and other health professionals. And the endpoint of all this activity must be some measurable change in behavior and attitude by the student, which is the goal of any educational endeavor. This will require, among other things, a different kind of laboratory exercise than that in the usual course in the curriculum and a different kind of evaluation in terms of behavioral outcomes and competencies on the part of the student.

In my judgment these challenges are not being met nor will they be completely met in a short period of time. Depending on the local situation and the attitude of our faculties, it will be some little time before this accreditation standard will be met to the complete satisfaction of our colleges and the accrediting council.

At the other end of the spectrum in pharmaceutical education is the problem of pharmacy supportive personnel, whether they be called pharmacy assistants, subprofessionals or technicians. Mere mention of the term in any group of pharmacists, whether they be practitioners, educators or both, is sufficient to generate argument that usually is more emotional than objective. It is not a question of whether such persons are in existence; they are, they have been and they will continue to be.

The contention and arguments revolve around the questions of how and where they should be trained, what should their function be, and most important and emotional of all, should they be given formal recognition.

There is no question in my mind that pharmacy supportive personnel can perform a useful function. They can free up the time of the pharmacist to do those things in terms of patient and physician education and service that only the pharmacist can do and should do.

I do not see, at the present time, the necessity to provide a formal, academic program for the education and training of such persons. To subject them to a two year academic program as some advocates would, in my opinion, be a misuse of time, effort and manpower. The environments in which such a person would be placed and the specific functions he would perform are of such diverse nature that a great deal of what might be included in a two year academic program would be superfluous and nonrelevant. Even after completion of such a program it would be necessary to provide him with an on-the-job type of training to equip him to perform those specific functions required in the place of practice in which he would find himself.

For the routine, non-judgmental kinds of functions that the pharmacy technician would perform, an organized, systematic on-the-job type of training should suffice. Many hospital pharmacies have demonstrated the adequacy of such training programs and there is no reason why it could not be done in the community pharmacy.

There are those who fear that the recognition and use of pharmacy technicians pose such a threat to the pharmacist that they might some day clamor for official recognition and licensure with the aim of taking over the functions of the pharmacist. My answer to them is simple. If the pharmacist is content to continue to do those routine, non-judgmental things that a technician can do and cannot or will not spend his time and effort in the more sophisticated judgmental functions of patient and physician education and service, that only the pharmacist can and should do, then he deserves the consequences that might result.

Let me now turn to another issue of great significance in pharmaceutical education and that is continuing education or, more specifically, mandatory continuing education. No one would deny the necessity for the pharmacists to keep up to date in his practice; over the years, our colleges of pharmacy have devoted a considerable portion of their resources, both human and financial, to providing programs of continuing education for his benefit. Until very recently, however, not more than ten percent of our pharmacists have taken advantage of such programs.

The advent of legislation in Florida a few years ago, providing for the pharmacist to present evidence of the completion of a minimum amount of approved continuing education as a requirement for relicensure has brought a whole new perspective to this issue. It also has set off a series of actions activities in many states that are cause for concern. In the past few years several states have followed Florida's lead and there are indications that a number of other states will follow. Thus, the bandwagon effect for mandatory continuing education is in full swing and it appears to be rapidly approaching the status of a fad.

Concurrently, where once the colleges of pharmacy were the main sources of continuing education programs, now a plethora of agents and agencies are getting into the act. These range from individual and corporate entrepreneurs to local, state and national associations with programs of varying and, in some cases, doubtful quality. The boards of pharmacy in the various states, who are responsible for administration of the requirement, are adding to the concern by their acceptance of almost any and all programs that are presented for approval, with little or no concern for quality control. The situation is analogous to that in the internship requirement. Some years ago I stated that it appeared that state boards of pharmacy were willing to accept as a preceptor for internship training any pharmacist who was for motherhood and against sin. Their standards for approval of continuing education programs seem to be about as high. To their credit, however, it should be noted that they are becoming aware of the problems of quality and steps are being taken toward more effective accreditation of programs that are being offered.

Meanwhile the game of mandatory continuing education rolls merrily along and any pharmacist who needs to meet the requirement has no trouble in finding his choice of many approved ways of satisfying the requirement at little inconvenience to himself.

But what does it all mean? As it so frequently happens, it seems to me that we are putting the cart before the horse. We need to ask ourselves some fundamental questions. What are the purposes and objectives of continuing education? Most of us would give the obvious answer-to insure the retention and improvement of the pharmacist's professional competence. But what are the competencies that the pharmacist needs and how can they be measured? To my knowledge, no individual or group has addressed this question and until we have a valid answer to it we will continue to spin our wheels in an aimless manner.

Having answered that question, the next one is how best can the pharmacist meet the need to retain and improve those competencies that have been determined as necessary for him. Is continuing education in a group situation the only way? Can it be assumed that requiring the pharmacist to complete a program of lectures or seminars will improve his competence? If so, what should be the content and format of such programs? It is at this point, and not before, that the accreditation of programs should be brought into the picture.

Is self-study to be ruled out as a possibility? What about the pharmacist who keeps up to date through continuous education on his own as he meets the need for it in his professional practice? Is he to be subjected to the same requirement to attend seminars and to engage in other types of continuing education activities that his less conscientious colleague is subject to? Should not he have the opportunity to demonstrate his achievement of the accepted standard of competence without meeting a legislated requirement that reduces all pharmacists to the least common denominator?

And that leads to the ultimate question. After all of the continuing education has been completed, whether it be by lectures, seminars, cassette tapes, prescribed reading, self-study, or by some other means, how do we determine whether it has achieved its objective; whether, indeed, the pharmacist has retained or improved his competence as measured against approved and accepted standards? The only valid way, in my opinion, is to require him to demonstrate his continuing competence by a challenge examination as a requirement for relicensure. With the present generally excellent caliber of graduates that our colleges of pharmacy are turning out today, I would suggest that our state boards of pharmacy might well de-emphasize and turn their time and efforts to development of a competency examination for licensure renewal. Unless we, as a profession and as individual members of that profession, are willing to commit ourselves and see it through to that extent, then we should quit kidding ourselves about mandatory continuing education and recognize that, in its present status, it is largely of window dressing value for our self-image and, hopefully, for our public image.

Continuing competence, not continuing education, is the fundamental professional issue. As you know, during the past two years an AACP/APhA Task Force on Continuing Competence in Pharmacy has been engaged in the study of this issue and its final report appeared a few months ago. That report and its recommendations have provided the profession with a well formulated blueprint for action and represents a challenge that will occupy the best minds of the profession, as well as a charge on its other resources, for some time to come.

Let me close with a brief reference to unity in pharmacy. As most of you know, when I was President of the American Pharmaceutical Association a few years ago, it was my hope and ambition to bring about a better, more effective organizational structure for all of American pharmacy. I was particularly concerned with improving the relations between the APhA and the National Association of Retail Druggists and harbored the hope that the two organizations might be brought under the same umbrella in a way that might result in a merger. No good purpose would be served by my recounting here the events that transpired, starting with high hopes for the unity conference in New Orleans in October 1972 and ending in complete and divisive disruption of communications between APhA and NARD some months later. Suffice it to say that my hopes were soundly dashed. I realized sadly that, although emotionally and by temperament, I am a great proponent of the frontal attack type of assault on a problem, that was not the way to go in this case.

But the idea and hope for unity did not die. While APhA continued its study toward a better organizational structure, and after the wounds had healed, two men of goodwill and compassion, William Apple of APhA and Willard Simmons of NARD, initiated quiet, private talks for the good of the profession. I don't know what all they talked about but it is apparent that they came to the mutual agreement that their two organizations have many more interests in common than they have differences.

Out of those talks and further discussions with and by their governing boards, there resulted the Committee on Pharmacy Economic Security (COPES). Although its title might indicate a narrow, restricted interest, I am sure that the leadership of both groups envision more than the title implies; in the words of Chairman William F. Appel of the APhA Board of Trustees, it is "the direct result of the efforts of both associations to give life to the desires of all pharmacists that the two major national organizations representing their interests live and work together with one common objective-the future welfare of all practicing pharmacists."

Obvious signs of goodwill and cooperation, of agreement in philosophy, and of unity in purpose and action have been abundantly apparent between APhA and NARD in the months since the formation of COPES. Any objective observer of the current scene would agree and would be greatly heartened by this development. Yet there still are self-annointed, carping critics among us who support neither organization and who apparently feel that their main mission in life is to engage in destructive criticism of both. They are best to be disregarded and the pharmaceutical press would be well advised not to give them space to spread their divisive comments.

In some recent correspondence with a colleague who participated, reference was made to the so-called "abortive" unity conference in New Orleans. I am more optimistic and like to feel that, rather than being abortive, the conference just may have been the ground in which the seeds of harmony, cooperation and unity were sown. Although the seed bed was rocky and barren for awhile, the current good climate between the two organizations has favored its germination. Again, in the words of Chairman Appel, "pharmacists have been given the opportunity through the good-faith efforts of NARD and APhA to take the beginning steps towards the idealized goal of pharmacy unity."

Perhaps all we can expect at this time is unity of purpose and action. But I will be so bold and optimistic as to predict that, if this favorable climate continues and I see no reason why it will not-there may well result a mutual desire and action by APhA and NARD to merge and thereby bring about organizational unity as well. There will then remain the challenge of bringing the American Society of Hospital Pharmacists under the organizational umbrella so that, at long last, pharmacy will indeed be able to speak as one voice.

Thank you all for sharing in this occasion. ■

1975 Remington Medalist

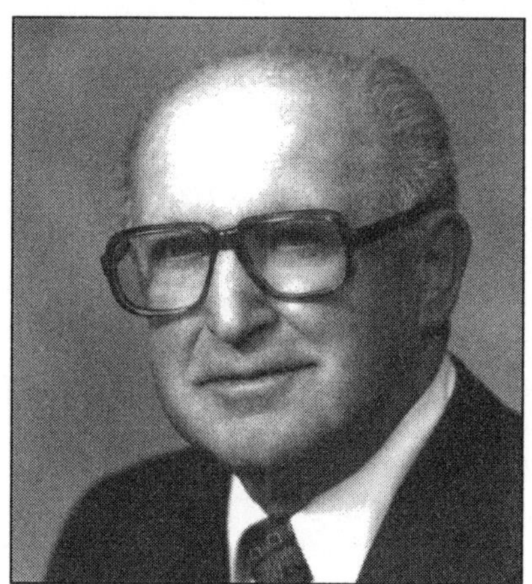

ALBERT DOERR
(1904-1985)

Albert Doerr was born in Lehr, North Dakota, and graduated with a B.S. degree in pharmacy from North Dakota State University in 1928. He purchased a pharmacy in Napoleon, North Dakota, in 1937, which he operated for 22 years. During this time he served on the Napoleon City Council, as president of the Foster School District Board, and as treasurer of the Logan County Red Cross. He was also owner of a funeral home and served for a time as Logan County coroner. In 1954, he was named executive secretary of the North Dakota Board of Pharmacy, and the following year he was named secretary-treasurer of the North Dakota Pharmaceutical Association. He moved to Bismarck in 1959 where he continued his organizational work until he retired in 1982. A member of the American Pharmaceutical Association, Doerr served as president of both the North Dakota Pharmaceutical Association and the North Dakota Board of Pharmacy, and honorary president of the National Association of Boards of Pharmacy. He was selected as the 1976 Remington medalist for the leadership he provided which resulted in the 1973 action by the U.S. Supreme Court holding constitutional a North Dakota statute requiring that majority ownership of pharmacies must be in the hands of registered pharmacists.

A Growing Profession in a Changing World

Albert Doerr

The 1975 Remington Medal was presented April 7, 1976, at the Marriott Hotel in New Orleans, Louisiana, during the American Pharmaceutical Association annual meeting April 3-8, 1976. Doerr's Remington address was not published, but an original manuscript was provided by William H. Grosz of Bismarck, North Dakota.

In this bicentennial year it is gratifying to see and hear the "corner drug store" often referred to as one of the great American traditions. We are pleased and proud that the neighborhood pharmacy on the city street corner, in the suburban business center, or on the main streets of rural America, has come to hold a prominent place in the affections of so many Americans.

But pharmacy today, and the pharmacies in which we practice, are a great deal more than museum pieces of a nostalgic era, delighting us with fond memories of less complicated times.

Changes are coming about rapidly in pharmacy, mostly for the better. Pharmacy has adapted successfully to change over the years, mostly through self-improvement. I am confident it will continue to do so. And I do not believe we have to do away with all of the basic fundamentals upon which we have built over past generations, and create an entirely new system under a whole new set of rules and philosophies.

Most of the pharmacies that survived and thrived during the past quarter-century are busier and more actively serving their communities today than ever before. If I may use my own state as an example, we did go through a period when there was a decline in the number of pharmacies, mainly because of population shifts, the mechanization of agriculture, and family farms giving way to larger operations requiring less people power. As with our farms, pharmacy too has found itself concentrated in larger establishments, serving larger population centers and the rural areas surrounding them. By the very nature of our state and its geography, big in square miles but sparse in population, rich in people resources but modest financially, we have numbers of small towns throughout the state with relatively small populations. Many of these are served by one physician and one pharmacist, and here is where we find a real one-to-one professional relationship. The pharmacist and physician frequently consulting each other, sharing a colleague to colleague mutual respect. And here, too, is developed a real people-to-people relationship between the pharmacist and patients, each needing the other.

Today, with the development of our state's coal, oil, water and other natural resources, we are predicting an increase in pharmacies to help care for the health needs of a growing population.

Locations where pharmacy is practiced may change with the times, but the tradition of service in helping to provide for the health care needs of our people remains firmly rooted in our profession.

Pharmacists throughout America today are providing more valuable services to their communities and more effective drugs for their patients. They are held in high professional esteem by the public and by their peers in the health professions. And yet we are troubled by a pervasive feeling of uncertainty throughout most of pharmacy-among pharmacy practitioners, wholesalers, and the pharmaceutical industry. This may stem in part from most of the planning that is being done for us in the bureaucracy and the political circles of a paternalistic Federal Government.

James Reston asked recently in his *New York Times* column, "In a world of increasingly powerful labor unions and multinational corporations at home, and centrally organized economies and cartels abroad, is it really reasonable to suppose that we will have less rather than more Federal control in the next decade?" Reston's observations could well apply to what is happening to pharmacy. We already are the nation's most regulated profession and industry. And all signs indicate that in the years ahead there will be even more Federal involvement in pharmacy practice, and in the business side of managing it.

It is doubtful that the Government agencies planning so much of our future are putting a very high priority on the economic well-being of pharmacists. What we have seen so far points strongly in the other direction.

There is DEA, and FDA, FTC, and OSHA. There is HEW, IRS, and ERISA, and our alphabet agencies seem to keep multiplying. We are all too familiar with the Federal government's involvement in our professional lives, its current role in Medicare and Medicaid, and its determined march toward totally Government-controlled national health insurance.

And, of course, we are about to have HEW's Maximum Allowable Cost regulations, scheduled to go into effect later this month, along with its estimated acquisition cost provisions which Government planners have promised would save millions by taking it out of the incomes of pharmacists. Thirty years ago, Leavitt Parsons editorialized in *The New England Apothecary,* "It is hard to picture how far our economic independence has already been compromised for an imaginary political security; no individual, nor any state, can accept continuous gratuities without paying for the offered security with either freedom or self-respect." Dr. Parsons' words, three decades ago, were indeed prophetic. It may well be that there is really nothing wrong with pharmacy that a little less Federal Government wouldn't help.

Certainly, it is not my intention to condemn our Federal Government. With all its excesses and deficiencies, it probably is the best in the world. But we should recognize that there also are two or three other political subdivisions-the states, the counties, and in most localities the city or town governments. They are not there by accident, but by design in recognition of the fact that for many purposes, governments closer to the people they serve can serve them best.

It has been my privilege for the past twenty-odd years, to serve the State of North Dakota's Board of Pharmacy. Serving on a board with outstanding pharmacist-citizens from throughout the State, one cannot help but observe the inherent benefits to both the public and the profession in having laws applying to pharmacy interpreted by pharmacists who live there, and rules and regulations adopted by pharmacists who know and understand their peers in the profession as well as the public they serve.

The 1973 Supreme Court decision which reversed the 1928 Liggett vs. Balderidge decision on pharmacy ownership has been mentioned in connection with tonight's ceremonies. Whether or not the honor you are bestowing upon me is deserved or appropriately placed, I think the greatest significance of that decision was that it reaffirmed that states do have the right to determine what in their judgement is best for their own citizens.

Our involvement with an ownership law did not originate, as might be supposed, as a crusade against the corporate ownership of pharmacies. When I became secretary of the Board of Pharmacy, I noted with some concern the number of pharmacies owned in the state by non-pharmacists. Clinics of two or more physicians, farmers, depot agents, widows of deceased doctors, bankers, radio technicians, jewelers, salesmen, lawyers, and morticians, these made up nearly 25% of the pharmacy ownership in North Dakota. Our state pharmaceutical association, through the legislative process, sought to assure the public that its pharmacy services would be under the immediate control of fully qualified pharmacists. The North Dakota legislature accepted this view and enacted its law requiring pharmacies in the state to be under the majority ownership of registered pharmacists. And it has been reaffirmed by the Supreme Court, without judging the wisdom of the law, that our states do have the authority to enact and enforce such laws. Whether or not they want them is, of course, a judgement to be made by the people in each of the states and their elected representatives.

With the rapid changes and advancements taking place in Pharmacy, many state boards have come to recognize that the pharmacy laws which they are responsible for administering are outdated. But a comprehensive revision of an entire pharmacy practices act is a herculean task, especially where it is important to assure consistency with other laws of the state, the Federal drug laws, and some degree of uniformity with the laws in other states. Fortunately for us all, help is on the way. A major project of the National Association of Boards of Pharmacy has been the development of a Model State Pharmacy Act for the use and guidance of individual states in renovating their own statutes. While the input to this Model Act has been nationwide, combining the best of ideas from many states and other sources, it avoids the rigid, inflexible aspects of a Federal statute. The Model Act is specific and helpful in stating areas which should be covered in the law, but will leave much to be spelled out in regulations by the individual boards to meet the specific needs of practitioners within their own states and the public they serve.

There is a great deal of work to be done yet on developing and refining the Model Pharmacy Act, but I am confident that when it is completed, it will be a significant step forward in modernizing our state laws. Not the least of its advantages will be its relative degree of uniformity in format and content to overcome the hodgepodge nature of fifty different state pharmacy acts, yet retaining the individuality of each of the states in meeting the specific needs of their people.

Through involvement over many years with the boards of pharmacy, one of my interests, quite naturally, has become the pharmacy internship as a prerequisite to registration as a pharmacist. The internship, as the direct descendant of the apprenticeship, is the oldest and most basic form of pharmacy education and training. Even with the sciences, social studies, and professional courses taught in our colleges today, the internship remains as a most important final touch to the pharmacist's preparation for his career and his service to the public. The added touch of professionalism is gained by the apprentice and journeyman working alongside the master craftsman. I wish I could say that all internships make an equally valuable and necessary contribution to the intern's skills and knowledge. Unfortunately, they do not. We may need improvement, as pharmacy examiners, in the requirements we place upon internships. We may need to advance the techniques of measuring and evaluating internships and their effectiveness as preparation for professional practice. These are problems with which the board of pharmacy must be concerned. And they are.

But we must also look at the responsibilities of the individual pharmacist as a preceptor, a teacher, the master practitioner preparing the novice for the career on which he is about to embark. We must think seriously about the preceptor's attitude toward his intern and the responsibility he has accepted as a teacher. As pharmacists we must regard the internship primarily as a learning experience. We must think first of the intern as a young person under the preceptor's charge who is there primarily to test his collegeacquired knowledge in an actual practice situation, and to polish his skills as a practitioner, not as just another semi-skilled employee who will meet one of the state-imposed requirements for licensure by working in the pharmacy for a specified period of time.

Technicians, in contrast to interns, are another matter. Opinion is greatly divided on the recognition, if any, which should be given pharmacy technicians, what training, if any, should be required, and who should be responsible for setting standards and providing their training. Of one thing we can be reasonably certain. Non-pharmacists are employed today in many pharmacies, and as the duties they perform go beyond clerical and janitorial, they will increasingly be called technicians and will require some training and preparation of a semi-skilled nature. The Millis Commission, in its final report said, "it seems highly probable that pharmacists' aides will be employed in ever increasing numbers." That may be, but I believe it should be accepted as a serious responsibility of the profession clearly to define the role of the pharmacist, and those functions which may be performed only by a pharmacist. We should also assure that dispensing of drugs and any related function is performed at all times under the immediate supervision of a pharmacist.

The serious responsibilities involved in the recognition and accurate dispensing of potent drugs, and awareness of the possible consequences of even minor errors or misjudgments, should remain uppermost in any decision to delegate these duties to anyone other than a fully qualified pharmacist.

It is recognized, of course, that the use of technicians in pharmacy, as in any other profession, is primarily to increase the productivity of the professional, freeing him from more routine duties to concentrate on those requiring his particular knowledge and skill. It really becomes an economic issue. But viewing it in that light alone, we should consider the economic needs of those who have invested substantially in time and money to become pharmacists. If the trend continues, as now appears to be the case in some areas of the country, toward increasing unemployment among qualified pharmacists, it would hardly seem to be in the best interests of the public or the profession to encourage extensive use of technicians in tasks beyond their level of knowledge, while pharmacists are forced to seek employment outside the profession.

I would like to turn away, briefly, from this inward look at ourselves in pharmacy, and consider our relationships with the public we serve. As more formal recognition is given the clinical aspects of pharmacy, pharmacists increasingly like to consider themselves "patient-oriented." I am happy to see the emphasis on clinical pharmacy in our colleges. But if I understand the term correctly, clinical pharmacy emphasizes the pharmacist's concern for the patient, and his physical and mental well-being, his assurance that the patient knows and understands how to take his medicine, and what to expect from it; that it has been ordered properly and will be taken in the correct dosage; and that there are no physical or therapeutic incompatibilities with food or other drugs the patient may be taking. This may be a grossly oversimplified view of clinical pharmacy, but it is what most pharmacists have been doing throughout my forty-odd years involvement with the profession-or at least were until prescription volume increased so much there no longer was enough time to be spent with the patient. We must continue and renew this interest in our patients and give them the full benefit of the pharmacists' knowledge. After all, they are the sole reason for the existence of our profession.

But besides being patient-oriented, we need to become more public-oriented. The public today is seeking answers to questions about drugs such as why do they cost so much? Aren't they all alike and isn't the cheapest just as good? What does the pharmacist do other than transfer labels on a bottle of pills? Why aren't prescription prices advertised? And many more. Chances are, most people won't ask. Instead they are getting answers, right or wrong, from consumer activists, from union leaders and politicians with axes to grind, from sensationalized headlines and articles in the lay press, anywhere but from the most logical source of factual information about drugs-the local pharmacist. The information the public wants and really needs is right there in the community pharmacy. Provided the pharmacist is accessible, and will take the time, and is willing to keep himself informed, and to involve himself in discussions which may require detailed and thoughtful answers.

The Study Commission on Pharmacy observed that our colleges of pharmacy may have to consider giving less emphasis to the physical and biological sciences and more to behavioral and social studies. Acknowledging the need for pharmacists' knowledge about drugs, the Study Commission said they must also have ready knowledge about people, about relationships and communications with them, and about systems and costs of service. This is exactly what we are talking about. I am not advocating that all pharmacists go back to school for post-graduate courses in applied psychology and the social sciences. What I do feel is necessary, though, is for the pharmacist to adopt an attitude of openness with his public to be accessible for frank discussions on drugs and health-related matters. When cost is the topic, put the emphasis on what pharmaceutical services and quality products will do for people rather than only defending their cost. Emphasize the importance of drugs and pharmaceutical services as a means of cost saving and their positive contribution to more economical health care.

We need to emphasize to the public that professionally selected drug therapy, combined with skilled medical care and pharmaceutical services, can be one of our greatest assets in controlling total health care costs. I began this talk with an optimistic view of pharmacy today. And I am confident that with its proven adaptability, its continuous improvement of knowledge and skills, and its ever-increasing contributions to the public good, pharmacy will be a shining light, for the good of mankind, far into the future.

Tonight, for me, marks one of the greatest highlights of a lifetime in pharmacy, and retirement is coming into view in the not too distant future.

In looking at the list of previous recipients and their contributions to pharmacy, I feel very humble alongside them. I accept this award with humility and assure you that it will be treasured by me and my family for the years to come. ■

1976 Remington Medalist

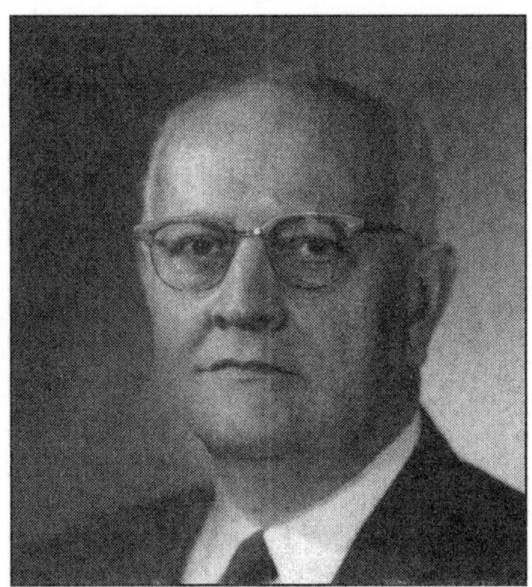

Melvin William Green
(1910-1991)

Melvin William Green was born in Bluffs, Illinois, and received a B.S. degree in pharmacy in 1932, and a Ph.D. degree in 1935 from the University of Pittsburgh. He then served as research associate at Mellon Institute in Pittsburgh 1936-1938; assistant professor of pharmacy at the Cincinnati College of Pharmacy 1938-1940, assistant professor of pharmacology at Georgetown University College of Medicine in Washington, D.C. 1940-1942, and associate professor of pharmaceutical chemistry at the University of Wisconsin School of Pharmacy 1949-1952. He served as a member of the USP revision committee 1950-1960.

A life member of the American Pharmaceutical Association, Green served as chief chemist for the APhA Drug Standards Laboratory 1942-1949, secretary of the Pan American Federation of Pharmacy and Biochemistry education section 1957-1960, and a consultant on pharmaceutical education to USAID for Vietnam 1968. Green was named director of educational relations for the American Council on Pharmaceutical Education in 1952, a position he held until his retirement in 1974, during which time he "sold the proposition that pharmacy is a professional school, the same as medicine and dentistry, and that is should be treated as such in the university."

I Wonder As I Wander

Melvin William Green

The 1976 Remington Medal was presented May 17, 1977, at the New York Hilton Hotel in New York City, during the May 14-19, 1977, American Pharmaceutical Association annual meeting. A brief summary of Green's Remington address was published in the *Journal of the American Pharmaceutical Association,* volume NS 17, page 406, July 1977, but the complete text of Green's Remington address was obtained from his widow, Mae Green of Cedar Rapids, Iowa.

Most of you are aware that the past 20 some years of my life have entailed travelling over a half million miles in the interest of pharmacy education. I often thought of the familiar song "I Wonder as I Wander" during those years and this prompts me to give these few remarks the same play on words as a title.

A younger pharmacist asked me recently, "How does one go about getting the Remington Medal?" I explained that it is really rather simple. The place to start is with the thoughtful choice of grandparents and parents. You then carefully select an empathetic wife who understands long absences from home in the interest of professional progress and who won't expect you to sew on your buttons, for she knows you will never be able to see eye to eye with the needle. You also have children in whom you have faith. Now that the homefront is secure you arrange to know and to work with the stalwarts in the field, and have a successor like Dan Nona whose youthful vigor and tact is bound to enhance your own efforts. It has been said that no man is a hero to his secretary or his valet. This may be true, but my secretary for many years, Miss Ella Lodgaard, is a hero to me.

I was fortunate to be able to learn from and to work with such people as Justin Powers, C.G. King, George Beal, Julius Koch, Ed. Reif, Robert Fischelis, Louis Zopf, Troy Daniels, Bob Swain, Pat Costello, Karl Bambach, Dick Deno, Edward C. Elliott, Grover Bowles, Paul Briggs, Fred Mahaffey, George Archambault, Linwood Tice, John Weaver, Bill Apple, George Hager, Jack Orr, David Krigstein, George Webster, Frank Dickey, Leib Riggs, Varro Tyler, Bill Selden, Louis Busse, Harold Hewitt, George Urdang, Arthur Uhl, Lloyd Parks, H.C. McAllister, Charles Bliven, Glenn Sonnedecker-the list has already grown so long that the risk becomes greater that I have missed more than I have named.

My father was a World War I veteran. Sometime after father's return from the trenches, the King of Belgium paraded in Pittsburgh where we were then living. My father took me to see him and when the King's car approached, father stood me on his shoulders so that I could see better. The man standing next to father said, "Young man, I hope that you will always remember that to really know what is going on you must stand on experiences' shoulders." That was a strange thing to say to an eight-year old, but tonight I recognize that these many experienced shoulders on which I stand stretch out like a pontoon bridge.

My career could scarcely have been launched in the 1930's without the research fellowship support of the *United*

States Pharmacopeia. Later the support of the American Pharmaceutical Association and the *National Formulary* made it possible to work in the important field of drug standards. In 1939 the APhA, the American Association of Colleges of Pharmacy and the National Association of Boards of Pharmacy started and contributed money and manpower to the American Council on Pharmaceutical Education which probably could not have supported a director if it weren't for the far-sightedness and appreciation of values of the American Foundation for Pharmaceutical Education and its then able Director Dr. W. Paul Briggs.

My first position after the Ph.D. was research on drug standards for the *USP.* This was at Mellon Institute in Pittsburgh at a time when many consumer products and technologies were being born. It was exciting to see ground work laid for permanent pressed clothes, tenderization of meat by shortening the hanging period in the presence of ultra violet light, development of such diverse products as latex paints and skinless wieners, control of mine acids in the bituminous coal fields, environmental sanitation, improved brick making, techniques for cleaning old oil paintings, evaluation of baby and infant foods and many others now considered to be commonplace.

In the drug standards field, I am proud to have been a part of many developments that now are taken for granted. The National Formulary Laboratories, which were supported largely by pharmacists, made many early significant contributions. The *National Formulary* was not only first to have standards for compressed tablets, they pioneered in weight tolerances for them as well. Working with glass chemists and the American Society for Testing Materials, we developed the first standards for glass containers, including prescription bottles, to hold and store drugs. We got to know statisticians who had developed statistical quality control, sequential analysis and similar techniques to assure the unusual uniformity of the munitions used at the Normandy Beachead and turned this knowledge to drug control use. Being conscious of the cumulative effect or possible effects of minute quantities of heavy metals such as lead and mercury, we strengthened the testing procedures for these elements in micro amounts a matter that is getting requisite attention by environmentalists only today.

As an aside, we once received a letter from someone claiming to have provided a definitive study of the ash content of Helonias and Aletris in which it was stated that the "figures tell the story." Since we could never quite read the story, Justin Powers and I bantered the letter about quite a bit. Gladys Powers who undoubtedly was the only living person who had every word of the *National Formulary* read aloud to her and with feeling said, "0, come on fellows, you know Helonias and Aletris aren't drugs, they are the two chaps who first swam the Hellespont!"

In many ways even though my total teaching time was rather short it produced many of the greatest satisfactions. To watch Allen Daniels turn from a trap drummer into a pharmacist and a state association secretary right before your very eyes is certainly nothing less than a minor miracle; to watch a shoe cobbler's son struggle to make ends meet and then succeed in becoming a prominent pharmacist physician carries a reward that really can't be topped.

But I would like to concentrate my remarks tonight on the phase of my career dealing with accreditation and related educational matters. In over 20 years of such activity, the many experiences could lead me to reminisce about many persons and events. Some of them would be amusing, some entertaining and some, perhaps, even instructive. But I would rather confine most of my remarks away from the past toward some concerns for the future.

If you look at pharmaceutical education today in terms of where you wish that it were, progress has been very slow. If you measure where it stands against where it has been, probably it has moved faster than any other professional discipline in the university. This forward thrust is the product of many hands and heads, supplemented by the dollars from many sources including what New York's own Dr. Nyquist calls that "money-splendored thing," the Federal Government. While I am proud to have been a part of this progress, I am jealous of the much greater contributions that many of you and my absent friends have made.

At the close of World War II, the status of pharmacy was at ebb tide or close to it. Please understand that this is not another funeral oration for pharmacy. I have lived long enough and heard so many such orations that I no longer attend pharmacy funerals. There was in the late 1940s little respect for the pharmacy faculty which generally was inadequately prepared by academic degree or current professional knowledge and experience; equipment was inadequate as were buildings; one school of pharmacy had dirt floors and students were characterized as being among the lowest on the totem pole. In one university a favorite saying was that dropouts from the school of education transferred to the school of pharmacy for the improvement of both. This situation had a deleterious effect on the profession on the outside for it meant that potential lawyers, doctors, school teachers, preachers, actors, artists, geologists, engineers, parents, and all kinds of educated people that make up a community left the university with a negative view of our profession. Clearly, something had to be done to change the picture, not only to affect public opinion but to restore our own confidence in ourselves.

Since by definition a university is supposed to be a community of scholars, a place to start was to put pharmacy on a scholarly level by strengthening the research and scholarly backgrounds of the faculty, increasing publication in the form of books and papers in scholarly journals, encouraging qualified students to go into advanced education and, with or without advanced degrees, to seek out and to accept positions in society that clearly indicated that pharmacists had expanded horizons too.

The size of current graduate programs, the dollar value of research funds, the active participation of pharmacists on programs of leading scholarly and research societies, all are indicators of success. I venture to say that on every campus today, pharmacy is placed in an elevated position by undergraduate students and faculties, generally. This means that all of these aforementioned university graduates return to the outside community with a respect for pharmacy which is deserved if the profession as a whole lives up to the pedestal that now has been structured for it.

This uplifting of pharmacy at the university level has been necessary and it has been exciting, but something has been missing. The missing link seems to have been the failure to recognize that pharmacy practice had not been moving effectively with the other health professions-in fact, the older pharmacy profession was like physical education, nutrition science, and many other fields, in a sense only tangentially related to the health professions. It was not only difficult to relate the important scientific aspects of pharmacy to prevalent practice, there was virtually no forward thrust to professional practice of the type that should come from a university-based discipline.

This is where we are now-in the midst of a revolutionary and evolutionary process of attempting to establish professional and social relevance. This is the meaning of the clinical approach to pharmacy practice. If these practical practice goals can be established on a firm scientific and technological base, we will have a winner. If we attempt to establish ourselves as consultants with no firm chemical, physiological, biological and social foundation to the consult, pharmacy and the public will again become losers.

There are today many unknowns in the likely pattern of health practice of the future. But one thing appears to me to be clear and that is that nearly all general health practice will take place at the community level, for the hospital is obviously too expensive a tool for the majority of illnesses. This to me means that the community pharmacist will retain his centrist position even though the character of his practice may change. It also means a rather desperate need for research on ways to make his community practice more effective. Procedures will have to be found, for example, to open up the patient's medical records to the community pharmacist approaching the character of such records in the hospital, if the pharmacist is to be in a position to make his expertise really effective.

We have just spoken briefly of where we have been and where we are, not eloquently, but in precis, and so you are no doubt expecting me to tell you where we are going, to put on the seer's robes and foretell the future. My friends, not to mention enemies, have repeatedly told me that I am not very wise, but even though short of wisdom, I am wise enough not to attempt to foretell the future in a rapidly changing social and professional scene.

If you will bear with my egotism for a moment-and by the way an egotist is one who wishes to die in his own arms-I would like to talk about some needs as I see them.

One of pharmacy's goals post World War II has been to get pharmaceutical education into the university setting-at least the stance if not the organizational pattern. It seems to me that the result is too often a splendid isolation under the university umbrella so that now the problem is shifting to one of getting the university into pharmacy.

Are we going to try again to emulate medicine or do we have both the courage and the ability to stand on our own feet? Some rainy day, when you have little to do, make a list of the drug-related knowledge that is not based on the physical and biological sciences. The most obvious is drug addiction and abuse, the former of which is at least partially biologic.

Economics plays a considerable role-not only the negative effect on pocketbooks, but also the positive effect of reducing absenteeism because of illness and many other factors. I feel certain that you are more aware than I of the numbers of prescriptions written by physicians and other qualified practitioners that are never dispensed. Why? What about the physician that prescribes medication to be taken before, after, or with meals with the expectation that the patient gets the medication 3 times a day without recognizing that there are people who, for one reason or another, eat once a day or the teenagers who eat continuously all day long? Then there are overpopulated areas in the world that have depended on illness and death to maintain demographic stability where penicillin and other drugs have upset this balance. There are the legal situations that revolve around package inserts, responsibilities relating to patient medication records, malpractice from failure to manipulate wisely biological equivalency and other situations. In some public school systems the teachers are expected to see that students who have chronic medical problems, including hyperactivity, take their medication regularly. This issue has pharmaceutical connotations worthy of our concern. You can fill in the blanks with many more matters which do not come into most of our pharmacy curricula.

To set up the missing new departments to represent these issues in our colleges with the several needed disciplines would not appear to me to be in the best interests. Such action would likely diminish the isolation of pharmacy in the university but would be unlikely to attract first rate scholars in these areas. While there are notable exceptions, there is a feeling of the need for a critical mass in every field and the undesirability of shielding such a scholar from a broader range of students.

On the other hand, in pharmacy there are subjects to interest non-pharmaceutical scholars. An example that comes immediately to mind is the interest of the economist in the fact that there are elements of pharmacy practice which are substantially free from the economics of the traditional marketplace.

While for the past few minutes we have focused on the need for broadening the education of the pharmacy student, it may be even more important to consider pharmacy's contribution to other phases of health education and, indeed, to the general education of the undergraduate university student body. In the pandemic of drug addiction and abuse problems on campus and in society, most pharmacy schools have either taught courses or were active in seeking solutions. But prior to this panic period, I can think of only two or three colleges of pharmacy that had formal classes in drug-related matters for non-pharmacy undergraduate students. Yet here are elements of personal health that touch everyone in which little systematic knowledge beyond hearsay and the *Readers Digest* is available. As important as is the drug addiction and abuse problem there are many other factors to which every educated person should be exposed. These days my wife and I live very close to a limited number of people nearly all of whom have some chronic health problems. Many questions beyond the obvious money problems that are asked about drugs suggest that general drug knowledge could and should be enhanced. That responsibility is largely ours. Another reason for involving more undergraduates in pharmacy-related health affairs is that present trends indicate the high probability of many more persons becoming actively involved in aspects of health affairs to an even greater extent, not only as consumers but as participants. We are not only speaking of the frequently mentioned paramedics, but the involvement of teachers, pastors, engineers, attorneys, social scientists, electronic technicians, chemists biologists, economists, politicians, administrators, and others in health affairs. Certainly these people should be better informed about pharmaceutical affairs both as undergraduates and in continuing education.

As the medical scenes move away from the limited medical concept to the broader health center concept, more universities might consider a general pre-health professional program in place of the traditional pre-medical, pre-pharmacy, pre-dental programs. Such approach is likely to place more square pegs in square holes.

Much has been said about broadening the education of the pharmacist by at least protecting the amount of non-science, non-professional courses in general education if not increasing the available hours. In this connection, it seems to me that the university and the liberal arts college have an obligation to recognize some of the roadblocks, such as the intense specialization of the faculties in the humanities, and subsequent difficulty students have of getting upper division courses without prerequisite courses which are often not truly prerequisite and germane. While we all recognize the value of developing the whole man, to do this either we will have to develop a strengthened broad primary education to achieve that objective, place professional education for such professions as pharmacy on a post-baccalaureate basis, or reevaluate the university structure to achieve these objectives more effectively than now is too often the case.

Assuming the concept of C.P. Snow that there are indeed two cultures the humanistic and the scientific it would seem to me that their separateness is inevitable. But I like to think of the scientific culture as dealing with problems that are soluble, albeit difficult, while the humanities deal more with situations that are likely insoluble and are concerned with the absurdities of life. Possibly one element of human growing up is the recognition that every problem does not have a solution and that absurdities of life are there to be confronted. If there is hope in these areas of living, it is likely to come from the humanities and their focus on values. I submit that some of pharmacy's problems are likely insoluble ones. Many do not lend themselves to quantification and the rigid logic of, let us say, physics. Possibly the problems exist in part, or at least appear to be so acute, because pharmacists of my generation received so little education in such value thinking.

The pharmacy professional curriculum has become stabilized now as a result of the studies of the Pharmaceutical Syllabus, the Dille pharmacology report, the Blauch-Webster study and other related studies. Many commonplace curricular elements are taken for granted as being necessary although they are based on specific needs of a time gone by which may or may not exist today. The need may still be there but there is a need for conscious assurance. Take physics for example. In times gone by, many high schools offered no instruction in physics and many, if not most, high school graduates did not take the course. The beginning college course of that period was little better than the high school course of today and today's college course has changed its character considerably as a result of nuclear and electronic developments. Without any implication of negativeness, I ask, "What are the purposes of physics in today's outlook? Why not study the question in more depth?"

Because of today's need for a greater knowledge of the organic chemistry of the heterocyclics and a rather specialized physical pharmacy, and the changing physical emphasis in basic organic chemistry courses, what is the right balance between basic organic chemistry and applied professional courses?

In short, we need to ask ourselves the really hard question of what does a pharmacist need to know to practice intelligently and professionally now and in the future as far as our foresight can take us? It should be distinctly understood that this is not a plea for the return to the mediocrity of the 1930s but rather for a stronger curriculum with more clearly defined professional purpose. In face of the knowledge explosion and the social revolution that has existed since World War II, we cannot afford to waste the student's time to prepare him for last decades professional battles.

As S. L. Washburn, professor of anthropology at the University of California says, "The universities are highly successful in vocational training: the production of professionals such as lawyers, doctors, business administrators, engineers, and professors proficient in research. The universities fail in putting knowledge into a form in which it can be used by the educated person. They fail in conveying to the public the progress in knowledge that is essential for democracy, for informed decision making. Obviously knowledge is growing at a fantastic rate, and techniques are getting more complicated. More departments will have to be formed and more specialities created. This expansion is a necessary part of progress and of human adjustment to a world of undreamed of possibilities. But at the same time there needs to be a different sort of progress, progress toward a general understanding of the nature of the world."

As a concerned citizen in a country that claims to have a broadly educated populace, I am a little ashamed of the level of public debate over most of our present critical issues. Logic is being dethroned in favor of pure, or really not so pure, emotion. We in education have a responsibility for that situation to exist. We will not correct it until we admit it.

Well, you can see there are lots of things to be done. I have had so much pleasure in doing the few things that I have done that I regret that I will have little, if any, opportunity to get into the fun that is to come. And fun it will be.

After all of these mutterings, possibly Robert Frost summed up what I have been trying to say much better.

"My object in living is to unite
My avocation and my vocation
As my two eyes make one in sight.
Only when love and need are one.
And the work is play for mortal stakes
Is the deed ever really done
For Heaven and the future's sakes." ■

1977 Remington Medalist

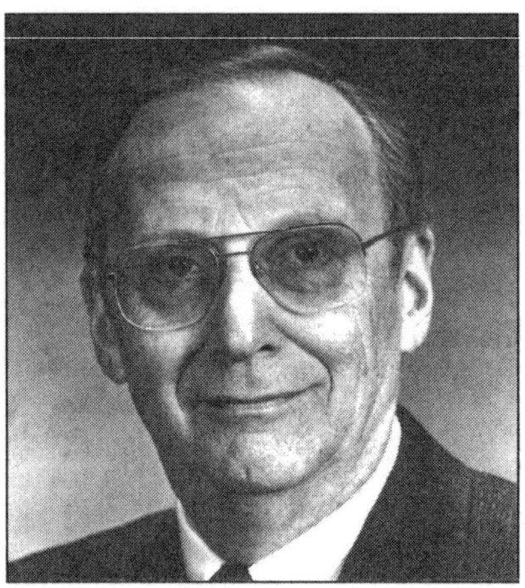

DAVID JACOB KRIGSTEIN
(1924-2003)

David Jacob Krigstein was born in Wilmington, Delaware, August 10, 1924. After service in the U.S. Army during World War II, he graduated with a B.S. degree in Pharmacy 1949 and an M.S. 1968, both from the Philadelphia College of Pharmacy and Science. He served as an instructor in pharmacy at his alma mater 1949-1952 before opening his own professional practice pharmacy in Wilmington, Delaware, which he operated from 1952 to 1976. During this period, he also served as executive secretary of the Delaware State Board of Pharmacy 1961-1971, and as a consultant to the Delaware Department of Health and Social Services 1966-1971. He then joined the Blue Cross and Blue Shield of Delaware serving as director of drug programs 1977-1979, as director of institutional services 1979-1980, and as vice president for health care services 1980-1983. Then from 1983 to 1989, he served in the dual capacity as senior vice president of the Blue Cross and Blue Shield of Delaware, and president of the Blues' subsidiary, The HMO of Delaware, Inc., with the responsibility of the operation of two health care centers in New Castle County, Delaware. He also served as chairman of the Delaware Governor's Council on Drugs 1978-1984.

Joining the American Pharmaceutical Association in 1953, Krigstein served as chairman of several APhA standing committees, as AMA's representative 1968-1976, as president 1968-1974 of the American Council on Pharmaceutical Education, and as speaker of the APhA House of Delegates 1974-1976. After 1990, Krigstein served as a consultant until his death on July 5, 2003.

Decisions and Professional Destiny

David Jacob Krigstein

The 1977 Remington Medal was presented May 16, 1978, at the Bonaventure Hotel in Montreal, Canada, during the American Pharmaceutical Association annual meeting, May 14-18, 1978. Krigstein's Remington address was published in *American Pharmacy,* volume NS18, pages 395-397, 1978, under the title of "A Call for Self-Discipline." However, we are using the title provided by the 1977 Remington medalist in his original text.

I accept the high honor of being inducted as the 51st Remington Medalist with deepest humility.

Let me commend the past presidents of the American Pharmaceutical Association for reaching into the ranks of the practicing pharmacists for their selection. The fact that they selected pharmacist Krigstein is of little significance when compared with their boldness in recognizing that the profession for better or worse is its rank and file practitioners.

By my own measure, my contributions to our profession are minute. But my love and aspirations for our profession are second to nobody's. One cannot be closely associated with an Apple, a Tice, an Abrams or a Parks, as I have been privileged to be, without being inspired to do everything one can to help pharmacy's star shine a little brighter in the health galaxy.

I also learned from these and many other thoughtful and dedicated colleagues in our profession that "Wishing will not make it so." The world we live in-and our society-is neither perfect nor just, and at times we have to make some hard and uncomfortable decisions.

It is this decision making process as practiced by our profession that I wish to visit with you about this meeting.

We are celebrating the 125th Annual Meeting of our national professional society this week. And even without citing any historical references, I feel comfortable in saying that throughout this century and a quarter, American pharmacists have been unwilling to resolve the professional vs. merchant paradox. You know all the pro and con arguments as well as I do, but the bottom line always comes down to "1 can't make a living by being a full-time professional."

Many of the pharmacists who have said this in the past, and many who say it today, really believe that the only choice of the majority in any generation of pharmacists is to be part-time practitioners. And whether we like it or not, this "gut" feeling of the majority is not, and has not been, without its economic foundation.

When Hubert H. Humphrey practiced pharmacy in Huron, South Dakota, forty years ago, the soda fountain and general merchandise made it possible for the Humphrey Drug Company to provide pharmaceutical service to the community. But that was forty years ago. Today, some pharmacists are making it economically by being full-time practitioners in rural communities smaller than Huron. They are making it because the profession has greatly extended the scope of pharmaceutical service. These pharmacists have come to recognize that they are qualified and competent to do more than dispense a prescription exactly as the physician ordered or ring up the register on an OTC sale. They have even come to recognize that some of their pharmaceutical service has to be performed at the bedside of their patients.

During the 1950s and 1960s it appeared that professional renaissance was well on its way toward a permanent change in the profile of American pharmacy. Although the movement toward full-time and comprehensive pharmacy practice made some important advances, it didn't, in my opinion, achieve its potential. I am sure that anyone who has given the subject any attention can offer a number of reasonable explanations as to why our success was limited. In my mind, there is but one basic reason. And that is the profession lacked a strong, unified organizational structure to lead the way.

Let me make it clear, I am not unappreciative of the growth and leadership of the American Pharmaceutical Association during the last two decades. I have been part of that leadership, and I am personally familiar with the obstacles APhA has had to overcome to achieve as much as it has.

Perhaps I can explain more precisely why I am so concerned about our profession's decision-making process, particularly its deficiencies.

Earlier I mentioned that we made some important advances in the 1950s, but we also suffered several major setbacks. In the first part of that decade we debated the Elliot Survey recommendation that pharmacy move from a four-year to a six-year academic program. Blind opposition by NARD, which was then pharmacy's largest and strongest organization, and vacillation by APhA permitted the educators to make a decision which more properly should have been made by an enlightened profession.

As you well know, the compromise was a five-year program which settled nothing and cost us dearly in precious time. APhA has articulated a forceful position this time around, and I can only hope that pharmacists give the APhA position their unequivocal support.

Some pharmacists recently took umbrage at the National Association of Chain Drug Stores and the National Wholesale Druggists' Association for their policy statements on this issue. I would remind these pharmacists that anybody has a right to speak out on this or any other pharmacy issue. The profession owes everybody who does speak out a courteous audience. But having listened, the profession cannot afford to be unduly pressured or improperly influenced. The profession's responsibility is only to the public it serves and itself.

It was also in the 1950s that pharmacists, in blind faith, supported the drug industry's campaign to enact antisubstitution laws. The original objective of stopping counterfeiting was noble indeed, but if the profession had gone about its decision-making process in an orderly and reasoned way-rather than acting out of blind loyalty-the results would have been considerably different. We could have supported legislation to stop nefarious counterfeiting without giving up our professional right to engage in legitimate drug product selection. We are spending the decade of the 1970s recovering a necessary professional prerogative. As we all know, it is costing us dearly and we may never fully recover what we so naively gave away.

I know that it is a very touchy issue with most educators, but again let me say for the record that we didn't do right by either the public or the profession on the manpower issue. The fact that our pharmacy school enrollments have dropped slightly the last two years is of marginal comfort. The oversupply of pharmacists we are generating in the 1970s is indefensible when measured by public cost benefit criteria. What concerns me even more is that the profession appears to be immobilized about deciding what it should now do to close the spigot far enough and long enough for the profession to recover. Perhaps it is simplistic thinking on my part, but we will have a manpower surplus until every competent member of the profession has an opportunity to be gainfully employed as a full-time practitioner. Except for brief war periods, that has not been the case since the turn of the century. Closing our eyes is not part of the decision-making process. We may feel more comfortable for a moment, but then comes the time when we must open our eyes.

My reason for singling out the manpower issue is not to open old wounds or to resurrect past controversy. Rather, this issue serves as a classic example familiar to us all regarding the two key points which I regard as the central theme of my comments this evening.

First, the profession must face up to reality and have the courage and conviction to make carefully considered, objective decisions; and

Second, the profession must have the foresight to recognize the long-range impact which will follow such decisions, and the dedication and persistence to stand by those decisions even though it means enduring short term hardships.

Capitation money was an attractive and tempting carrot waved by the government in front of money-starved pharmacy schools. It is very understandable that college administrations would eagerly reach out to grasp this immediate remedy for ailing budgets.

But, in the process, precious little thought was given to the long-term projections. Today we are graduating highly qualified, sincerely motivated young people who are unable to find employment in their chosen profession. As in reading production reports from the auto makers in Detroit, or even statistics from the Communicable Disease Center in Atlanta, it is too easy for us to think of these as just abstract numbers. But each of those numbers represents a human being, a young man or woman, a dedicated pharmacist who is now frustrated and disillusioned.

Under the best of prospects, new pharmacist faces a lifetime of marginal employment and under utilization. And even worse, many of them will have the hard choice between no employment or taking a position in some alien field outside the profession.

This situation was not of their making, but of ours. The leadership of American pharmacy was responsible for determining the nature of the curriculum, the number of pharmacy schools, and the size of the student enrollments. The easy-road decisions made during the late 1950s and 1960s are now coming home to haunt us.

Our decision-making behavior in the past should suggest at least it does to me that we have been too preoccupied with the immediate rather than long-range future.

In the early 1960s we failed to see the handwriting on the wall and got left out of Medicare. We came to our senses rather quickly, but our effort to add an out-of-hospital pharmaceutical benefit was out of synchronization with other national goals to which Congress gave priority attention.

We have made a number of critical and epochal decisions in the last ten years, and our track record suggests, again at least to me, that we are starting to learn something about the process and what our objectives should be.

Whatever its weaknesses, whatever its shortcomings, APhA's decision-making process has been working quite well in recent years. Time and again, the profession as a whole has come around to accept positions and embrace philosophies reflected in APhA policy decisions which, a few years earlier, were thought of as radical, unpopular or controversial. In other cases, concurrence is given either grudgingly or in name only.

APhA's positions on the MAC program and on Actual Acquisition Cost fall into this latter category. These proposals did not fail because they were unsound or wrong, but because much of organized pharmacy and many individual pharmacy practitioners refused to accept short-term hardships and preferred the comfortable, easy route. Only too late will they learn that they have chosen the road to economic disaster and professional oblivion.

This brings me to the final point which I would leave with. Being right is important but it is not enough.

APhA, as the national professional society, can adopt the best of policy positions, but unless it has the broad-based support of the profession-both organized groups as well as the collective body of grass roots practitioner-its effectiveness is severely blunted and diminished. It is policy existing in a vacuum.

Pharmacists love to think of themselves as an independent bunch, even to the point where they delude themselves. But, ironically, to achieve and to retain independence requires a willingness, albeit voluntary to accept and to accede to the decisions democratically arrived at by the majority.

At the time of the American Revolution the colonists wanted independence from England. But their success directly depended upon their willingness to subjugate their desire for personal independence to the broader task of collective independence. History tells us that a favorite analogy used by colonial leaders was to compare the strength of a stout piece of rope to the fragile weakness of its individual strands of fiber. And less than a century later, Abraham Lincoln reluctantly went to war saying that "A house divided against itself cannot endure." So it is for all areas of life including the health professions.

There are just about as many dentists in the United States as there are pharmacists. They are distributed about as evenly throughout the country. Moreover, they are similar in many other respects such as their level of education. However, since World War II, dentistry has made much greater strides than pharmacy with regard to average income, public image perception, maintaining a favorable environment of practice, and general selfesteem.

In my analysis, I am convinced that there is one single underlying reason for this success. The American Dental Association has a membership of over 95 percent of the country's dentists and an affiliated structure which includes all state and local associations. When ADA speaks, everyone knows that American dentistry is speaking. The result is that ADA is listened to and its views carry enormous weight.

American dentists are also an independent breed. But they also know professional self-discipline. Hence, when ADA has adopted policies or issues that were highly controversial at that time within dentistry such as fluoridation of public water supplies, or extending its seal of acceptance program to include dentifrices members did not rebel; they did not drop their membership in protest; they did not form new organizations.

And although they did continue to debate the issues within their councils and house of delegates, the ADA remained strong and, because of such strength, its voice and its policies continued to have great public impact.

There is a lesson here for us. Had pharmacy followed the same course thirty years ago, we could enjoy the same economic rewards, the same power and the same prestige.

Now it is late. But not too late. There is a mass of uncommitted pharmacists spread across the United States; they also lack professional self-discipline. We can reach them; we can convince them; we can convert them. But first, we must convince and convert those who would be their leaders. Many of them are in this room.

And so, that is the challenge and the hope I leave with you. ■

1978 Remington Medalist

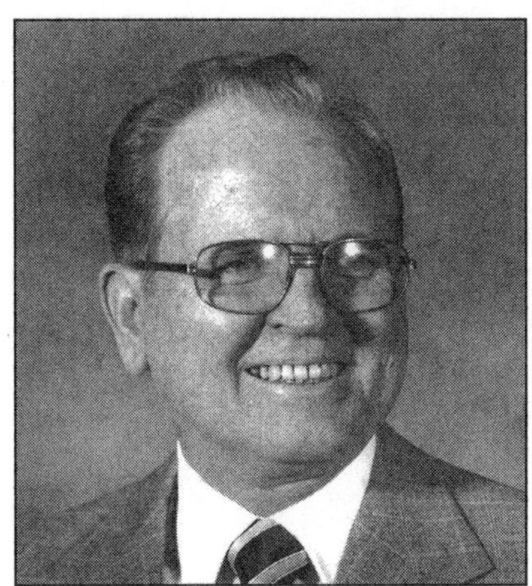

EUGENE VADEN WHITE

Eugene Vaden White was born in Cape Charles, Virginia, on August 13, 1924, and received a B.S. degree in pharmacy from the Medical College of Virginia in 1950. He served as associate community pharmacist 1951-1953, a partner in community pharmacy in Front Royal, Virginia 1953-1956, and in 1957 he purchased his own pharmacy in Berryville, Virginia. On April 9, 1960, he introduced the patient medication system into community practice, and in November 1960 he transformed his typical "drugstore" into a patient-oriented professional pharmacy with a professional office setting and a private consultation area, the first of its type and design in the U.S. A prototype of the "Pharmaceutical Center" was unveiled at the 1965 American Pharmaceutical Association annual meeting by U.S. Vice President Hubert H. Humphrey.

White introduced the pharmacotherapy home follow-up concept in 1970, and authored in 1978 *The Office-Based Family Pharmacist* describing the new concept of pharmacy practice. The "Eugene V. White Distinguished Lecture Series" was established in 1998 at the Bernard J. Dunn School of Pharmacy in Winchester, Virginia. After 48 years of pharmacy practice, 38 years of which were in his pharmacy office setting, White donated his Berryville office pharmacy to the Shenandoah University where it was replicated as a teaching museum in the School of Pharmacy.

The "And Others" Profession

Eugene Vaden White

The 1978 Remington Medal was presented April 25, 1979, at the Disneyland Hotel in Anaheim, California, during the April 21-26, 1979, American Pharmaceutical Association annual meeting. White's Remington address has not been published, but the address has been preserved as a manuscript in the APhA Archives.

Tonight I accept this honor on behalf of my wife, Laura. No one is more cognizant than I that any achievements that may have occurred in Berryville, Virginia, have not been through my efforts alone.

Not only have I been blessed with encouragement and assistance from my wife, she has also contributed many ideas and many hours of her time and talent on behalf of the pharmacy profession and few within or without it have demonstrated greater zeal toward its improvement than she. I also acknowledge with thanks my mother's suggestion of the challenging profession of pharmacy when I was in a quandary as to career selection.

Nevertheless, it was through the dedication of a loyal team that nebulous dreams and ideas were transformed into hard realities. The six years of signal performance by my former associate pharmacist, Carl F. Emswiller, Jr. of Leesburg, Virginia, in fostering the concept of an office practice of pharmacy to the people at a critical time in its evolution played a significant part in assuring its success. This dedicated pharmacist is one of pharmacy's unsung heroes and recognition of his work is long overdue. Carl's wife, Jewel, is also a strong advocate of the concept and has expounded on it many times. Two staff members, Doris Ann Ladd and Eloise Denney Yerger, were dedicated to conducting the practice on a very personal basis. Bruce D. McWhinney, Pharm.D., as a teenaged delivery boy at the founding of the concept played his part in its success. Though the professional atmosphere is vital as a part of the concept and it required teamwork to insure its success, in the final analysis; however, all of our efforts would have been fruitless had the people of Clarke County, Virginia, rejected these "radical" ideas at the beginning.

Some of you may be puzzled by the title I have selected for this address. I know pharmacists in particular are aware of its connotation for how many of us in recent years have not read or heard reference to our profession in journals, at meetings, and especially in the news media in this ranking: "Medicine, Dentistry, Nursing and others?" And others. That's us! Nearly 30 years ago when I graduated from pharmacy school, the major medical professions were listed as "Medicine, Dentistry, Pharmacy and Nursing." Nursing, then only a three-year course, was last, but why did it forge ahead of pharmacy-which has had at least a five year curriculum for 19 years-and why is pharmacy so often slighted? Could it be that the nursing profession discovered for itself what Thomas Jefferson stated: "Dependency begets subservience?" Nurses balked at being known as the "Physician's handmaiden." The nursing profession increased the length of its curriculum, expanded its role, and is assuming responsibility for its own actions. Simply stated, they realized medicine could no longer do it all or take credit for all, and they are taking advantage of the opportunity.

What did the pharmacy profession do during these three decades? In the academic and institutional areas, it progressed, but, I regret to say, in the community area it retrogressed. The creeping cancer of commercialism has virtually destroyed our professional identity in the community. Who would have dreamed just a few years ago that the term "grocery store pharmacist" would be in our vocabulary? Probably most of the pharmacists who work in these grocery stores don't like the idea anymore than I do, but they may feel trapped and that they have no other choice. There is even a movement afoot to develop a "professional approach" discount image for the small retailer.

As long as we attempt to function as professionals with shelves behind us, displays to either side of us, a counter in front of us, a cash register at hand, and in a standing position, we are going to remain the "and others" profession. If we are to survive as a profession, we must get the pharmacist out of the "store" and the "store" out of pharmacy. When one surveys the contemporary community pharmacy scene across this nation, I know this appears to be an impossible dream, but, in my view, it can and it will be done. The time has come for some radical thinking and a new approach to pharmacy practice in the community. The optometrists established a precedent for us when they separated from the jewelry store-and where do they practice? In most instances, in an office environment. They, too, were told separation would never happen.

One of pharmacy's giants, the late Remington Honor Medalist Dr. Donald E. Francke, described the typical American drugstore as a "commercialized jungle" and stated:

"We cannot continue to grasp simultaneously at the best of the professional world and at the best of the business world. In attempting to grasp both we lose both. We must decide either to follow the paths of the other health professions and concentrate our efforts on the health needs of the people, or to follow the paths of the entrepreneur."

Perhaps there has been little demand from the grass roots for change because pharmacists acquiesce to what they see in community practice. Isolated from the main stream of pharmacy thinking, they may feel they are powerless or helpless to do anything about things which may be negative for the profession. But there is a way to escape the tentacles of commercialism the office practice of pharmacy concept. Many of you may be unaware that for nearly 19 years I have been completely disassociated from commercialism. I have practiced my profession full-time without sidelines; without merchandising; without a single display of any product; without a penny spent on radio, newspaper, or billboard advertising; without sale promotions; without deceptive gimmicks; and without attending one wholesaler's Christmas gift show. Who is to say society will not support us as full-time practitioners? I would wager 90 percent of the community pharmacists would prefer practicing in an office setting and they can if that is their desire and goal.

The commercial interests in recent years have raised the hue and cry that the education obtained by the new graduates is irrelevant and useless for community practice, and that the educators should "face the realities of the marketplace" and provide business and marketing-oriented courses for students. But if we have determined that to continue on the path of commercialism pharmacy as a profession will perish, of what possible value is it to abide by the dictates of the commercial interests? I feel that as long as the commercial interests complain that the pharmacy curriculum is irrelevant to their needs, then the educators should rest assured that they are on the right track.

In my view, the key to the entire problem is not to make the present pharmacy curriculum relevant to commercialism in community practice but to change community practice so that it is relevant to what is taught students in pharmacy schools. What is taught the students can be made relevant by establishing a professional setting in the community from which the expertise and value of the competent pharmacist and Doctor of Pharmacy can be demonstrated to the public which will then in turn demand and expect this type of service because they feel they are entitled to it.

We now have the opportunity to upgrade the private practitioner's involvement in patient care to such a degree that the product/profit-oriented pharmacist cannot possibly compete with what the patient/ pharmacotherapy-oriented pharmacist is achieving for his patients. If only the educators could agree to discontinue teaching the few remaining commercial courses in the colleges of pharmacy, what the students currently observe in community practice would not be reinforced and I would hope the students would then be more willing, enthusiastic, inspired, and motivated to help make the changes that are so necessary to eliminate commercialism for our environment and make us truly a profession, thereby aiding in removing the stigma of the "and others" profession.

Little did I dream when I wrote a letter to the editor of the *Virginia Pharmacist* 25 years ago predicting the future role of the pharmacist as prescriber that the side effects of that thinking would lead me to the Remington Honor Medal. The shockwaves of that prediction have subsided somewhat and now prominent people are beginning to give it serious thought and consideration. But also little did I dream 25 years ago that two then unconceived physician extenders-the physicians' assistants (PAs) and the Nurse Practitioners (NPs) would now be a threat to the future role of the new breed of pharmacy practitioners.

If all kinds of task forces and surveys have revealed the extent of irrational and inappropriate prescribing by physicians and dentists and their deficiencies in the fields of pharmacology and pharmacotherapy, how can anyone justify or claim that the even less qualified PAs and NPs should have the legal right or prerogative to prescribe potent drugs? Yet, without fanfare the PAs and NPs in some states are already legally prescribing all but Schedule II controlled drugs under so-called supervision of physicians, and in some areas that supervision consists of a pad of signed prescription blanks. One pharmacy publication editorialized that allowing PAs to prescribe "places the pharmacists in a position of making sure that a physician really signed the prescription." In my view, the editor in trying to protect us may have missed the cardinal point. Our prime concern should not be who signed the prescription but why the PA is allowed to be in the prescribing role at all. Why do we acquiesce by our complacency while others are engineering for themselves our place in the sun?

Once organized medicine began delegating the prescribing role to the PAs and NPs and assisted in lobbying efforts to amend State statutes to legalize it, medicine relinquished its prescriptive prerogative and can never again bombard the pharmacy profession with the admonition, as it so often has in the past, that no one-but no one-is qualified to prescribe potent drugs except licensed physicians and dentists. We must be aware that today, as in the past, the apparently self-serving pharmaceutical industry has been a tremendous force and power in zealously protecting the medical profession from encroachment of its prescribing prerogative. The industry has vigorously opposed, and continues to oppose, proposals for expanding the pharmacist's role in the direction of a decision-maker in drug therapy.

Just as it required the support of the people to help us to amend the anti-substitution laws, the pharmacy profession may have to bring the incongruity and peril of allowing prescribing by the PAs and NPs to the public's attention to convince them that the pharmacist-the one professional who has years of concentrated study on drugs-should have the legal right to prescribe. No other medical team member has the expertise equal to that of the new pharmacy graduate to make judgmental decisions on drug therapy and the capability to correlate the information on adverse reactions, drug interactions, toxicities, excretion rates and the whole gamut of therapy from the vast resources available to him. Increasingly, the physician in diagnosing and treating is making greater utilization of the pharmacist and his knowledge of the pharmacokinetics of drugs. The physicians and dentists have neither the time, resources, or the background knowledge to thoroughly research new drug products or new drug problems, and even less so the PAs and NPs. With inexpensive quality generic drugs appearing on the market, physicians are showing a renewed interest in office dispensing and, in fact, in some states they are attempting to amend statutes to permit it.

I think that we should be forewarned that the next assignment to the PAs and NPs by the physicians may well be the dispensing of medications from their offices all properly recorded, serialized and labeled to meet all pharmacy board regulations and/or the delegation of patient counseling and educational roles on the use of medications, for example, explaining patient package insert information. If this occurs, just what remains for the future pharmacist to do? Does anyone in this room know of any alternative role for the skilled pharmacy clinician? Remember, at least three courts have already ruled that the "counting and pouring of medications" is not a professional endeavor or function, though our State Boards of Pharmacy decreed it so for years. While we are busy "minding the store," the PAs and NPs just may assume our future role. Ironically, pharmacy educators are involved in the teaching of pharmacology and prescribing to those who would preempt the pharmacy profession. I know pharmacy has been at the "crossroads" for centuries, but for sure, this is one of the most critical periods in our history. I think it's high time we raise our voices in unison and strongly object to and resist efforts of the PAs and the NPs to be involved with pharmacy at all, much less prescribe potent drugs, or else we may not even retain the "and others" professional status.

For years I have envisioned the future pharmacist practicing primary care along with the physician in a common office complex, not as a mid-level or second level practitioner, but on a joint, equal, independent and unsupervised basis where he has ready access to all patient records and an opportunity for close interaction with other health-care professionals. I am firmly convinced that if we allow this opportunity to develop a new role on the heath-care team to elude us, our demise is certain.

Cognizant of the critical physician shortage in an expanding population, the busy physician must become aware that the pharmacist is not out to compete with or threaten his position on the health-care team. He should realize the pharmacist has uncovered a great void in the health care system-the lack of a specialist in pharmacotherapy and that the pharmacist feels he is the most logical and the best qualified person to fill this void. The pharmacist sees an opportunity to practice on a level that can greatly benefit the patient, and provide the physician with more time for functions that only he can perform.

But few of these goals can be achieved without unity. How many more Remington Honor Medalists must address this issue? "A branch cannot bear fruit away from the vine." The American Pharmaceutical Association must be the vine and accept the responsibilities inherent in that role of leadership. I realize there are many branches in American Pharmacy but the branches die unless they remain attached to the vine. Unless pharmacy has a vine to supply support and nourishment, the branches cannot bear fruit. All of us need continually to learn new skills, utilize our talents, be creative with new ideas and always be on the quest for excellence in all that we do. The APhA should continually provide strength, direction, assistance, and encouragement for its members.

Pharmacy desperately needs a common goal. If we do not have ideals and goals for the future which are necessary to develop a common direction for the profession, we become subject to the ideals and hopes of others who will determine for us what our future will be. If we decide our own future, the progress we then make will be in accordance with our own needs and aspirations.

In a personal vein, there is only one sad note for me on this happy occasion, nine years ago this very day my father died suffering from cancer. But thinking of my father also brings back fond memories of him, one of which I should like to share with you tonight. I vividly recall his annual Spring ritual of plowing his garden. He would implant into the ground the end of a rake handle, and then from the opposite end of the garden, using the rake as his guide and goal, start plowing the row. Setting off rows with a hand plow is not an easy task and often wire grass, roots, rocks, or other obstacles would cause him to falter but with an eye on his goal, he persevered and plodded onward. I always knew what to expect when he reached the rake and stopped. Wiping his brow with his red bandanna handkerchief, and with a faint smile of satisfaction and pride on his face, he would look back at his handiwork, always the straightest of furrows.

I think pharmacy needs to implant its "rake" and strive for the goal of eventually qualifying all pharmacists as pharmacotherapy specialists and then we, too, can look upon our achievements with a great sense of satisfaction and pride-all to the benefit of our patients and the health-care team. It is then that we will cease to be the "and others" profession. ■

1980 Remington Medalist

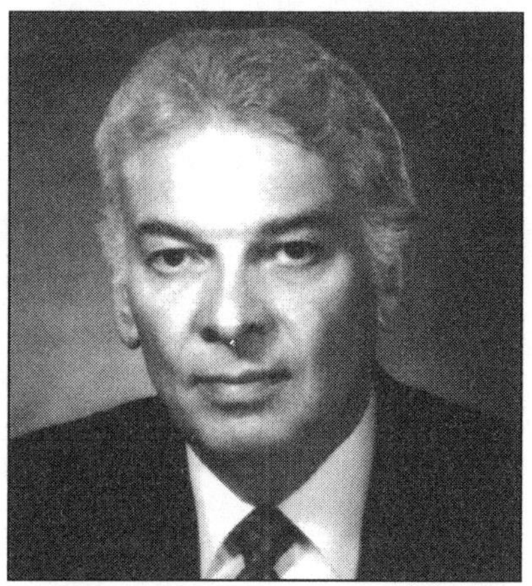

JOSEPH DALTON WILLIAMS

Joseph Dalton Williams was born in Washington, Pennsylvania, August 15, 1926. After active duty in the U.S. Navy submarine service during World War II, he received a B.S. in Pharmacy in 1950 from the University of Nebraska. Immediately following his graduation, he joined Parke-Davis as a sales representative working out of the Kansas City branch office. He was promoted to field manager in 1951 and was transferred to the Parke-Davis executive offices in Detroit in 1952 where he served in various capacities in market research. He was elected a Parke-Davis vice president in 1970, and upon completion of the merger with Warner-Lambert, he was elected executive vice president in 1971, and president of Parke-Davis in 1973. He was transferred to the corporate headquarters in Morris Plains, New Jersey, in 1976 as president of the Warner-Lambert Pharmaceutical Group. He became president of Warner-Lambert in 1979, and chairman of the Board and chief executive officer from 1985 until his retirement in 1997.

A member of the American Pharmaceutical Association, Williams served as Pharmaceutical Manufacturers Association chairman 1984-1985, founded and chaired the pharmacy relations committee, and was president of the International Federation of Pharmaceutical Manufacturers 1987-1988. He also served as president of the New Jersey Commission on Higher Education, and a member of the board of directors for AT&T, Eckerd Drug, Exxon, J.C. Penny, and Therapeutic Antibodies, Inc.

ONCE A PHARMACIST, ALWAYS A PHARMACIST

Joseph Dalton Williams

The 1980 Remington Medal was presented April 20, 1980, at the Washington Hilton Hotel in Washington, D.C., during the American Pharmaceutical Association annual meeting April 19-24, 1980. Williams's Remington address was not published, but a transcript has been prepared from a tape recording.

I feel like I just won the gold medal at the Olympics. Since its beginning in 1918, the Remington Honor Medal has been the most coveted award in American Pharmacy. For almost a century, Remington's *Practice of Pharmacy* has been as familiar to pharmacy students, just as Gray's *Anatomy* has been to the medical students.

Joseph P. Remington left an indelible imprint on our profession and to even be indirectly associated with this famous pharmacist is indeed an honor. My Dean, Rufus A. Lyman, became the 25th Remington medalist while I was a student at the University of Nebraska. So my appreciation for this honor is longstanding. I accept this very, very special award with humility and, of course, with pride. I want to especially thank the past presidents of the American Pharmaceutical Association who selected me. I thank and commend them for recognizing that management, as well as practice, research and teaching, is a role in which pharmacists can make meaningful contributions to our public health and also to the pharmacy profession. As all of you know, the pharmaceutical industry in the U.S. had its origin in pharmacy. Despite our periodic and episodic differences, the profession and industry have enjoyed a symbiotic relationship for almost two centuries. It is only natural for us to focus on recent events; and in the last 15-20 years we have done a lot of finger pointing at one another. APhA leaders have not been reticent in criticizing the industry, but I also know from first hand experience, APhA leaders give their first priority to resolving the problems that confront them. They recognize that the right to criticize brings with it the obligation to participate.

I have observed that even during the most difficult periods of industry profession relations, our national professional society has respected the integrity of the pharmacists and scientists employed within the industry. Research and development is one of the major building blocks of the worldwide pharmaceutical industry. And I am proud of the contributions that the APhA Academy of Pharmaceutical Sciences is making in furthering the science of pharmacy.

However, the U.S. pharmaceutical industry did not establish its world leadership through research and development alone. U.S. excellence in management, technology, quality control, production, and marketing completes the successful formula. There are some people in our country who would punish the industry for its worldwide leadership and success. This is the kind of negative thinking that contributes to our current economic woes. Last week APhA Chairman Mary Munson Runge addressed the Pharmaceutical Manufacturers Association annual meeting. If they didn't fully understand the profession's aspirations and problems before then, I can assure you that my colleagues in the industry do now. I was particularly pleased to hear Mary say that APhA is not only concerned with the economic survival of the profession, but that APhA is also concerned with the economic survival of the industry. Mary appropriately pointed out, "The profession cares about the economic survival of the industry because the profession recognizes that pharmaceutical products are a key element in the health care equation as well as the prime physical component of pharmacy dispensing practice."

Chairman Runge didn't leave the PMA meeting without challenging the industry. As you know, for years our industry has routinely made certain low-volume products available as service products. Many firms, because of economic conditions, are having to make crossroads decisions about continuing this practice. Mary asked us to look again and she supported her plea with a logical argument that anything that keeps the bigfoot of federal bureaucracy out of the field of drug development, production, and manufacturing could be a sound, longterm business decision.

Fellow pharmacist FDA Commissioner Goyan has also challenged the industry to address the problem of orphan drugs, drug therapies of great potential, which do not realize that potential because of limited commercial value.

I remember just a few years ago the White House enlisted the industry to overnight respond to the flu vaccine emergency. For a few weeks we were national heroes. For years we will be paying for our patriotic response, taxpayers included. I mention these items only in passing to indicate to the profession that life in the pharmaceutical industry today is anything but a bed of roses. I also want to reinforce your recognition of our interdependence. We not only need to know how much we need each other, but we need to work harder at helping each other.

In 1967, the Remington Medalist said, "Medicine, pharmacy, and the pharmaceutical industry are inseparably joined in the common challenge of serving sick people. Each much act according to its own conscience. Pharmacy always stands ready to cooperate with medicine and industry, but the profession must speak for itself." Bill Apple, whom I just quoted, has not only spoken ably for the profession for many years, but he has also respected those who spoke for medicine and for the pharmaceutical industry.

Several years ago in Michigan, I developed a dialogue with Robert C. Johnson who later served as an elected president of APhA. Bob, along with Bob Gillespie who was then APhA president, and Lou Sesti, urged me to become involved in the dialogue between the profession and the industry. It was good advice and helps account for my presence here today.

I would be remiss if I didn't point out that the effort to improve communications among ourselves is a team effort. Many of the members of that team are pharmacists who specialized in management. Men whom you all know, men like Mike Bongiovani, John Huck, Milt Hendricks, Irwin Lerner, Larry Hoff, Fred Lyons, Gene Step, to mention only a few, are well known to you. I know that I speak for every pharmacist in the industry when I say that regardless of our current assignments, once a pharmacist always a pharmacist. In honoring me you have honored all of us. We do have mutual problems. We have mutual opportunities to further improve our working relationships and our team efforts to serve the American people. I pledge you my continuing efforts and thank you very much. ■

1983 Remington Medalist

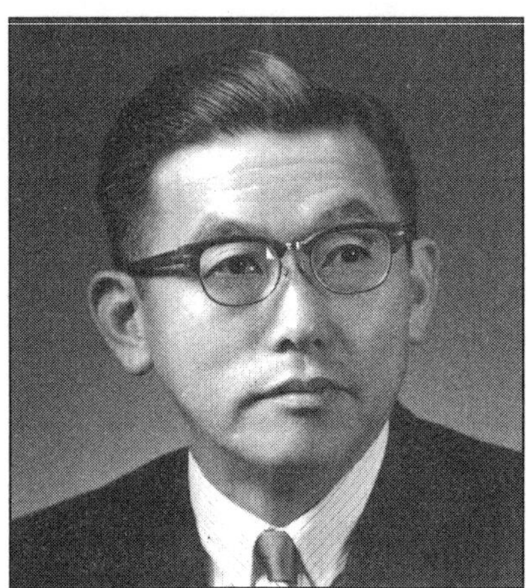

TAKERU HIGUCHI
(1918-1987)

Takeru Higuchi was born in Los Altos, California, and received an A.B. degree in chemistry from the University of California Berkeley in 1939, and a Ph.D. degree in physical and organic chemistry from the University of Wisconsin in 1943. He commenced his professional career as a research chemist in the synthetic rubber program at the University of Akron, Ohio 1944-1947. He then joined the faculty of the University of Wisconsin School of Pharmacy as assistant professor 1947-1949, associate professor 1950-1953, professor 1954-1963, and Edward Kremers professor of pharmaceutical chemistry 1964-1967. He then joined the faculty of the University of Kansas School of Pharmacy as regents distinguished professor of chemistry and pharmacy, during which time he also served as director of the Alza Institute of Pharmaceutical Chemistry 1968-1972. He established INTERx Research Corporation in 1972, serving as its president until the firm was merged with Merck Sharpe and Dohme Research Laboratories in 1980. At the time of his death, Higuchi was serving as chairman of the board of Oread Laboratories, a corporation established in 1983 to commercially develop biotechnology created at the University of Kansas.

Higuchi was a founder of the American Pharmaceutical Association's Academy of Pharmaceutical Sciences, serving as its first president 1965-1967. He was the recipient of such APhA awards as the Ebert Prize in 1954, the first Research Achievement Award in Physical Pharmacy in 1962, the Justin Powers Award in Pharmaceutical Analysis in 1964, the Stimulation of Research Award in 1967, and the Kolthoff Gold Medal in Analytical Chemistry in 1977. In 1981, the Academy established the Takeru Higuchi Research Prize and Endowment Fund to recognize the highest accomplishments in pharmaceutical sciences.

A Deserved Recognition to Takeru Higuchi

The 1983 Remington Medal was presented April 10, 1983, in New Orleans, Louisiana, during the American Pharmaceutical Association annual meeting April 10-14, 1983. Higuchi's Remington address was not published, and neither a copy of the manuscript nor a tape recording of his presentation has been located. In the absence of Higuchi's Remington remarks, we are publishing Edward G. Feldmann's "Editorial" appearing in the April 1983 issue of the *Journal of Pharmaceutical Sciences*, volume 72, page 329, 1983, which was devoted in its entirety to scientific papers authored by some of Higuchi's more than 200 students and research associates.

Over the years, the field of pharmacy has been generously blest with its share of outstanding scientists. These men and women through their immediate research, or through guiding and directing their scientific research associates, have made significant contributions that have advanced our knowledge of drugs: their identification, their mechanism of action, their strength or potency, their relative effectiveness, their stability, their toxicity, and so on.

In many instances, such information not only added to the body of knowledge in pharmacy, but also to that in other fields of science, including biology, pharmacology, botany, physics, mathematics, and toxicology.

Rarely, however, does the individual who is noted for making major or even landmark achievements in the area of scientific research also have a significant impact on changing the course or direction of professional practice in pharmacy.

That perhaps, is what most sets Takeru Higuchi apart from other contemporary pharmaceutical scientists-even the great ones. And, undoubtedly, that characteristic probably was an important factor in the deliberations of this year's selection committee for the Remington Honor Medal. The Remington Medal is referred to as "the highest award" that the profession has to bestow, and generally it has gone to someone having a close identity with the profession in its broadest sense: education regulation, standards establishment, administration, literature, manufacturing, or clinical practice.

Consequently, the very recent announcement of Dr. Higuchi as the 1983 Remington medalist acknowledges his broad contributions to pharmacy practice, and may well serve as the capstone to his career and his honors. But in this column, it would be especially appropriate to take note of his contributions to the pharmaceutical sciences.

Although his personal education and training were in chemistry rather than pharmacy, Dr. Higuchi became identified with pharmacy early in his career when he accepted a faculty position at the University of Wisconsin's School of Pharmacy. And, as an individual of strong personal loyalty, once he made that commitment, he did so wholeheartedly and with complete conviction and dedication.

While many of his academic colleagues including those whose roots were in pharmacy-minimized their pharmacy connections, Higuchi proudly identified himself with the profession. Moreover, he greatly supported the growth of the pharmaceutical sciences by presenting his research results at scientific pharmacy meetings and by submitting his papers for publication in scientific pharmacy journals. In addition, he preached what he himself practiced. Namely, he encouraged his numerous graduate students and colleagues to follow his example in their presentations and publications.

The quality of the scientific programs at the spring and fall meetings of the APhA Academy of Pharmaceutical Sciences, and the international recognition and stature of the *Journal of Pharmaceutical Sciences,* both are due in a very large measure to Higuchi and his disciples. They constitute viable testimonials to the impact that this man has had in advancing the cause of the sciences in pharmacy.

Numerous things could be written in praise of the man whom many of us fondly call "Tak." (This writer's personal acquaintance goes back over 31 years to December 1951, when he had a long discussion with the then young professor in his office regarding the merits of graduate study at the snowbound campus of the University of Wisconsin.)

However, we will limit our remaining remarks to just two interrelated matters which in themselves are unusual tributes to Dr. Higuchi.

First: A special full-day symposium in honor of Higuchi was presented during the APS national meeting in November 1981 in Orlando, Florida. All the papers presented at that symposium were authored by present or former students of Professor Higuchi-over 200 doctorate and post doctorate people took their training under him as their major professor.

Subsequently, most of those papers were considered for publication in the *Journal of Pharmaceutical Sciences,* and those that were eventually accepted are collected together in this April 1983 issue-along with several other papers by Higuchi students-as a special issue in tribute to him and in recognition and appreciation of his tremendous contributions to the journal.

Second: At that same meeting in Orlando, Higuchi's friends and colleagues, in conjunction with the APhA Academy of Pharmaceutical Sciences and the APhA Foundation, announced that a new award was to be established in honor of Dr. Higuchi. This new award would carry with it a very substantial monetary prize and would be intended to honor those who have made broad and pioneering contributions to the pharmaceutical sciences. Hence, it would not be limited to any special field of the pharmaceutical sciences, nor would it be intended to recognize any single achievement no matter how noteworthy.

Through the work, support, and generosity of many participants, the Takeru Higuchi Research Prize is now coming to fruition, and plans are underway to present it initially this fall.

The significance or importance of any award is a very nebulous thing, and it can be judged in various ways. However, in many respects, named awards tend to reflect the stature of the persons for whom they are named and are intended to recognize.

In this light, the Higuchi Prize immediately assumes rather gigantic proportions aside from any other considerations, including the amount of the monetary component.

Many years ago, one of Dr. Higuchi's students nicknamed him "The Little Giant," because of his rather diminutive physical stature coupled with his very large presence on the scientific research scene.

We are indeed pleased to see this current "coming together" of such a variety of honors-Remington Medal, special Journal issue, major new research award in recognition of The Little Giant's enormous contributions to the pharmaceutical sciences. ■

1984 Remington Medalist

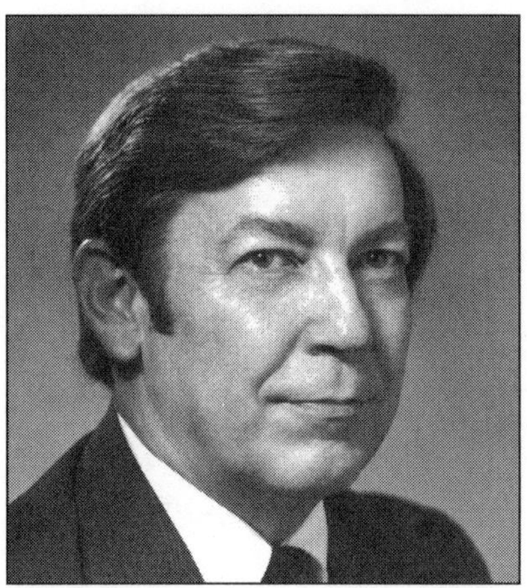

William Mohn Heller

William Mohn Heller was born in Orrville, Ohio, on March 15, 1926, and received a B.S. degree in pharmacy from the University of Toledo in 1949, an M.S. in 1951, and a Ph.D. in 1955 from the University of Maryland. After service in the U.S. Army, during which time he attended the University of Indiana 1943-1944 and Biarritz American University in France 1945, he interned in hospital pharmacy at The Johns Hopkins Hospital 1949-1951, and practiced as a relief community pharmacist in Baltimore 1949-1954.

Heller joined the faculty of the University of Arkansas School of Pharmacy serving as assistant professor 1954-1960. He was chief pharmacist of the University of Arkansas Medical Center 1955-1966, and was chief investigator of the research team that developed and demonstrated the first hospital-wide unit doses dispensing system. He was the first editor of the *American Hospital Formulary Service* 1955-1963, and joined the staff of the American Society of Hospital Pharmacists in 1966 serving as director of the department of scientific services. He was appointed executive director-designate of the U.S. Pharmacopeial Convention in 1968 and served as executive director until his retirement in 1990. As USPC executive director, Heller relocated the headquarters to its own building, negotiated the acquisition of the *National Formulary* and the APhA Drug Standards Laboratory, and broadened the basis of support for USPC with the introduction of both the *Pharmacopeial Forum* and *USP Dispensing Information*. In retirement, Heller serves as the member-at-large of the U.S. Adopted Names Council; senior advisor to the USP Expert Committee on Nomenclature and Labeling; and member of the board of grants and consultant to the Board of Directors of the American Foundation for Pharmaceutical Education.

An Unparalleled System of Volunteers

William Mohn Heller

The 1984 Remington Medal was presented May 6, 1984, in Montreal, Quebec, Canada, at the Opening Session of the May 5-10, 1984, American Pharmaceutical Association annual meeting. Heller's Remington address has not been published, but the remarks have been preserved by both tape recording in the APhA Archives and a manuscript provided by the medalist.

I have just a couple of minutes for remarks before the show starts. It has been suggested to me many times over the years that we ought to put a centerfold in the *United States Pharmacopeia* to liven it up. But to follow my talk with thirty dancing girls is more than I could have bargained for.

I am sure that every Remington medalist has been deeply grateful for this recognition, as I am. And I am sure that each medalist had hoped to be both profound and thankful in their remarks. But few other Remington medalists have had as much reason to be so thankful to so many people who have been co-workers along the way.

Gloria Niemeyer Francke, who captured me as a graduate student to work on her comprehensive bibliography on hospital pharmacy, and taught me to appreciate the pharmaceutical literature.

Ken Barker and 26 other pharmacists who made our unit-dose dispensing system work at the University of Arkansas.

Joseph Oddis and George Provost who enticed me to join the American Society of Hospital Pharmacists headquarters staff, and who showed me that there was life for a pharmacist outside of a pharmacy.

Lloyd Miller and Mary Griffiths who persuaded me that if working on the USP committee of revision was interesting, work as part of the *USP* staff would be fantastic.

Ken Barker and Joseph Valentino who proposed that the *USP* should help advance pharmacy practice by getting into the dispensing information business. Keith Johnson and his staff who conceived and brought to fruition the patient advice part of the dispensing information. Tim Grady and his staff who brought drug standards back to the practice level. And Robert Henry and Alice Kimball who made you like it all.

Finally, George Archambault, the most inspiring, unpaid, dollar-a-year man anyone has ever had as a confidante.

I had the good fortune of working in a system of volunteers who are unparalleled in the concentration of decision-making expertise which helped the *USP* better serve pharmacists, physicians, and the public of both the U.S.A. and Canada.

Most of all, I am thankful to our forbearers, including Joseph Remington, for passing on to us this remarkable organization called *USP* which is unique in the world.

Someday, I hope that each of you has an opportunity to visit the *USP* offices in Rockville, Maryland. When you do, I want to show you what happened when Professor Remington became chairman of the committee of revision in 1901, a position he held until his death 17 years later.

Charles Rice, a hospital pharmacist, had been chairman of the *USP* committee of revision for two decades. All of the correspondence between committee members, and the entire record of *USP* revision was written by hand in a beautiful and elaborate script. Page after page of this huge book, 18 inches long, 12 inches wide, and five inches thick, are filled with beautiful script. Then when Remington took over, he wrote his first committee circular on a typewriter.

Now here we are at another time in history where the demarkation is sharp, and perhaps just as painful to those of us who have helped bring about this change. Computers are replacing the typewriter as our vehicle for communications. And communication information is replacing compounding and packaging as our primary service to our patients.

Our successors at *USP* and at the American Pharmaceutical Association will be looking back to see what we did with our opportunity. Truly, it is a time for a new beginning for all of us, as organizations and as practitioners. We look forward to working with you to make them proud of us. ■

1985 Remington Medalist

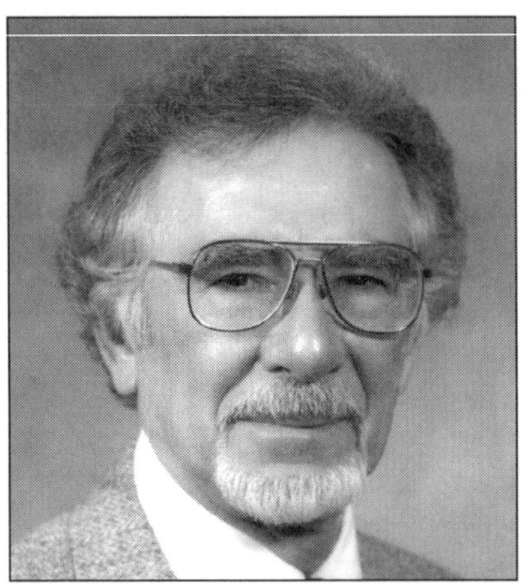

WILLIAM LEONARD BLOCKSTEIN
(1925-1995)

William Leonard Blockstein was born in Irwin, Pennsylvania, November 11, 1925. After service as a hospital corpsman in Okinawa and China during World War II, he received a B.S. degree in Pharmacy 1950, M.S. 1953, and Ph.D. 1959, all from the University of Pittsburgh. He was an instructor at his *alma mater* 1953-1958; assistant and associate professor 1959-1964 at Wayne State University College of Pharmacy; associate professor 1964-1967, professor 1967-1987 and Edward Kremers professor 1987-1991 at the University of Wisconsin School of Pharmacy; and clinical professor of preventive medicine at the UW School of Medicine 1972-1991. In 1969, he became the first statewide program chairman of the University of Wisconsin Extension health sciences unit. He served as American Association of Colleges of Pharmacy section of teachers of continuing education chairman 1964-1965; and as Rho Chi Society secretary-treasurer 1961-1967, vice president 1967-1969, and president 1970-1972.

Blockstein served as APhA Michigan Branch president 1958-1959, chairman of the APhA public relations committee 1962-1963, editor of the APhA annual meeting *Daily Bulletin* 1963-1964, director of public relations for the APhA Academy of Pharmaceutical Sciences 1966-1968, staff director of the APhA Task Force on Pharmacy Education 1981-1983, and pharmacy editor of the APhA *Handbook of Nonprescription Drugs* (ninth edition, 1988-1990). Blockstein served as professor emeritus at the University of Wisconsin School of Pharmacy until his death on February 19, 1995.

On Association

William Leonard Blockstein

The 1985 Remington Medal was presented February 20, 1985, at the American Pharmaceutical Association annual meeting February 16-21, 1985, in San Antonio, Texas. Blockstein's address was not published, but the text of the presentation has been provided by the Remington medalist.

One of my favorite speakers usually began his sermons, saying, "Before I start, I want to say something."

Well, I want to say something. I want publicly to thank Dr. Charles J. Sih, the F.B. Power professor of pharmaceutical chemistry at the University of Wisconsin School of Pharmacy for his leadership in nominating me for this high distinction. When Dr. Sih told me of his plans, I told him how warmed I was that a world-class scientist such as he would take time from his own research efforts to prepare a nomination for me. That effort was reward enough. And to think that his efforts and those of the others who nominated me have brought us to this moment. I, truly, am touched, honored and grateful to all.

In remarks given when I accepted the Rho Chi lecture award, I spoke about "A Majority of One." I made the point that one person could make both a contribution and a difference. On this occasion, I want to discuss "Association." There are two points that I will develop. First, that associating allows many to make a difference, and second, that associations are capable both of introspection and of change.

Almost a century and a half ago, Alexis de Tocqueville, the French patrician and statesman, observed our young democracy as only an outsider could. He wrote,

"Americans of all ages, all conditions, and all dispositions constantly form associations." Continuing, he said,"... I have often admired the extreme skill with which the inhabitants of the United States succeed in proposing a common object for the exertions of a great many men and in inducing them voluntarily to pursue it." Americans form associations for the smallest undertakings and seem to regard association as the only means they have of acting in a democratic society.

De Tocqueville commented that America, the most democratic country on the face of the earth, represented a contrary fact. Because all citizens were independent, they were feeble; they could do hardly anything by themselves. None of them could oblige his fellows to lend him assistance. He observed that "feelings and opinions are recruited, the heart is enlarged, and the human mind is developed only by the reciprocal influence of men upon one another." De Tocqueville suggested that in a democracy, those influences for good can best be accomplished by associations.

Let's consider five associations and their most recent or forthcoming reports that have the potential greatly to influence the course of events for our profession, for health care and for the general development of our American society.

First, the Task Force on Pharmacy Education, created by the American Pharmaceutical Association. The Task Force Final Report has already begun to recruit feelings and opinions, enlarge the heart and develop the human mind. Individuals, policy review groups, and entire associations are considering the implications of this, the fifth major pharmacy study this century. Task Force observations about changing responsibilities and differentiated roles of today's and tomorrow's pharmacists, the resolutions calling for evolution to the desired goal of the six year Doctor of Pharmacy degree for entry level pharmacy practice, swift action on the external degree issue, appropriate use of precious human and material resources, and the notion that association through consortia will provide relief for pharmacy education's problems have a potential for good as we prepare for a bright future of professional service.

The Association of American Medical Colleges (AAMC), an association of medical deans and faculty members recently reported on "Physicians for the Twenty-First Century." This is the association's first major report on medical education in just over fifty years. The AAMC report lists recommendations and strategies to improve the effectiveness of instruction, to promote learning and aid in the personal development of each medical student. The AAMC report has already stimulated broad discussion among medical school faculties and their disciplinary societies about present and suggested philosophies and approaches to medical education and college preparation for medicine. If the report's recommendations were adopted, physicians in the 21st century would be much different from their predecessors.

Pharmacy practice and pharmacy education can learn from the AAMC report. Competition to get into medial school, depersonalized and even anonymous relationships between professors and students, a better system for evaluating student's clinical experiences, the notion of premature specialization, and a broadened preprofessional general education for professional school admission are issues common to both professions.

I've had an opportunity to review and comment on a document slated for 1985 release in final form by the Western Inter State Commission for Higher Education (WICHE). WICHE represents yet one more association: public agencies, schools, and colleges working together by sharing resources for a collective good. The report, "Pharmacy Manpower and Education in the West" will demand the attention of educators, practitioners, legislators, and policy makers not only in the western states, but also from all other locales. The report highlights two points: first, supply of pharmacist practitioners through schooling, population immigration, or other life changes. And second, demand for pharmacists by population groupings, or urban/rural centered geography or shifts in age categories of those needing pharmacy services. Today's imperfect pharmacy manpower forecasting demands immediate improvement if the nation is appropriately to allocate for our valuable health resource. Pharmacy manpower projection efforts will be improved in significant ways, as scholars and planners address the issues highlighted in the forthcoming WICHE report.

"Adult Learners: Key to the Nation's Future" is the title of a position paper just released by the Commission on Higher Education and the Adult Learner. The commission was organized by the American Council on Education, the higher education lobbying association which serves some 23,000 key people in the field of post-secondary education.

Twenty years ago, I bet my life and my professional career that there was a significant future in adult and continuing education. It's nice to have a commission report that validates my bet. The report tell us what needs doing in the way of a national policy, including: developing or renewing employability for the unemployed; maintaining and enhancing occupational and professional skills; providing equal access; and developing a knowledgeable citizenry. The commission report points out barriers to meeting these needs. They include: lack of public awareness; inappropriateness of present institutional structures, generally not designed to serve adult learners; new level of learner awareness; and, of course, the inadequacy of funding for adult education.

A blue ribbon panel, the Committee on Investor-Owned, For-Profit Health Care, of the Institute of Medicine of the National Academy of Sciences (TOM) is examining several issues in the contemporary health care arena. These include quality and cost of care, range of services provided and type of patients served, as well as the public policies and economic forces that are contributing to the expansion of investor-owned for-profit management of medical caret I suspect that the forthcoming report will touch on existing and future considerations of the not-for-profit-health care sector as well. The future of the health care marketplace is important to each of us; this TOM report will certainly recruit feelings and opinions and develop yet another level of public dialogue.

In this brief overview, I've exemplified de Tocqueville's observations about our democratic society. By associating through associations, individual voices gain strength and credibility so as to assure the clash of ideas and the circulation of opinions. The second point I've developed is that associations are capable of keen observation and a willingness to put forth ideas that have the potential of improving present circumstance. Both points put forth my view that unselfish promotion of both the general welfare and individual good makes progress possible.

Now, I want to close by saying something else.

The news of the Remington Honor Medal was difficult for me to absorb. Those close to me know how moved I was, and how I couldn't even talk about it with them. I've adjusted, somewhat, to the news now. I want you to know how much I am indebted to my dear wife, Liesl; to three unique persons, our children: David, Susan, and Michael; to countless friends, teachers, colleagues, and students for the many ways in which their lives have touched mine. Each person and each institution where I have served has helped to shape a part of my life and career.

Finally, I wish to pay tribute to a very special class of people whose names I don't even know. They are those, who through the years, have been nominated by their colleagues for the Remington Honor Medal. Each year since the award was first given in 1919, deserving people are set aside, perhaps for a moment, or for a longer time. To those nominees, the profession of pharmacy owes much. For all of us here, whose condition in the profession is good and getting better, I salute those nominees. I trust that, in appropriate ways, their contributions to the practice, science and art of pharmacy will receive the recognition due them for the good that they have done. ■

1986 Remington Medalist

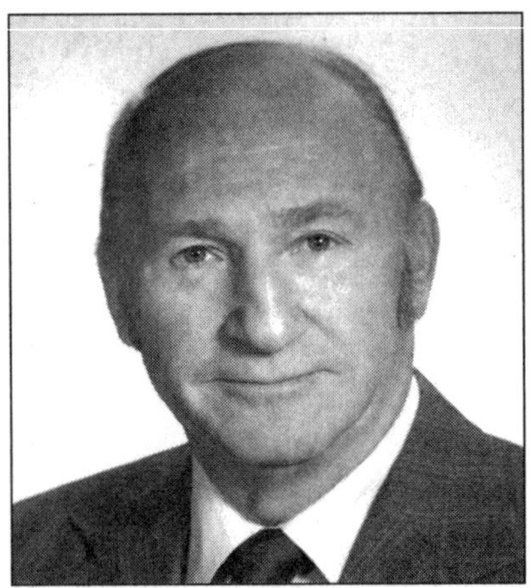

IRVING RUBIN
(1916-1998)

Irving Rubin was born in New York City on April 7, 1916, and received a Ph.G. degree from the Brooklyn College of Pharmacy in 1936. After practicing pharmacy in New York City and serving in the U.S. Army during World War II 1942-1946, he commenced an unparalleled career in pharmaceutical journalism first as pharmacy managing editor of *American Druggist* and editorial director of the *Blue Book* 1938-1960. He joined Romaine Pierson Publishers in 1961 as editor of *American Professional Pharmacist* whose title was changed in 1969 to *Pharmacy Times*. He became corporate vice president in 1980, editor-in-chief in 1987, and editor-at-large until his death on March 13, 1998. He served as president of the American Pharmaceutical Association New York Chapter 1955-1956, president of the Brooklyn College of Pharmacy Alumni Association 1946-1948, and council member of the American Institute of the History of Pharmacy 1975-1978.

Rubin is especially noted for his leadership in many national campaigns including the administration of a Pharmacist's Oath at graduation in 1961; publication of *The Pharmacy Graduate's Career Guide* in 1970; efforts to obtain a U.S. postage stamp honoring pharmacy that was achieved in 1972; establishing a full-time pharmacist in the U.S. Capitol pharmacy in 1979; and increasing pharmacists' awareness of drug abuse prevention in the 1970s and 1980s.

ONE SYMBOL FOR U.S. PHARMACIES

Irving Rubin

The 1986 Remington Medal was presented March 16, 1986, at the Moscone Convention Center in San Francisco, California, during the March 16-20, 1986, American Pharmaceutical Association annual meeting. Rubin's Remington address was published in *Pharmacy Times,* pages 34-36, April 1986.

There are many reasons why I gratefully accept-with humility and happiness-the 1986 Remington Honor Medal. However, the most unique reason involves Dr. Hugo H. Schaefer who following the death of Dr. Joseph Price Remington in 1918 conceived the idea of the Remington Medal. A longtime leader in Pharmacy, Dr. Schaefer was also dean of my pharmacy school-the Brooklyn College of Pharmacy-now called the Arnold and Marie Schwartz College of Pharmacy and Health Sciences. In addition, it was Dr. Schaefer's personal recommendation which enabled me to start working in national pharmacy journalism. Thus, I owe a great debt to the person who conceived the idea of the Remington Medal.

My 45 years as a full-time pharmacy editor have given me a rewarding and enjoyable opportunity to work on behalf of our profession. It has been exiting to meet and know top people in Congress, in the White House, in the governmental agencies, and in the professions-across the nation. For example, how can I describe my reaction to The White House request-in 1983-for me to write a letter to be signed by President Reagan and Nancy Reagan? I cannot. The letter was designed to summarize the pharmacist's importance in the fight against drug abuse. I wrote the letter, and was delighted that it was accepted exactly as written.

In reviewing the challenges involved in projects for the nation's pharmacists, I note that there is a common thread which ultimately led to victory in many of these activities. Somewhere along the way, success also entailed discouraging developments, severe setbacks, near failures, and out-and-out failures. But, persistence plus the active support of many people were the key factors in converting impending failure into success-especially with respect to the Pharmacy Stamp project in 1971.

Quite naturally, it is pleasant to look back and review past victories. However, Baseball's Babe Ruth once said: "You can't win tomorrow's ball games with yesterday's home runs."

And so why don't we discuss-right here and now-how we can win one of tomorrow's ball games for Pharmacy? The ball game involves a suggestion I made-which failed urging that there be one symbol to identify Pharmacy in the United States. In this connection, here are salient portions of my December 1970 editorial in *Pharmacy Times.*

"The only real evidence of uniformity is a lack of uniformity.

"This statement summarizes the fact that American pharmacies do not display any single symbol or emblem to identify themselves as pharmacies. Even a perfunctory study of the exteriors of pharmacies clearly reflects the countless and often-confusing ways that they are identified as places where prescriptions and health-related products and services are available.

"Identifying symbols are employed by pharmacists in a number of other countries. From personal conversations with practicing pharmacists in [several of] these nations, I have learned that identifying symbols are helpful not only to the public and to other professions, but to Pharmacy itself. A symbol is an important piece in the jigsaw puzzle of professional recognition for Pharmacy.

"By working together and creating 'One Symbol for Pharmacy"-which would be displayed prominently on the exterior of all pharmacies-we will perform a constructive service for the public and the professions including the pharmacists of America."

Incidentally, not one of some 60 European pharmacists I questioned in France, Spain, and West Germany could give me a single disadvantage of the "One Symbol" concept.

Up until now, projects like getting the Pharmacy Stamp approved and highlighting the need for a pharmacist in the U.S. Capitol pharmacy have generally meant requesting something from people outside of our profession. In contrast, the "One Symbol for Pharmacy" involves Pharmacy leaders agreeing among themselve on one symbol for all.

One of the intraprofessional problems often experienced in the past was lack of cooperation between some national pharmacy associations. This lack of teamwork was a roadblock back in 1970 to implementing the "One Symbol" suggestion. However, the climate has now changed and happily teamwork appears to be the order of the day.

By the way, the "One Symbol for Pharmacy" effort in 1970 was also sidetracked by the start of the all-out successful drive for the Pharmacy Stamp early in 1971.

In any event, it's logical today for the national pharmacy associations to implement the "One Symbol" concept.

In leaving this cooperative project to the associations, may I offer one basic thought? Pharmacy should work very closely with its mutually-supportive systems manufacturers and wholesalers. In applying this suggestion to the "One Symbol for Pharmacy" concept: (a) The Symbol itself must be fully approved by pharmacy associations, (b) The artistic aspect of the Symbol might be assigned to manufacturers and their advertising agencies, and (c) The distribution of the Symbol might be made by wholesalers.

However, the final decision on the Symbol and all related matters must be in the hands of the national pharmacy associations. And now, let's wait and see what will happen to this idea of "One Symbol for Pharmacy."

Looking ahead at the pharmacist's prospects for the next few years, I am greatly encouraged. There is a growing respect for the pharmacist's expanding role as a national health-care resource by the public, by other professions, and by government. But, still more needs to be accomplished in this area-and I have great confidence in effective Pharmacy leaders backed by alert and well-informed pharmacists. Yes, there will be discouraging developments, severe setbacks, near failures, and out-and-out failures. But, doing what is right for the public-backed by cooperation, persistence, and political whack-will help to win the day for Pharmacy. Basically, it is what the individual pharmacist does-multiplied over and over and over that will make the real difference!

In conclusion: Even as a longtime editor, I really can't find words to express my gratitude for receiving the Remington Honor Medal. Many, many people-too numerous to mention-helped bring victory to several Pharmacy projects I was privileged to work on over the years. Without their help, many of these efforts would have been failures instead of successes.

During World War II, Sir Winston Churchill-in describing his nation's gratitude to the Royal Air Force for helping to win the Battle of Britain-made this statement: "Never ...was so much owed by so many to so few."

In describing my gratitude for the Remington Honor Medal, may I editorialize Sir Winston's words by saying: "Never was so much owed by someone to so many."

Thank you very much! ■

1987 Remington Medalist

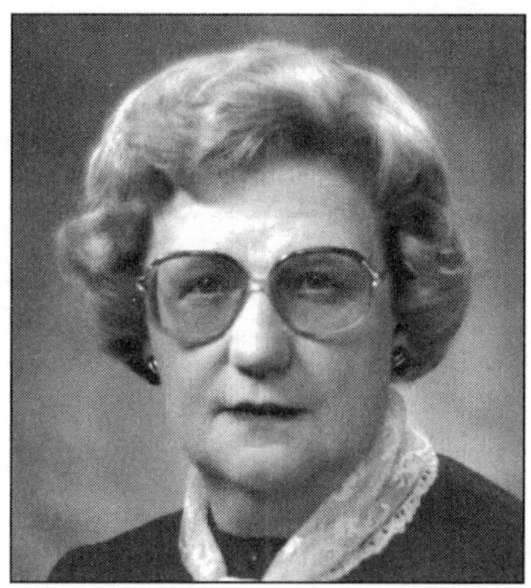

Gloria Niemeyer Francke

Gloria Niemeyer Francke was born in Dillsboro, Indiana, April 28, 1922, and she earned a B.S. in Pharmacy in 1942 from Purdue University, and a Pharm.D. in 1971 from the University of Cincinnati. Following service as a community pharmacist in Dillsboro, Indiana 1943-1944, and as assistant to the chief pharmacist at the University of Michigan Hospital 1944-1946, she became assistant director of the APhA Division of Hospital Pharmacy 1946-1956, executive secretary of the American Society of Hospital Pharmacists 1949-1960, and research associate for the Audit of Pharmaceutical Service in Hospitals 1956-1964. She then served as drug literature specialist at the National Library of Medicine 1965-1967; as clinical pharmacy teaching coordinator for the Veterans Administration Hospital in Cincinnati, Ohio 1967-1971; secretary of the American Institute of the History of Pharmacy 1968-1978; and chief of the program evaluation branch, Alcohol and Drug Dependence Service, Veterans Administration 1971-1975. She rejoined APhA staff 1975-1985 and was elected APhA honorary president in 1986. Gloria Francke's journalistic achievements include service as assistant editor of the *Journal of the American Pharmaceutical Association* 1946-1947; associate editor of the *American Journal of Hospital Pharmacy* 1944-1964; co-author of *Mirror to Hospital Pharmacy* (1964), and *Perspectives in Clinical Pharmacy* (1972).

The Danger of Scattering Our Forces

Gloria Niemeyer Francke

The 1987 Remington Medal was presented March 28, 1987, at the opening session of the American Pharmaceutical Association annual meeting March 28-April 2, 1987, in Chicago, Illinois. Francke's address was not published, but the text of the presentation has been provided by the Remington medalist.

To receive the Remington Honor Medal is beyond my greatest expectations. I thank all of you, members of APhA and our past presidents. An occasion such as this deepens our feeling about the profession we all love and nurture. It can move us toward the kind of commitment which led one medalist to refer to Joseph P. Remington as "a man of remarkable tenacity of purpose." I pay special tribute to Professor Remington whose name will live forever in American Pharmacy.

Back in what some may call the "ole days," the Remington medalist was given an entire evening for felicitations, congratulations, speeches by their long-time colleagues, and then a long address by the medalist. I remember one speech, indeed a very good one, was so long that it was published in three parts in the Association's Journal. I enjoyed those times, a chance to see the "greats" in pharmacy, an evening in New York City, and the midnight coach (and I mean train not plane) to Washington so that I could be back to 2215 for a day's work, not so fresh, but inspired and instilled with an overwhelming confidence that I had chosen the right way to make a living and spend my lifetime.

Fortune has it that my life has been surrounded by Remington medalists and by others who knew medalists, beginning with the first in 1919. I have read their speeches and know something of their roles in American Pharmacy. Perhaps I should not mention names because there are so many. But I must recall that I worked with seven medalists from Jenkins, my Dean at Purdue, to Fischelis, Sonnedecker, Francke, and Apple. Bowles and Heller were my co-workers early in their careers. I knew many others over these past decades. And I wish there were time to tell you about the first medalist James Hartley Beal, and the second, John Uri Lloyd. I learned to know both through their writings, their children, and even grandchildren. All of these pharmacists influenced my thinking about what Pharmacy ought to be. We again pay tribute to them, along with all who have worked hard to protect and build our profession through this American Pharmaceutical Association.

At moments such as this, there is a tendency to look back to yesterdays. But, in the words of Gibran, "Life goes not backward nor tarries with yesterday."

Were I to present a medalist's address today, I think that I would talk about the "burden of leadership" or perhaps "the danger of scattering our forces." My observations would be based on total immersion in pharmacy for more than a half century. At times, I fear that the burden of leadership prevents most of us from taking responsibility for the destiny of Pharmacy. We dare not hold back and merely "hope for the best for tomorrow." We must position ourselves to control the future of our profession, not only looking at the issues which benefit us today, but those that endure and will affect pharmacy practice tomorrow.

Pharmacy is a proud profession with great resources. No one denies that our numerous organizations, councils, and boards, with opportunities abounding, are part of this wealth. Yet, I have a deepening fear that we may be scattering our forces and that pharmacy's future may be the poorer for it.

It is difficult to imagine what tomorrow will be like. But one central thought keeps returning to my mind. We must have the ability to generate leaders, many leaders, who have a genuine commitment to the profession of pharmacy and to the men and women pharmacists who practice, who teach, who manage, who manufacture, who write and edit, and who do research. I am not thinking much about "power and politics;" rather, I am thinking about bringing about a common view that transcends our area of practice. There is only one thread which ties us all together we are pharmacists.

In closing, I say thank you to the hundreds of pharmacists who have touched my life, to my teachers represented here today by our Honorary Board Chairman, Dr. Donald Brodie. Recently referred to as the "Premier Scholar of our Profession," Mr. Brodie (as I knew him) exemplifies all the good teachers I have had throughout my life. I owe a debt of gratitude to a host of mentors who have contributed immeasurably to making my life's work full and satisfying. To my families, the Niemeyers and the Franckes, who have supported and sustained my seeming "craze" for pharmacy, a thank you.

With all of you, the honor of the Medal is shared. ■

1988 Remington Medalist

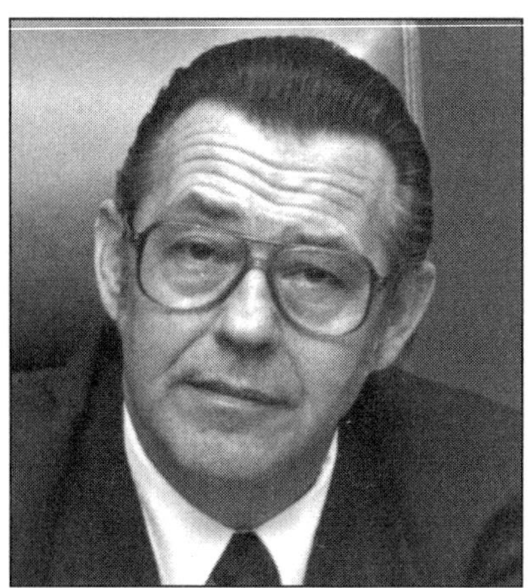

PETER PAUL LAMY
(1925-1994)

Peter Paul Lamy was born in Breslau, Germany, December 14, 1925, and he received a B.S. in pharmacy 1956, M.S. 1958, and Ph.D. in biopharmaceutics 1964, all from the Philadelphia College of Pharmacy and Science. Alter service in the U.S. Army 1958-1961, and as instructor in pharmacology at the Women's Hospital in Philadelphia 1960-1962, he joined the faculty of the University of Maryland serving as assistant professor 1963-1967, associate professor 1967-1972, and from 1972 until his death on March 21, 1994, as professor at the School of Pharmacy, research professor in epidemiology and preventive medicine, professor of family medicine at the School of Medicine, and founding-director of The Center for the Study of Pharmacy and Therapeutics for the Elderly. He served variously as vice chairman of the University of Maryland task force on aging, chairman of the American Association of Colleges of Pharmacy task force on aging, and as special consultant to the 1981 White House Conference on Aging.

A member of the American Pharmaceutical Association, Lamy served as editor of *APhA Contemporary Pharmacy Practice* 1978-1982. He also served as pharmacy editor of *Maryland Pharmacist* 1974-1976, editor of a column on geriatrics and gerontology for *Drug Intelligence and Clinical Pharmacy*, column editor for the *Journal of Gerontological Nursing*, a member of the editorial board of *Geriatric Medicine Today*, author of *Prescribing for the Elderly*, and editor of *ElderCare News*.

The Elderly: Challenge and Opportunity

Peter Paul Lamy

The 1988 Remington Medal was presented on March 12, 1988, in Atlanta, Georgia, at the opening session of the American Pharmaceutical Association annual meeting March 12-16, 1988, held in the Georgia World Congress Center. Lamy's remarks were not published, but a transcript has been prepared from a tape recording and from Lamy's recollections.

It is a pleasure to accept this award, the highest in American pharmacy. I accept it with great pleasure, as it gives me an opportunity to recognize those who have made this possible and those who have helped me throughout my career. I want to extend my appreciation to my peers who voted me recipient of this medal. Let me express my special thanks to my family, my wife Angela, my daughter Margaret Luise, my son Rudolf, and my son Carl, all of whom, incidentally, worked very hard helping me with my book *[Prescribing for the Elderly]* and all of whom have supported me throughout these last four decades. Let me also introduce my son-in-law, James Lachowicz, a Lieutenant Commander in the U.S. Coast Guard. It heightens my appreciation and pleasure to receive this medal in their presence.

Of the many colleagues who have helped me and supported me in my goals, three stand out, three who made it possible for me to receive this valued award. They spearheaded the effort, they were the driving force. They are Mrs. Madeline Feinberg, director, Elder Health Program, of the University of Maryland; David Banta, executive director of the Maryland Pharmacists' Association, and Dr. Philip Gerbino, professor at the Philadelphia College of Pharmacy and Science and director of the Philadelphia Geriatric Institute.

It is most important for me to extend my appreciation and thanks to Parke-Davis for supporting my efforts and my Center. Specifically, I would like to recognize Joseph Dilger of Parke Davis and Walter Weglein from Warner Lambert for their unstinting support. Of course, there are many others from the School of Pharmacy, University of Maryland and the Philadelphia College of Pharmacy and Science and many organizations who, over the years, have helped me to pursue my interest in the elderly and their needs.

I like the elderly. Why do I like them? I like the elderly because they are a nice group of people, often with a wonderful sense of humor. Recently, President Reagan said, "finally, I am on a national network, and I want to say something." Well, today, I want to say something about the elderly who represent a challenge and an opportunity to pharmacy and pharmacists.

The elderly, often with multiple diseases receiving multiple drugs, need help. The National Institute on Aging has called for an interdisciplinary community-based system for the care of the elderly, in which we, as pharmacists and drug experts, must participate. We have not yet achieved in helping to set up that system and participating in it.

Let us look at what others are doing. The internists have gotten together and asked "are we doing the right thing?" Are we teaching our students so that they can practice 30-years hence? And what type of practice will there be 30 years from now? It is not going to be institutional practice. It is going to be ambulatory practice without the humongous backdrop that we have in the hospital. It is going to include information centers using the latest in high technology. We need to teach our students that, and we haven't done it yet.

What does the American College of Physicians tell us? Last year they reported that unfortunately physicians do not participate in home care, and this year they tell us that we are doing a poor job in practicing for the elderly. Why are we not pushing the federal government to provide pharmacy with the same kind of federal support which is available to psychologists, psychiatrists, physicians, dentists, and nurses?

In December 1986, there was a meeting in Baltimore co-sponsored by pharmacy and the National Institute on Aging to evaluate clinical pharmacy and geriatrics. The conclusion was that the teaching of physicians is often accomplished by pharmacists, but we do not have support to teach a clinical pharmacist. Instead the federal government turns to regulations. Starting in 1990, there must be an outside expert for every nursing home who checks to see if I am using psychotherapeutic agents correctly.

What can (and must) Pharmacy do? Let's look at the changes in the health care system. The old and traditional boundaries of pharmacy are changing. There is no longer a clear delineation between community pharmacy, chain store pharmacy, and hospital pharmacy. These boundaries are blurring and disappearing. The site of care is changing, based on patient demands and cost considerations. We now deal with preventive care, acute care, and chronic care. Seventy percent of all prescriptions dispensed are chronic care drugs, to be used not only in nursing homes, the "traditional" site of longterm care, but to the six million elderly in home care and the three-quarter of a million elderly in assisted care. We need to develop systems of outcome-oriented pharmacy care for these care sites.

And if we are too slow, we will, no doubt, be told what to do. Last October, the *Federal Register* published new regulations under the heading of OBRA 1987. Under these regulations, pharmacists will be held responsible to monitor psychotropic drug use, especially antipsychotropic drug use in nursing homes and the use of unnecessary drugs. We will need to monitor that it not only is the right drug for the right patient at the right time, but that it is the right drug prescribed for a specific diagnosis and with a therapeutic outcome specified. We will need to monitor whether the outcome is reached.

Thus, we will need pharmacists well-trained in these concepts and care procedures. We will need to have schools of pharmacy adjust their curricula, and we need to convince our pharmaceutical organizations to keep convincing legislators and insurers that pharmacists are, indeed, the drug experts badly needed in the care of elderly.

In any case, I appreciate the high honor. To those of us who were welcomed to this country with open arms, it is nice to be able to give something back. For this I thank all of you. ■

1989 Remington Medalist

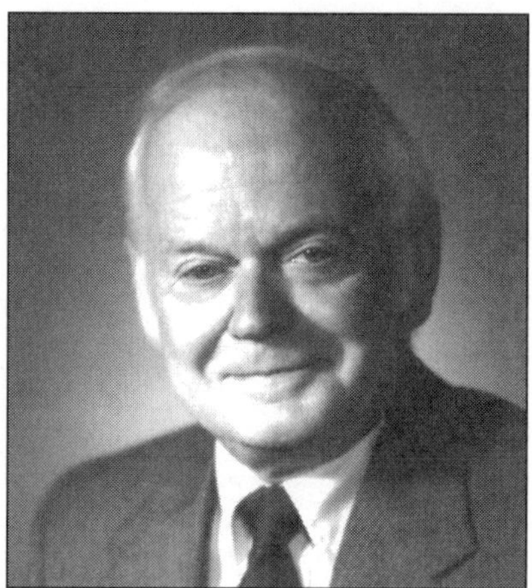

Lawrence Clayton Weaver

Lawrence Clayton Weaver was born in Bloomfield, Iowa, on January 23, 1924, and served in the U.S. Air Force as an instructor-pilot and in the China-Burma-India theater of operations during World War II. He then received a B.S. degree in pharmacy from Drake University in 1949, and a Ph.D. in pharmacology from the University of Utah in 1953. He joined Pitman-Moore Company serving as pharmacologist 1953-1958, pharmacology laboratories director 1958-1960, and head of biomedical research 1961-1966. During this period he also served as Butler University adjunct faculty member at 1954-1964, and University of Indiana lecturer in pharmacology at the 1954-1961. He then served as University of Minnesota College of Pharmacy dean 1966-1984 and 1994-1996, as director of drug information and education at the University of Minnesota 1973-1979, and Pharmaceutical Manufacturers Association vice president for professional relations 1984-1989. He served Minnesota Governor's Health Planning Task Force chairman 1967-1969, American Association of Colleges of Pharmacy president 1973-1974 and American Foundation for Pharmaceutical Education vice chairman 1980-1981.

Weaver served as APhA Academy of Pharmaceutical Sciences Section on Pharmacology and Toxicology chairman 1972-1973, and the APhA Academy of Pharmaceutical Sciences president 1981-1982. He remains active in international affairs in his capacity as dean emeritus at the University of Minnesota College of Pharmacy, and as president of Larry Weaver Associates with a continuing interest in people with rare diseases.

A Federation of Pharmacy Organizations

Lawrence Clayton Weaver

The 1989 Remington Medal was presented April 8, 1989, at the Anaheim Hilton Hotel in Anaheim, California, during the April 812, 1989, American Pharmaceutical Association annual meeting. Weaver's Remington Address was published in *American Pharmacy,* volume NS29, page 479, July 1989.

My romance with the profession of pharmacy began 50 years ago when I started working at Fent's Drug Store in Bloomfield, Iowa, while attending high school. It has been my good fortune that my career has exposed me to pharmacy practice, pharmacy education, the pharmaceutical industry, and a national pharmacy organization. I have been privileged to have been involved in most of the issues facing our profession over the past three decades.

I have been involved in much of the change affecting the profession during a period when significant advances have been made. But that advancement has not been enough and it has occurred much too slowly. I believe several areas need immediate attention.

Within a few weeks the American Pharmaceutical Association will have new leadership. APhA and the environment in which the Association exists have changed a great deal over the past decade. We as members must let it be known what we want APhA to be in the next decade. I believe that substantial-even radical-change is in order.

We have long talked about a single voice for pharmacy. Such a goal is probably unattainable but surely we can improve on the present situation. APhA is different from other pharmacy groups in that it serves as a representative for all pharmacists. My hope is that APhA will lead in the formation of a federation that can serve the profession as the umbrella group within which all the specialty groups in pharmacy can address issues affecting the profession and our abilities to carry out our goals and objectives.

This would require a departure from its past. No longer would APhA serve individual pharmacists. Present members would and should find a home, and many already have, in one or more of the pharmacy specialty organizations. The specialty organizations together would, while retaining their independence, be the members of the new federation truly representing a new voice for the profession.

The structure of the Federation of American Societies for Experimental Biology could serve as a model. A federation of associations of pharmacy would evolve that would be limited to the United States initially but be structured to respond to global pharmacy as needs develop in the future. The influence and power of such a federation would make possible many of the needed changes in pharmacy.

Much of our early expertise was imported from Europe. Throughout the years we have been innovators in pharmacy and have gained support from many parts of the world. Now we need to share our knowledge and expertise, especially with our counterparts in developing countries.

The globalization of health care has been going on for more than a decade. An early sign was the use of the developed countries' expertise to build and staff new health facilities for, and deliver health care to, people in the oil-rich countries of the Middle East.

Although differences still exist as part of our different cultures and traditions, we do see the exchange of ideas bringing about change. Progress can be expected as the International Pharmaceutical Federation (FIP) redirects many of its services and activities, but more can be done. The bottom line is that the profession must follow pharmacy education's lead toward greater participation in the world systems of health care.

We must form an alliance with pharmacists wherever they exist. During the past few years, generic drugs, substitution, and other conflicts familiar to all of us have occurred in Europe. A "United States of Europe" will move toward reality in 1992. In lesser developed countries the pharmacist and the physician are part of the educated component of the society. We need to make sure that these people have access to knowledge about health care and the best systems for its delivery to their patients. Through this knowledge exchange we strengthen our relationships. One of the most effective approaches can and should be to support the enlightened thrust of the present leadership of FIP. Let us not lose this opportunity to make great strides.

A serious problem that this profession must deal with in a more aggressive way is managed health care. The most serious concern is how fast the authority to select drugs for patients is being lost by the professions to the non-health-professional healthcare manager. The result is that the patient has no real assurance that the best drug will be used, because it may not be available to the physician. Also, the pharmaceutical industry has a greater difficulty gaining use of new products even if they represent very significant advances in therapy.

To regain control of drug-product selection and use, the partnership between the physician and the pharmacist must receive priority attention. Every effort should be made to support a physician-pharmacist team to assure safe and effective drug-use control. The pharmaceutical industry can and should play a supporting role for this partnership and not tolerate isolated attempts to bring conflict to these two historically dependent health professions.

Health professional manpower supply and demand operates very much like the ups and downs of a roller coaster. It is rarely in equilibrium. This is particularly a problem now. Some believe there is a surplus of physicians, many know that there are shortages in pharmacy, and both academe and the pharmaceutical industry are facing crisis shortages in scientists for a number of disciplines. The extent of these shortages is, at best, a guess. For some answers we must wait for the results of a pharmacist manpower study supported by all the major units of the profession now in the early stages of implementation.

In addition, a manpower database for scientist needs now and in the future, particularly in the pharmaceutical industry, should be developed and maintained. Often the response to a shortage in a discipline (e.g., pharmaceutics) is made worse by the hiring of faculty members from educational institutions by industry, thus weakening the program and decreasing the quantity and quality of new graduates. Ensuring an adequate supply of pharmacists, scientists, and new drugs in the future depends on identifying future needs with an optimal database now under consideration by the Pharmaceutical Manufacturers Association. This comes at a time when other influences (e.g., biotechnology) increase demand for scientists.

It wasn't too many years ago that the profession became involved in the clinical component of education and practice. Many of our pharmacy schools were reluctant to include clinical education in their pharmacy curriculum. Some of this reluctance was due to a lack of resources to implement this kind of education. To overcome this, the federal government established legislation to provide funding support to pharmacy schools providing that they initiate clinical programs.

Today we have a wealth of experience and the clinical component in education is continually being improved.

A similar situation may be facing us today with regard to pharmaceutical services. They are inadequate. Despite the education that pharmacy students get today, our practice has not kept pace. Too many, if not the majority, of pharmacists do no better than a mediocre job of delivering quality pharmaceutical services. The new Medicare Catastrophic Coverage Act may serve the federal government as a lever in requiring a minimal level of pharmaceutical service to patients, but it seems to me that a responsibility of the pharmacy profession is the development of standards for pharmaceutical services that optimally serve the patient and assure that practitioners are qualified.

Perhaps a first step in the resolution of this problem is to look carefully at how we use our professionals. Can and should we give the pharmacist supportive personnel in order that the pharmacist might better use his/her knowledge? I think so. Is there a need to develop and implement more demanding standards of pharmacy practice? I think so. There are other constraints for each of us wherever we practice; they should be identified, defined, and resolved.

In one of my dreams about the profession, all sectors of the profession were sitting at a roundtable. There were no hidden agendas and no ranks. Everyone present was known for high ethical standards. The agenda contained issues that affected each in a different way. Everyone was committed to present their organizations' position in a frank and open manner. Unfortunately the alarm clock sounded before I knew how the meeting came out.

In real life I have seen and participated in meetings not too dissimilar to the above in which one or more of the components were absent. More effort needs to be directed toward strengthening relationships between various pharmacy national organizations, so that we can offer a unified front.

I suspect that my concerns and recommendations are not new to you. I suggest to you that they can serve as an agenda for developing a better profession and for identifying, developing, and implementing risk plans. I sincerely believe that if, in all cases, the target for our action is the patient's needs, we will be successful in fulfilling our professional responsibility and continue our place with pride as a part of the health team. ■

1990 Remington Medalist

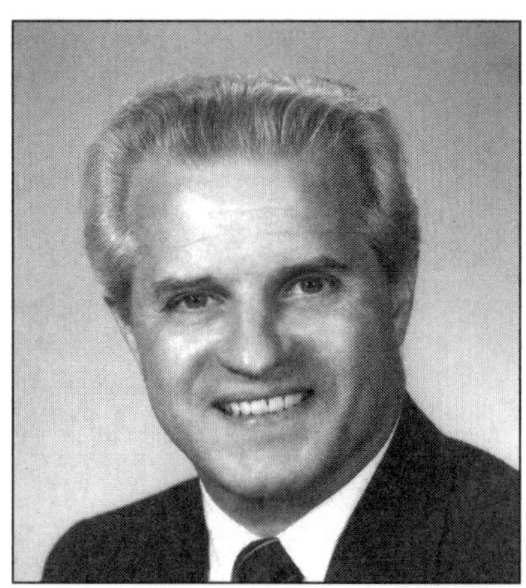

Joseph Anthony Oddis

Joseph Anthony Oddis was born in Greensburg, Pennsylvania, on November 5, 1928, and received a B.S. in pharmacy from Duquesne University in 1950. He then served as staff pharmacist at Mercy Hospital in Pittsburgh 1950-1951, and assistant chief pharmacist 1953-1954 after military service. He then served as chief pharmacist at Western Pennsylvania Hospital 1954-1956, and on the staff of the American Hospital Association 1956-1960. Coming to Washington, D.C., in 1960, he served as director of the American Pharmaceutical Association's division of hospital pharmacy 1960-1962, and as executive vice president of the American Society of Hospital Pharmacists from 1960 to 1998. He served as secretary of the National Council on Patient Information and Education 1982-1985.

Oddis gained international fame as president of the International Pharmaceutical Federation (FIP) Hospital Pharmacy Section 1977-1981, FIP vice president 1984-1986, and was the first American to serve as FIP president 1986-1990. He is an honorary member of pharmaceutical societies of Australia, Canada, Great Britain, and Israel.

REVISITING THE STRENGTHS OF PHARMACY

Joseph Anthony Oddis

The 1990 Remington Medal was presented March 11, 1990, at the Convention Center in Washington, D.C., during the March 10-14, 1990, American Pharmaceutical Association annual meeting. Oddis's Remington address was summarized in *American Pharmacy,* volume NS3O, page 346, June 1990; and was published in its entirety in *American Journal of Hospital Pharmacy,* volume 47, pages 1985-1988, September 1990.

Here it is-we've just entered a new decade, and already I have to wonder, Is there any professional experience that can top this?

No, that's highly unlikely. Of all the activities in which the Remington Medalist participates, this luncheon address is one I've been looking forward to with particular enthusiasm, for I knew that many who would be in this room number among the most important people in my life.

When you think about what you want to say to friends, loved ones, and close colleagues on any occasion like this, you tend to get a bit philosophical yes, and a bit nostalgic, too. I hope you'll be indulgent as I share with you some of the thoughts and memories that this great honor has awakened in me.

First a few memories.

The year is 1945. World War II is winding down. I'm finishing high school in Muse, Pennsylvania, and I visit Duquesne University, accompanied by a local priest who is a loyal alumnus. I'm visiting Duquesne to learn about the school of music, but an unplanned encounter with Hugh Muldoon, the dean of the school of pharmacy, leaves me so impressed that I determine then and there to study under him.

It's now 1946. I'm a freshman at Duquesne, and I bump into Sister Gonzales, a childhood Sunday school teacher of mine and now a fellow pharmacy student who is two years ahead of me. From this reacquaintance comes an invitation to work in the pharmacy at Mercy Hospital in Pittsburgh, which I do during my four years of school.

So, as you can see, one coincidence led to my entry into pharmacy school, and a second one introduced me to institutional practice.

Now, one more memory.

The year is 1953. I am recently back from the Army, working as a pharmacist at Mercy Hospital, and Dean Muldoon has just received the Remington Medal. With much pride, I head over to Duquesne to hear an encore presentation of his Remington Address, which he gave earlier in New York. This was the first of many Remington addresses that I would be privileged to hear in the years that followed.

Those are some of the recollections, the images, that have occupied my memory lately.

Somehow, it's now 1990-the "nineties" still has a strange ring to it, doesn't it-and here I am, following in Dean Muldoon's footsteps. How much my life has changed since those days in Pittsburgh. But how great an honor it is to receive the same award as did my early mentor.

Recently I put my hands on Dean Muldoon's Remington Medal address. Entitled "The Strengths of Pharmacy," it has the same eloquence, grace, and clarity as the man himself. Remarkably, much of what it says about pharmacy is as relevant in 1990 as it was in 1953. In fact, in its declaration of pharmacy's collective values, it may be a timeless statement about our profession's strengths.

Speaking, as he was, during the depths of the Cold War, he said this about his era's young pharmacists, of which I was one: "They are not unrealistic idealists. They desire only what we are confident they will have an opportunity to earn in a fear free democracy a modest living for themselves and their families, practicing worthily the profession for which they have been trained."

Certainly, American pharmacists of my generation have been so blessed. And now, thanks to recent events, perhaps the next generation of Eastern European pharmacists will be equally blessed. Today the West rejoices as the Cold War's bleak chill gives way to democracy's warming potentialities. We rejoice as the freedoms that we almost take for granted are won, tortuously, one country at a time. May the people of Eastern Europe and elsewhere around the world speedily obtain what Dean Muldoon held dear for us: the opportunity to make a living in security and freedom.

The dean concluded his address by stating, simply and confidently, that pharmacy is strong. He predicted that it would continue to be strong for five reasons: 1. Because of pharmacists' character and motivation, 2. Because of public trust based on age-old, faithful, and intelligent service, 3. Because of the profession's respect for education, 4. Because of pharmacy's awareness of its problems and its willingness to face them, and 5. Because of pharmacy's deep concern for the future.

The dean's conclusions in essence, his five bases for optimism in the profession we've inherited led me to my own ruminations about the strengths of pharmacy today.

For the next few minutes, let's see how American pharmacy in 1990 stacks up against Dean Muldoon's five criteria.

First, Dean Muldoon praised pharmacists' character and motivation. If I were allowed only one reason to explain why I, too, am optimistic about our profession's future, it would be because of the men and women who people our profession.

I believe that pharmacists share a passion for continual improvement-improvement in their practice skills and in the systems through which they deliver pharmaceutical care. Throughout America, pharmacists are fighting to raise the level of services provided in all practice settings. In one way or another, pharmacists are looking for ways to maximize their value to their patients, to their health-care colleagues, and to their communities. This is to our profession's great credit.

So I wholeheartedly agree with Dean Muldoon that pharmacists' character and motivation augur a strong future for the profession.

Next, we turn to the dean's perception that pharmacy enjoys the public trust.

I am sure you have all noted Gallup polls of recent years in which pharmacists were found to be America's most honest professional-more so than teachers, lawyers, physicians, even members of the clergy. This, no doubt, is partly a result of the positive attributes of pharmacists that I just mentioned and partly a result of public disillusionment with those other professionals.

But, to be frank, isn't the pharmacist's high standing largely a reflection of the public's low expectations of us-of what we should offer them as head professionals? Are we really doing enough to justify the public's trust? Or, to pose a more fundamental question: Are we helping people make the best use of their medications? I'm afraid that indicators such as the high incidence of adverse drug reactions and poor patient compliance suggest that we still have a way to go to live up to a number-one ranking with the public.

There is a way, however, for us to justify Americans' high opinion of us, and that is to channel our knowledge into patient care.

There is a way for us to hold onto our patients' high opinion of us, and that is to let go of traditional methods of practice that squander our skills and to embrace opportunities that the changing health-care scene provides.

Let me give you one example: managed care. With today's cost-containment pressures, community pharmacists are increasingly being brought into the nation's proliferating managed-care systems. This is a tremendous opportunity for these practitioners to broaden pharmaceutical services beyond the dispensing of prescriptions.

Individual pharmacists can offer to perform drug-use reviews for health-plan administrators and to provide patient consultations as a plan benefit. They can offer to help a health plan's medical staff develop a formulary. In concert with the medical staff, they can develop policies and procedures for ensuring the quality of drug therapy.

Providing such services is within our grasp today. It is in providing such services that we can preserve the trust Americans have in their pharmacists.

The third strength mentioned by Dean Muldoon was pharmacy's respect for education.

In what is an interesting coincidence, he referred to a debate then under way about whether to extend pharmacy education in all colleges from four to five years; some colleges, he noted, already had five and six year programs. An echo of that earlier topic now reverberates throughout the profession. The question of the moment is, should the American Council on Pharmaceutical Education (ACPE) revise its accreditation standards to focus on the doctor of pharmacy (Pharm.D.) as the only professional degree program?

This is bound to be one of pharmacy's most prominent issues in the nineties, and that is well and good. For pharmacy education is the foundation on which strong pharmaceutical services are built. We in the nineties are every bit as certain of that proposition as was my dean in the fifties. Perhaps a difference is that, today, we need to consider education in the context of pharmacy work force needs as a whole, including the issues of technical personnel and specialization. As a corollary to our reassessment of pharmacy education, we need to study the most appropriate way of regulating pharmacy practice for the future. It should be unnecessary for state boards of pharmacy to be highly prescriptive about the manner in which pharmacies provide services. Instead, a state board's focus should be on the outcome of those services.

ACPE is embarking on a crucial mission for our profession an exploration to determine the appropriate educational standards for practice in the twenty first century. In the months of discussion that lie ahead, I urge all sectors of pharmacy to participate in a spirit of cooperation, open-mindedness, and objectivity. And after we have all had our say, I urge the profession to base its decision on an image of the role pharmacy should be fulfilling for society.

The Pharm.D. issue is only one among many major challenges facing the profession as it heads into the twenty-first century. You'll recall that Dean Muldoon found strength in pharmacy's awareness of its problems and its willingness to face them.

How does pharmacy today compare on this score with the profession in the fifties? Very well indeed, I believe. In today's increasingly complex health-care environment, simply keeping tabs on pharmacy's problems is no mean feat.

Consider the broad range of functions performed by today's pharmacists in this rapidly changing environment, and you begin to appreciate why Dean Muldoon saw the ability to confront problems as an important measure of pharmacy's strength. You also begin to appreciate the need for pharmacy to address its problems systematically and strategically. That's one of the things the joint Commission of Pharmacy Practitioners (JCPP) helps us do.

Pharmacy took an important leap forward when JCPP came into being 13 years ago. This group, which embraces all sectors of the profession through pharmacists' national organizations, provides a forum for the profession as a whole to discuss issues large and small.

With JCPP, when unanimity is not reached, understanding is still advanced. When professional interests are threatened, pharmacy speaks with one voice and achieves strength through unity.

Finally, said Dean Muldoon back in 1953, pharmacy will remain strong because of its deep concern for the future.

Can anyone doubt that pharmacy in the nineties takes its future very seriously? Somehow, despite a history that may extend back as far as ancient Babylonia, contemporary pharmacy is anxiously planning for its future.

For example, in 1985 and again last October, members of all sectors of the profession looked the future square in the eye at a conference called Pharmacy in the 21st Century. The purpose of this conference was to identify critical issues the profession will have to wrestle with as it positions itself over the next 15 to 20 years. The basis for the meeting was a belief that the same set of factors will influence each facet of the profession, to one degree or another, in the years ahead.

Participants at the 1989 meeting scored the importance of 112 issue statements that grew out of workshop sessions. Receiving almost unanimous agreement and the highest score was this statement: "There is a need for pharmacy to actively demonstrate and communicate its value in health care."

If Dean Muldoon had been in attendance, I'm certain he would have agreed strongly with this statement, for he actually anticipated it in his Remington remarks of 1953. He said, "Many think of the pharmacist only as a businessman, not as the conscientious guardian of the health of the people he really is. It is time to turn the full beam of the spotlight of public attention on pharmacy." The dean then emphasized-and here I paraphrase-that informing the public about what we do is not a one-or two-day task, but a multi-year process. As you and I well know, this is a process that continues to this day and so it should, indefinitely.

Only when we convey to the public, and only when we convey to other health professionals, our value in health care, will pharmacy manifest the strength many in this room have fought hard to build. But have no doubt: That time will come.

Meanwhile, we in pharmacy can be genuinely glad that there is-as someone once put it-"enough work to do, and strength enough to do the work." ■

1991 Remington Medalist

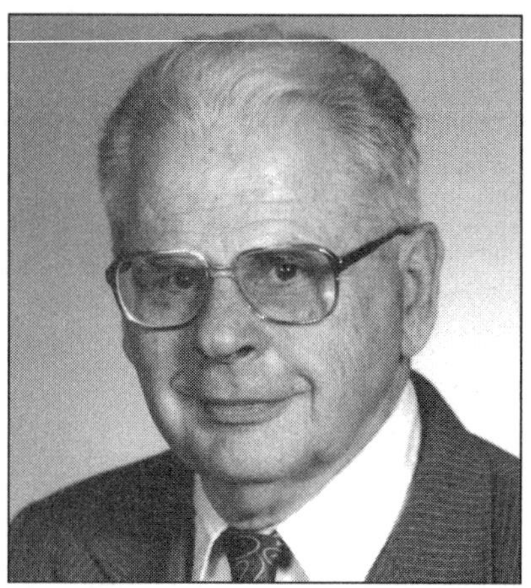

GEORGE BERNARD GRIFFENHAGEN

George Bernard Griffenhagen was born in Portland, Oregon, June 9, 1924. After 2-1/2 years service in the U.S. Army Combat Engineers in North Africa and Europe during World War II, he graduated with a B.S. degree in Pharmacy 1949 and an M.S. 1950 from the University of Southern California. While serving as curator of the Smithsonian Institution's division of medical sciences 1952-1959, he also served as American Pharmaceutical Association annual meeting coordinator and archivist commencing in 1953. After joining APhA as a full-time staff member in 1959, he served as director of communications 1959-1986, editor of the *Journal of the American Pharmaceutical Association, Practical Pharmacy Edition* 1962-1976, creator and editor of the *APhA Handbook of Nonprescription Drugs* (1967, 1971, and 1973 editions), APhA House of Delegates interim secretary in 1989; and APhA honorary president 1990-1991. In his capacity as APhA director of international affairs, Griffenhagen served as secretary of the organizing committees for international pharmacy Congresses held in Washington, D.C., in 1954, 1971, and 1991, as well as the 1987 joint Japan-U.S. Congress in Honolulu, Hawaii. He also served as Pan American Federation of Pharmacy vice president 1963-1991, Academie Internationale d'Histoire de la Pharmacie treasurer 1971-1994, and various capacities in the International Pharmaceutical Federation. He has authored more than a dozen books on pharmacy history and pharmaceutical philately, including *150 Years of Caring: A Pictorial History of the American Pharmaceutical Association* (2002). Since his retirement in 1989, Griffenhagen serves as executive secretary of the American Institute of the History of Pharmacy, and as an APhA consultant.

WHO ARE THESE REMINGTON MEDALISTS?

George Bernard Griffenhagen

The 1991 Remington Medal was presented March 10, 1991, during the American Pharmaceutical Association annual meeting in New Orleans, Louisiana, March 9-13, 1991 An excerpt of Griffenhagen's Remington address was published in *American Pharmacy* (volume NS31, pages 418-419, 1991); the complete text is published here from an original manuscript.

The first Remington medalist, James Hartley Beal, told those gathered for the 1919 Remington dinner, "No words at my command can adequately express my appreciation of the honor of having been selected as a Remington medalist. I can only assure you that I am very deeply sensible of the distinction which you have conferred."

These remarks of James Hartley Beal so eloquently express my present feelings, and the list of those who have been honored with the Remington Medal has so impressed me, that I want to share with you a sense of the tradition established by Joseph Price Remington and some of the thoughts of our Remington medalists.

All but two presented remarks following their receipt of the Remington medal. Only about half of the Remington addresses have been published in full. But fortunately others exist as tape recordings or as published summaries.

Gloria Francke, the first woman to receive the Remington medal, described in 1987 how "the Remington medalist was given an entire evening for felicitations, congratulations, speeches by their long-time colleagues, and then a long address by the Medalist." Gloria continued, "I enjoyed those times-a chance to see the 'greats' in pharmacy, an evening in New York City, and the midnight train to Washington so I could be back at 2215 for a day's work-not so fresh, but inspired and instilled with an overwhelming confidence that I had chosen the right way to spend my lifetime."

Rufus Lyman, first editor of the *American Journal of Pharmaceutical Education,* explained in his 1947 Remington address how his dinner was planned. Hugo Schaefer, who was responsible for creating the Remington Medal, and himself the 1951 Remington medalist, met with Lyman and exclaimed, "Rufus, the matter of the Remington program must be settled at once, and that means right now. There will be several speakers who are well qualified to tell of your efforts, and then you will make a speech in which you will deny what all previous speakers have said."

Hugo Schaefer then shook his finger, and said: "Rufus, you must remember one thing; this will be your swan song."

Although I have not attended as many Remington dinners as Gloria Francke, I was also inspired by these experiences. And I found some of the Remington dinners as entertaining as they were inspirational. I recall in particular how long-time U.S. Commissioner of Narcotics, Harry J. Anslinger, described his feelings in receiving the 1962 Remington medal. He said: "This is one of the few times during my slide down the banister of my career that the splinters have pointed in the right direction."

Since 1979 when the Remington

presentation was moved from a dinner arranged by the APhA New York Chapter to the APhA annual meeting, Remington medalists' responses were significantly limited and only a few of the extended remarks have been published. But thanks to the original proposal of Remington medalists Bill Blockstein and David Krigstein, and the current efforts of APhA executive vice president John Gans, plans are now underway to publish all Remington addresses in a single volume.

Over the years, many Remington medalists paid tribute to Joseph Price Remington. A few offered anecdotes like Samuel L. Hilton, 1935 Remington medalist, who described how he participated in meetings with Remington which often lasted until 4:00 a.m.

But it was 1931 Remington medalist E. Fullterton Cook, co-editor of *Remington's Practice of Pharmacy,* who provided the most intimate anecedotes. He described Remington's apprenticeship to Philadelphia community pharmacist Charles Ellis and his subsequent employment by Dr. E.R. Squibb. Remington loved to tell of an incident when Squibb and Remington were inspecting a laboratory operation. They discovered that a trusted workman unintentionally used an excessive amount of alcohol in the menstruum for a fluid extract of Cinchona. Dr. Squibb ordered the worker to pour it all into the sewer. Afterward, young Remington protested and suggested that he could have recovered the alkaloid. But Squibb replied: "Joseph, the influence on that man is worth the cost; he will never again make this mistake."

Cook also described an incident which occurred when Remington had just completed the first edition of *Remington's Practice of Pharmacy* illustrating the care which Remington took in all of his endeavors. Despite having exactingly checked every statement and figure, several typographical errors were subsequently found in the textbook, and this made Remington so sick that he was bedridden. When Mr. J.B. Lippencott heard of this, he sent a note telling Remington not to be downcast because this was a common experience of all authors. Lippencott wrote that the first edition of *Webster's Dictionary* went to press without including the word "dictionary."

The experience led Remington to be exacting in his demands upon his associates which won their loyalty and affection, and to strengthen his passion in Pharmacy and his confidence in its future-of which we can all be proud.

Linwood Tice reminded us in 1971 that it is traditional for a Remington medalist to give a blueprint of the future." And some Remington medalists even made predictions of things to come. In 1972, Remington medalist Glenn Sonnedecker presented a retrospective future of American pharmacy. Speaking from the vantage point of the year 2072, he observed: "A forgotten historian of the late 20th century [Glenn Sonnedecker] often expressed conviction that the value of history did not preclude prediction. Yet, he was not above the whimsy of looking at the future retrospectively. Probably he would not be surprised (if he could know) that things turned out quite differently from what he imagined."

What subject do you think most frequently served as a blueprint for Remington addresses? If I told you that nearly one-third of all Remington medalists were pharmaceutical educators, it would be easy for you to guess. It is pharmaceutical education which, according to 1963 Remington medalist Glenn L. Jenkins, "holds the key to the future advancement of our profession."

The second most frequently discussed subject by Remington medalists involves pharmacy practice. From James Hartley Beal in 1919 to Eugene White in 1979, Remington medalists routinely sought to resolve what David J. Krigstein (1977) called "the professional versus merchant paradox," and what Donald E. Francke (1970) described as the elimination of "commercialized jungles called drugstores."

Remington medalist Hugh C. Muldoon summed it up in 1953 in one of the most eloquent and comprehensive Remington addresses ever presented. He said: "We admit, regretfully, that there will always be men engaged in pharmacy who differ in their choice of values. There will be profit-seeking traders who will flaunt their disloyalty to an ancient calling and scoff at imperatives of professional ethics. But the great majority will aggressively support their profession, understanding its primary purpose, aware of its past accomplishments, and proud of their own professional activities that promote the common good."

The third most frequent theme of the Remington addresses dealt with pharmaceutical science, the development of drug standards, and the role of pharmacists in industry. Remington medalist K.K. Chen summed it up in 1965 by observing that "a professional must be founded on a solid, scientific base; otherwise it will lose ground and may eventually disappear."

Far down on the list of most frequently discussed subject by Remington medalists is international relations. In fact the first to even mention international relations Hugh Muldoon who applauded "Pharmacy's steadily developing international outlook." But international relations came to the forefront in the 1980s. Remington medalist Irving Rubin gave us an example of how we can learn from our overseas colleagues by proposing in his 1986 Remington address that the U.S. should also adopt a standard symbol to identify pharmacy. Three years later, Lawrence Weaver emphasized the need for "greater participation in the globalization of health care."

My interest in international relations commenced during my 33 months of World War II service in North Africa and Europe. My subsequent interest in philately, collecting postage stamps of the world depicting drugs and pharmacy, taught me much about the world in which we live.

My first official role in international pharmacy relations was service as secretary general of the Fourth Pan American Congress of Pharmacy held in Washington, D.C., in 1957. I learned much from Congress chairman Robert A. Hardt.

But I also recall how I had come to Bob Hardt's aid during the Congress when he introduced Pan American Federation president and Brazilian pharmacist Antenor Rangel Filho as "Dr. Filho." I had to discreetly slip a note to Bob Hardt suggesting that he address our Brazilian colleague as "Dr. Rangel," explaining that "Filho" is the Portuguese word for "junior."

When Bob Hardt received the 1964 Remington medal, he predicted, "The profession of pharmacy in the U.S. will assume a greater role in world leadership." And indeed it has, thanks to the leadership of Remington medalists Donald E. Francke and Joseph A. Oddis. I am especially pleased and honored to note that FIP general secretary Jan Martens and FIP Congress Coordinator have traveled all the way from their homes in Holland and Germany to be with us this evening. I also wish to recognize the presence of Pan American Federation of Pharmacy (FEPAFARBIO) Section of Professional Pharmacy president Fernando Soto.

When FIP held its first Congress outside of Europe, I tried to convince the Pan American Federation to meet with the 1971 FIP Congress in Washington, D.C. But neither FTP or FEPAFARBIO were then ready for such a joint venture. Now, 20 years later, this goal will be achieved at Pharmacy World Congress to be held in Washington, D.C., the first week of September. To give you an idea of the scope of Pharmacy World Congress, as of last Wednesday we had received 266 contributed abstracts from pharmacists in more than 40 countries, and the deadline is not until April 1.

Hopefully Pharmacy World Congress can now achieve yet another objective-that of providing a "healing balm" to be compounded by the several thousand pharmacists of the world who will converge on Washington, D.C., the first week of September. This now becomes possible as we re-focus our attention from enforcing international law and order in the Middle East to that of promoting international health around the world.

The conflict in Persian Gulf is reminiscent of that described by APhA secretary Robert P. Fischelis in his 1943 Remington address.

He said: "The events of December 7, 1941, galvanized our people into a united force with a single objective. We are all proud of the achievements of our military forces."

To show this pride, Remington medalist H.A.B. Dunning unveiled a memorial at APhA headquarters in 1948 which is dedicated to all pharmacists who served in the U.S. military from the Revolutionary War to World War II. A flagstaff rises from a marble and granite base with a sculptured bronze drum depicting six uniformed pharmacists spanning 200 years. Also pictured are formulas for alcohol (the preferred pharmaceutical solvent during the Revolutionary War), ether (the anesthetic of choice in the Civil War), sodium hypochlorite (disinfectant of World War I), and penicillin of World War II.

As a World War II Army combat engineer, I am mighty proud of this memorial in APhA's front yard. Also speaking as an ex-combat engineer, I have noted that conspicuous absence of U.S. Army Engineer units in the first troops to come home from the Gulf. Just as my World War II engineer battalion continued clearing out mine fields while the infantry was taking R&R, those Army engineers in the Gulf are still today clearing out mine fields in Kuwait. We all know that they too will soon return home to receive a resounding welcome, and some of them may enter pharmacy as I did. And with them will come the pharmacists who have distinguished themselves in the Gulf.

What better time is there for making an appeal on their behalf? Let us add another bronze panel to the APhA memorial recognizing those pharmacists who served in Korea, in Vietnam, as well as in the Persian Gulf. I hope that potential sponsors will be lining up to offer their support for installing such a timely memorial panel.

Virtually every Remington Medalist paid tribute to those who shared in their achievements. 1920 Remington medalists John Uri Lloyd acknowledged "his absent friends and silent co-partners." And noted explorer Henry Rusby described the influence of teachers and others who contributed to shaping the life which led to his selection as the 1923 Remington medalist.

But William S. Apple said it best in his 1967 Remington address. He said: "A teacher affects eternity; he can never tell where his influence stops. I have had the good fortune of being exposed to many wise and stimulating teachers, both inside and outside of the classroom. They taught me that men who attempt to preserve the status quo march to battle on a treadmill. And they taught me that nothing is so perfect that it can't be improved."

Just as Bill Apple said it in 1967, I repeat it tonight. "To all my teachers, both inside and outside of the classroom, wherever they are, I say-thank you!" And a very special thanks to my mentor, Edward S. Brady.

Bill Apple also recognized the APhA headquarters staff by noting: "Those of you who have come in contact with APhA understand and appreciate the dedication and competency of the men and women who work at 2215 Constitution Avenue. Their efforts form the mold out of which this year's Remington medal was cast."

I too pay tribute to the dedicated men and women who have worked at, and those who are presently serving at, APhA headquarters.

Remington medalist Grover Bowles recently told me that his interest in Remington medalists over the years had led him to conclude that most have had a supportive spouse who deserves much credit for keeping the recipient on track. No spouse of a Remington medalist has done this any better than my dear wife, Joan. And I also owe much to the support I have received from my wonderful family.

APhA secretary Evander F. Kelly concluded his 1933 Remington address with these words which represents my own sentiments: "The receipt of such a high honor has led me to a rather searching appraisal of myself and of the calling to which my working life has been given. The working life of the individual is, at best, but a comparatively short period of time. To those who live with purpose, it seems entirely too short to those who merely live, time is of little importance.

"During this brief period we make our contribution. There can be no repetition, no opportunity to correct omissions or mistakes. The working life is the most precious possession that the individual can give to any cause."

As E.F. Kelly concluded, I too conclude that "Pharmacy has been kind and considerate to me." Thank you for helping to make this possible, and God bless. ■

1992 Remington Medalist

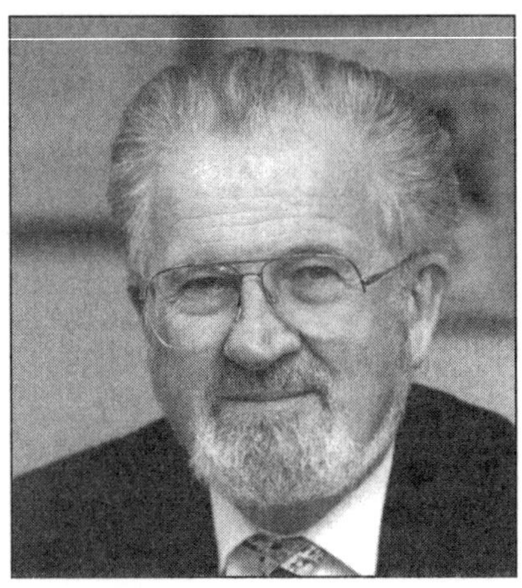

Jere Edwin Goyan

Jere Edwin Goyan was born in Oakland, California, on August 3, 1930, and attended Humboldt College 1948-1949. He graduated with a B.S. degree in pharmacy from the University of California School of Pharmacy in 1952, and subsequently earned his Ph.D. degree in pharmaceutical chemistry from the University of California, Berkeley, in 1957. He began his career as a pharmaceutical educator at the University of Michigan College of Pharmacy 1956-1963, and joined his *alma mater* as associate professor 1963-1965, as professor and chairman of the department of pharmacy 1965-1967, and as dean 1967-1979 and 1982-1993. He served as president of the American Association of Colleges of Pharmacy 1978-1979, was elected a member of the National Academy of Sciences Institute of Medicine in 1978, and served as commissioner of the U.S. Food and Drug Administration 1979-1981.

An American Pharmaceutical Association member since 1949, Goyan served as a member of the APhA Committee on Education 1968-1969, as chairman of the APhA Policy Committee on Organizational Affairs 1969-1970, and as APhA's representative to the United States Adopted Names (USAN) review board 1970-1979. Goyan now serves as president of Goyan and Hart Associates in Kingwood, Texas. He is chairman of the board of directors of Sciclone Pharmaceuticals, and serves as a member of the Board of Emisphere Technologies, Penwest, Inc., the Institute of One World Health, and four non-publicly trade companies.

The Rational Use of Drugs

Jere Edwin Goyan

The 1992 Remington Medal was presented March 15, 1992, in San Diego, California, during the American Pharmaceutical Association annual meeting March 14-18, 1993. Goyan's Remington address was not published, but an original manuscript was provided by the recipient. Goyan's presentation included video scenes from the University of California School of Pharmacy, but they are obviously excluded from the following lecture.

When I learned that I would be the 1992 Remington Medalist, I reacted in ways that I suspect mirror the reactions of previous recipients. First, I was shocked, but that quickly gave way to delight. Then, almost immediately, I began reminiscing about all the people I have known during my 45 year association with the profession of pharmacy who have had some part in my being here tonight. Because I am someone who believes that every interaction with another human being changes me in at least subtle ways, my list of mentors includes just about every pharmacist, educator and scientist I have known. Given that, there is simply no way in which I could begin this presentation, as would seem appropriate, by acknowledging all of those individuals who have contributed to whatever it is that has earned me the Remington Medal. I hope, therefore, that everyone from whom I have learned will forgive me for simply saying thank you; I could not have done it without you.

My involvement in pharmacy began as a delivery boy for a community pharmacy in Eureka in 1943, and has included practice in community pharmacy, teaching and research in two major universities, service as commissioner of the United States Food and Drug Administration, and for the longest period of time and the richest both in terms of personal reward and challenge-25 years as dean of the School of Pharmacy at the University of California, San Francisco.

Looking back, I have come to realize that one way or another, I have devoted my career to two concepts, the rational design of drugs and the rational use of drugs. I confess that, to a large degree, my role has been analogous to that of the driver of a chariot. I have been blessed with a team of powerful beasts who have their own notion of where they want their hooves to go but who have left the course and ultimate destination up to me, insofar as I have been light on the whip and generous with the oats. And what a wondrous race we have run together, indeed, the innovations that have taken place in both areas over the past three decades still seem to me incredible, and I feel privileged to have played a small role.

During the early part of my career I was constantly troubled by what I saw as the vague connection between education and practice, as illustrated by an exchange that actually took place between a professor of pharmaceutical chemistry and a student in a classroom at UCSF in 1957. It seems that the professor had just completed a detailed description of the spectrophotometric method for determining the quantity of atropine in belladonna extract when a student asked, "Is there an alternate method for analyzing atropine, one that, perhaps, does not require a spectrophotometer?" "Why do you ask?" the professor queried, cautiously. "Well," the student said, "you just never know when the spectrophotometer in your pharmacy is going to break down."

What the student was really asking, of course, was what the spectrophotometric analysis of atropine had to do with the practice of pharmacy. That question was not unusual. Indeed, it was symptomatic of the science-dominated pharmacy curricula of the time and it could have been asked during almost any lecture in almost any course in any of the nation's then 73 schools of pharmacy. What, indeed, did spectrophotometry, partition coefficients, the Henderson Hasselbach Equation, structure-activity relationships, chemical nomenclature, drug synthesis and a whole host of others, have to do with the daily requirements of pharmacy practice?

The fact of the matter is that all pharmacists who graduated from our programs between the late forties and the sixties entered practice knowing far more about chemistry and the physical sciences than they did about drug therapy and the biological sciences. Interestingly, this was also the period during which pharmacists were widely asserted to be the nation's most overtrained and underutilized health professionals, a cliche so splendidly ambidextrous that it was deployed to advantage by friend and foe, alike. Friends used it as the basis of a plea for greater respect and influence. Foes used it as a prime example of the misguided excesses of the educational institutions, one bordering on conspiracy, an argument that I note has been resurrected of late by some of those who oppose the universal Pharm.D. degree.

Regardless, both friend and foe were wrong. Overeducation implies excessive education, and that was simply not the case. In actuality, pharmacists were undereducated when it came to assisting prescribers in coping with a problem that had grown for years and was beginning to compromise the quality of drug therapy. The problem, of course, was the information overload that attended the entry into the marketplace of hundreds of new drug products annually. Although slow to react, it was the pharmacists' science training that eventually provided them with the tools to compartmentalize the problem and nibble at it from its edges inward. Patient profiles came first and from them, many other concepts developed which would collectively come to be called "clinical pharmacy."

During much of the period in which curricula and practice were changing so radically, basic transitions were also taking place in the pharmaceutical sciences which, to my amazement at least, have brought science closer to practice than it was in the past, although some of its practice implications are still ahead of us.

Most of us remember when new drug research consisted of producing a hundred or so analogs of a substance already known to be an active drug. Today, because of the blossoming of molecular biology, we are in a position to explore the mechanism of action of many drugs at the molecular level. For example, we can now determine how the drug interacts with some receptor on a protein, and from an understanding of that receptor, what sort of a molecule might achieve a better fit and therefore be a more effective agent with potentially fewer side effects. This is hardly a new idea. It was, after all, the central theme of Ehrlich's lock and key hypothesis. However, science today makes it possible for us to do the things of which Ehrlich only dreamed.

On more than one occasion, when discussing the rational design of drugs or the rational use of drugs, I have been told that these were simply ivory-tower visions with no possibility of fulfillment. At such times, I have often recalled what Cervantes wrote about his experiences while attending dying soldiers in Africa:

"These were men who saw life as it is, yet they died despairing. No glory, no gallant last words... only their eyes filled with confusion, whimpering the question: 'Why?'

"I do not think they asked why they were dying, but why they had lived. When life itself seems lunatic, who knows where madness lies? Perhaps to be too practical is madness.

"To surrender dreams–this may be madness. And maddest of all, to see life as it is and not as it should be."

Although the quest for rational drug design and rational drug therapy will probably never end, we are nearer to our destination because of men and women who saw things not as they were, but as they should be. It has been my privilege to be one of them and I accept this high honor on our behalf. ■

1993 Remington Medalist

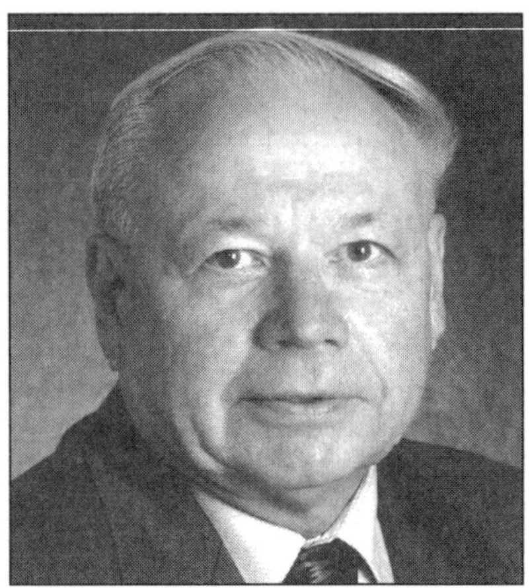

Robert Charles Johnson

Robert Charles Johnson was born in Detroit, Michigan, August 24, 1935, and received a B.Sc. in 1958 and M.Sc. in 1962, both from Wayne State University. After serving two years as manager of McUmber Pharmacy in Trenton, Michigan, he became field director 1959-1962, and executive director 1962-1968 of the Michigan Pharmaceutical Association, and editor of *Michigan Pharmacist* 1963-1969. He then became executive director of the California Pharmaceutical Association 1969-1990, turning organizational chaos into a California symphony of coordination. During this period, he also served as executive officer of the Nevada Pharmaceutical Association 1980-1985, and editor of *California Pharmacist* 1969-1990. Johnson then served as chairman and chief executive officer of PCS, Inc., as well as corporate vice president of McKesson Corporation 1990-1995.

Johnson served the American Pharmaceutical Association as vice chairman of the APhA House of Delegates 1969-1970, APhA vice president 1972-1973, and APhA president 1974-1975. He has also served as the National Council of State Pharmaceutical Association Executives president 1976-1977; Stanford Home Foundation president 1982; California Society of Association Executives president 1984-1985; American Council on Pharmaceutical Education vice president 1986-1988; and the Board of Medic-Alert Foundation International chairman. More recently he served as Scottsdale Healthcare System board chairman 2000-2003; and Midwestern University College of Pharmacy assistant dean since 1998.

MISSED OPPORTUNITIES

Robert Charles Johnson

The 1993 Remington Medal was presented March 21, 1993, at the Hyatt Regency Hotel in Dallas, Texas, during the American Pharmaceutical Association annual meeting March 20-24, 1993. Johnson's address has not been published, but the text of the presentation has been provided by the Remington medalist.

To say that I am deeply honored in being selected as a Remington Medalist would, indeed, be the understatement of my lifetime. Nothing gives me greater honor than to be selected; first, by a screening committee of distinguished professionals and then by my peers the past presidents of APhA.

As a past president, one of the great privileges I cherish (you have very few when you become a past president), is the opportunity, each year, to be involved in the selection of the Remington medalist. For seventeen years now, I have cast a ballot for distinguished members of our profession; and to now be included among this list is one of the greatest honors I could ever hope to achieve.

When I left my life-long career as a pharmacy association executive in 1990, I was certain that the Remington Medal would no longer be a recognition that I could ever hope to achieve, especially since I was leaving to take a position in managed health care, an occupation that many people only love to hate. But, fortunately, there are those who understand my goals, to advance the practice of pharmacy in managed health care and also remember over thirty years of dedication to advancing pharmacy; to those I will be eternally grateful.

I have had the opportunity throughout my career of listening to approximately twenty-five Remington addresses. Each of them had sage advice to offer. Each set forth either observations of the present or visions for the future. I hope my message can blend the present with the future; share some concerns for what might have been and the opportunities that lie ahead, if we can only move quickly enough to seize them.

Two persons who influenced me very early in my career were my Dean, Stephen Wilson and Dr. William Blockstein. Dean Wilson encouraged me to seek a masters degree in Pharmacy Administration recognizing, obviously, that my talents were more administrative than scientific. Bill Blockstein monitored my graduate work and provided the encouragement to complete my Masters Degree at a time when I was also accepting the responsibility to take over the management of the Michigan Pharmacists Association. At that time, I was immediately thrust into the controversy of the decade of the 60s affiliation between APhA and state associations. Dr. Blockstein served on the Michigan Task Force that was studying that hotly-contested political issue and we spent many hours together, discussing the pros and cons of reciprocal membership requirements.

This was also the issue that brought me close to another early mentor in my career, Dr. William Apple. It was a relationship, that in many respects, was not unlike a marriage. We fought and argued, vehemently at times, over issues on which we disagreed; at other times, the strength of our relationship provided leadership and direction for the future.

It was Bill Apple who first taught me what leadership was all about, including the price that one had to pay to be a leader. Bill Apple visited Michigan in 1961, when I was preparing to assume the Michigan Pharmacists Association executive director's position at age twenty-six. The affiliation issue was being hotly debated and he reminded me that if I were going to be the head of the Michigan association, I needed to decide whether to be a leader or a follower and admonished me that you couldn't be both and be successful. He also advised that to be a leader meant taking positions that would not always be understood or accepted, and one had to be strong enough to accept the criticism and attack that is often directed toward those who dare to speak out for their beliefs. This conversation with Bill convinced me to no longer debate the issue of affiliation within myself, but to take a position and then do all in my power to achieve it.

While I still carry the scars of the many battles over affiliation and then later the unification wars that were waged in California, I have always been grateful to Bill for encouraging me and teaching me what leadership was all about; and I never regret the decision I made. To be a leader, you must have vision; you must be willing to accept change; you must endeavor to convince others to accept change and above all, you must have courage and not fear reprisal for standing up for your beliefs.

Regrettably, our profession is bleeding today as a result of insufficient vision, too little leadership and too many who are unwilling to understand and accept the changes that are occurring in the health care system. I cannot help but think where pharmacy might be today if the concepts of unification, as embodied in the affiliation movement, had been universally accepted.

The abandonment of the reciprocal membership requirement in the late 70s accompanied by a growing lack of interest in the relationship between national and state associations, significantly weakened the profession and resulted in the floundering dilemma that prevails to this day. Too many Neros have been fiddling while the profession was burning.

It was becoming apparent in the early 80s that the American health care system was in turmoil and required drastic surgery. In fact, in 1981, Alain Enthoven, who was then President Reagan's health care advisor, addressed the APhA annual meeting in St. Louis. Dr. Enthoven said that competition among providers must increase, which would result in fewer numbers of health care providers serving larger numbers of patients.

While more than a decade has passed without overall reform of the system, as advocated by Enthoven certainly significant changes have occurred. Hospitals were forced to accept DRGs which has lowered hospital bed occupancy and forced some hospitals to close or convert to long-term care facilities. Physicians have accepted group practice as a way of life and are signing up to participate in HMOs, PPOs, IPAs, and accepting the reduced fees that health care buyers are negotiating.

The formation of the business-labor coalitions in the early 80s made it appear obvious that payors were going to force change to avoid the continuing escalation of health care expenditures. The handwriting on the wall was pretty clear, and it was only a matter of time before these changes would affect pharmacy.

In 1983, in a University of Texas centennial address, I urged the pharmacy associations, APhA, NARD, ASHP, and NACDS set aside their differences and come together to form a "think tank" for American pharmacy to not only seek an understanding of the changing health care system, but more importantly, to develop a strategic plan that would ensure pharmacy's integration into that changing system. Most regrettably, this Texas address was met with either defensive responses or simply ignored. Now, ten years later, the profession is still without a strategic plan and little has happened to ensure pharmacy's role in the evolving health delivery system.

There was a tremendous opportunity in the decade of the 80s, to reshape pharmacy practice from a distribution function to one of managing drug therapy. This regrettably hasn't happened.

Let me endeavor to describe pharmacy practice as it is perceived by those major buyers of health care today. They see prescription drugs as mere commodities that one should attempt to buy at the most competitive price. When we discuss the value-added service provided by pharmacists such as consultation, avoidance of drug interaction, and selection of the most cost-effective therapy, the response is usually a blank stare or disbelief. It is not uncommon to hear a major payor comment that he never sees his pharmacist except behind the glass wall and consequently, hasn't the foggiest idea of what a patient consultation should consist of or what its value might be.

We all know pharmacists who do practice in a very useful and professional manner, and some who even make their patients aware of the valuable services they render. Unfortunately, this is overshadowed by all too many who are content to stay behind the glass wall and perform essentially those functions that could and should be performed by a technician.

The profession is faced with the challenge of demonstrating the value of the services that pharmacists provide and at the same time convincing those practitioners who are not willing to accept patient management responsibilities to seek other career pursuits.

Time is running out. In my 1974 APhA Presidential address, I stated "we have won the battle of drug product selection, we now must turn our attention to the selection of drug therapy." This address was delivered in Chicago and the aftershocks were felt down Michigan Avenue at the AMA headquarters. I was the subject, at the time, of more than one uncomplimentary article in various medical publications.

Bill Apple, who was a little nervous over that presidential address, said later, "well, at least you got their attention." While I may have gotten medicine's attention, it didn't register with pharmacists; and today, almost twenty years later, the selection of drug therapy is passing to Formulary P & T Committees and Drug Utilization Administrators.

The responsibility to interchange the drug product as allowed by all fifty State Pharmacy Practice Acts, is only occurring 30 percent of the time; much of that being forced by third party benefit plans.

Pharmacists today have the pharmacological and clinical expertise to assume the responsibility for selecting the most appropriate and cost-effective drug therapy for their patients. It will take initiative on the part of the pharmacist to communicate with the physician and advise as to the most appropriate therapy.

Physicians are becoming extremely conscious that their patients' benefit plans are seeking cost reduction. Doctors are under the gun to an even greater extent than pharmacists, to date at least, to select less costly treatment. Therefore, if approached properly, most will cooperate and accept the pharmacist's advice as to the least costly, most effective drug regimen. If this responsibility is not sought and assumed by the pharmacists, what then can the pharmacist expect to do as high-tech takes over in health care delivery.

Drug distribution is also changing dramatically. We are much closer, in this country, to unit-of-use packaging than many believe. This was borne out in Steve Schondelmeyer's report at the recent *USP* Unit-Of-Use Conference. Despite this there are those that are advocating the status quo-to count and pour. That simply will not last. In most countries throughout the world today, prescription drugs are dispensed in unit-of-use packaging, increasing numbers of drugs are dispensed that way in America, as Dr. Schondelmeyer reports. What then will pharmacists do if they are unwilling to assume the responsibilities for drug therapy selection and management?

Today, 50 percent of all prescriptions are being paid by a third party. That number will increase to 80 percent before the end of this decade. Third party payors are insisting on acquiring drugs at the least possible cost. Consequently, if drugs are available in unit packaging, will the dispenser of those drugs remain the pharmacists?

Over the past two decades, the advancement of clinical pharmacy has occurred.

Pharmacists are educated and trained today to fulfill a much more responsible role in patient care. Regrettably, what our educational institutions have not done is prepare the pharmacists with an understanding of health care economics. So much emphasis has been placed on clinical pharmacy which is critically important, but failure to prepare the student for the changing dynamics of health care reform, has been a great disservice. I served six years on the Accreditation Council and my colleagues on the Council grew tired of my pressuring for curriculum inclusion of pharmacy administration; not as we knew it in my day, but as it must be taught today to prepare the student for the health care environment that exists today and as it will evolve tomorrow.

It should be clear that missed opportunities can no longer be tolerated, for the very future of the profession is at risk. The health care industry is moving to hightech and as we all know, the high tech industry moves very rapidly. We are on the threshold of transmitting medical information electronically at the point-of-service. I envision the day will soon arrive when a patient is seen by a physician and before leaving the doctor's office, information will be transmitted to a managed care administrator (such as PCS Health Systems), where eligibility will be determined and the diagnosis, along with the prescribed therapy, will be reviewed to assure the most cost-effective medication is prescribed. The prescription orders will then be transmitted to the pharmacist and medication will be available by the time the patient arrives. What then will be required of the pharmacist? We have already acknowledged that the drug will be prepackaged; but how valuable is the medication if patient compliance does not occur?

Pharmacy practice changed very dramatically in this century when compounding was replaced with pre-fabricated drugs. Before the century ends, another dramatic change will occur. The opportunity has been presenting itself for more than a decade, but it hasn't been seized upon. Will it now? I can only, once again, urge the leadership to unite and architect pharmacy practice for the 21st century. This will require abandonment of the traditional and carving out a totally new mantle upon which the profession of the future can be built.

While I have suggested that utilization review and therapy selection are likely to be in the hands of the managed care administrators, there is still opportunity for pharmacist practitioners to assume this responsibility and most assuredly, the patient management/compliance requirements, which are going unmet today, provide opportunity for pharmacists to utilize their clinical skills.

It will be extremely difficult for many pharmacists to replace the distributive function with the clinical; but most assuredly, there is no future for pharmacy if it is based primarily, as it is today, on the repackaging and distribution of the product. This is not to say that product distribution can't remain under the jurisdiction of the pharmacist because these are dangerous chemical entities; they require supervised distribution, but, that must become the secondary responsibility. The health system today will not, in fact, is not willing to pay the price for highly skilled and educated persons to dispense drugs. I believe, however, that the system will pay for the appropriate selection and use of these drugs, and it is that responsibility upon which the future of this profession must be built and built quickly. Pharmaceutical manufacturers should have an interest, as well, in assuring that their products are being properly utilized, and more importantly, that the expected results are being achieved.

The future of medical care is outcome oriented. We cannot continue to spend excessive sums for treatment without being more assured of the results and their timeliness. Manufacturers may well be required to accept risk in guaranteeing the results of their products if their products are to be included in the health plan's formulary. It would behoove manufacturers to compensate pharmacists to monitor patients for compliance, in order to determine the real effectiveness of their products.

It is likely that the price of drug products in the future will be negotiated between manufacturer and payor or the plan administrator on behalf of the payor. It is also conceivable that the pharmacist will not have to invest capital to pay for these products. The pharmacist's compensation then will come solely from the payor and/or manufacturer for the consultation, monitoring, and compliance responsibilities. This makes it imperative that the profession demonstrate the value of these services, so that a fair and reasonable fee structure can be determined.

When I accepted the position to become the CEO of PCS Health Systems, it was because I had a vision for what the future practice of pharmacy must be if, in fact, it will be at all. I have been disillusioned with the profession for not planning and restructuring. However, there may be opportunity through a consortium of health care buyers, concerned manufacturers, and professional leaders, to demonstrate the value of a significantly different role for pharmacists in the rapidly-changing delivery system. With McKesson's support, I have made that commitment and despite the inability of some to understand the efforts we are making, I am determined to see this vision through.

Because of a decade of neglect, we must face the realities of today's marketplace that is unwilling to pay for anything more than the product. We must also understand that as President Clinton and government forces restructure the health system, based on a managed competition philosophy, pharmacists like physicians and others in the system, will find that they must practice in a different environment than they have in the past. Competitively-based practice networks are the reality of today's marketplace and are the cornerstone of the evolving system being designed by the Clinton Task Force and with the support of Congress and Corporate America. To fail to understand the realities of this current situation and be unwilling to learn to adapt to it, will most assuredly result in extinction. The system is changing rapidly in the managed competition direction and it simply isn't going to be reversed. Corporate America, Congress, and the Administration will see that it doesn't.

Time is critical and drastic change is in order. If small and medium size chains and independents are going to survive, it will only be through the formation of Managed Care Networks. These local networks of pharmacies must be prepared to negotiate at competitive prices. At this particular time, price or cost is all that is of concern to the large buyers. Consequently, to stay alive, very competitive price negotiations must occur between Managed Care Networks of pharmacists and plan administrators.

In some instances, such as Medicaid, pharmacy networks will need to form and negotiate with hospitals and physicians, since many state laws only recognize groups of physicians and hospitals for the purpose of treating Medicaid patients. Unless pharmacy keeps its foot in the door by forming networks and negotiating competitively, there will never be the opportunity to seek compensation for the value-added services.

I have observed the responses from pharmacy to the health care reform initiative currently underway. In many respects, it has been too little too late. Some responses are more in the order of preserve what is, protect what is, and, prevent what will be.

APhA's response appears to recognize the dramatic changes taking place, but it does not seem bold enough to get the attention of those charged with reforming the system. For example, in addressing reimbursement for pharmaceutical care, the emphasis continues to be on product with additional compensation for ill-defined services that today's buyers are not convinced of. To get attention, compensation for pharmacists' services should address such cost-effective measures as increased generic usage, formulary utilization and therapeutic appropriateness.

Keep in mind, cost-reduction is what is on everyone's mind. If compensation addresses how cost-efficiencies can be achieved through pharmacist intervention, there will be a much better chance of acceptance of pharmacy's position.

Recently, I attended a breakfast of the National Health Council in Washington D.C.; Senator Jay Rockefeller was the speaker, and he admonished the audience of health care representatives not to come with the same old theories. He said "there is no time left for that, instead, come to us with bold new approaches for that is what the health system in America is badly in need of."

I would encourage American pharmacy to listen carefully to what is being asked and respond more forcefully with a different approach. To receive attention, pharmacy's bold new approach should include Managed Care Networks of pharmacies that will accept performance standards, based on cost-saving techniques such as I have just described, and intent on providing the value-added services of the pharmacists that will improve the overall delivery of health care.

PCS, if it too will survive, must respond to marketplace demands. We will seek to include, whenever possible, pharmacy networks consisting of those committed to performance standards that will result in cost-effective health care. It is also our intent to undertake demonstration projects, to determine the value of the pharmacists' clinical services. Some predict that my vision for pharmacy will not be fulfilled. Recently, a good friend, the senior executive of one of our largest customers, commented to a mutual friend, "I know what Bob's beliefs are for his profession and I know how badly he is aching to make those beliefs become reality I'm only afraid it's too late." I cannot accept that fate. Things often have to become very bad before they become better. I think we are at that stage. Will the redesign of pharmacy practice occur? This is essential if the future is to be assured. Only if vision and a united leadership begin to prevail. You have heard my commitment to making it happen. I am anxious for pharmacy to respond.

Nearly 500 years ago, Machiaveffi offered this admonition: "It must be considered that there is nothing more difficult to carry out, nor more doubtful of success, nor more dangerous to handle, than to initiate a new order of things. For the reformer has enemies in all those who profit by the old order, and only lukewarm defenders in all those who would profit by the new order, this lukewarmness arising partly from fear of their adversaries, who have the laws in their favor, and partly from the incredulity of mankind, who do not truly believe in anything new until they have had actual experience of it. Thus it arises that on every opportunity for attacking the reformer, his opponents do so with the zeal of partisans, the others only defend him halfheartedly, so that between them he runs great danger." I have experienced this more than once in my career.

In closing, I want to thank Tina and my two sons, especially, for always sharing in my dreams, often not understanding why it was necessary to take so much time away from home, but never complaining. Tina served as mother and father during the boys' early years, while I served the profession at both the state and national level. They shared in my moments of triumph and accepted my few moments of despair without complaint. When I had no one else to share my frustrations with, Tina was always willing to listen and lend her encouragement. I could not have achieved success without my family, without my associates who served with me on the staff at the Michigan and California associations, and now at PCS, and without faith in the Supreme Being who has always somehow steered me in the right direction.

When I left Michigan in 1969, at the end of the first stage of my career, I borrowed a quotation from Adlai Stevenson. It seems appropriate to repeat that quote as a closing thought:

"I have said what I meant and meant what I said. I have not done as well as I should like to have done, but I have done my best, frankly and forthrightly. No man can do more and you are entitled to no less." ■

1994 Remington Medalist

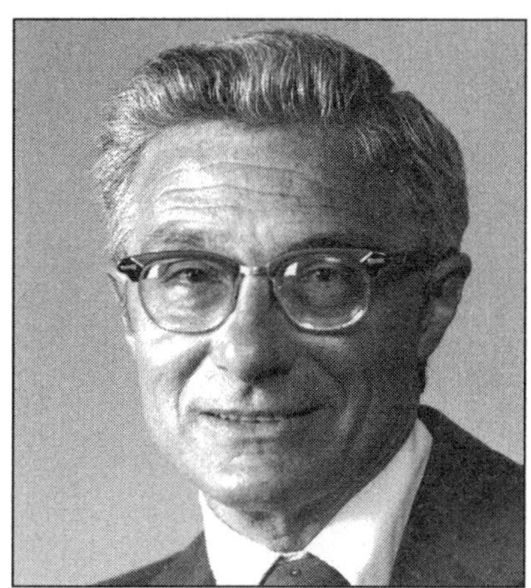

JAMES THOMAS DOLUISIO

James Thomas Doluisio was born in Bethlehem, Pennsylvania, September 28, 1935, obtaining his Bachelor of Science in 1957 from Temple University School of Pharmacy, and his Ph.D. degree in 1967 from Purdue University. He served as assistant and associate professor from 1961 to 1967 at the Philadelphia College of Pharmacy; as professor and assistant dean from 1967 to 1973 at the University of Kentucky College of Pharmacy; and as dean and Hoescht-Roussel professor from 1973 to 1998 at the University of Texas College of Pharmacy.

Doluisio served as American Pharmaceutical Association president in 1982; as American Association of Pharmaceutical Scientists president in 1988; as USP Board of Trustees chairman from 1990 to 1995; and as International Pharmaceutical Federation (FIP) vice president from 1995 to 1998. He served in 1974 as a member of the U.S. Office of Technology Assessment Drug Bioequivalence Study Plan; from 1976 to 1978 as chairman of the HEW Health Care Financing Administration Pharmaceutical Reimbursement Advisory Committee; and from 1976 to 1983 as a civilian consultant to the U.S. Air Force Surgeon General.

WHAT COULD BE

James Thomas Doluiso

The 1994 Remington Medal was presented March 20, 1994, during the American Pharmaceutical Association annual meeting in Seattle, Washington, March 19-21, 1994. The lecture was not published in the *Journal of the American Pharmaceutical Association*. The text of the presentation is preserved in the APhA Foundation Archives.

I am greatly honored to be the 1994 Remington medalist. I have had the good fortune to know many medal winners and I am in awe of their accomplishments. I have concerns about my worthiness for this medal. First, I feel that my accomplishments do not measure up to those of other recipients. Second, I feel my best accomplishments are ahead of me, not behind me.

It was on a quiet evening that I read the material submitted for my nomination. The comments of people I greatly respect were very important to me. Just to know that these people judged me as a candidate was honor enough. I am a teacher and it was especially important to me that Dan Hussar, a student of mine at the Philadelphia College of Pharmacy and my first Ph.D. graduate, led the nomination effort. All the nominators were generous, but the words of 1971 Remington medalist Linwood Tice, my dean at the Philadelphia College of Pharmacy and the person who most influenced my dual life in professional affairs and scientific affairs, were especially important to me.

No one does anything alone. If I have excelled, it is because my wife Phyllis has given me the support needed in good times and bad times. If I have excelled, it is because the University of Texas College of Pharmacy excels. In many ways, what I have attempted to accomplish has not been done by me. It has been done by the faculty, by the staff, by the students, and by the alumni.

I owe much to where I was educated at Temple University and at Purdue University, and I owe much to where I have taught at the Philadelphia College of Pharmacy and Science, at the University of Kentucky, and at the University of Texas. I have been dean for 20 years at Texas, and it seems like a much shorter period because we have developed a very successful program. For all of you who have been my teachers, or my students, or my professional colleagues, I say "Thank you?" This medal is as much yours as it is mine.

Lyndon Johnson once stated, "The hardest task is not doing what is right, but to know what is right." As I reflect on the many times that I have come to the fork in the road that called for a decision, I have tried to know what is right for our profession and the public we serve. However, knowing what is right on controversial multi-dimensional issues is not easy. In some cases I was in conflict with good friends who disagreed with my views. I considered those differences of opinion as cause to re-examine my motives and make certain that I have properly listened to the opposite point of view.

I greatly value the friendship of many who had (or may still have) different views, but respected my views and continued our friendship. From some who have extended congratulations to me there has been an impression that this award signifies an excellent conclusion to my career. I am afraid I am going to disappoint these individuals because I consider that I am still in mid-career and there is much to be done in these critical times. From others who have extended their congratulations there has been an acknowledgment of sustained leadership. Many of you know me and know that I have never thought of myself as a leader. In fact, I have often been skeptical of people who viewed themselves as leaders. I view myself as a "teacher." To be a "teacher" one must also be a "learner." This constant cycle of learning and teaching has always sustained my activities that may have caused me to get out in front of concepts in which I believe.

There are two different stories that are told about leadership during the French Revolution. In one story, a young activist saw a mob running down the street. He raced to the front of the mob and yelled, "Tell me where you are going so I can lead you." To me, this person is a false leader who is controlled by the mob and without his own principles. There is a second story that occurred during the French Revolution. The French army was doing badly during a battle and a young lieutenant rushed to give his general the latest battle report. He said, "General, all is lost. The enemy has us completely surrounded." The general excitedly jumped to his feet and with enthusiasm proclaimed, "Finally we have the advantage. We can attack in any direction." I have always enjoyed the lesson of leadership in that story. The optimism of the general is demonstrated by his development of a positive strategy when others saw only defeat.

Hopefully, whatever leadership I provide is closer to that of the optimistic general rather than the mob leader.

I have been surrounded daily by the most talented leadership we have in all of pharmacy, student leadership. I have thrived on interacting with students. They are bright, creative, energetic, and they have no concept of the impossible. They are driven by the truth and by what they perceive as right. Although this student environment continues to energize me, it also brings one of my disappointments in pharmacy. It is the failure of many of these exceptional student leaders to emerge as state and national leaders within our profession when their time comes.

However, I am eternally optimistic. Some point to our future in pharmacy and say it is dependent on the implementation of pharmaceutical care. That is partly true! Some point to our future and say it is dependent on an improved educational system. That is partly true! Some point to our future and say it is dependent on the cost effectiveness of pharmaceutical services and reimbursement policies. That is partly true! But our future is also dependent on is the quality of people who enter and sustain our profession. Lyndon Johnson had a theme of the Great Society during his presidency. He stated:

> "The Great Society asks not how much
> but how good;
> not only how to create wealth
> but how to use it;
> not only how fast we are going
> but where we are headed;
> it proposes as the first test for a nation
> the quality of its people.

The greatest factor that will catalyze the future of pharmacy is the quality of today's students. Today our College has four qualified applicants for every student we admit to the program. The students we reject are very good, while the students we admit are exceptional. The 1985 to 1995 graduates will be the best and brightest of any ever graduated. This single factor gives us our greatest opportunity for the future. Our challenge will be to keep these pharmacists motivated. With reasonable opportunity they will transform our profession.

Clearly, the 20th century was America's century. We entered the 20th century as a young energetic nation with significant potential. During the century we became world leaders in education, technology, wealth, and politics. We began new and fresh with the belief that anything was possible and we often achieved our potential. Perhaps it was World War II that was a turning point for us. Our nation demonstrated a resolve, a military, and a technology that signified to all that we had arrived and had become the most dominant nation in the world. No longer could we surprise people with our energy and creativity; we were expected to perform as a world class nation should perform.

Will the 21st century also be America's century? Maybe, but many have concerns. My concerns focus around a worldwide economy, especially in a field that is critical to the development of pharmacy: namely, new drug product development. I am concerned that our electronics industry, steel industry, lumber industry, and oil industry have difficulty competing worldwide. I see signs that the U. S. pharmaceutical industry has increasing worldwide competition affecting our current prominence. It is possible that it is only a matter of time until we see the energy, vitality, and national commitment of the Japanese, the Chinese and others challenge our nation's preeminence.

I have heard it said that today's students may be the first generation of Americans who will likely have a lower standard of living than their parents. I hope not! That is the American dream that you and I have lived, and the American dream that motivated us must be passed on to succeeding generations. I have had the opportunity to visit with pharmacy students and pharmacists around the world. I have been in Third World countries where the life expectancy is 46 years. Inexcusable! I have been in Eastern Europe during the Cold War and saw the smothering effects of communism and socialism.

Intimidating and scary! I have talked to bright pharmacy students in India who knew they lived in a class society that did not reward success due to education and hard work. Frustrating! Americans undervalue our society. It has and will always reward the well-educated, the creative, and the hard-working. It rewarded us and it will reward future generations.

I have beard some say that young people simply have too many options, that they have never been hungry, and that they are not motivated to excel. These are not the young people I see studying pharmacy. What I see instead are students who are bright, have great communication skills, and have a social commitment to embrace and deliver clinical pharmacy and pharmaceutical care. But how we educate them in our colleges and what opportunities we give them in our profession are critical factors. Finally, I would like to address some Issues in the areas of drug discovery, pharmacy education, and professional practice.

I am a strong supporter of the research-intensive pharmaceutical industry. Those of you who know me in professional affairs might be surprised that I have been an active scientist. I take special pride in drugs that I have worked on that are valuable therapeutic agents; drugs like doxycycline, dicloxacillin, and more recently through my long association with the Hoechst Medical Department, furosemide, cefotaxime, pentoxifylline to name a few. Actually my scientific interests overlap with my professional interests because I believe that the professional growth of the profession is very dependent on the development of high tech pharmaceutical services that will be necessary for new high technology drug products and devices.

My concern about the pharmaceutical industry is that they are not as research intensive as I would like to see them. It seems that commitments to research for new products greatly diminished after the thalidomide incident. Commitments diminished even further by concerns over generics, and now seem to be diminished even more because of concerns about health care reform. Recently, Nobel Prize winner Steven Weinberg identified what he called problems in our national intellectual infrastructure. He commented, "It seems that financial rewards of those who work in American companies grow in direct proportion to how far one is from the actual design of products or means of production, reaching a maximum for those who merely manipulate corporate finances."

Today the pharmaceutical industry is restructuring. In that restructuring I have concern about the emerging priority for the research that supports the development of new drugs. Often financial managers and marketing-oriented pharmaceutical executives seem to dominate industry decision making, tending to have short-term priorities to the detriment of long-term priorities necessary for new product research and development.

In my view, the true success of the pharmaceutical industry will not be altered by health care reform or changing tax incentives. The future of the great American pharmaceutical industry, and it is great, is linked with the sustained quality of its research. The industry should partner with the aggressive biotech industry and partner with the basic research at the National Institutes of Health and universities. But it should not delegate its fundamental strength of research to others. The industry will be diminished if it stops being research intensive and becomes development intensive and service intensive.

Shortly our profession's performance may catch up with our rhetoric and we may truly be a clinical profession. I am excited by the advancement that pharmacy education has made in adjusting the programs for the advancement of clinical pharmacy and the implementation of pharmaceutical care. However, one concern I have in this area is that pharmacy education seems to be adopting medical education as its prototype. I have never been a fan of medical education. What I admire is the excellent students that medicine has attracted for decades. Great students will make a modest program look great. The implementation of extensive internships and rotations in patient care settings may have been appropriate for an earlier low tech era. But in terms of today's resources, high tech alternatives must be considered. Computer assisted, problem-based learning, computer technologies utilizing virtual reality, and other technologies are here today and available. But we seem to be hooked on the medical model of education that is expensive, heavily dependent on broad networks of patient care facilities, and very oriented to specialty practice rather than primary care. It is likely that patient care facilities will soon question their commitments of resources to the medical education process.

We are seeing clinical pharmacy clerkship sites that once were voluntarily committed to pharmacy education now asking for reimbursement. Health reform will soon hit the funding of medical residents and fellows. Health reform advocates state that medical education and practice are overly specialized and have not focused properly on primary care. Thus, as we look to the medical model, what we may be missing is that the nursing professional that is moving aggressively into primary care. It may surprise you that the University of Texas College of Pharmacy is in discussion with our nursing program to determine if pharmacy/nurse practitioners trained individuals might be a valuable primary care provider.

Pharmacy education and the profession misread our opportunities in nuclear pharmacy. As a profession we are fortunate that nuclear pharmacy is a relatively small percentage of professional practice. I see signs that we may be misreading our opportunities related to high tech, biotech type drugs. The education of future pharmacists must involve molecular biology and biotechnology. Pharmacy practice must look beyond the stable, solid-state oral dosage forms such as tablets and capsules. We must realize that future high tech drugs will dominate therapy and will involve short-term stabilities, extemporaneous compounding, and will often be parenterally administered and infusion pump controlled. If community pharmacies move away from these complexities they will likely be turning away from their future.

If there is a current theme in health care that is certain to continue is one of cost effectiveness. It appears that boundaries will change between health professionals and those changes will promote the lowest-cost professionals providing the highest level of services of which they are capable.

Because of this trend we can expect that some duties being done by physicians regarding drug use, administration, and control will become mainstream activities of others; perhaps some by nurse practitioners and some by pharmacists.

Similarly, some duties currently performed by pharmacists will drop down to the activities of pharmacy technicians. The key issue for our profession may be to gain new responsibilities as we lose current responsibilities. My confidence in our profession and in our educational system is such that I cannot bring myself to defend our profession on the basis of "counting and pouring." These tasks can and should be done by technicians. In the near future they will be done by computer-interfaced robotics, and in many cases, by the manufacturer of unit-of-use packaging systems. We are a clinical profession, a knowledge-based profession, and our current services and our future services should revolve around our professional knowledge and our communication skills.

It is disappointing to see the current spectrum of performance of pharmacists and pharmacies. Our best are excellent; our lowest 20 percent are inexcusable. There are some who believe that what these pharmacists require is a more appropriate or better education.

I strongly disagree! These pharmacists are not providing poor pharmaceutical services because they lack a quality education. The solution is not to provide them with more education. My philosophy has always been to work to make the best better, to set higher standards, and to have the main body of the profession adopt those higher standards. What do we do about the practitioners who do not adopt reasonable contemporary practice standards? My view is that we strengthen our state board regulations and mandate a higher standard since voluntary adoption of reasonable standards has not occurred.

We may have just lost an ideal period to adopt higher standards for our profession. We seem to be ending a brief period of pharmacist shortage. During a pharmacist shortage period, pharmacist recruitment tends to be, in part on salary and in part, on professional environment. But there are signs that there may be a softening of the job market for pharmacists. Pharmacists searching for job opportunities may tend to enter job environments that are less than ideal. Our task for the profession will be to aggressively pursue new professional roles that excite young pharmacists and expand our profession. The elements of pharmaceutical care, the involvement of pharmacists in patient assessment, the selection of certain classes of therapeutic agents by pharmacists, and having more authority for the renewal of maintenance drugs are all within our reach if we have the professional will and commitment.

I remember when I entered this great profession in the 1950s. Some call it the golden era of pharmacy. Most prescriptions were dispensed by independent pharmacy owners. There was no such thing as a third-party prescription plan, no Medicaid or Medicare, no mail order pharmacy, and everybody liked "Old Doc." In actual fact, the 1950s were not that great. The pharmacist was being reduced to a distributor of a product and was told not to advise the patient. But out of this era was born the concept of clinical pharmacy and patient related pharmaceutical services. Education has moved more rapidly than practice in implementing these concepts. Our rhetoric is strong but reasonably uniform performance is lacking.

The differences are too great between what often "is" pharmacy service, what "should be" pharmacy service, and what "could be" pharmacy service. But we are gaining on it because we have certain dreamers in our profession who keep pushing us forward. As an academician I have a fondness for dreamers. I believe each of us should listen once a year to Martin Luther King's great speech with the theme "I have a dream." I happen to be an admirer of President John Kennedy and of Robert Kennedy. When Bobby Kennedy was running for President, he stated, "Some see things as they are and ask 'why?' Others dream things as they could be and ask 'why not?'" As we enter the 21st century, during the era of health reform, I believe it is important for pharmacy as a profession to dream of things as they could be and ask "why not?"

Our profession and industry are fortunate to have its share of idealists and dreamers. They should be honored by our profession. They should be our conscience and our guide. The 1967 Remington medalist William S. Apple was one of our dreamers who raised our standards of practice through his lifetime of outstanding contributions. He served APhA with distinction from 1959 to 1983. When I served on the APhA Board of Trustees and as APhA President in 1982, he taught me much about our profession and the society we serve.

Recently I had occasion to read several of Bill Apple's speeches. When Bill became APhA Executive Director in 1959, pharmacy was a confused profession which had lost its confidence. Bill ignored all the negative signs and charted a path for our profession that was based on the needs of the patient and appropriate drug use. He changed our terminology, the very way we addressed each other. It was Bill who stressed, "We are not druggists, we're pharmacists. We serve patients (not customers) in our pharmacies (not drug stores)." He fought for expanded pharmacist responsibilities like drug product selection and he caused pharmacists to again take pride in our profession.

In a 1976 speech Bill Apple made a statement about his being called a dreamer: "Some people who view my efforts in a less positive light have called me a dreamer. I appreciate their unintended compliment. Yes, I dream of a profession that has done its homework on how it can help bring about a more effective and efficient health care delivery system. I dream of pharmacists taking time to talk with patients. I dream of a public and government expressing its appreciation of the pharmacist's contributions through equitable and adequate compensation. Yes, I dream of all the good things that can and should happen. Then I awake and spend my days trying to make my dreams come true."

We should greatly value the highly regarded and important nature of pharmacy. And I hope in each of us will become a dreamer who spends at least part of his/her day trying to make those dreams come true.

I have attended Remington Award ceremonies since the 1960s when the banquet was held in New York City. I have had the pleasure of personally knowing many Remington medalists. Perhaps all medalists were dreamers like Bill Apple. I know that I am, and I am very proud and honored to be the 1994 Remington medalist. ■

1995 Remington Medalist

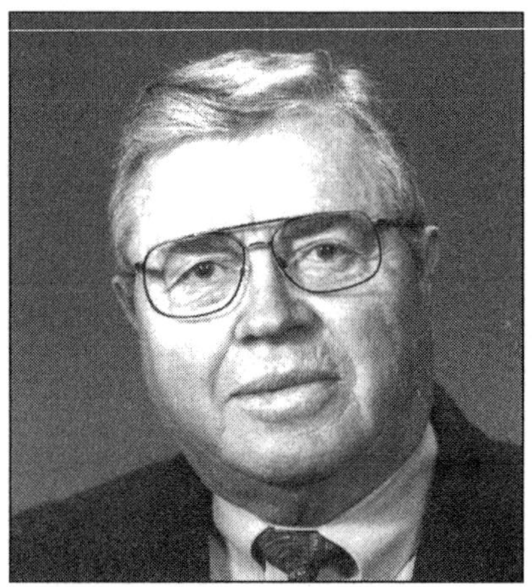

Max Ward Eggleston
(1922-1997)

Max Ward Eggleston was born in Waverly, Iowa, on August 4, 1922, and received a Bachelor of Science degree in 1947 from the University of Iowa College of Pharmacy. He served as Waverly, Iowa, community pharmacist from 1948 to 1984, and as owner of the Pharmacy Sales and Management Company from 1984 to 1997. He served as Iowa Pharmacists Association president from 1960 to 1961; as Iowa Pharmacists Association House of Delegates chairman from 1965 to 1966; as Iowa Interprofessional Society president in 1966; as a member of the Iowa Board of Pharmacy Examiners from 1975 to 1982; and as Iowa Pharmacy Foundation president from 1990 to 1992.

Eggleston served as American Pharmaceutical Association president from 1968 to 1969; as APhA Board of Trustee chairman from 1969 to 1970; and as American Council on Pharmaceutical Education president from 1978 to 1982. His volunteer leadership in his community included founder and chairman of the Waverly Community Chest, the forerunner of the Waverly United Way; as chairman of the Waverly Industrial Development Commission; and as chairman of the Waverly Chamber of Commerce. He died November 6, 1997, in Waverly, Iowa.

Reflections

Max Ward Eggleston

The 1995 Remington Medal was presented March 19, 1995, during the American Pharmaceutical Association annual meeting in Orlando, Florida, March 18-22, 1995. The lecture was not published in the *Journal of the American Pharmaceutical Association*. The text of the presentation is preserved in the APhA Foundation Archives.

Receiving the Remington Medal is a wonderful experience. Like a trip to the moon, it was nothing I expected to happen in my lifetime. From a nomination through a screening committee to an election by your peers erases from my mind the slightest doubt that all things are possible.

My life in pharmacy started well before a decision was made about my pursuing a pharmacy degree. I grew up in a family that operated a pharmacy. I was first the maintenance man and then became a quality soda jerk, a position I was awarded at the age of twelve, and stayed with it through high school. I learned how to bank a fire and cleanup the store to get it ready to open by 7:30 a.m. I graduated from high school in 1940, and my mother told me that if I was going to college I would have to study pharmacy. There was no discussion and it never occurred to me that she didn't have the right to make that decision. I started in the fall of 1940 at the University of Iowa, graduated, and became licensed in 1947. On Christmas Day 1944, while I was in the service, I married sweet Lorraine. This past Christmas we celebrated our 50th wedding anniversary. Lorraine has always made it easy for me; I could pursue my interests in pharmacy and she stayed home and raised the family. We have three children and three grandchildren.

In 1947, I started working as a licensed pharmacist in the family store and in the first year filled about 100 prescriptions. We never had any idea of the diagnosis or illness our medicine was supposed to cure because we were not supposed to ask the patient. This is when I became acquainted with a nearby dispensing physician. His office assistant could count but she couldn't make gentian violet solution, so that responsibility was given the pharmacist. I spent the greater part of that first year blue-stained. Another prescription we were lucky enough to get was for a nosedrop, made by mixing menthol and camphor crystals which liquified in a eutectic state, and then adding mineral oil. You didn't have to be much of a genius to know that wasn't the best nosedrop in the world.

The professional situation that I found in Waverly made it extremely important for me to be active in our local pharmacy association. It convinced me that there were many problems that needed to be addressed by the profession. The start of my professional career was stymied by the fact that 80 percent of the physicians in Iowa dispensed medication. When we attempted to put a pharmacy in a local physician's clinic, the clinic responded by hiring their own pharmacist. I then realized that I had to get involved in an organized effort to help change the professional situation that existed.

During my second year in Waverly, I started attending all the pharmacy meetings that I could, and I tried to become as involved as the system would allow. In 1956, I became the second vice president of the

Iowa Pharmaceutical Association, in a lockstep system to be president in 1960. Robert Gibbs, who subsequently served as executive secretary of the Iowa Pharmacists Association, preceeded me as president.

I attended my first APhA convention in 1958. It was there that I heard Robert Abrams describe the professional fee system for prescription pricing. It appeared to me to be the proper way to get paid for professional services since it largely took the product out of the procedure for determining the prescription price. I used that pricing process from the early 1960s until I sold my pharmacies in 1984, and I championed that concept while I was involved in leadership at APhA. Although many in pharmacy today unfortunately still question the wisdom of that initiative, I truly believe that the system is essential to our long term survival if we are to be considered a valued part of the health care system. Why is it that some in our profession continue to believe that our worth as health care professionals should be measured by the markup on a product price determined by a manufacturer? What better time than now when we must identify a means of receiving adequate payment for cognitive pharmaceutical care services?

In an open letter to our community, I announced in 1964 that our pharmacy would no longer be selling cigarettes. It seemed to be an obvious thing for the profession to do by convincing the consumer that we were serious health care professionals. I recognized that other pharmacists might not immediately join this initiative because they feared the loss of income. Today, more than 30 years later, this should be a dead issue, but unfortunately, many in our profession continue to cloud our image in search of short term economic gain.

Throughout my leadership career in pharmacy, I have been concerned about the issue of one voice for pharmacy. This is still a major impediment to pharmacy's success today. My contention was then, and is still today, that pharmacists need to speak with one voice on behalf of the profession and its practitioners. We have that voice in APhA. While many may disagree, I never believed that NARD [now the National Community Pharmacists Association] was a voice for pharmacy practitioners. They only spoke for the owner of drug stores. Nonetheless, they said they spoke for community pharmacists. They were joined in this task by the National Association of Chain Drug Stores (NACDS) who took an interest in trying to speak for chain drug stores. Specialty organizations effectively speak to the special interests of certain segments of the profession, but they can do no more. Only one organization can and does speak for all pharmacists, regardless of practice or degree. That organization is APhA.

It was always difficult for me to understand or justify pharmacist membership in both APhA and NARD. They were diametrically opposed on many issues and it was impossible for a pharmacist wearing their health care professional hat to support both organizations without being somewhat corrupted by the conflicting views. Supporting both agendas confused the one voice concept since the goals of the pharmacist as a health care professional were often usurped by the needs of the retailer.

In the early sixties, J. Curtis Nottingham, the former director of the Virginia Pharmaceutical Association, became the architect of the affiliation movement; if this had been fully developed it could have created the one voice concept. As state associations started to affiliate with APhA, the voice APhA used to speak for the profession was truly strengthened. However, the reciprocal membership requirement of the affiliation agreement was abandoned in the early 1980s, and that loss significantly self-destructed the organizational strength of the profession. I would only hope that the elected leadership can reconstruct the original affiliation movement so that APhA can assume its rightful position as the voice for all the nation's pharmacists.

Clearly it is time for the profession to reassess whether organized pharmacy is optimally structured to provide unity of purpose for all of pharmacy. The numerous positions and postures assumed by all of the groups supposedly speaking for the profession have created tremendous confusion for both those in the profession as well as all others who come in contact with pharmacy. It is little wonder that government agencies, legislative bodies, managed care organizations, and the public in general are often unsure of where pharmacy stands on any given issue. In the process of this re-examination, the organizational egos of both the staff and volunteer leadership must be checked at the door. To do otherwise will surely doom us to continuation of the problems that have plagued us for the past forty years.

Imagine an all inclusive affiliation system where each state organization and all the national pharmacy organizations would have membership in the APhA House of Delegates. This would create the parliamentary mechanism that would collectively define the professional needs that all pharmacy organizations should be addressing. This would be but one of the many innovative approaches that could be employed to truly bring pharmacy together and allow it to present a united front and a unified voice.

I first met William S. Apple in 1961 in Cedar Rapids, Iowa. His approach to the problems of the profession was easy for me to digest. He had my wholehearted support in his efforts to instill in the profession the need to solve its own problems and develop the kind of practice environment to which the profession aspired.

As time went on, it was my fervent hope that we could convince Bill Apple to help select his successor and then retire to the mountain top and be the Moses of Pharmacy. My hopeful expectations had little support and when the time came, APhA was wholly unprepared for his departure. The leadership proceeded to fail in its responsibility to the profession. I hope that lesson will stay fresh in our minds and that the necessary protection will be built into the system so that this kind of chaos does not happen again. Failure to learn from the past is inexcusable.

Leadership has many responsibilities. Let me offer two illustrations of the overriding importance of good leadership. Staff members of pharmacy organizations have a difficult role in enlisting knowledgeable volunteers who can and will evolve into a strong corps of electable leaders. It is not sufficient for an organization to merely nominate and elect somebody for every office; the individuals nominated and ultimately elected must understand, and agree to support, the programs that are in place. Any existing conflict of interest or disagreement must be addressed and resolved before the election process proceeds so that the elected board's credibility will not be in jeopardy.

Leadership also has the responsibility of identifying good ideas regardless of source. Once a course is agreed to, leadership must insist that the ideas be followed through to their conclusion. I remember clearly when, in the mid-1960s, the APhA Board of Trustees agreed to set aside $200,000 for a study of computer needs for our professional society. We let it hang there, never insisting that the study be conducted. I believe we may have done a long term disservice to the association because we did not follow through. Had we become involved in a significant way at that time with computerization, one can only wonder what kind of an information powerhouse APhA could represent today.

I have always been grateful to APhA president Kenneth Tiemann for appointing me in 1975 to the board of directors of the American Council on Pharmaceutical Education (ACPE). Being allowed to participate in that forum is the best way to get a handle on what happens in the accreditation process. It was always obvious to me that any improvement in professional education led not only to improved self-esteem but better remuneration.

While I served in ACPE leadership, they had representatives from the National Association of Boards of Pharmacy (NABP), the American Association of Colleges of Pharmacy (AACP),and APhA. Talk at that time started about increasing the representatives on the ACPE. The ASHP and the National Association of Chain Drug Stores

(NACDS) were spirited in their efforts. The American Society of Health-System Pharmacists (ASHP), because of its affiliation with APhA, was always represented. NACDS requested membership on ACPE professing they were entitled to participate because they represented so many pharmacists. Nothing could be further from the truth; their drugstore chains hired many pharmacists but NACDS certainly did not represent these pharmacists. NACDS also suffered from a conflict of interest that could be exhibited in the kind of curricular requirements that they would suggest for pharmacists that their chains were planning to hire.

The ACPE proposal for accrediting only those colleges of pharmacy that offer a Pharm.D. degree as the entry level degree brought out the negative as well as the positive elements of the profession. In the beginning, and even now, there are factions within the practice and academic communities in pharmacy that are opposed to the Pharm.D. program. It always seemed to me that everyone in the profession should be in favor of the long-term improvement of the education of the pharmacist. Frankly, I was always surprised by the lack of unanimity in academia as well as in how the profession seems to set the agenda for academia.

One of my long held tenents, that does not currently have much support, has been that a practicing pharmacist should always be the president of ACPE. Neither the regulators (NABP) nor the educators (AACP) should hold that position. The profession has to be held responsible for enhancing the position of the pharmacist and one of its primary responsibilities is to continue to improve the educational level of the pharmacist.

During my first accreditation visit, it became perfectly obvious that the procedures plainly identified the good, the bad, and the indifferent. I was amazed at how quickly the strengths and weaknesses appeared during an accreditation visit. The educational institution was always the primary benefactor of the process. The American Council on Pharmaceutical Education under Dan Nona's leadership immeasurably improved the accreditation process. How fortunate the profession is to have the capabilities of ACPE to insure that our continuing education providers are also subject to ongoing reviews that guarantee quality.

One of the major concerns today in curriculum development is the need to maintain the necessary core of general education. The need for strong professional education is a given, but for pharmacists to function in the best interest of the society they serve requires that they receive a broad-based general education. Gaining that broader background is very difficult in our professionally-based educational process. The hours devoted to general education are constantly under attack by forces developing additional professional education. General education requirements should be protected and expanded when the opportunity is presented.

In the early 1960s the potential for group practice and office practice seemed to exist. Eugene White's conversion from a standard drug store to an office practice was a pretty gutsy thing to do and he was applauded and admired by the profession for his efforts.

McKesson got excited about trying to create a turn-key conversion package, but as is often the case, they made it so expensive that a lot of potential office practice proponents were talked out of it because of the cost. Fear of the new and unknown took care of many others. The profession, especially APhA, did a lousy selling job and a new method of practice virtually died before our very eyes.

The profession has embraced pharmaceutical care and it seems to be the proper step for the practicing pharmacist to follow. In my entire professional life, the drug product was an essential part of pharmacy practice. I hope that throwing out the drug product with the bath water, as some in the profession appear to believe, doesn't negatively affect our survival in the future. We need to maintain our franchise for controlling and managing the drug distribution system, but we can no longer allow these tasks to be our sole professional focus. Drugs are what differentiates pharmaceutical care from medical care, but we must concentrate on caring for patients, not manipulating drugs.

Pharmaceutical care is a visionary new method of practice. Many in the profession are concerned about how they will convert their practice and adopt this new philosophy. If everyone was already meeting the existing requirements of the Omnibus Budget Reconciliation Act of 1990 (OBRA) by insuring that the patient has all the information he or she needs about their drug therapy, pharmacy practitioners would have a big lead on closing in on the totality of pharmaceutical care as the basis for all pharmacy practice. Once a pharmacist truly adopts a patient, instead of a drug product, they should be able to convert from a standard dispensing pharmacy practice to the prototype of the new system without devastating the existing practice module. The profession did a miserable job of selling the office practice concept, a mistake we cannot afford to repeat with pharmaceutical care. Let's make it possible for interested people to convert to a pharmaceutical care system that suits them without throwing up mega barriers that may slow or stop the process.

Calvin Knowlton recently indicated that the profession is experiencing the "in-between times" -- the times between what was and what will be. Pharmaceutical care is our way out of the "in-between times." Its impact is certain to extend our professional life line. If we don't accept this opportunity, our demise will become a reality.

One of the distinguished current elders of the APhA Board of Trustees, Robert Gibson, recently wrote that he is disheartened to see pharmacists that seem happy to be blissfully ignorant and fail to understand the winds of change swirling around our profession. He pointed out that we are facing a cultural revolution within the profession. Organized pharmacy may need to mount a fierce, unrelenting, perhaps ruthless, campaign to make pharmacists understand that if they don't change, others in the health care system are out there ready and willing to take over our responsibilities.

A future practitioner in pharmacy, Michael Hogue, suggested steps pharmacy students could take to pioneer these changes. Hogue urged students to take their enthusiasm to the work place, encouraging preceptors/employers to allow them to practice pharmaceutical care. Together pharmacists and students can increase patient satisfaction and improve patients' drug therapy outcomes. Students should hold their peers accountable, understanding if some students make pharmaceutical care a standard expectation at internship sites and work places, others would follow suit. Those who do not participate in the activity will be held accountable for slowing down the professional journey that will benefit all of us.

John Gans asked me to give my vision of the future as I see it. Currently my only vision at my age today is trusting in the daily sunrise. We have always fought to maintain our identity but the battles of the past will be "Mickey Mouse" compared to what we will experience in the future unless we grab hold of pharmaceutical care and assure ourselves of continued involvement in providing the best drug therapy and patient care in the overall medical care programs in this country.

I am reassured by what I see. The leadership has adopted a direction and hopefully can speed up the process. Our young pharmacists and pharmacy students will not approve of a procedure that holds them hostage while their future passes them by. We must move with assured haste.

You have been listening to a professional who spent most of his life practicing pharmacy, caring for patients. While I was given many opportunities to serve the collective interests of the profession, I always returned to my practice and my patients. I never tried to escape to something perceived to be more rewarding. I am grateful for my life in pharmacy, and I am happy to have been able to serve the profession over the past 48 years. I thank each of you for sharing with me the happiest occasion of my professional life. ■

1996 Remington Medalist

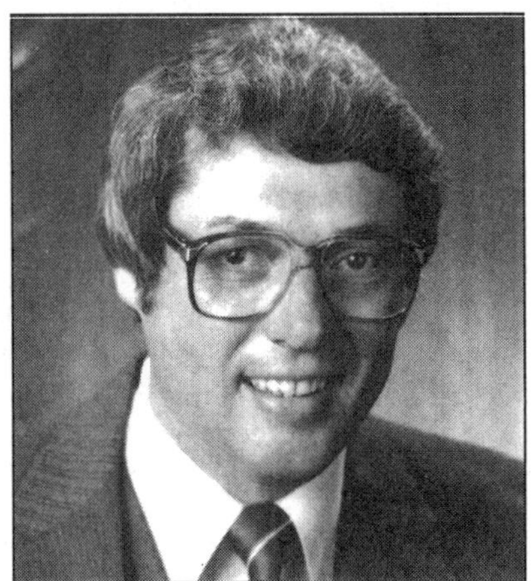

Maurice Quinn Bectel

Maurice Quinn Bectel was born in Muskegon, Michigan, on July 9, 1935, and obtained his Bachelor of Science degree in 1960 from Ferris State University School of Pharmacy. From 1963 to 1983 he was owner of Bectel Pharmacy in Muskegon, serving as Western Michigan Pharmacists Association president from 1963 to 1965, and Michigan Pharmacists Association president from 1971 to 1972.

Bectel served as 1983 American Pharmaceutical Association president and as 1983-1984 chief operating officer. He then served as president of the Pharmaceutical Research and Manufacturers of America Foundation from 1986 to 1997, and as vice president for pharmacy affairs of the Pharmaceutical Research and Manufacturers of America from 1989 to 1997. He also served as treasurer of the Pan American Federation of Pharmacy from 1992 to 1994.

ONE JOURNEY TOWARD THE FUTURE

Maurice Quinn Bectel

The 1996 Remington Medal was presented March 10, 1996, during the American Pharmaceutical Association annual meeting in Nashville, Tennessee, March 8-12, 1996. The lecture was not published in the *Journal of the American Pharmaceutical Association*. The text of the presentation is preserved in the APhA Foundation Archives.

I begin my remarks with probably one of the most overworked literary references known. I do so for two reasons: First, because I believe it sets an appropriate context for what I want to say. Second, because I want to establish at the outset that I am not above using a well-worn cliche to present my thoughts.

The quotation to which I refer is the first sentence of Charles Dickens' novel, *A Tale of Two Cities*, that reads: "It was the best of times; it was the worst of times."

For those of you currently involved as providers or suppliers in what is commonly referred to as "The Health Care-System," Dickens' words ... or at least the last half of them ... should strike home. We need not go far or wait long for someone so involved to express the view that maybe, this is the "Worst of Times." However, I would suggest that in other ways, this may be viewed as the "Best of Times." This evening, I want to address both aspects of the situation in which we now find ourselves as they relate to our future.

In light of the honor accorded to me as the 67th Remington Medalist, I should not have to remind this audience that I am a pharmacist by education, by training, by experience, and by commitment to my profession. Nor will I burden you with a detailed chronology of my 36 years as a member of this profession. I should note, however, that for the first 25 years I was like many of you, a practicing pharmacist dealing directly with patients. For the past eleven years I have been associated with the research intensive pharmaceutical industry in funding the education and training of young medical and pharmacy students while continuing to foster improved relations between industry and pharmacy. Consequently, I believe that I am in a position to offer some perceptions that have their origins in both areas of my professional career.

I hope these perceptions will provoke thought, discussion and, possibly actions that will benefit all involved in the development and delivery of pharmaceuticals and furthering the concept of pharmaceutical care.

It is beyond argument that the health care-system has undergone and will continue to undergo profound changes in its economic structure, its technical development, in who or what will exercise control over the delivery of health care and, finally, in the actual delivery of those health care services to the patient. Let me illustrate each of these propositions with examples from recent pages of the public press.

An article discussing a report of a committee of health experts notes that young Americans who want to become physicians should think twice about doing so. This is because an increasing surplus of doctors and strict controls on health care costs, may, and I quote, "make it hard to earn a living." The same article takes note of the recent report of the Health Profession's Commission that recently jarred the health professionals' world. It not only describes the existence of a surplus of physicians, but also a surplus of nurses and pharmacists.

Another recent article pointed out in the context of America's increasing reliance on health maintenance organizations and "managed care" to control health care costs, that the vast majority of employers evaluating HMO plans for their employees place the issue of cost far above issues relating to the quality of health care services. This article is one of a series, examining the goals, promises, and realities of the managed care concept including the fact that the annual salary of the CEO of one of the largest managed-care companies exceeds six million dollars.

Finally, among the series of managed care articles to which I refer, there were a number of what we might call "horror stories" involving patient access problems, restrictions on physician and pharmacist professional judgment, treatment failures and worse, resulting from health care services provided -- and in a number of instances apparently not provided -- to patients in managed care programs.

I do not propose to "beat a dead horse" with regard to the concerns and the examples that I cite here, because I believe that each of you could present your own litany of examples and concerns. In what direction should these examples propel us in the profession of pharmacy and in the pharmaceutical industry? To the protection and maintenance of the status quo? I think not.

First, I do not believe that the current health care-system status quo is one that either the pharmaceutical industry or the profession should perpetuate, and returning to the system of a decade or two ago is not an option. Therefore, it is mandatory that dreams of the past be put aside; that unattainable goals be put aside; that intra- and interprofessional posturing be put aside; and the disputes that have divided and continue to divide pharmacy and the pharmaceutical industry be put aside. We must recognize a mutual obligation to avoid skirmishes that threaten to damage, if not destroy both sectors. If they occur, they can only inure to the benefit of others. Our historic mutual reliance must not further evolve into an adversarial relationship.

Now, as the upheaval continues in the nation's health-care system, I urge both pharmacy and the pharmaceutical industry to recall our past, how importantly we have served one another and how collectively we have contributed significantly to improved patient care. As health care moves toward a shared-risk system, we have so much to offer one another. Pharmacists have frontline access to the patient and are held in high regard by the consumer. The pharmaceutical industry should recognize that trust and partner with pharmacy to assure that the most appropriate drug therapy is provided.

Further, we must not overlook how valuable the pharmacist can be in achieving patient compliance, through appropriate drug therapy management, thus helping the industry's products achieve their desired outcome. Pharmacists, in turn, must look cooperatively to the industry for information on disease management as well as educational support to assist the pharmacist in fulfilling a new clinical role in the evolving integrated health-care system.

What should that new role be? The Pew Charitable Trusts Health Commission recently projected that a reduction of 40,000 pharmacists would needed for the future, supporting their contention that one-fourth fewer colleges of pharmacy would suffice. I believe the PEW Commission was predicting their data on the historic and traditional role of the pharmacist as a dispenser, rather than as a drug therapy manager practicing comprehensive pharmaceutical care.

There are several exciting initiatives that are currently underway encouraging the practice of pharmaceutical care:

- The APhA/NWDA Concept Pharmacy Project is being showcased at this 143rd APhA Annual Meeting. This Project is designed to assist and encourage pharmacists to change their practice to that of pharmaceutical care.

- The American Center for Pharmaceutical Care has been established by APhA and state pharmacy associations as a separate entity and is being supported by many Pharmaceutical Research and Manufacturers of America (PhRMA) member companies to advance the reengineering of pharmacies and train pharmacists in the principles of providing pharmaceutical care.
- Faculty training programs in pharmaceutical care are underway through APhA and the American Association of Colleges of Pharmacy.
- NARD (now the National Community Pharmacists Association) has launched a program that is dedicated to improving patient outcomes through pharmacist-directed disease and wellness programs. And,
- ASHP has initiated Project Catalyst to advance the practice of pharmaceutical care.

Unfortunately, these initiatives alone won't suffice. Change must be initiated by individual practicing pharmacists. Pharmacists cannot wait for leadership to do it for them because it won't happen. It will take large numbers of practicing pharmacists to move the process.

Pharmacy must also change the public perception of the profession's capability to contribute in a new and expanded role. It is imperative that the profession develop and implement a nation-wide educational and public relations campaign to shift public opinion.

The image of the pharmacist as a dispenser must be replaced with an image of the pharmacist exhibiting a more intellectual contribution to health care as a care giver specializing in drug therapy management. I am encouraged by American Medical Association's recent media blitz regarding the value and benefits of pharmaceutical care.

Pharmacy cannot operate in a vacuum. Other members of the drug therapy management team, physicians, nurses, the research-intensive pharmaceutical industry, and others all have a role to play and an interdependent relationship with pharmacy. The name of the game is collaborative drug therapy. Associations of both the pharmaceutical industry and pharmacy must also become leaner in terms of their organizational structures so that their respective interests can be represented more effectively in the health-care system debates. There can be only one goal for both the profession and the industry: To achieve a full and rewarding role in the health-care system to the greatest possible extent in the face of numerous contending interests pursuing the same objective. Now is the time to resolve our differences and acknowledge that single goal.

Early in our nation's history, when the 13 colonies were struggling for independence, there were many debates in which they had great difficulty in reaching agreement. Eventually, however, they were able to present to the world their Declaration of Independence.

On that occasion, Benjamin Franklin informed his colleagues that "We must all hang together or assuredly we shall all hang separately." Franklin's message was not lost on his listeners. Despite many deep-seated differences among the colonies, they managed to get their act together. Although rooted in history, Franklin's proposition regarding the need to unify those with basically similar interests, and march together for the common good, is timeless.

Today, for the profession and industry to maximize their future opportunities, each must recognize that it has been a natural ally of the other and that this natural ally relationship does and must continue to exist. The "ties that bind" have been strained at times and often for legitimate reasons. The point that we should all appreciate is that neither perceived or actual right or wrong is attributable wholly to one interest or the other.

What also must be recognized is that both the pharmaceutical industry and pharmacy will continue to witness profound internal and external changes. We should not overlook or underrate some of the most significant changes that have already occurred.

During the past decade, the research-intensive pharmaceutical industry has undergone significant consolidation and downsizing. Since I joined the PhRMA Foundation in 1985, seventeen companies have ceased to exist. Strong incentives for mergers within the industry continue to be present, and it is possible -- if the merger trend continues and is projected into the next century -- the research-intensive pharmaceutical industry will consist of six to ten multi-national, highly-diversified pharmaceutical companies with multiple specialized subsidiaries. Similarly, the wholesale drug segment in the past decade has also witnessed its numbers diminishing from 150 corporations to fewer than 60 today.

Despite population increases, the total number of pharmacies has remained relatively constant, although we all know that many independent pharmacies in that number have been replaced by mass merchandisers and other types of chain organizations. I could give you a litany of statistics, but suffice it to note that radical consolidation is now beginning to take place within the chain drug industry itself, and the percentage of pharmacists who are employees as compared to those who are self-employed continues to rise.

With consolidation rampant throughout, can associations ignore the economic pressures driving their respective constituencies? Only at their peril, I believe. Just as they have done themselves, pharmacy and the pharmaceutical industry should be assured that their respective organizational structures are capable of representing their interests as efficiently and effectively as their resources will allow. With the current nationwide focus on increasing efficiency and output in the face of shrinking resources, it is apparent that this is not the time for pharmacy or the pharmaceutical industry to be swimming against the tide. This is the time for a close examination of association structures, and for serious consideration of the potential benefits of consolidating professional and industry interests into a smaller number of more effective organizations.

This is not a new proposition. I well remember the efforts of the late APhA President, William S. Apple, and other pharmacy leaders to encourage the creation of "one voice for pharmacy." Those efforts failed, not because of any inherent weakness in the "one voice" concept, but because of the impossibility of reaching consensus as to whom would be the "one voice."

Why then do I now suggest that the profession should attempt to breathe new life into a concept that most in pharmacy probably think is long past? I do so because of my commitment to the profession, and because I believe that making its organizational structure collectively more effective is one of the many steps essential to creating a reasonable assurance of pharmacy's continued viability.

I do not propose what optimum number of organizations might best represent the profession or which organization or organizations should survive. My strong conviction, however, is that there is an important role for pharmacy in tomorrow's health-care system. I am equally convinced that such a role is not likely to be developed if, and so long as, the profession is divided according to particular practice interests. Today, it is increasingly difficult to differentiate between the constituents of the many pharmacy organizations. The economic resources of the profession cannot be wasted by maintaining an organizational structure that no longer effectively represents the profession.

The issue I have raised in the pharmacy context is very similar to the issue that is being faced by the pharmaceutical industry. You should be aware of the extent of consolidation and downsizing within the industry, but the numbers that I mentioned earlier do not tell the entire story. I am sure that many pharmaceutical industry observers still think in historic terms of the industry being comprised of two separate and distinct segments, the "brandname pharmaceutical industry" and the "generic pharmaceutical industry."

As the industry continues to consolidate,

this historic pattern of basic and often diverse interests within the industry has become a delusion of conventional wisdom. Without reciting statistics, let's observe that a large number of brandname companies produce generic product lines. Most generic manufacturers have been acquired by brandname companies, and the entry by foreign manufacturers, alliances, and the increased marketing of former prescription products into the OTC marketplace are examples of dramatic changes in the pharmaceutical industry.

All of these realities should disabuse industry observers, and certainly the pharmacy profession, of the belief that the historic differences between "brandname" and "generic" pharmaceutical manufacturers still exist as they did in the past or that the interests of "brandname" and "generic" manufacturers continually conflict rather than come together.

Moreover, the business of pharmaceutical manufacturing and drug development is becoming more and more a global activity. Issues relating to the "harmonization" of international standards for pharmaceutical products have become a substantial practical and economic concern for the industry as this trend continues.

It is true, that organizationally, the pharmaceutical industry has not yet come together but it is heading in that direction. Given what undoubtedly will be a continuing consolidation of the pharmaceutical industry, will it serve the industry's interest to maintain multiple trade associations identified with segments of the industry that no longer exist as a practical or meaningful reality? Do the current or future interests of the companies that make up "the pharmaceutical industry" require their maintaining and supporting separate interest groups? Or should the consolidation that is occurring within the industry itself be mirrored by similar consolidation of the organizations that currently represent the pharmaceutical industry?

With appreciation and due respect for all of the organizations and individuals who have devoted their efforts to representing the industry as it has existed, I predict that, in the not far distant future, the pharmaceutical industry will redefine its own organizational structure to bring it in line with current realities.

Coming back to pharmacy, I respectfully suggest that each of my perceptions about the pharmaceutical industry is equally applicable to the profession of pharmacy and its organizational structure, with one major exception. Unfortunately, given the history of prior efforts to unify the profession, I lack the confidence that I have expressed about the pharmaceutical industry when it comes to predicting the outcome of current or future efforts to unify and consolidate representative organizations.

I recognize that individual personalities will play a more prominent role within the profession and its current organizational structure than might occur within the industry and industry organizations. I also recognize that the profession's "turf" is divided into a greater number of identifiable segments than within the industry. Finally, I recognize that a number of organizations within the profession have existed for much longer periods than organizations within the pharmaceutical industry.

Perhaps these differences between pharmacy's organizations and those of the industry are principally reflective of the differences between professional associations comprised of individual practitioners and trade associations comprised of corporate members. All of these factors may make the profession's organizational restructuring task more difficult than that of the industry. However, in my view, they do not make the task impossible.

I look forward to a health-care system that will offer the pharmacist an opportunity to build on initiatives involving collaborative drug therapy management through pharmaceutical care.

I am also optimistic that expanded opportunities will exist for pharmacists as important contributors to the discovery and development of new therapeutic agents within the pharmaceutical industry. I continue to believe in a rewarding future for pharmacy and the pharmaceutical industry. However, we must devote our efforts to guaranteeing that future and time is of the essence.

One thing should be clear for both the profession and the industry. What the future will bring does not lie wholly within the profession's or industry's hands. However, the future does lie in large part within the profession's and industry's hands. How those hands are put to work in determining the future will be critical.

For our profession, I have two essential aspirations. First, I want to see pharmacy's future determined with recognition of its real and vital contribution to public health and welfare. Second, I want to see pharmacy's future positively influenced by its ability to come together and expend its resources and energy to preserve and enhance that future.

I conclude this 67th Remington Lecture with a best of times note. There is no doubt in my mind that the pharmaceutical industry and pharmacy will have an essential role in the health-care system of the future. My most fervent wish for the pharmaceutical industry and pharmacy is that they will work together to enhance their relations and develop a strategic alliance which will respond effectively to the challenges presented by a changing health-care system.

When we look back from the vantage point of the 21st century to the period of the 67th Remington Lecture, I want and expect them to say, remembering and paraphrasing Charles Dickens, "They may have seemed like the worst of times, but they have proven to be the best of times."

For me, and for my family, my being the recipient of the 67th Remington Honor Medal certainly makes this the "best of times." I am grateful for the honor and look forward to being an active participant in bringing about a "bright new day" for pharmacy and the pharmaceutical industry. ■

1997 Co-Remington Medalist

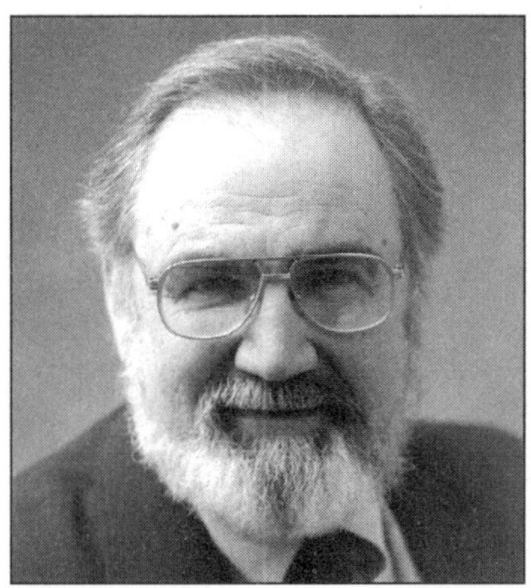

CHARLES DOUGLAS HEPLER

Charles Douglas Hepler was born in Newton, Massachusetts, December 18, 1936, and received his B.S. degree from the University of Connecticut in 1960, his M.S. in 1965, and his Ph.D. in 1973, both from the University of Iowa. He served as practicing pharmacist in Waltham, Massachusetts 1960; U.S. Public Health Service assistant chief of pharmacy service 1961-1963; Duke University Medical Center associate director of pharmaceutical services 1965-1966; University of Iowa College of Pharmacy instructor 1966-1973, assistant professor 1974-1979, associate professor 1979; Virginia Commonwealth University School of Pharmacy associate professor 1979-1988; University of Florida College of Pharmacy professor and chairman of the department of pharmacy health care administration 1988-1998, and since 1995 as director of the DuBow Family Center for Research in Pharmaceutical Care.

Hepler served as a member of the American Society of Hospital Pharmacists council on education and manpower 1981-1984; American Association of Colleges of Pharmacy commission on implementing change in pharmaceutical education 1989-1996; National Patient Safety Foundation research committee 1998-1999; and the International Pharmaceutical Federation (FIP) committee on good pharmacy practice 1989-1993, and FIP Board of Pharmacy Practice 1995-1999.

FOUR VIRTUES FOR THE FUTURE

Charles Douglas Hepler

Two 1997 Remington Medals were presented March 9, 1997, during the American Pharmaceutical Association annual meeting in Los Angeles, California, March 7-12, 1997. Hepler's address was published in the *Journal of the American Pharmaceutical Association*, pp. 470-473, July-August 1997.

I accept the honor that this medal bestows with gratitude and humility. Even to have been considered far exceeds my greatest expectations. Thanks to Mike Schwartz and Lowell Anderson for nominating Linda Strand and me, and the selection committee and past presidents of APhA for selecting us. It is encouraging that APhA has chosen to award the Remington Medal to two academics who have tried to join theory to practice. I hope that this will encourage others to collaborate in this challenging area.

Linda and I owe a debt to Don Brodie, upon whose very considerable life's work we built our efforts. Someone recently commented that, if clinical pharmacy came from California, pharmaceutical care came from the heartland of Iowa and Minnesota. Don Brodie was born and raised in Iowa, but was a father of clinical pharmacy in California. So we all spent time in the Midwest and here we are, back in California. Life includes a lot of cycles like that.

The last ten years have been by far the most challenging of my life. This is probably because ideas about professional practice are much more interesting when we implement them. Implementing ideas about patient care involves many people whom I have not met. They take an idea, shape it to their own template, and make it work. Truly wonderful and amazing.

I have felt accomplishment beyond my expectations, just as receiving this award is recognition beyond my expectations. But I also have experienced feelings of failure, sometimes quite painfully. Still, overall, the trend is toward successes, and we must continue. After all, as we try to create this new practice, failures do not count against us except to tempt us to discouragement. It helps me to remember that we are not in a mine field where we can lose everything from one error. We are not in a game that we can lose if our failures outnumber our successes. We are like the pilot in the first chapter of Tom Wolfe's *The Right Stuff*. We need to keep trying until we find what succeeds, at each step in the struggle. We are succeeding.

I want to discuss four virtues that I believe can help us to achieve our potential. These are faith, hope, charity, and honesty. The greatest of these is charity, but I will begin with hope.

Pharmaceutical care is a wonderful idea. However, it existed, in one form or another, in the minds of many people, in the late 1980s when Linda and I wrote our paper on "Opportunities and Responsibilities in Pharmaceutical Care" that was presented as the keynote address at the Pharmacy in the Twenty-First Century Conference in Williamsburg, Virginia, October 11-14, 1989]. I think part of the answer is in a remark made by Robert Kennedy made in South Africa. Kennedy said:

> "Each time a person stands up for an ideal, or acts to improve the lot of others, or strikes out against injus-

> tice, he sends forth a tiny ripple of hope, and, crossing each other from a million...centers of energy and daring, those ripples build a current which can sweep down the mightiest was of...resistance....Like it or not, we live in interesting times. They are times of danger and uncertainty, but they are also more open to...creative energy...than any other time in history."

We have stood up for this ideal in times and places when it was not quite acceptable. David Angaran can tell you a story about my trying to explain pharmaceutical care to a Delta ticket agent at 2:00 a.m., which I admit is over the top, even for me. Perhaps our willingness to talk about pharmacists and patient care is a part of the answer. I'm not complaining; nobody made me do this and it has been great fun.

Pharmaceutical care gives us hope that our profession can restore its past greatness, not by our becoming chemists again, but rather by our making a commitment to outcomes that are valuable beyond price to our patients, in a health care environment that is being stood on its head by rapid change. It gives us hope of being able to do what most of us came into pharmacy to do, which is to make a decent living by helping people make the best use of medicines. Most importantly, it gives us hope that we can find our way out of our present difficulties, into an apparently more secure and satisfying future. We are on the way. The transformation of pharmacy's professional aspirations is quite far along. What remains is the transformation of community practice, which is just beginning. However, there is a catch.

Of course, there is always a catch. The catch is, we have to take the initiative. As Calvin Knowlton put it, "first get the outcome, then get the income." So hope leads us to charity. Not charity in the sense of giving to the poor, but charity as *caritas*, caring for those who suffer.

The health care marketplace is more structured and much tougher than the one in which most of us grew. It is a lot better at controlling inputs to the system, like the "drug benefit," than at really producing the outcomes that we all want for our patients. Because the market has squeezed so much excess capacity out of community pharmacy, practically nobody has time to play around with pharmaceutical care. Very few can participate in the sort of study that would prove our worth to patients. I know this because I have tried repeatedly to do such studies in community pharmacies. They are difficult to set up, but so far they have been impossible to sustain.

I personally hate to fail, but I have to admit that we have not yet succeeded. Hanne Herborg and her group in Denmark have finished one outcomes study using the University of Florida model, with very encouraging results. Others are underway in Canada, Holland, and Spain. Most American community pharmacists, however, as much as they might like to be involved, are just too busy surviving, or at least they think they so.

I do not think that this problem of not having time for pharmaceutical care is a business problem. I reject the reasonable-sounding motto of "I won't do it until they pay me to do it." We keep looking for business solutions, somebody to pay for pharmaceutical care, but maybe we are not going to find one until we solve our own moral problem. I think that we are allowing the market to ride us into the ground, and it will continue to do just that until we are used up or until we stand up. Martin Luther King once said that anybody can ride you when you are bent over, but nobody can ride you when you are standing tall. What would happen if most pharmacists decided to stand up for patients and their need for pharmaceutical care?

When someone becomes ill or dies from mismanaged drug therapy, it does not make a real difference whose fault it was. Usually there is plenty of blame to go around. Standing up for patients means that we will do what we can to prevent injury and death, no matter who may be at fault. If we see a serious problem that we can fix, we fix it,. If we were standing on the curb of a busy street, and a child stepped into the street, we would not ask whose job it was the rescue the child. We would see that an accident was about to happen and we would try to prevent it. We should make a commitment to our patients to do the same for them.

What if most pharmacists refused to ask patients to sign OBRA-90 waiver forms, but instead really offered to counsel and to make sure of three things: (1) that the patient is getting (or will get) the medicine correctly, including proper use of administration devices like syringes or inhalers; (2) that the medicine is having the desired effect; and (3) that the medicine is not having an undesired effect, either on clinical outcome or on the patient's quality of life. What if most pharmacists insisted on standards of practice that required those three simple things from every community pharmacist? What if most pharmacists insisted on getting paid for providing those services? That's what I mean by finding a moral solution.

Nobody has a right to ask a pharmacist to fill so many prescriptions, just to survive economically, that patient welfare is put in danger. But they do ask us, and we acquiesce. That's an interesting word, by the way, acquiesce. It means, at its root, to become quiet or to accept passively. And that's exactly what most of us are doing.

Peter Senge, in his book, *The Fifth Discipline*, tells a story that is useful to explain resistance to change. It is called the "boiled frog" parable. A frog was placed in a pot of cool water, and he was comfortable so he didn't jump out. Then someone turned on the heat, but as the water slowly heated up, the frog never quite got around to jumping out. Finally, the water became so hot that the frog could not jump out. Thus the frog was boiled through his own acquiescence.

Many people will ignore this as something that is easy to say if you happen to be a tenured professor. But forget for a minute who is saying it and ask yourself, don't you wish our profession had stood up for patients ten years ago, when we still had the capacity to try a promising new practice model like pharmaceutical care? Don't you think our patients would wish it, too, if they knew how large an impact we can have? Don't you wish we had done that five years ago? Aren't we going to wish, five years from now, that we had done it this year? Are we doomed to be like the frog in the parable?

Some people will say that they are powerless. If they practice this way, somebody else will underprice them in a very price-conscious business. True enough. One thing that I have learned about pharmaceutical care is that we really can't succeed alone. Our profession must raise its minimum standards, and then we must tell the world what we have done, and why. We have to encourage our state pharmacy boards to regulate for outcomes, not for the benefit of pharmacists but for the public benefit they are sworn to serve. None of this will be easy, and it might not completely succeed, but sitting in this pot of hot water, labeled "I won't do it until they pay me to do it" is not working either.

Hope for a better future and commitment to our patients requires faith. Faith in ourselves, faith in the social power of professions, and faith in the principle that in a free society, or at least a free market, the people eventually get their way. Actually, since the fall of the Soviet Union, we can see that even in societies that are not so free, the people eventually get their way.

If we decide to stand up for our patients, we will need faith in ourselves, that we can help patients make the best use of medicines or at least that we can learn how. Enough pharmacists have been trained to provide pharmaceutical care by now that this question is settled. There is a way to train community pharmacists to provide pharmaceutical care in a reasonably short time. We should be willing to implement and evaluate programs and to publish the results.

If we decide to stand up for our patients, we can expect them to stand up for us, not out of affection or gratitude but because they need help with drug therapy. We all know the statistics on preventable drug-related injury and death. We all read the surveys that show that patients are dissatisfied with health care when nobody listens and nobody addresses the problems of daily living caused by illness and therapy. And they trust us more than any other profession year after year. What are we waiting for?

If we decide to stand up for our patients, we can expect to find allies everywhere. Pharmaceutical care involves a natural overlap of interest among patients, practicing pharmacists and practicing physicians (politics notwithstanding). While we could misunderstand this as competition, we can more usefully and accurately think of it as cooperation. Let's remember the power of the professions to speak for patients. Let's also remember that we have the same enemy, drug-induced disease and all the random things that can go wrong in therapy.

Honesty is, at its root, belief in and respect for reality. Every sane person bases his beliefs and actions on observable reality. As a life long academic, I am committed to a logical structure that is based on formally observable reality. Therefore, we should encourage pharmaceutical care systems only if we have some evidence that they produce more optimally cost-effective outcomes than the programs they would replace. But I wonder if pharmacists have taken this principle too far.

When I look around at the world of health care management, I see a double standard for evidence. We tend not to question the conventional wisdom, for example, that we can lower total costs of care with formularies or with prescription expenditure caps. But we demand impossible levels of proof for proposals that contradict the conventional wisdom, or that might change the status quo. Let me provide two examples.

Recently, Susan Horn and her colleagues published a paper evaluating the effect of formularies, as they were used by five managed care programs nationwide, on costs of care. This elaborate large scale study suggested that formularies, as used by those managed care programs, did not result in lower cost. Use of formularies was associated not only with higher drug costs but also the cost of physician office visits and emergency room visits. A storm of criticism resulted, and still continues. Most of it concerns details of the study's methodology, yet some of it is personal and vicious. Some of the methodological criticism might be valid, but all of them beg the question of "the emperor's new clothes."

The critics tend to assume that there is plenty of rigorous scientific evidence showing that formularies do control costs in managed care. However, the truth is, the emperor is parading in the nude. There is practically no such evidence, certainly none that would meet the standard of Horn's critics. Even the literature on the effectiveness of formularies in hospitals, which is a much simpler case, is quite mixed. But a paper that contradicts the conventional wisdom is held to much higher standards than the conventional wisdom itself.

For another example, Steven Soumerai and colleagues at Harvard showed that a prescription cap imposed on Medicaid recipients in New Hampshire backfired in a particularly nasty way. Although the cap reduced prescription numbers and expenditures, it increased nursing home and hospital admissions. Therefore, it increased total costs many times more than prescription cost savings. In addition, the policy dislocated many poor elderly people who were not able to return home after the cap was abolished. One would think that there followed a nationwide movement away from prescription caps, but that did not happen. These studies seem to have been ignored by at least six state Medicaid programs, and I don't know how many private insurance programs. Prescription caps continue.

Now, we should not jump into such flawed decision making with flawed research. But that would be totally unnecessary in any event. Studies have been appearing regularly for years that show the cost effectiveness of cooperative drug therapy management systems. However, many pharmacists, including many managers, do not know about these studies. Some who do know about them say that they are reluctant to argue in favor of pharmaceutical care systems because each study has some imperfection. In other words, we are oppressing ourselves.

We have trapped ourselves in a box, in which we need evidence to justify the studies needed to provide the evidence. Meanwhile, the world goes forward with other programs that are based on far less evidence than we have. In addition to the two examples from community practice, let me ask the hospital pharmacists, do they think that new nursing programs are adopted because the nurses have perfect research showing cost effectiveness? Does the director of nursing refuse to advocate proposals because the evidence is not from randomized clinical trials?

So, what is honesty? Does it require proof beyond any doubt? Perhaps the double standard that I described could be used to fend off pharmaceutical care programs. However, typically we have not even gotten that far. Perhaps the primary line of resistance to pharmaceutical care is our own lack of education in systems and lack of willingness to make a decision based on "imperfect" evidence. Perhaps we require another virtue, courage to advocate what we believe in, even if we cannot absolutely prove we are right. One of William Blake's *Proverbs From Hell* says, "if you lack the courage to be a hammer you will get the role of the anvil."

When the Florida Therapeutic Outcomes Monitoring project developed a method to set up pharmaceutical care in community pharmacy, we assumed that the main problem would be teaching pharmacists how to do it safely, effectively and consistently. If we could do that, we assumed that pharmacists would find a way to get paid, and the practices would prosper. We have done that, but few practices have changed, because the pharmacists were not paid for their services. It's not that they submitted bills which were refused. They did not bill. In a manner of speaking, they did not believe in the demand for pharmaceutical care.

Then we made a similar mistake by approaching third-party payers and trying to convince them to pay for pharmaceutical care. In a manner of speaking, the payers did not believe in the supply of pharmaceutical care. So evidently, we must recognize that a market requires three things: supply, demand, and a way to transact business. These three elements develop only in an interaction with each other. It would be no better to create demand without supply, even if we could, than to create supply without demand.

So now we see a way forward. We should create demonstration projects as temporary micro-markets involving a third-party payer, a group of community pharmacists trained to provide pharmaceutical care, and a simple payment mechanism. The payer would offer an experimental member benefit to high-risk patients, including those in whom drug-related morbidity is especially expensive. A university research center would train the pharmacists, then collect and analyze the data. Trained pharmacists would provide and be paid for comprehensive care. Everybody would share risk. We would keep this artificial micro-market going long enough to find out whether pharmaceutical care in community pharmacy can be cost-effective. After that, perhaps the researchers bow out and the market takes over.

Imagine for a minute that, all over the United States, practitioners, educators, state association executives, and managed care representatives have gotten together and developed such programs. Imagine that there are ten or even fifty such demonstration programs going on right now. Suppose that each of these practitioners and educators courageously advocates whatever these studies show is good for patients. How could we fail to change our profession? Also, if different programs used different models and approaches, we might also be able to test some of our passionately held theories about which approaches works better.

In conclusion, pharmaceutical care has seized our hearts and minds. It has given us hope for ourselves, our profession, and our patients. Many of us can never go back to old ways of thinking about drug therapy. But we are still just beginning the transformation of community pharmacy practice, and after that, of the drug use process in community practice. The way forward requires basic virtues of hope, commitment to others, faith in ourselves and our system, respect for reality, and the courage to speak out. So we come back to old truths. As T. S. Eliot explained in his *Four Quartets*:

> We shall not cease from exploration
> And the end of all our exploring
> Will be to arrive where we started
> And know the place for the first time. ■

1997 Co-Remington Medalist

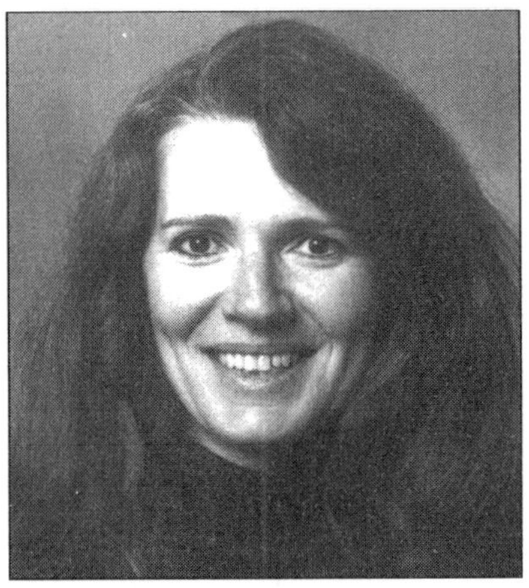

Linda Mae Strand

Linda Mae Strand was born in Hutchison, Minnesota, on May 2, 1953, and received her B.S. in Pharmacy in 1972, Pharm.D. in 1977, and Ph.D. in 1983, all from the University of Minnesota College of Pharmacy. She practiced community clinical pharmacy at the Riverside Pharmacy in Minneapolis 1979-1983, and then joined the faculty of her *alma mater* serving as assistant professor 1982-1983. She then served on the faculty of the University of Utah College of Pharmacy 1983-1988; the University of Florida College of Pharmacy 1988-1990; returning to the University of Minneapolis to the present. She also has served as Potchefstroom University Department of Pharmacy Practice in South Africa visiting professor 1996, and as adjunct associate professor at the University of Toronto Faculty of Pharmacy in Canada since 1990, and the University of South Australia School of Pharmacy and Allied Medicine since 1997.

Additional positions held by Strand include Food and Drug Administration clinical consultant 1978-1980; St. Paul Ramsey Medical Center clinical research associate 1981-1983; Pharmacy Practice Consultants president 1985-1988; and consultant to the University of Illinois 1984; University of Michigan 1986-1988; University of Pittsburgh 1988; Albany College of Pharmacy 1990; Stanford University Hospital 1991-1992; Brooklyn Veterans Administration Medical Center 1993, and University of Puerto Rico School of Pharmacy 1993.

Re-Visioning The Profession

Linda Mae Strand

Two 1997 Remington Medals were presented March 9, 1997, during the American Pharmaceutical Association annual meeting in Los Angeles, California, March 7-12, 1997. Strand's address was published in the *Journal of the American Pharmaceutical Association*, pp. 474-478, July-August 1997.

Thank you all very much. This is such a great honor and a surprise for me. I am humbled by your recognition. And, like all others who get here, I have many to thank for the privilege. I wish to thank my very special family, and so many who helped to develop the ideas and complete the work we are focused on this evening. Michael Smith, Albert Wertheimer, Harold Wolf, Don Perrier, Doug Hepler, and of course, Larry Weaver, all helped me in such significant ways. Two others who helped me more than anyone deserves are my colleague and spouse, Peter Morley, and my dear friend and colleague, Robert Cipolle.

I would like to thank two gentlemen who helped me greatly from a distance, Donald Brodie, and Eugene White. Not only were the ideas of these two men important to me, but their character, their integrity, their honesty, and their humility, all helped me to define the way I wanted to approach my career. How does one say thank you for all of that?

It should not come as a surprise that, as Doug [Hepler] aptly observed, pharmaceutical care came from the heartland of Iowa and Minnesota. It is a very unique place. We have long-cold winters in Minnesota, and this year was worse than most. Snow piles up and bitter winds chill us to the bone. On days when even the hardiest among us despair, we grit our teeth and, mumbling our daily mantra, "layers, layers, layers," we encase ourselves in numerous pieces of shapeless clothing and head for the door. So, winter in Minnesota is a time when the landscape is dotted with snow covered "Michelin men" struggling to make sense out of life. Little comfort is found in endless discourse on the subject of adaptation. Even the birds have the good sense to bask in the Florida sunshine. Why did I ever leave?

But, not all is lost in the midst of our harsher moments. Winter can also be a time of reflection. I have spent a great part of the winter thinking about the profound, and often perplexing, changes that surround us, and often appear to sweep us away in one wave of despair after another. I am not a pessimist or a cynic by nature, and so I see these forces as challenges, to engage in critical discourse, and find meaning in what appears at times to be total madness.

I would like to share with you some of my thoughts about a value I hold very dear, that of pharmaceutical care. I would like to examine our progress toward making this pharmacy's *raison d'etre*. Then I would like to proposed an amended definition for pharmaceutical care that takes into account many of the things we have learned since 1990. Finally, I would like to leave with you a few suggestions of what it will take to realize the goals implicit in this amended definition.

So, is pharmaceutical care alive and well? Or is it fettered by external forces such as tradition, a lack of imagination, and unwillingness to take risks? In my view, pharmaceutical care, as a concept, is alive and well.

We have taken the first step, perhaps the most important step, toward making pharmaceutical care our reason for being.

However, the health status of those engaged in such a discourse has yet to be determined. I am concerned that we might be "stuck" here when there is a great distance to go. And the most dangerous aspect of this is that I believe this first step to be the easiest of all the steps we need to take before patients actually receive, and benefit from, pharmaceutical care.

I say that agreeing on this mission is the easiest step for many reasons. First, pharmaceutical care is the right thing to do, so it is easy to agree with it. Second, it is what pharmacy has been searching for. And third, it serves our own best interest. So, accepting the concept of pharmaceutical care has been relatively easy.

The next few steps will be much harder because they will require that we change our actual behavior. Therefore we will have to change views of ourselves, and we will have to change traditional structures. We will have to change other people's views of us. And, perhaps of most consequence, we will have to take the next steps, not for the benefit for ourselves, but for the patient's benefit. But there is some very good news. I believe we have learned enough to warrant an update of the original definition that Hepler and I offered in 1990. I think this updated definition will help us see, and then take the next difficult steps.

A major part of this discourse spins off the early (prototypical) definition of pharmaceutical care enunciated by Hepler and Strand in 1990. We offered a foundational starting point that defined pharmaceutical care as "the responsible provision of drug therapy for the purpose of achieving positive patient outcomes."

Clearly, the stage was set, and the concept described specifically enough. However, I now believe we have learned enough to warrant an extension to this initial description. Thus, I propose the following definition for your consideration: "pharmaceutical care is a practice in which the practitioner takes responsibility for a patient's drug therapy needs, and is held accountable for this commitment."

As I said, winters in Minnesota can do strange things. Sometimes, even when we finally get warm, we turn up the heat. Let me try to make you comfortable with my revisionism. One key element here is what for the present I will term its assertive, prospective tone. This is basic. Also, it is quite clearly firm in its resolve to act, to take responsibility, and recognize and accept the full weight of accountability. A full acceptance of all that entails is essential to move forward. Moreover, I am firmly convinced that unless and until we take the responsibility for patient care as the focus of our responsibility, and are prepared to be held accountable for our actions, we will not meet the standards and expectations of those in health care who have already reached this "crossroad," and have chosen their path wisely.

I see pharmaceutical care as a philosophical world view with a strong normative content capable of liberating us from the fragmentation and discord that still exists in pharmacy. This becomes clearer when we introduce the concept of practice into our discourse. Aristotle asserted that good practice is derived from practical wisdom. This sounds like a good place to begin. Practical wisdom brings about the good in social, political and personal life, and has a strong ethical/moral content.

Furthermore, as the German philosopher Hans Gadamer avers, practical wisdom not only provides us with a dominant moral sense, but it also provides practitioners with a sense of identity. Identity is realized through the making of choices, choices about how a particular good can be achieved. Discourse concerning the nature of "the good life," "a good death," or a "good practice," allows us to develop a "reflective practitioner," someone who has examined conceptions of the "good practice," and through outer and inner dialogue, has concluded the journey with a sense of purpose, and a strong sense of who she or he is. For some, this might sound a bit optimistic. But, I remain firm in my conviction that this is a good place to begin. Only individual agents can determine the outcome, and by their actions they will write our history.

Perhaps the most important contribution made to a theory of practice is that put forward by Alasdair Maclntyre. He says that by a practice he means "any coherent and complex form of socially established cooperative human activity through which (moral) goods internal to that form of activity are realized in the course of trying to achieve those standards of excellence which are appropriate to, and partially definitive, of that form of activity..." This results, he adds, in "excellence, and human conceptions of the ends and good involved, are systematically extended."

William May, a distinguished ethicist, helps to clarify things. He draws our attention to a very important distinction made by Maclntyre who has "distinguished between the (moral) goods internal to a practice, such as the arts of lawyering, healing, and preaching, and the goods external to the practice, such as fame, reputation or fortune that a practice may generate". It is the (moral) goods internal to practice that should presently preoccupy us, and shape who we are. Practice as a whole system of meanings, not just the technical skills, should be our focus. Fame, reputation, and fortune (that is to say, reimbursement) will follow.

Practice is also about culture. Culture is "the symbolic expression of shared perceptions, valuations, and beliefs." Therefore, as Philip Selznick states when we speak of "organizational culture" we refer to "the creation of common understandings regarding purpose and policy." Selznick also brings to our attention a frequently ignored characteristic of organizational culture if it is weak and superficial, or fragmented, and discursive; then it is not likely to be of much use by its members or those it purports to serve. Hence, a practice, if it is to have any meaning at all, should have a strong culture with goal-defining norms and values. As Maclntyre says, practice should be a coherent whole, and not simply a "patchwork quilt" of technical skills and multiple realities." Practice cannot be left to those who simply say, "its what I do."

Defining practice through a prism of assorted activities, and *pro forma* job descriptions, is simply far off the mark. I cannot emphasize enough how important it is to place practice at the center of all we think and do. All practice must be intentional and purposive. It must draw upon conceptual theory and, in turn, feed back into, and modify theory. What we learn within the context of a practice leads us to reformulate thought and action.

It is for the above reasons that I strongly define pharmaceutical care as the development of a specialty practice. While this claim for a generalist receives common acceptance in all health professions, but for some unfathomable reason, pharmacy continues to believe otherwise. Yes, there are many who cling to the idea that a specialty practice stands on its own devoid of a general foundation, or the need for a logical progression from general to particular. Such a fantasy does little to establish a unifying consciousness of professional identity and purpose.

Should pharmacy drift further into a state of fragmentation, exemplified by the nature of systems specialists, organ specialists, drug specialists, delivery system specialists, and others, without an integrative foundational conceptualization of a general practice, then we will at least have provided an entirely new meaning for "nuclear pharmacy." When one adds to this confusing array of "experts" those identities derived from "sites," the picture becomes even more frustrating and puzzling to onlookers in other health professions.

If pharmaceutical care is to have any palpable value, any currency in the exchange of ideas with other health care practitioners, then we need a common ground. There is an immediacy, an urgency attached to this matter, and it demands our attention more than at any other period in our history. To "seize the time," and not stand firm in our resolve to integrate our struggling factions, can only result in dissolution and loss. Too extreme? I think not! The need for pharmaceutical care is very real, and will continue to be highly visible. The real "extreme" is to be found in the prevailing winds of change that are presently fanning the imaginations of other practitioners outside of pharmacy. On a daily basis I am confronted by enthusiastic individuals, drawn from numerous health care professions, who want to understand pharmaceutical care. For what purpose, you may ask. I will leave that to your imaginations.

Pharmaceutical care is an idea "whose time has come;" what we do with it can and should be foundational to who we are and what we can offer. Personally, I think our direction is clear and remarkably simple. We must commit to building practices of pharmaceutical care one patient at a time, and in so doing establish once and for all that we all share a fundamental understanding of our collective enterprise.

I am happy to report that with the help of many practicing pharmacists, we have created a practice that meets these expectations. It is a practice that begins with a patient's drug therapy needs. It incorporates goal setting, problem identification, problem solving, and value formulation. It is comprehensive. And in a real sense, it is bounded, rational action packaged in a patient care process that is understandable. It is a foundational practice upon which a specialty practice can be built when patients' needs dictate. Pharmacists are practicing it and students are learning it, so don't reinvent the wheel and don't hide behind not knowing. All of this is to say that the practice portion of the new definition should present no problems for us as we take the next step.

The revised definition states that pharmaceutical care is a practice in which the practitioner takes responsibility for a patient's drug therapy needs and is held accountable for this commitment. So let us now focus on the relationship that allows the practitioner to take responsibility for the patient.

Pharmaceutical care is also relational. It is not simply the authoritative allocation of the pharmacist's facts and values. Rather, it is a practice that derives a large part of its strength and legitimization from the partnership, or alliance, formed between the practitioner and the patient. We call this alliance the therapeutic relationship. To this end it is collaborative, and multi-vocal. The patient is at the center of all things therapeutic. I see this last point as an imperative that cannot be ignored. In an authentic, viable, pharmaceutical care practice, we focus our attention on a whole person, not a product, not an organ system, or not a disease state. Even medicine has moved, albeit slowly, away from the biomedical reductionism in *extremis* that for so long was their mechanistic (and some might say dehumanizing) focus.

As an aside, I must say that I find it puzzling and perplexing that disease-state management, born from the loins of the pharmaceutical industry as a marketing device, and embraced by managed care as an administrative technique with which to report costs and control expenditures, should for an increasing number of pharmacists, become confused with pharmaceutical care. Without entering into a protracted debate on possible ethical and sociocultural transgressions, there are numerous questions that such a fragmented, disembodying, unempowering, Cartesian conceptualization of "practice" presents. While time does not permit me to expound further on this matter, I feel it necessary to make my position, and that of my colleagues Morley and Cipolle, quite clear. We categorically reject this disturbing example of "misplaced concreteness," and urge others to do likewise.

While some may consider my case for the centrality of the whole patient to be a mere shibboleth, I can only reiterate what I have said here and elsewhere. Patients are whole persons in all their complexity, and it is dehumanizing and wrong to see them otherwise. Other health care providers accept this conception of human personhood, and we should do no less. Respect for personhood is central to pharmaceutical care practice.

The relational nature of pharmaceutical

care requires that we respect the patient's autonomy, preferences, and needs. Such a partnership requires that the pharmacist earns the trust of the patient and does what is best for that individual. There is no room for self-interest. All negotiation is governed by the principle of beneficence-in-trust, and in a strong respect for patient wishes. In a real sense we must identify empirically-based needs, and then interpret patient wishes, and incorporate these into our judgment and recommendations.

This raises another important consideration that hinges entirely on our willingness to take responsibility for patient care seriously: patient advocacy. Within my conceptualization of pharmaceutical care, I see the role of patient advocacy as axiomatic. Our first responsibility is to the patient, and we must at all times respect this commitment. Pharmacists should act on behalf of patients even to the point of challenging traditional authority in all its manifestations whether it be physician or nurse driven, or the increasingly powerful influences of assorted accountants, or economically obsessed members of the managerial elite.

We must proactively serve the needs of patients rather than reactively subordinate our therapeutic judgment, and the wishes of patients, to the authority of other health professionals. Of course, it goes without saying, that all dissent, and all advocacy, must be conducted with civility and respect for all concerned. Advocacy, within the context of pharmaceutical care, requires our total commitment to the critical examination of all patient medications. Are they appropriately indicated? Are they the most effective agents for this patient? Do they represent the safest modalities for treatment? And, before we can even consider issues related to patient compliance we must decide whose interests we represent, and address them in a professionally meaningful manner.

Patient advocacy requires the pharmacist critically examine the judgment and prescriptive decisions of others as they affect the well-being of the patient. Remember, in relationships such as those typically found in pharmaceutical care, the pharmacist is the patient's agent, not the unquestioning enforcer of any other authority. This is the essence of the covenant.

With the rise of consumerism and consumer authority, we will find greater emphasis placed on patient needs identified outside of traditional patterns of authority. Consumer authority, self-care, and the dissolution of traditional professional boundaries, will most certainly require a clearer demarcation of roles and responsibilities, as defined by us, and not by external legislative fiat as in the past. Solidarity, and a unified practice, are essential prolegomena to our social recognition, and our survival as a practice profession with health care as our primary purpose. The patient *qua* consumer will ultimately decide our worth. But, first we must present a picture that speaks for itself and requires little or no deconstruction on the part of those who are seeking assistance on drug-related matters.

The blurring of professional boundaries, combined with increasingly discursive health seeking practices, can and will produce levels of mystification heretofore unheard of. Increasingly, degrees of legitimization and authority are extended to practitioners previously considered marginal and of questionable efficacy, or social value. Presently, complementary, or alternative health practices, are a "growth industry," and do not appear to be a passing fad. Some will doubtless vanish as a result of disenchantment or litigation. However, many more will continue to attract the hearts and minds of numerous consumers. New Age cultural realignments are already diffusing throughout a broader population, and are increasingly becoming subject to allopathic interest.

In this post-modern world we are all "ethnic," to the extent that traditional boundaries of identity, self, and cultural positioning, are increasingly breaking down, to be re-formulated in the next grand narrative of human progress. Cultural diversity is the present in America, and it is against this cacophonous plurality of beliefs and practices that the next stage in pharmacy's evolution will unfold. All the more reason for this beleaguered profession to sort out its identity, promulgate its commitment to a "way of practice," and boldly grasp its responsibilities to meet the needs of patients, and confront the ineluctable forces of change.

It is against this backdrop of change that I urge serious consideration, and the adoption, of a more active, participative definition of pharmaceutical care. This commitment to act and willingness to be held accountable, provides a foundation that serves the best interests of patient or consumers, and permits professional identity and purpose to be solidified on grounds that transcend self-interest. Indeed, I hope to persuade you that a professional identity forged on the anvil of public interest will better serve its constituents, and make a significant contribution to the public good and human well-being. We cannot keep talking about it; we must move on to accomplish these high ideals.

As I said at the beginning, long Minnesota winters provide ample time for reflection, and inner dialogue. While the cold can at times be numbing, it can also stimulate, two qualities that I may have brought with me to this occasion and unleashed upon you. But, spring is in the air, and I feel the warmth of other issues drifting in across the fields surrounding me. I would like to close basking in the warmth of things to come, things that need to be done before the summer heat provides that sleepy comfortable feeling that things can wait. I leave you, then, with a few questions to reflect on, some more dyspeptic than others.

Can we reach a general agreement that we must have a commonly held foundation of practice which is not branded as the Minnesota, the Michigan, the APhA, or the Comprehensive model, but instead, pharmaceutical care?

Can you accept the need for a generalist practice as a place to begin so that we can reconfigure clinical pharmacy practice to serve as specialist practice?

Can you present a unified professional identity to other health care professionals, or will you depend on them to integrate the pieces, and define who you are, and what you do?

Do you continue to be defensive and reactive and seek solace in the past, that "golden age," that nostalgia for the "good old days" when we felt little need to confront troubling questions, and even more, troubling people?

Can you let go of the past and welcome the uncertainties and insecurities of what could be (paradoxically) an exciting future?

Are you prepared to compete in the "marketplace" of practice concepts, and processes, as these impact patient care?

Can you move from product to person as your primary focus?

Can you present a strong argument that your services, in any sense, are socially valuable and worthy of remuneration, by a patient?

Can you document and justify, your claims to the satisfaction of those accustomed to processing information derived from more traditionally recognized practitioners?

Can you become secure enough, certain enough, and committed enough, to pharmaceutical care, to display the passion that most administrators are looking for, under the guise of data... data... data?

Do you really understand how much hard work it takes to make a legitimate claim to a common practice?

It is my fervent hope that we can continue to call upon everyone here to participate in critical discourse and contribute to the shaping of our profession. We must call upon educators to teach the practice of pharmaceutical care, and we must expect them to address relevance and meaning in a patient care practice profession.

We must hold our leadership responsible for making bold pronouncements for a clear direction and to map out a course that is courageous and filled with enough passion and certainty to propel us in the right direction to take calculated risks.

We are free to chose, and I am reminded of the words of the philosopher William Barrett who declares that the best argument for freedom "is the horror of the world without it." And chose we must to meet the new millennium with new ideas and courage to carry them out. Let us choose pharmaceutical care as a practice in which the pharmacist takes responsibility for a patient's drug therapy, and is held accountable for his commitment. It is our re-vision, and resolve, that will see us through. Thank you very much for this great honor. ■

1998 Remington Medalist

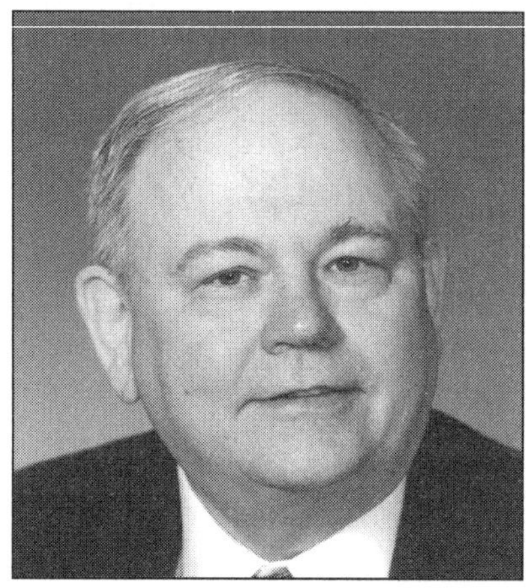

Kenneth Neil Barker

Kenneth Neil Barker was born in Spring Valley, Ohio, on March 25. 1937, and received his B.S. degree in pharmacy 1959, his M.S. degree and a residency in hospital pharmacy 1961 all from the University of Florida, and his Ph.D. at the University of Mississippi 1971. He joined faculty of the University of Arkansas Medical Center serving as project director of drug systems research 1962-1969 where he introduced the "unit dose" medication distribution system to hospitals which greatly improved the safety and accuracy of the drug dispensing and administration process. He then joined the *United States Pharmacopeia* as director of administrative research 1970-1972, and continued to serve the U.S.P. as chairman and project director of the National Coordinating Committee on Large Volume Parenterals 1971-1980. He returned to academia at Northeast Louisiana University as associate professor 1972-1975, and in 1975 he joined the faculty of Auburn University School of Pharmacy in Alabama as associate professor. Since 1976, he has served as professor in the department of pharmacy care systems, and in 1998 he was elevated to Sterling Distinguished Professor and director of the Center for Research on Pharmacy Operations and Design at Auburn University.

On Pharmacy Practice Theory and Quilt Making

Kenneth Neil Barker

The 1998 Remington Medal was presented March 22, 1998, during the American Pharmaceutical Association annual meeting in Miami Beach, Florida, March 21-25, 1998. Barker's address was published in the *Journal of the American Pharmaceutical Association*, pp. 426-429, July-August 1998.

During the general session of the APhA meeting, I was given the opportunity to acknowledge the many persons who, through their guidance, inspiration and support, have been important in my professional career. My family could not attend, so I would like to recognize them now: Louise, Brad, Linda, and Doug.

It has been my good fortune to have been associated with outstanding leaders, working in stimulating and supportive environments. That leaves one with the nagging feeling that with all that going for you, you had better do something!

But how can I hope to cope with the challenge of presenting remarks, in the shadows of giants such as Joseph Remington, John Uri Lloyd, and James Hartley Beal, or those recent recipients of the Remington medal? Well, for one thing, I was given just 15 minutes and I'm sticking to that. My strategy is to fight quality with brevity as the old saying goes.

My career has been focused on research in pharmacy operations to help solve the problems of pharmacy practitioners, first in hospitals, later in community pharmacy, and today in managed care. My dad was a community pharmacist and I grew up hearing about such problems as the impatient patients, unreachable doctors, long hours on your feet, and varicose veins.

As a student, work in a hospital pharmacy introduced me to another world of problems. The practice of compounding, for example, where nurses mixed intravenous drug admixtures for your veins while pharmacists had to stick to their ointments, just scratching the surface of their potential.

Then, in graduate school I needed a thesis topic. My dispensing teacher at Florida, William Husa, told me that pharmacists were responsible for preventing errors and I wondered how many there were. The psychologist on my committee asked, "Why don't you go up and look?" So I observed nine nurses as they gave medications, and I compared what they gave against the chart. The discrepancies were astounding, one error per each patient, each day. As a solution, my advisor, Warren McConnell, urged me to get a research grant to try out an idea which he called the unit-dose concept.

I wrote and submitted three major grant proposals. One was for research on medication errors, and the second was on unit dose. The third was different, a fellowship for a Ph.D. in health systems research. The two proposals for over a million dollars to conduct such research was funded, but not the one to learn how. That was my introduction to the wacky world of grantsmanship. So, I learned by trial and error. It was a wonderful learning experience, and I got hooked on research.

I read that the subject most frequently addressed by previous Remington award winners was devoted to pharmacy education: the second was pharmacy practice. I have always thought of myself as a practitioner who went into academics to learn how to help solve practice problems. I was encouraged by leaders like David Knapp and Melvin Green who told us back in 1977 that nearly all general practice would take place at the community level; that the community pharmacist would retain his centrist position even though the character of this practice may change; and there would be a "rather desperate need for research on ways to make community practice more effective." Research on pharmacy practice became the central focus on my career.

The ultimate purpose of research is to contribute to theory. I'm now going to talk about the development of pharmacy practice theory, and how it relates to quilt making. I know something about the former. I knew nothing about the latter until I married a quilter. In a good marriage you learn from each other, and I have learned a lot from my wife, Louise. Do you picture little old ladies doing handiwork on quilts by candlelight? Get with it! Today's quilters sit at their computers in the evening, and use a program called "Interquilt" to trade patterns worldwide.

My "honey, I'm home" is greeted by my wife's report that New Zealand is just checking in, and a quilter in Iceland needs help. If you sneak up behind a quilter and look over her shoulder as she works on her computer, you might read about tricks for hiding the quilt pieces from "DH" (dear hubby). My favorite, "keep them in the deep freeze, labeled meatloaf." Quilt makers also talk funny. "Batting" has nothing to do with baseball; it's the cotton stuff that they put in the middle of a quilt. "Fat Quarters" is a way of measuring fabric, involving math that only quilters understand.

My theme is simply this. The work of Donald Brodie and the Millis Commission began a new theory of pharmacy practice, whose construction is well under way. I propose to explain why I think it will work, and why things will turn out Okay. Quilt making isn't easy. It involves considerable geometry and rigor. For example, the points have to be sharp. Not all of the points of our developing theory of pharmacy are sharp yet, but we're working on it. And we need it badly, for protection from the "cold," turf wars threatening the patient pharmacist covenant, and the warmth of that mutual trust.

During my career, it has been my privilege to observe some of our best quilt makers at work. In constructing a quilt, the squares are made first, and finally they are all sewn together. Those I have watched and the squares they have contributed to modern pharmacy practice theory include the following.

1. Don Francke: The conceptualization of a very new role.
2. Donald Brodie: Speak up for the need for a theoretical base to our practice.
3. Bill Smith: First quantify the cost effectiveness of the new "clinical practice."
4. William Heller: On the formulary system, our role in compounding admixtures and reformulating the *USP*.
5. Bob Bogash: Anticipating automated dispensing video.
6. Allen Brands: Re-engineering the pharmacist-patient interface in the Indian Health Service.
7. Paul Parker: Marketing the development of our new pharmacy practice.
8. William S. Apple: The pharmacist role in healthcare economics.
9. Richard Penna: Positioning pharmaceutical care in the politics of healthcare.
10. Fred Eckel: On the role of research in professional practice.

11. Robert C. Johnson: Developing ("synthesizing") a new model state pharmacy organization.
12. Joseph Oddis: The design and synthesis of a great national professional organization.
13. Carl Trinca: The design and synthesis of a great national academic organization.
14. Lloyd Allen: The resurrection of compounding in pharmacy.
15. Sam Kidder: The "square" for consulting pharmacy.
16. Doug Hepler and Linda Strand: Conceptualizing how to put all this theory into practice, under the label of "Pharmaceutical Care."
17. John Gans, Lucinda Maine, and Lyle Bootman: Collecting and presenting the evidence on why patients need our new role.

Speaking of presenting evidence, we pharmacists present our results at APhA annual meetings. Quitters take their quilts to their own convention where thirty thousand women gather to show and see quilts. Hotel rooms are sold out three years in advance, and they spend eight to ten million dollars on quilting. If you think we have a problem of listing co-authors on our research reports, keep in mind that quilters may have 20 or more persons working on a single quilt.

What do we need to do now? Pharmacy's quilt pieces are done, and it's time to bring them together. For many in pharmacy it's cold. They are in danger of being frozen out, and the old quilt of regulatory protection has worn thin. Our young pharmacists and students are looking to us for help.

I'm optimistic. I believe we can implement our new theory of pharmacy practice now for some very good reasons. Our external environment has changed. The famous marketing book, *Positioning*, makes the point that it does no good to tell your story until somebody's ready to listen. The market is now ready and listening. I believe we are prepared to offer what every survey, namely that they show that the public most wants a health professional who is effective and accessible, and someone they can trust. We command the most effective drug therapy; we are accessible; and we are first in the public's trust.

I have seen the evidence. In the last five years, our department at Auburn has been involved in re-engineering projects involving hospitals, health maintenance organizations, and drug chains. The charge has been to redefine the role of the pharmacist, and redeploy them for maximum value. Our model is "Pharmaceutical Care." It has not been easy. The points had to be "real world" sharp, but it is really working. Colleges of pharmacy are finding the same. The "Pharmaceutical Outcomes" projects are supporting this movement.

In closing, I urge three things. The first is to recognize where we are in the process since most of our squares are done. The second is to remember who we are as we bring it all together. When quilters travel, they e-mail ahead, and the quilters in the next city meet and take care of them. I asked my wife, "You climb into a car with a stranger? Aren't you afraid of muggers?" She said, "Mugged by a quilter?"

This reminded me that pharmacy has been like that. Go anywhere, and a pharmacist will help you. Gloria Francke in her Remington address spoke of that "thread that ties us all together; we are all pharmacists." We need fellowship to work together better. We have had some exceptional leaders in pharmacy. But like many Americans, we can be poor followers, uninformed, and then unforgiving. Today, the leaders of our pharmacy organizations are bringing this quilt together in an unprecedented way. Never have I seen pharmacy so unified in self-concept, nor our leaders so deserving of our support.

My last point is for my fellow academics. Our new unified theory of pharmacy practice is a "quilt" designed to be used. This is no academic exercise; it is about the core of our practice. As Jordan Cohen points out, the objectives of education and practice have never been better aligned. The quilters have a little poem for baby quilts about this:

We expect you to lie on your quilt.
If you hurt, you may cry on your quilt.
On a cold rainy night, Don't you fret, you're all right;
You'll be snug, warm, and dry on your quilt.

Our new quilt won't keep us from pain, but it can keep us together and warm in the knowledge of who we are as we grow into our new role in health care. There are many pharmacy quilters who have contributed squares to our quilt. I myself will be happy to be remembered as one who contributed a few squares. ■

1999 Remington Medalist

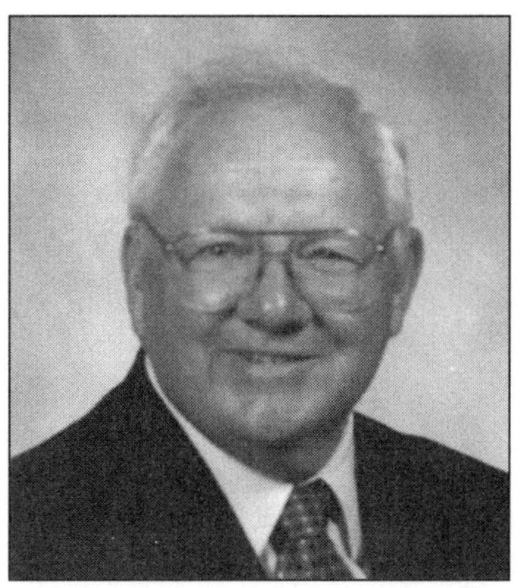

Carl Franklin Emswiller, Jr.

Carl Franklin Emswiller, Jr. was born in Washington, D.C., October 21, 1935, and graduated with a B.S. degree in Pharmacy 1962 from the Medical College of Virginia. The same year, he joined Eugene V. White in Berryville, Virginia, as an associate pharmacist. In 1968, he purchased his own pharmacy in Leesburg, Virginia; in 1974 he moved his practice to the Jackson Professional Building in Leesburg converting it to a clinically oriented office practice which he operated until his retirement in 2000. He served as associate clinical professor for his alma mater's clerkship program 1973-2000; Northern Virginia Society of Pharmacists secretary-treasurer, vice president, and president 1963-1966; Virginia Pharmaceutical Association executive council 1965-1968; Virginia State Board of Pharmacy chairman 1991-1993; and American College of Apothecaries vice-president, president, and Board chairman 1990-1994.

Emswiller joined the American Pharmaceutical Association in 1962, serving APhA Academy of Pharmacy Practice executive board 1975-1979; *American Pharmacy* editorial advisory board 1977-1982; APhA Educational Affairs Committee chairman 1980; reviewer for several editions of the *Handbook of Nonprescription Drugs*; and was elected in 2001 to the APhA Foundation board of directors. He was also inducted into the National Academies of Practice in 2000 serving as Pharmacy Section vice chairman.

A ROAD LESS TRAVELED

Carl Franklin Emswiller, Jr.

The 1999 Remington Medal was presented March 7, 1999, during the American Pharmaceutical Association annual meeting in San Antonio, Texas, March 5-9, 1999. Emswiller's address was published in the *Journal of the American Pharmaceutical Association*, Supplement 1, pp. 1-3, July-August 1999.

I have been fortunate in my career by having been associated with extraordinary people. The first was my dean, Warren E. Weaver. The second was Eugene V. White, a community pharmacist in Berryville, Virginia. The third is George Archambault, the 109th president of the American Pharmaceutical Association. These three have had a profound impact on American Pharmacy and it has been my good fortune to have known all of them on a very personal basis.

The 1999 Remington Honor Medal is the most significant recognition and honor that I have ever received. I was fortunate to have been a participant in the Remington Honor Medal program in April 1979 when the 1978 recipient, Eugene V. White, was honored. Having been an associate of Gene's for six years, I did not think I would ever be happier or more proud than I was for Gene that night. And I must admit, it was not a road that I ever thought of as one which I would ever travel.

I chose the title of my address, "A Road Less Traveled," based on the poem by Robert Frost entitled *The Road Not Taken*. In this poem, the speaker approaches a point where two roads diverge, and he chooses the "one less traveled," rather than the "road not taken."

The very first good thing to happen to me after I passed my state boards was to become associated in practice with Eugene White in Berryville, Virginia. Gene had already converted his pharmacy into an office practice when I joined him in 1962. His tutelage and leadership in the profession of pharmacy would set examples and standards for me that are still in place some 37 years later. Early in my career, through Gene's leadership and contacts, I was exposed to many other top leaders in pharmacy. It seemed like the whole world of pharmacy came to Berryville to see this new way of practice Gene had created.

For those who could not come to Berryville, the APhA and McKesson and Robins collaborated and built a prototype of what was then called "The Pharmaceutical Center" which premiered in 1965 at the APhA's annual meeting in Detroit. Seven pharmacists who were already practicing in this environment staffed the exhibit to explain the various areas of the practice in an office setting. I was assigned to the patient medication records area to explain the information pharmacists should collect from patients in order to use these records in practicing "clinical pharmacy" or "pharmaceutical care."

It was an exciting time in pharmacy. The profession was charged; you could feel it in the conversations at that meeting. Many pharmacists waited in long lines for hours to go through the exhibit again and again. Those of us who staffed the exhibit literally talked until we began to lose our voices. I can remember being especially impressed when one pharmacist told me, "This is my third time through this exhibit and I've got just one more question." Just think of the hours this pharmacist waited to ask one more question. Now I realize that we were just beginning to learn what patient information we needed to gather and how to organize it and use it in a meaningful way.

Computers were still not in wide use, and the records we kept and used were manually transcribed.

Upon return from that exciting meeting in Detroit, Gene and I had conversations that led us to believe that all of community pharmacy practice would be in an office setting by the year 2000. After all, why not? Wasn't this a new opportunity to practice pharmacy as so many pharmacists said they wanted to practice? Wasn't this yet another road to travel?

I believed it was, and so in 1968 I left Berryville to purchase my own practice in Leesburg, Virginia. While the practice I bought was a traditional pharmacy, from the first day I took over I used patient medication records. It took some time for patients and physicians to understand how what I did in my practice could benefit them, and little by little they accepted the benefits. In 1974 a medical office building was constructed near the local hospital in Leesburg. Many of the physicians relocated their practices into this building, and they encouraged me to move my practice into the building. I did and made it an office practice. Nothing commercially on display. A truly professional environment.

I also added one more thing that I considered vitally important, a private area to talk with patients. This consulting office has been and is being used for various patient monitoring activities, such as blood pressure, glucose and cholesterol screenings. It has become a patient education area as well as a private consulting area.

I continued to develop and revise patient information forms that would help me to become a stronger and more useful part of the triage between the pharmacist, the patient, and the physician. While some of these forms are still used, there is no doubt that the use of computers has increased our capacity to perform important functions for the patient.

Now we are on the eve of the new millennium, but not all of community pharmacy practice is in an office setting. I have to wonder why? Was it that we did not really believe we could perform these new functions? Were we not educated enough in patient care to practice differently than we had in the past? Did all pharmacy practitioners, as well as academia, and industry, really believe this was the future of community practice?

If we did, then I am at a loss to explain where we are in community practice on the eve of the new millennium. We had 30 years to make beneficial and useful changes, yet it seems it was not until OBRA laws demanded that we perform certain functions that we even began to prepare for practice in the next century.

Pharmacotherapy should be our forte today, and I now believe that it will be in our future. It will happen as we continue to educate and train for it, and it is a natural progression of pharmacy practice. Our success may come down to convincing managed care payers that we are the very best there is in performing that function. I am convinced, however, that we will meet the challenge and overcome the obstacles.

I have now been in my current practice setting for over 25 years. I have been there because I chose to be there. I have been privileged to do what I have been doing and it gives me a great sense of pride to say that I am a community pharmacy practitioner. But not all pharmacists have traveled the same road. I am particularly saddened by those young pharmacists who after only a year or two in practice are so disillusioned that some even say, "I hate pharmacy."

Let's examine some of the reasons young pharmacists are disillusioned with their profession after only a short time in practice. "Not enough time." "The workload doesn't allow me to counsel patients about their medications like I know I can." I hear these comments from young pharmacists nearly every day.

Managed care has said that reduced fees can be made up in volume. However, this practice only allows the pharmacist less time per patient and so we begin to take away the opportunities of what we are training pharmacists to do. The beginning of frustration!

Next, transmitting medication claims electronically sounds good until you can't get a claim through because of a returned electronic message that reads, "Patient coverage terminated," or "NDC not covered," or "Refill too soon," or "Use alternate brand," or "Brand name not covered." These are only a few of the reasons for unsuccessful adjudication of claims but each takes important time away from the pharmacist. Then there is the situation of a change in the patient's co-payment that no one has been advised of, or the patient has ignored, or is unaware of.

You can guess the conversation that occurs when a patient expects a $5 or $10 dollar co-pay and is met with a $20 co-pay. Again, pharmacist's time is taken up with dissatisfying functions. The result is, again, frustration. This is only compounded further by management and managed care both saying, "do more volume." But the economics of it say you must do it with less help because the economics of it does not allow for the help that is required. A frustrating situation. This situation must change and I believe it will. Managed care and insurance companies will eventually recognize the pharmacist's value and proper payment for these services will have to follow.

I am saddened also by what the pharmaceutical benefit managers, insurance companies, and managed care companies have done to our profession. I am concerned about the negative effect these forces have on health care in general. Patient's feel they are just a number and health care is no longer important.

While I do not pretend to know the ultimate road health care will travel, I do hope pharmacy will never lose sight of the fact that good health care, and, yes, good pharmacy care has and always will be a one-on-one situation. Whatever path we take to get us from where we are to where we are going will always require our efforts to be one-on-one.

That, I believe, is our great opportunity. It is a challenge, to be certain, with all that is going on within our profession, but it is also an opportunity. And that is where we can become very excited about the future of this profession. What is there to be excited about in the future? To name a few:

- Disease State Management: Asthma, diabetes, cholesterol, hypertension and anticoagulation management are but a few of the things in which pharmacists are becoming involved. While Mississippi is the first state to have Medicaid pay for the pharmacist's work in these areas, I am convinced others will follow. The next logical step is for private insurance to also cover these services.
- Prescribing Authority: Twenty-three states already allow pharmacists to write and change prescription orders under a physician's supervision. Nineteen other states have it under consideration. We have the documentation that proves we can save money in the health care system and can provide better patient care at the same time. But it cannot be done the way managed care is currently leading us. We must, therefore, take another road.
- Compounding: This has always been an exclusive legal right of this profession. We got away from it as manufacturers continued to proliferate, but there will always be a need to have a pharmacist individualize medications. Each person is different and so are their needs. Again, pharmacists have the skills to maximize medication outcomes necessitated by individual patient needs.

I believe that the opportunities for pharmacists in the next millennium will be exciting. I experienced that kind of excitement over 30 years ago when I entered this profession. Now I am near the end of my career, but if I were just starting out I think I could get just as excited now as I was then. There will be challenges and new destinations, and there will be new roads to get us there, but I truly believe the best is yet to come.

I would be remiss at this time if I did not acknowledge the support, encouragement and love rendered me by my wife, Jewell. She has always been there and enabled me to do so many of the things in life that I have done. In many ways, she has been one of pharmacy's strongest advocates. She knew the story and never hesitated to tell it like it was. I am very thankful to her for the road we have traveled together. ■

2000 Remington Medalist

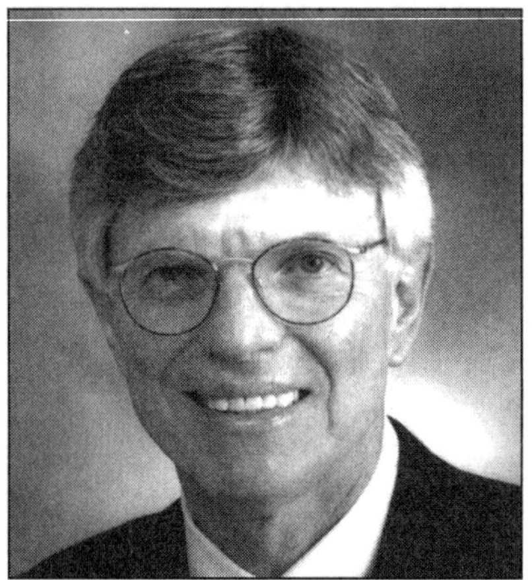

Daniel Aloysius Nona

Daniel Aloysius Nona was born in Chicago, Illinois, November 12, 1935, and received his B.S. in pharmacy 1958, M.S. in 1963, and Ph.D. in pharmaceutics in 1967 all from the University of Illinois. After service as a hospital pharmacist at the University of Illinois Hospitals 1958-1962, he joined the faculty of his alma mater as assistant professor 1967-1970, associate professor 1970-1973, and professor 1973-1974. He also served as Argonne Laboratories research associate 1967-1973, and Illinois State Board of Pharmacy member 1968-1974 and chairman 1971-1974.

Nona became American Council on Pharmaceutical Education executive director in 1974 where he served until his retirement in 1999. During this period, he provided leadership for reform in pharmaceutical education, including the stimulus for change in standards that resulted in the Doctor of Pharmacy degree as the sole entry degree. He also instituted a program to assure pharmacists of quality continuing education program including certificate programs. Following his retirement, he served as American Council on Pharmaceutical Education senior fellow 1999-2000; University of Illinois professor emeritus he was given in 1974, and AACP executive director emeritus since 2000.

ACCREDITATION STANDARDS FOR PHARMACEUTICAL EDUCATION

Daniel Aloyius Nona

The 2000 Remington Medal was presented March 12, 2000, during the American Pharmaceutical Association annual meeting in Washington, D.C, March 10-14, 2000. Nona's address was published in the *Journal of the American Pharmaceutical Association*, Supplement 1, pages S19-S24, September-October 2000.

When John Gans presented me with the option of three past recipients of the Remington Honor Medal to be master of ceremonies, I indicated that I would be privileged to have any one them serve. However, I offered a fourth possibility, if he would be willing, that of Grover Bowles, a past president of the American Council on Pharmaceutical Education (ACPE), and a long-time friend and mentor.

Grover is known as a man of few words. But his words, I have learned, are acute and incisive. Early in my tenure with the Council, Grover and I were walking through the hallways at a meeting, when we overheard a passerby remark to his colleague, "There, with Grover Bowles, is that young, upstart executive director of ACPE. We need to keep an eye on him." After a decent interval passed, Grover observed: "It's extraordinary how soon one gets known in pharmacy." The Remington Honor Medal is, indeed, a great honor. A personal honor, for sure, but also, a collective honor for the ACPE, its members and staff, both past and present.

Shakespeare wrote that we are authors of ourselves. If this is true, it should be understood that this author has plagiarized from many sources, for this recognition simultaneously honors many who have been a part of who I am, and what I may have contributed. In the preface to my master's thesis completed now so many years ago, I cited a saying attributed to Francis Bacon, which I have attempted to follow throughout my professional life. Bacon states that professionals are debtors to their profession; for as members of a profession seeking to receive countenance and profit, so too ought they of duty, to endeavor themselves by way of amends to be a help and ornament.

I am, indeed, a debtor to several exemplary practitioners who suggested that a youthful high school boy consider pharmacy. Professor Martin Blake urged me to pursue graduate studies, and Fred Mahaffey, then executive director of the National Association of Boards of Pharmacy, encouraged me to pursue the position with ACPE, in a curious, but memorable way. When Fred detected that I was Hamlet-like in deciding on continuation of teaching, knowing my love for students, or embarking upon a new and uncertain career pathway, he recalled the wisdom of that distinguished philosopher, Mae West, whom he quoted as saying, "Between two evils, I always pick the one I never tried before."

A debtor, certainly, to ACPE member Harold Godwin and former Council member Mike Schwartz, who toiled so hard to make me look good in the Remington selection process. I want, also, to acknowledge my colleagues at ACPE, Jeff Wadelin, Kimberly Werner, Ulric Chung, Dimitra Vrahnos, and Lynn Moen, who have contributed so much. And, I extend good wishes to my successor, Peter Vlasses; to present Council members (John Mauger, Bob Osterhaus, Judy Christensen, Ted Matthews, Mary Anne Koda-Kimble, Dennis Helling, Terry Short,

Paul Boisseau, Mike Hart, and Whit Moose); to all the past Council members, with particular recognition of those courageous members, particularly Tip [Varro] Tyler, Mary [Munson] Runge, and David Krigstein, who, in 1974, took a chance on a young professor, rosy in outlook but green in experience; and, of course, to family members and to special friends and counselors, Henri Manasse and John Russell.

A debtor, for sure, but with regard to being an ornament, I think of Oscar Wilde's observations as he toured the wild west of the 1890s, where in a raucous saloon he noted a sign reading "Please do not shoot the piano player, he is doing his best." Like that piano player, I tried my best.

To be added to the list of past recipients of this award since 1919 is daunting. But I maintain perspective by noting that of these 70 medalists, almost one third have been associated with ACPE at some point in their professional lives. So my being here may not relate so much to any contributions I may have made, but rather, to my wise career choice and the statistical edge offered by affiliating myself with ACPE.

A collective honor, too, in that any individual achievement realized is also a reflection of the work of the entire profession through the agency of ACPE. It takes many elements to produce a distinguished profession and establish national educational standards. An accreditation process enabling public decisions regarding adherence to the standards so set, is clearly one of them.

While standards and accreditation may be easily presented as quality assurance and quality enhancement, it involves a complex process, often little understood by practitioners and academics alike. A process that is, at once, a fortress of steel and a house of cards, with an outcome that is dependent upon the involvement and acceptance of pharmacy's community of interests. Its high passion necessitates a low profile, adding to perceptions of mystery and magic. Standards and accreditation rest on ideas and words such as professional, appropriate, adequate, judgment, and quality. In dealing with a process that hinges on such soft terms, it is easy to imagine the difficulties in mediating differences among people who do not agree on what it is that they do not agree, and on which they often disagree vigorously and emotionally. Indeed, a love-hate relationship appears to exist for standards and accreditation, recalling the Woody Allen story about the man who complains about his eccentric brother who thinks he is a chicken. The man would like to have the brother put away somewhere, but he has come to depend upon the eggs.

But where would our profession be without the eggs? I believe we can answer the egg question with succinct consideration of our educational standards as they evolved, and the impact of those standards on pharmaceutical education and pharmacy practice. Accordingly, I have chosen to tell a brief history of the present, which, in fact, is a story of progress in pharmaceutical education, and fundamental to progress for pharmacy practice. I have chosen the accreditation standards to be our storyteller since standards, by derivation, encompass, across the spectrum of time, everything and everyone in the profession of pharmacy: individuals, practitioner and academic organizations, policies, resolutions, key studies, and task forces. All, for the most part, represent a consensus, at a particular point in time.

Giving off-stage voice to our story is a Greek chorus of past Remington medalists whose comments, culled from their acceptance addresses, are intended to serve as surrogates for the great number of leaders who have contributed so much for so long. It should be underscored that this record of progress is presented, not as a history lesson, but rather as a guide for the future. For, in my view, trying to plan for the future without a sense of history, is like trying to plant cut flowers.

We begin our story in 1932, with a call by the profession to establish standards for colleges of pharmacy, *vis--vis*, the convening by the profession of an organization called the American Council on Pharmaceutical Education, or ACPE as it is affectionately known, to serve as the standard setting, accrediting agency.

The first standards for colleges of pharmacy were developed during the years 1932 to 1937. These standards were strongly influenced by a broadly based study of the profession, conducted during the 1920s by W. W. Charters. This study culminated in a report entitled *Basic Material for a Pharmaceutical Curriculum*. This study was initiated, in large measure, as a result of the profession's concerns for the lesser role and rank given to pharmacists in the armed services during the first World War.

The Surgeon General's low opinion concerning the pharmacist as a professional was influenced by the negative impression of pharmacy's educational requirements. The curriculum study of Charters provided the stimulus for sweeping changes in pharmaceutical education and pointed pharmacy practice in a new direction. The study uncovered the broad health care activities and responsibilities of the pharmacist who was seen as an autonomous health care practitioner with patients who have various needs, and who was accountable to the public served.

Of critical importance, the Charters study related pharmacists, as professionals, to the quality and quantity of their education. A four-year collegiate-based program was seen as an important beginning for the profession. Accordingly, the first standards codified the educational essentials set forth, stating that the baccalaureate in pharmacy degree, and that degree only, should be given for the completion of the new four-year course of study.

The first standards reflected a professional revolution, with replacement of the two-year (Ph.G.), and three-year (Ph.C.) programs. In addition, the lingering debate of the merits of requiring a high school diploma for entry to the profession was laid to rest. For curricular content, the new standards relied on practitioner documents already in existence, namely the *Pharmaceutical Syllabus* and the *Basic Material for a Pharmaceutical Curriculum*.

Other standards focused upon the development of a solid collegiate infrastructure to support the curricular content and its delivery, such as: organizational requirements for an independent college or as a college that was part of an institution; the development of a faculty of adequate size and quality; appropriate class sizes; collegiate admission requirements; and adequate equipment and physical facilities. With little or no infrastructure of note in many cases, adherence to these standards necessitated much work on the part on many for a long period of time.

Revisions of standards continued during the 1940s and early 1950s. These refinements took into account the momentous *Pharmaceutical Survey* of 1948, produced under the leadership of Edward C. Elliott, and with the assistance, once again, of W. W. Charters. This survey provided a blueprint for the advancement of pharmacy practice and, its correlative, the further development of pharmaceutical education. In partial response to the Elliot Report, the revised standards adopted specific curricular content, with deletion of curricular guidance previously offered by the *Pharmaceutical Syllabus* and *Basic Materials* documents.

Acceptance of the Elliott report's recommendation that the American Foundation for Pharmaceutical Education provide funding for ACPE adequate to support a full-time staff officer was, from my perspective, also an important development. While the Elliott Report's observation regarding the desirability of a six-year program leading to the professional doctoral degree was left to another generation to wrestle to the ground, it did spawn further professional study and debate. The standards revision of 1960 considered this debate, and incorporated the compromise position of a five-year baccalaureate in pharmacy program and a doctor of pharmacy degree based upon a four-year professional program, preceded by two years of pre-professional studies.

The *Pharmaceutical Curricula*, a report prepared by Lloyd Blauch, of the U.S. Office of Education, and George Webster of the University of Illinois, concluded that during the first half of the 20th century, pharmaceutical education moved from a chaotic condition to a fairly well-organized and standardized system. Moreover, it stated that the steps forward were usually opposed, but in spite of this, progress was made. These authors foresaw an important role for ACPE to play in the future progress of the curriculum, as if observing that the standards setting process of the profession now had plenty of teeth, although for the moment, were still buried, as in a newborn's gums.

A critical issue during these formative years was the need to achieve acceptance, not only of the standards, but also of the often difficult accreditation actions based upon them. This meant allaying fears of deans, faculties, students, alumni, practitioners, and boards of pharmacy. Toward this end, the acceptance of the standards and accreditation decisions benefited from the relentless support of the profession's leaders who may be represented in our story by the wisdom sung by the Greek chorus of past Remington medalists.

The 1933 medalist, Evander F. Kelly, referred to the importance of education as presented by W. W. Charters, especially the pharmacist's role in public health. J. Leon Lascoff, the 1937 medalist, a practitioner and chair of the first edition of the *Pharmaceutical Recipe Book*, promoted standards development as "one of the most constructive things ever undertaken in our field." It is, he proclaimed, "certain to better our teaching institutions and is bound to produce better educated and thus better qualified pharmacists." Lascoff continued, "These factors are fundamental and certain to result in elevating the standards throughout the field."

Subsequent medalists, including 1943 medalist Robert P. Fischelis, and the 1944 medalist Harvey Evert Kendig, promoted improved education through better standards. The 1947 medalist, Rufus Lyman, urged the continued development of our educational standards, and with frustration wrapped in dark humor, opined, "What pharmacy needs most is the funerals of a lot of deans." While occasionally tempted to yield to such sentiments, we will see that the profession has been able to make progress without anyone going away, at least not that far. Indeed, in 1949, medalist Ernest Little, stated with pride the progress made in pharmaceutical education since the formation of ACPE, and discussed the future impact upon standards as a result of following the Elliott report.

In 1952, medalist Patrick Costello predicted that the development of educational standards for accreditation may well become an important factor, if not the dominant one, in determining the future contributions of pharmacy as a member of the health professions. 1953 medalist Hugh Muldoon, in discussing the then instant issue before the profession of a five or six year program, noted that the programs were of four years' duration since 1932, and advocated curricular changes. Muldoon noted that ACPE had an enormous influence in promoting the development of our colleges, physically, academically, and professionally, and referred to ACPE as a milestone in modern pharmaceutical education, whereby university administrations and boards of pharmacy rely on ACPE judgments and accept its decisions.

The standards adopted in the mid-1970s presented a transforming basis for pharmaceutical education. Standards for two separate and distinct entry-level, professional programs were presented: the baccalaureate in pharmacy program, customarily five years in duration, and the doctor of pharmacy program, customarily six years, although a post-baccalaureate manner of admission of one or two additional years was enabled for those baccalaureate in pharmacy graduates wanting to purse additional professional education. Curricular standards for the baccalaureate in pharmacy program required sound science underpinnings as well as practice experiences in patient care areas, community pharmacies, and institutional pharmacies. Now, for the first time, the curriculum in pharmacy was required to include practice experiences, then called clerkships and externships, under the supervision of a preceptor, or coach, who corrected wrong moves and required that right ones be made.

In tandem with the substantive changes in baccalaureate in pharmacy programs, the doctor of pharmacy program option was defined as a practice-oriented curriculum, rather than as a graduate program; this was an organizational and jurisdictional factor important to the future of the program. The program was enriched with biomedical knowledge and clinical experiences significantly beyond that provided by the baccalaureate in pharmacy program. Development of the two professional programs in pharmacy, in keeping with these standards, required accommodation of the new by alteration or elimination of the old.

Once again, our standards needed to deal with foundational and infrastructure changes, particularly the identification and development of practice facilities. Moreover, delivery of the curricula required the acquisition of substantial numbers of a new breed of faculty, namely full-time pharmacy practice faculty and voluntary practice faculty, or preceptors, resulting in a mix of science and practice faculty, thereby creating a significant cultural change in our colleges. The inclusion of an experiential component in the baccalaureate in pharmacy program, then but 400 hours or the equivalent of an academic quarter, prompted comprehensive curricular editing and reform. The new type of faculty, with expanded faculty voting rights and other governance changes, began to shape the future. This growth process, however, was not always pretty.

Once again and at a critical time, the profession's leadership supported the standards. Greek chorister and the 1973 Remington medalist, Grover Bowles, urged improvement in preparation of graduates for the humanistic responsibilities of professionalism and spoke to the need for continuing education and its inculcation during the formative years of the student. The 1974 Remington medalist, Lloyd Parks, noted the challenges that the new standards presented and urged our pharmaceutical science faculties, to whose vested interests the new standards represented a threat, to exhibit educational statesmanship. In 1975, medalist Melvin Green proffered that these new standards would better relate our education to that of the other health professions; the 1976 medalist, David Krigstein, lamented the lack of decisiveness on the part of the profession by not accepting the Elliott survey recommendation regarding timely movement to the doctor of pharmacy program.

The revisions of the 1980s refined the baccalaureate in pharmacy standards and expanded upon curricular expectations for the doctor of pharmacy program by adopting, in large measure, guidelines formulated over the previous years. In addition, accountability was formalized through the interplay of process and outcomes. Indicators for student achievement and educational outcomes were set forth so as to demonstrate, with appropriate evidence (such as performance on standardized licensure examinations), the success of the program in attaining its objectives. While somewhat ahead of their time, these standards also encouraged colleges of pharmacy, which offered a doctor of pharmacy program, to explore and contribute to the development of external and other non-traditional programmatic approaches to award the degree for baccalaureate-degreed pharmacists already in practice.

The idea of the doctor of pharmacy curriculum as the sole program continued as the elephant in pharmacy's tent, unspoken, but not unnoticed. During the revision process of the 1980s, several commentators suggested that the time had now come to complete the transitional system of two entry-level programs and develop standards by which the doctor of pharmacy program would become the sole professional degree program.

The 1985 medalist, William Blockstein, cited the APhA Task Force on Pharmacy Education calling for evolution to the doctor of pharmacy degree for entry to practice, noting the changing responsibilities of tomorrow's pharmacists. However, the standards, adopted in 1985, did not reflect this point of view, sensing that the timing for such a change was not yet right. Distinctive standards for the two professional programs were maintained. The issue continued to be discussed by both educators and practitioners, emerging as an "if" rather than a "when" proposition. The when, for some, was preferably long after they were safely in the grave.

In September 1989, ACPE issued its intention to propose new standards that would consider the convergence of historical initiatives, current practice developments, and future practice challenges. The revised standards would be proposed in a manner that would merge the two programmatic standards with a focus on a doctor of pharmacy program. The wording "a doctor of pharmacy program" was stressed, rather than "the doctor of pharmacy program," to signify the opportunity to re-imagine the system of pre-service pharmaceutical education and to symbolize the goal of curricular reform. Wholesome discussion and full airing of differences of opinion were expected and welcomed as a part of the time-tested forum of the standards revision process. Rather than another narrow or abstract debate about "two degrees" or about the length of the curriculum, this long-standing issue was intended to be reviewed within the constructs of the customary dialog surrounding the periodic revision of standards, with a stepwise, multiyear procedure.

Well, dialog there was, but customary it was not. As with James Bond's martini, the profession was shaken, not stirred. While standards setting often serves as a target for professional differences, this revision process included a strong contingent from the "fire, aim, ready" school of marksmanship. However, the strength, inclusiveness, and tenacity of the long-term process enabled the balancing of competing interests and concerns. The process, while arduous, achieved a consensus and a widely accepted outcome, as may be attested to by the fact that over 90 percent of the colleges are ahead of the implementation date of July 2000. The remaining colleges are right on schedule, and none are behind. To many students, and prospective students, this issue is already ancient history.

As in the earlier part of our story, professional leaders weighed in on the directions of pharmaceutical education, and particularly, the need for accreditation standards to reflect and foster the changes they forecast. These sentiments are reflected by the comments of 1989 Remington medalist Lawrence Weaver, and emphatically by 1990 medalist Joseph Oddis, who heard echoes from medalist Muldoon, marking improved standards as the foundation of our profession. Joseph Oddis noted that the revision process, then underway, was a part of a crucial mission for our profession, an exploration to determine the appropriate educational standards for practice in the 21st century. Medalists Jere Goyan (1992) and Robert C. Johnson (1993) were forceful advocates for educational preparedness for all students at the doctor of pharmacy level.

While outcomes for standards adopted since 1932 can be demonstrated in various ways, it is apparent to all that the profession has succeeded in standardizing our educational processes, and has enabled the most effective licensing system in the health professions. The standards have uplifted pharmacy education within the higher education system, becoming jewels among the academic units of the universities, both in professional education and in scholarship. While the standards have supported uniformity of process, space has been provided for faculty creativity in the development and delivery of the curriculum. The physical plants of our colleges and schools have emerged from basements to, in some instances, Taj Mahal knockoffs. And fundamentally, our graduates possess the professional competencies necessary to enter the profession, bringing to their practices stronger communication skills, new confidence, and assertive behaviors in support of their patients.

The successful outcomes registered for pre-service education engendered confidence and formed the profession's basis for the development of an accreditation process for providers of continuing education and, recently, for providers offering certificate programs. Deployment of the accreditation process has provided a uniform basis for the selection of quality continuing education offerings; has demonstrated the effectiveness and relationship between continuing education and continuing competence; and has provided a systematic process for improvement.

What progress might we reasonably predict from our new standards, those leading to the doctor of pharmacy degree? While nothing is as uncertain as the future, we can anticipate, with some certainty, that our new educational degree structure will ensure fairness to our students and assure the status deserving of our profession, our practitioners, and our patients. Also, we can, with a degree of certainty, predict that the curriculum will support the scope of contemporary practice responsibilities as well as emerging roles that ensure the rational use of drugs in the individual care of patients and patient populations. It can be said, too, that the curriculum will provide the professional competencies necessary to the delivery of pharmaceutical care in all practice settings, including and importantly for our future, in community pharmacies.

The new standards are concerned with what is presented as well as with how it is taught with assurances that it is learned. The new ways and means of teaching expected by the standards should not only be more effective, but also should yield happier learners, who, in turn, will relish lifelong learning and apply the good teaching they experience to counseling and educating patients. The increased involvement of practitioners in the governance of the colleges as well as in the design and teaching of the pharmacy practice component of the curriculum should ensure appropriate practice preparedness. New expectations for student services should foster leadership qualities, self-assuredness in students, and facilitate professionalization. Expectations for critical thinking should inculcate in the practitioner the need to expect the unexpected, to move beyond the search for black and white answers, and to understand the gray areas incumbent upon practitioners.

Emphasis on ethics should reveal that the secret to care of the patient is in caring for the patient. An environment for teaching and learning should be fostered that does not just tolerate but also celebrate the diversity of people, enabling pharmacists to practice effectively with every colleague and every patient. The educational design should support the wholeness of the science and art of pharmacy practice. Within that wholeness, the cataract may fall away, yielding a new clarity that is a humanistic practice. In this practice, patient and practitioner come together in a caring relationship; disease states become illness; curing becomes healing; business becomes service. Helping is not just extended from practitioner to patient, but also from patient to practitioner. Indeed, if our professional standards lead to a successful future, they will in effect have given our students the advice veteran circus performers give to those learning to perform on the flying trapeze; throw your heart over the bars and your body will follow.

Not a history lesson, I said, but a history engine to guide our profession's future. The standards now in place, along with those changes to follow, offer but a professional plan, an architectural design. Achievement of aspirations for competent and effective practitioners of the future, as envisioned by the standards, will require the profession in all its components not only to dream it, but also, to do it and to be it. Thank you all for this great honor. ■

2001 Remington Medalist

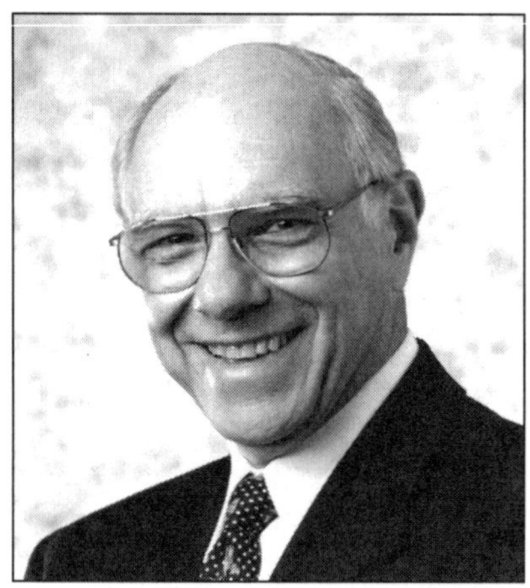

JEROME ARTHUR HALPERIN

Jerome Arthur Halperin was born in Paterson, New Jersey, February 21, 1937, receiving a 1958 B.Sc. in Pharmacy from Rutgers University; a 1962 Master of Public Health from Johns Hopkins School of Hygiene and Public Health; and a 1974 M.Sc. in Management from the Massachusetts Institute of Technology. From 1958 to 1983, he served as a U.S. Public Health Service commissioned officer variously in California, Illinois, Kansas, Massachusetts, New Mexico, New York, and finally in Washington, D.C. with the U.S. Food and Drug Administration. He subsequently served from 1983 to 1989 as vice president-technology for CIBA Consumer Pharmaceuticals, a division of CIBA-GEIGY.

Halperin then served as the U.S. Pharmacopeia chief executive officer and USP Convention secretary from 1990 to 2000. He has also served in various positions with the American Foundation for Pharmaceutical Education, the International Pharmaceutical Federation (FIP), the National Council for Patient Information and Education, the Pan American Health Organization, and the World Health Organization. In 2001, he became president and chief executive officer of the Food and Drug Law Institute, a position he still holds.

PHARMACY: A REPORT FROM THE 22ND CENTURY

Jerome Arthur Halperin

The 2001 Remington Medal was presented March 18, 2001, during the American Pharmaceutical Association annual meeting in San Francisco, California, March 16-20, 2001. A handout provided by Halperin and distributed at the Remington Dinner was published in the *Journal of the American Pharmaceutical Association*, Supplement 1, pp. S20-S24, September-October 2001. However, the following text as provided by Halperin is the actual presentation that was delivered.

I am Jerry Halperin. C3 is my designation as a third generation clone. I was created in the late 21st century and I am a pharmacist practicing in the year 2101. I was invited by the Jerry Halperin to report to you on the status of pharmacy in the 22nd Century. His Remington address provides his view of what would be necessary for pharmacy's success in the 22nd Century. I am here to tell you how it came out.

First, I should tell you a little about myself. I said I am a third generation clone. You may like to know how that came about. To celebrate the second millennium and APhA's sesquicentennial, APhA executive vice president John Gans inaugurated the Remington medalist DNA Bank to preserve genetic material from all living Remington medalists. He believed this would be a valuable contribution to pharmacy's posterity and a good revenue source for APhA.

As the first Remington medalist of the 21st Century, Jerry Halperin was given the honor of being the first contributor to the DNA Bank. Although human cloning did not become legal in the U.S. until 2035, APhA obtained special permission to create the first clone to begin the program in 2005. Barbara Halperin (C1), my "great grandmother," was offered the opportunity to gestate her husband's first clone. She declined. I believe her words recorded on the occasion were, "Thank you, but I've been carrying him for over 40 years already." A surrogate mother was recruited, a February *Playmate*....I forgot the year.

My father (C2) was cloned in the mid-21st century. By that time, transgenic technology had progressed to using other species for human gestation. By the time I came along, technology had progressed to ectogenesis, a technology of gestational pods, each essentially an artificial uterus to gestate a clone or an in-vitro fertilized egg.

In 2101, reproduction is considerably different than it was one hundred years ago. The dominant mode is procreation without pregnancy. Prospective parents now have choices. They can choose cloning, or they can order an *in-vitro* fertilized embryo with specific genetic qualities, such as enhanced intellectual or physical capacities or appearance. A surprising number of couples choose the 21st century method of reproduction which is still highly prized for its physiologic and recreational qualities.

Human cloning and genetic predetermination are not without controversies, even in 2101. They continue to pose significant challenges to our moral, social, and legal values. Civilization may value the contributions of another Leonardo da Vinci, William Shakespeare, Wolfgang Mozart, or Marie Curie, but it would feel quite differently about another Stalin, Hitler, or Pol Pot. Perhaps we have been lucky. We were concerned that parents would opt for athletic prowess or physical attractiveness, but parents who have selected genetic predetermination for their children have tended toward more socially valuable qualities, including intellectual honesty, compassion, and emotional intelligence.

There are twice as many of us living in the United States in 2101 (571 million) as compared with 2001 (281.4 million). We are also a more diverse society, and we are living longer too. Life spans for males increased from 74.1 years in 2000 to 88.0 years in 2100. Female life spans increased from 79.7 to 92.3 years over the same period.

The dominant medical technology in 2101 is Nanotechnology, the science of machines with self-replicating, reversible, variable speed motors, a trillionth of the size found in children's toys. We use therapeutic regenerators to heal wounds and burned skin. Most surgery has been replaced by noninvasive procedures employing nanotech assemblers and dissemblers to effect manufacture or repair at the cellular level. These nanotech devices are more accurate than their human counterparts for surgical procedures. They are also faster, less traumatic, and less expensive than surgical procedures. They have reduced and sometimes eliminated hospital stays. Nanotech robots ("nanobots") are in common use to prevent and repair problems before they become serious enough to be diagnosed and they serve as sophisticated drug delivery systems. Ultrasensitive nanotech sensors routinely read chemical base sequences of the DNA of individual molecules. It is interesting to note that the plans to build these devices and their modes of locomotion and action were first described in a textbook published in 2000.

The "one-size-fits-all" approach to 21st century medicines has been replaced entirely by a "one-size-fits-one (or few)" concept. Our medicines are based upon genomic concepts for individual patients and their personal genotypes. They have highly predictable and controlled onsets and durations of action. Most are entirely free of side-effects, helped by the presence of full genetic profiles on each person predicting the probability of side effects.

Most dosage forms are transdermal and have nanotech carriers. The Food and Drug Administration approved the first nanotech "drug" in 2033. Vaccines were retired in the 2040s when the diseases that required them were eradicated through genetic procedures that prevent the disease from developing or being transmitted. In the 2050s, implanted microcapsules with nanomechanical valves detect proteins from cancer cells and release just the right amount of anti-cancer drug at the exact location. AIDS was conquered in the 2020s, but before successful countermeasures appeared the disease claimed tens of millions of lives in Africa alone.

Inborn errors of metabolism, autoimmune diseases, deafness and other diseases and disabilities have been virtually eliminated. For the most part, diseases and congenital conditions are prevented, cured, or compensated for before conception or prevented or repaired in-utero or in the early months of life. Modern health technologies are genomic, robotic, or implanted. For example, about 60 years ago, we developed an artificial eye and an occipital lobe implant to correct blindness. We are virtually a disease free society, but, when genetic mutations in humans or other species result in new diseases, we have the technology to eliminate them, or at least curb potentially fatal conditions.

Consumers have also benefited from these changes. We no longer have problems of access to and payment for health care services. In this age of ultimately personal medicine, consumers have access to knowledge and services that are readily available, of high quality and free.

Pharmacy services now include routine visits by holographic pharmacists. The visits, available through home holographic imagers, may be programmed by a pharmacist or physician upon demand of a patient or consumer whenever necessary to monitor symptoms and progress. The results of these sessions are immediately transmitted to the patient's comprehensive medical record to alert the health care team of changes required in the medication regimen and to schedule follow-up visits.

We have fully exploited the genomes of humans, as well as food-producing animals and plants. Using this knowledge, we have maximized food production; bred healthier cattle, swine, poultry, and other food species; we have also created transgenic factories for medicines. By the middle of the 21st century, we found that it is more efficient and considerably less costly to grow protein (animal and vegetable) in cell culture. Through this technology, we have virtually abolished famine around the world and have ended forever concerns of animal diseases like the bovine spongiform encephalopathies (BSE) that plagued Europe 100 years ago.

The health professions went through considerable soul-searching and transition throughout the last century. They had grown closer through shared knowledge and use of expert systems used in practice. By the end of the second quarter of the 21st century, the combination of virtual reality and artificial intelligence technologies completely revolutionized education and teaching. This made it possible to balance the curricula scientifically, clinically, and culturally. Together, they eliminated the need for memorization, which had been necessary for professionals to master their disciplines.

During this transition, shared knowledge bases combined with shared training and interdependence in professional practice resulted in the individual professions treading on each other's turf. Each profession had a difficult time demonstrating its unique contributions to health care. For many years, efforts were made to combine the professions or create new ones. However, each profession steadfastly resisted, and medicine, pharmacy and nursing managed to retain their individual identities, but none is exactly like it was a century ago.

By 2065, English and Mandarin were the only languages in general use in science, commerce, and diplomacy. These two languages, coupled with the use of the global "UniNet" by more than 80 percent of people around the world, greatly facilitated global education and communication between health professionals and consumers, leading to better health services and improved health.

Good planning and concerted action throughout the 21st century enabled pharmacy to recognize that the profession was capable of much more than dispensing medicines and counseling patients. In 2001, pharmacists knew that they could do more. In addition to formulating and delivering new drugs, they knew they could also provide healing interactions, care, and reassurance.

In the 20th century, clinical pharmacy was thought to be that difference. It wasn't! In that same era, the concept of pharmaceutical care emerged. It had the potential to become that difference and pharmacists liked the way it sounded, but it still took three generations of pharmacists before they felt comfortable with the concept.

The attempt at defining pharmacy's unique contribution in the 21st century was the pharmacist-scientist who used genomic technologies to create the unique drugs and dosage forms for individual patients. Like nuclear pharmacy before it, however, this too became a niche practice, albeit an important one. It was neither unique to pharmacists nor broad enough for all to fit under its umbrella.

Nanotechnology opened new opportunities for pharmacists to merge that technology with genomic technologies to create drugs and dosage delivery mechanisms for the Age of Nanomedicine. Coupled with the expanded concept of pharmaceutical care, nanotechnology served as the uniting force with which pharmacists use their scientific, clinical, and cognitive skills to serve individual patients and their unique needs.

Twenty-first century pharmacy recognized that its challenge for success in the 22nd century was to determine its most valuable contribution to human health, and to bring that contribution into reality. That realization of the need to find its unique contribution awakened the profession.

Pharmacists recognized that they must make their contribution not just to one patient at a time, but also to humanity as a whole. Opportunity for humanitarian service became easier throughout the 21st century as the work decreased. Our work-week averages about 22 hours, while the work-week in your time averaged about 37.5 hours, and we now have more opportunity for humanitarian pursuits.

The *U.S. Healthy People 2010 Objectives* process established two overearching health goals for the U.S. in the first decade of the 21st century: longer years of life and elimination of health disparities. The U.S. policy paralleled the World Health Organization's *Health for All* vision which called for greater health equity, reflecting humanity's evolving perceptions of human rights.

American pharmacists joined together in addressing these overearching goals. They addressed questions about needless drug-related mortality and morbidity by joining the global dialogue examining legislative and regulatory requirements for placing and maintaining drugs on the market. Pharmacists advocated adequate testing, especially for the potential for serious or fatal adverse consequences. They sought better defined and more objective methods of determining appropriate benefit/risk ratios for drugs. They demanded mandatory protective mechanisms, including the skin tests to identify those persons who may be at risk of serious adverse reactions and must avoid the use of particular drugs.

Closer to home, pharmacists scrutinized their own practices and established procedures and safeguards to make them as free as possible from medication errors. Virtual reality, artificial intelligence, and new technologies have eliminated pharmacist-caused medication errors. Pharmacists also joined with other health professionals to guarantee equity in the cost of the delivery of health care. They recognized that only those people living in enlightened societies had a chance for long, healthy, productive lives.

To prepare for the challenges of the 22nd century, pharmacists in the 21st century addressed the need for pharmacy to have a clear, strong vision of its future. The prophet Isaiah said, "Without vision, the people will perish." But, merely having a vision is not enough. Pharmacy's vision requires continual tuning to assure that it stayed focussed on its Polar star so the profession knows where it is heading and why.

Pharmacy needed a vision of that strength to address its contributions to humanity and to invest each pharmacist with the understanding and satisfaction that he or she is contributing to creating structures and behaviors that will endure and serve humanity well. Pharmacy succeeded in creating a vision of such power and, in doing so, preserved and insured its future and its role in the service of humanity.

Your generations accomplished this feat in a creative way. Your leaders throughout the 21st century led a series of decennial conferences, held at the midpoints of the decades from 2005 through 2095. These decennial conferences established goals for the 22nd century in these areas:

(1) Pharmacy's unique contributions to humanity; (2) Content of pharmacy's knowledge base; (3) Commitment to adapting and employing new technologies in education, teaching, practice and research; (4) Pharmacy's contributions to ensuring optimum health outcomes; (5) Safety, equity, and cost-effectiveness in the provision of pharmacy services; and (6) Continual stretching of the profession's horizon to assure that it continues to aspire.

The French statesman Georges Clemenceau once said, "Generals cannot be trusted with anything, not even war." There were some that believed that this sentiment might also have applied to pharmacists' ability to envision their preferred future and to establish and achieve the goals necessary to attain it. They were wrong.

Pharmacists in the 21st century probably believed that they could have planned their future alone, but they were wise enough to know that they should not. Instead, pharmacists convened the decennial conferences, but they did not dominate them. Wisely, they included social scientists, ethicists, futurists, economists, legislators, biomedical scientists, and other health professionals.

Your leaders had a global view, recognizing that planning for pharmacy's future in the United States was important, but insufficient. Pharmacy is a global profession and its service to humanity knows no borders. American pharmacists engaged their colleagues around the world to join the efforts. They enlisted the World Health Organization, the International Pharmaceutical Federation, and other international and national organizations to join with them. Their efforts resulted in other countries beginning their own national planning efforts and joining into the global effort. These efforts led to another, parallel, system of international conferences held at the end of each decade to create a global vision and plan. These efforts also met with success and pharmacy was united and strong as the 22nd century dawned.

Your efforts throughout the 21st century extended pharmacy's horizons and energized the profession so that it entered the 22nd century better organized, surer of its place in the global health system, and confident of its contributions to humanity.

I have tried to describe pharmacy and its place in health care at the beginning of the 22nd century. If you like what you heard and want it to become reality, you have the knowledge and the capacities to make it happen. You only need the will.

It is now time for me to return to the Jerry Halperin whom you have honored with the Remington medal. There are many people who have been my mentors and without whose help I would not have received this honor. There are a few people whose influence on my career has been so profound and so valuable that I am compelled to express my appreciation to them.

George F. Archambault recruited me into the Public Health Service in 1958, and he provided guidance, leadership, and mentoring throughout my Public Health Service career. Jim Doluisio, who was chairman of the first U. S. Pharmacopeia Board on which I served, continues to be a valued mentor. William Heller, under whom I served for nine months, showed me what quiet leadership could accomplish. Clement Bezold, director of the Institute for Alternative Futures, guided my understanding that the future can be anticipated, forecasted, planned with alternative outcomes. J. Richard Crout, with whom I served as his deputy for six years, taught me who to inspire people to achieve personal goals that they did not believe they were capable of achieving. And Larry Weaver paid me the greatest compliment when he asked if he could nominate me for the Remington Honor Medal.

A special thank you to my wife, Barbara, and my daughters, Alicia and Rachel, who continue to be my resources and my encouragement to aspire. Truly, they have been the wind beneath my wings. They have all made this day one of the most memorable of my life. ■

2002 Remington Medalist

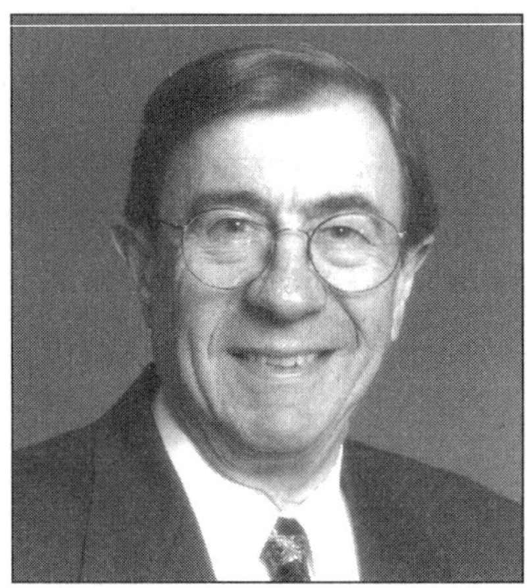

RICHARD P. PENNA

Richard Paul Penna was born in Palo Alto, California, September 7, 1935, and graduated with a B.S. Pharmacy in 1958 and Pharm.D. in 1959 from the University of California, San Francisco. He was a community pharmacist in Redwood City, California, 1959-1966, and assistant clinical professor at his alma mater 1961-1966. He served as Peninsula Pharmaceutical Society president 1960-1961, San Mateo Pharmaceutical Association president 1965-1966, and *California Pharmacy* pharmaceutical editor 1964-1966. He joined the staff of the American Pharmaceutical Association in 1966 serving as executive secretary of the Academy of General Practice of Pharmacy 1966-1973, director of professional affairs 1973-1983, director of the APhA *Handbook of Nonprescription Drugs* 1975-1980, secretary of the Board of Pharmaceutical Specialties 1976-1983, and vice president for professional affairs and Academy of Pharmacy Practice executive secretary 1983-1984. He also served on the National Health Council board of directors 1973-1980 and vice president 1977-1980.

Penna joined the staff of the American Association of Colleges of Pharmacy in 1985 serving as associate executive director 1985-1995, and executive vice president 1995-2002. He also served as Federation of Associations of Schools of the Health Professions treasurer 1998-2002. During his tenure at AACP, he helped to reshape pharmacy education to meet the changing needs of the profession.

Views From a Worker in Pharmacy's Vineyard

Richard Paul Penna

The 2002 Remington Medal was presented March 17, 2002, during the American Pharmaceutical Association annual meeting in Philadelphia, Pennsylvania, March 15-19, 2003. Penna's address was published in the *Journal of the American Pharmaceutical Association*, Supplement 1, pp. S10-S17, September-October 2002.

The American Pharmaceutical Association has recognized 73 Remington Honor Medalists since 1919. Their backgrounds span a spectrum of activities, duties, and responsibilities within the profession. There have been deans, faculty members, manufacturers, regulators, practitioners, and pharmacists from other sectors of our profession. A relatively small minority served their profession as staff of one of its professional societies, organizations, or trade groups. Many in this group served in the capacity of chief executive officer. The remaining, a very small minority (Justin Powers-1959, Gloria Francke-1987, and George Griffenhagen-1991), served as professional staff within organized pharmacy. Coming from this latter group has provided your 73rd recipient a rare opportunity not only to observe, but also to participate, in many of the momentous events that shaped our profession over the past three-and-a-half decades.

Laboring in pharmacy's vineyard during this prolonged time has allowed me to witness the profession debate, grow, expand, mature, fail, regroup, try again, succeed, revitalize itself, and then finally change its fundamental mission in serving the public. These observations have been invigorating, instructive, and sustaining. They stimulated and facilitated the maturing of my outlook on the profession in these later years, and they may be instructive to others as well.

Consequently, I have outlined, in no order of importance, a variety of issues and observations that may prove interesting and provocative.

Most professions, including the health professions, enjoy and employ throughout their existence a single mission that is the central core of their service to society. Changing their missions usually entails substantial disruption, and possibly disintegration of the profession. Within the past 20 years, pharmacy, optometry and, perhaps, nursing expanded their missions. However, pharmacy is unique among all the health professions in that this is the second time in our history that this has occurred. In the beginning, pharmacy's mission was to gather, assay, store, and distribute crude drugs for public use. Pharmacy also had the responsibility of fabricating dosage forms containing these drugs that were palatable, stable, and effective.

During the span of years between 1880 and 1900, the pharmaceutical industry grew up from a scientific base created by a growing pharmacy profession and assumed the responsibility of preparing dosage forms for public use. The profession maintained responsibility for drug standards and the science of drug development and product formulation. Pharmacists began to become involved with drug distribution. This created safe, efficient, accurate, and novel drug distribution systems to assure the public that dangerous and potent medications were stored safely and available when needed.

Seeds of pharmacy's third mission were sown in colleges and schools of pharmacy in the 1950s when pharmacology and expanded pharmaceutical chemistry courses enabled and encouraged students to critique drug action and compare therapeutic options. We saw signs of these curricular changes in the late 1960s when practitioners began to express their desires to help people make the best use of prescription and nonprescription medications. It wasn't long before pharmacy schools experimented by placing a practitioner in a nursing unit of a busy teaching hospital. This not only gave birth to the concept of clinical pharmacy, but also focused debate within the profession about how the profession should continue its evolutionary expansion.

Of course, the area into which pharmacy was expanding was considered the physician's realm, and organized medicine looked upon pharmacy's foray with mild amusement to outright contempt. Paradoxically, physicians teaching or training in those health centers in which pharmacists were practicing clinical pharmacy had nothing but praise for what these new practitioners were adding to the quality of pharmacotherapeutic decisions. Pharmacy still struggled with philosophical questions of roles, ethics, responsibilities, and relations with other health professions. At issue in early clinical pharmacy practice was that pharmacists advised and consulted with physicians regarding drug therapy. Pharmacists were not held responsible for their decisions; the profession had not professed a covenant between pharmacist and patient. These struggles came to a head in 1989 when Hepler and Strand articulated the philosophy of pharmaceutical care. The profession embraced the concept completely and expanded its mission to encompass the responsibility for outcomes of drug therapy and a commitment to patient care.

It is important to note that the profession has not abandoned product formulation and drug distribution as areas of professional responsibility. These remain critical and important functions. Our colleges and schools of pharmacy continue to prepare pharmaceutical scientists and generate new scientific knowledge in our academic research laboratories.

Over time, the profession expanded its responsibilities from product formulation to embracing drug distribution expertise and later to accepting the responsibility for pharmacotherapeutic outcomes. During each of these two transition periods, the profession engaged in intense discussions and debates related to whether all professionals must accept and practice according to the new paradigm. Recent debates related to the use of technicians and robotics in medication dispensing illustrates this tension resulting from our most recent expansion.

The profession has adopted pharmaceutical care as its new mission, and our colleges and schools have adapted and expanded their curricula to support this mission. However, we have only just begun this expansion. The profession has much further to go to *internalize* pharmaceutical care as an integral part of our professional *raison d'etre*. Some individual practitioners may provide pharmaceutical care, but the practice cannot be said to be profession wide. Moreover, pharmacy as a profession has not yet begun to behave like a profession of providers of pharmaceutical care. The public is quite aware of these deficiencies.

Two national and well-publicized reports from the Institute of Medicine (IOM) outlined in tragic detail the harm that medicines, inappropriately used, are inflicting on society. Of course, we in pharmacy were not surprised at these findings. Years before the IOM reports, our own research had documented the high personal and economic costs of drug-related illness. The trends in pharmacotherapy have been very clear. For the past 50 years, each new drug product approved for use has been more potent, more selective, more risky, and more expensive than the one it replaced. The explosive growth in direct-to-consumer advertising is achieving its goal of increasing drug use by U.S. patients. Switches of prescription medication to nonprescription use have increased the availability to the public of an array of effective, but potentially dangerous, treatments. Recent highly publicized market withdrawals of very useful, but dangerous medications, indicate that our drug use system increasingly is incapable of assuring patients that they will receive the best medications for their diagnoses.

Our medication use system is disintegrating before our very eyes. A pharmacotherapeutic leadership vacuum exists in our health care system. A profession needs to step forward to take leadership responsibility for designing and instituting safe and efficient medication use systems. There is no profession better positioned to initiate this leadership than pharmacy. We know drugs, how they work, their vast benefits, their dangers, their costs, and the complexities of their distribution. All the prescribing professions need to be involved in creating a new medication use system, but pharmacy is the profession that has the most comprehensive knowledge and experience to take the lead. Pharmacy took a major step in this direction when it developed the concept and adopted the policy of collaborative prescribing. Unfortunately, organized medicine and nursing have yet to appreciate the vast potential for the public good that this policy entails. We must convince them otherwise.

Recently, Kansas City pharmacist Robert Courtney pleaded guilty to diluting chemotherapeutic medication. The public's outcry over this terrible breach of trust reveals its profound feeling of betrayal by a health professional. The profession's response to this tragedy was timid and defensive. Society is waiting for pharmacy to step forward. If we are to achieve public confidence in pharmaceutical care, we must demonstrate publicly that we care deeply and passionately about how pharmaceuticals are used in society by individual patients.

All this having been said, a sea of change has taken place in pharmacy over the past 100 years. We have expanded from being concerned with the preparation of quality products to being concerned with and responsible for the patients who take these products. And pharmaceutical education played major roles in facilitating those expansions.

In other health professions, the relationship between the practice and educational sectors is an adversarial and contentious one. Not so in pharmacy. This is not to say that there is perfect harmony between practice and academia. On the contrary, there has always been a healthy tension between the two, but an active and respectful dialogue has also existed. That tension and dialogue have been responsible for many of the profession's advances over the past 100 years. The dialogue has resulted in a significant element of trust. Academic pharmacists alongside their practitioner colleagues have always played major roles in formulating policies and initiatives for the profession. As a result, academicians consistently are elected to responsible positions in practitioner organizations. For example, APhA president-elect Janet Engle and three of the past five APhA presidents are academicians. Half of the American Society of Health-System Pharmacists (ASHP) presidents during the past ten years have been from pharmaceutical education. At the American College of Clinical Pharmacy (ACCP), all but three of their presidents over the past 22 years have been from academia. This phenomenon is unique to pharmacy. It simply does not exist in other health professional practice organizations. The close collaboration has made it possible for advances in academic pharmacy to be quickly and efficiently translated into the practice arena. At the same time, it has made it possible for practice views to become part of the curriculum.

When pharmacy adopted pharmaceutical care as its mission, pharmaceutical education promptly initiated the process of creating a curriculum to prepare students to provide it. In 1992, pharmaceutical education made a momentous decision to expand and revise its curriculum from a traditional academic baccalaureate to a professional doctorate course of study.

The decision did not come without active and protracted debate. Indeed, we talked about, discussed, and debated the issue for over 40 years. The adoption of pharmaceutical care by the profession convinced the majority of schools and their faculty that the time was right for curricular revision and expansion. Academics quickly realized that we needed a curriculum to prepare practitioners who could deliver pharmaceutical care competently and efficiently. The short period of time between 1989, when pharmaceutical care was first articulated, and 1992, when the American Association of Colleges of Pharmacy (AACP) voted to support the Pharm.D. as the entry-level degree, was a time of intense reflection and self-scrutiny for academic pharmacy. The AACP Commission to Implement Change in Pharmaceutical Education provided key analyses, rationale, and recommendations to achieve this outcome. Our practice colleagues through APhA, ASHP, the Academy of Managed Care Pharmacy (AMCP), ACCP, the National Association of Boards of Pharmacy (NABP), and the American College of Apothecaries (ACA) provided valuable assistance, guidance, encouragement, and support.

If the time immediately before 1992 was filled with debate and questioning, the time following was characterized by the commitment of pharmacy school faculty not only to revise and expand the pharmaceutical curriculum, but to institute changes in teaching methods so as to create practitioners who are caring, knowledgeable, skillful, collaborative, and communicative decision makers, professionals, and leaders. Academic pharmacy's success at achieving this goal in a relatively short period stands as vivid testimony to the dedication and resourcefulness of these committed professional educators. It demonstrates clearly why academic pharmacy has always been, and remains today, a valuable and critically important asset to the pharmacy profession.

Over the past 35 years, the number of pharmacists in the United States grew 66 percent from 120,000 to 200,000. During this same time period, the number of organizations representing practitioners grew from five to nine, an increase of 80 percent. These numbers do not include changes in the numbers of those professional and trade organizations that exist in the periphery or in support of the profession representing scientists, regulators, educators, pharmacy benefit managers, third-party pay health programs, accreditors, and manufacturers. However, the conclusion that the growth of organized pharmacy merely has kept pace with the growth of the profession may be simplistic. An examination of the new organizations that sprang up over the past 35 years reflects the expansion of the profession into evolving practice areas such as long-term care, clinical pharmacy, managed care, and compounding. In essence, the growth and expansion of organized pharmacy has mirrored, quite accurately, the expansion of the profession. At the same time, existing professional organizations also have expanded their missions and scopes into areas such as nuclear pharmacy, oncology, nutrition support, and pediatrics to reflect the changing nature of the profession.

A number of commentators have remarked about the disadvantages of pharmacy's multiple organizations, especially with regard to their apparent inability to agree on national agendas or collaborate in common strategies. These commentators contrast organized pharmacy with organized medicine, nursing, dentistry, and other smaller health professions that have strong, national associations with the apparent support of the profession.

It is true that the pharmaceutical profession is populated by a variety of national organizations; and it is true that in some highly visible cases, we have not been able to agree on national agendas or strategies. Also, with so many organizations, no single organization has had the resources to tackle effectively those trans-professional issues that all professions must address such as work force studies, professional standards, and the creation and maintenance of a national database of practitioners.

However, it does pharmacy no value to compare our organizational structure with those of other health professions. We are not they, and they are not pharmacy. Pharmacy is unique in so many ways and our organizational structure is only one aspect of our uniqueness. The growth and dynamics of pharmacy's organizational structure mirrors the growth and dynamics of the profession. We need to take the time to understand and appreciate the true nature of organized pharmacy, and begin to appreciate and capitalize on our strengths, as we understand our weaknesses.

New pharmacy organizations came into existence because pharmacists practicing in expanding areas of the profession perceived a need for networking and education that were not available from existing societies. Notwithstanding how any of us may have felt when one of these new organizations began, we must admit today that they provide a highly focused educational experience for their members, and they generate abundant new knowledge related to their disciplines for the public good. On balance, the growth and expansion of organized pharmacy has been an asset within the profession and a positive force in public health.

Data on individual membership in the profession's organization are difficult to acquire and analyze. Of the 200,000 pharmacists in the country, one cannot determine if the percentage of pharmacists who belong to a pharmacy organization is greater or lesser today than in 1965. One fact appears certain, however; those who are members of pharmacy's organizations today appear to be more active and to demand more services than they did 35 years ago. This may be due to the fact that pharmacists are engaged in practices that are more involved in patient care than they were earlier and, as a result, desire the opportunities for networking and learning that only professional societies can provide.

One critical fact that stands out is that the resources that professionals are devoting to their organizations are much greater today. The number of pharmacists employed, as a proxy for a measure of the expenditure of resources, provides a glimpse into this phenomenon. In 1966, there were approximately 28 pharmacists employed in state and national pharmaceutical societies and organizations. That number was approximately 90 in 2001, an increase of over 200 percent. Clearly, the profession has seen it as worthwhile to invest heavily in its societies and organizations. Because these groups are continuing to prosper and grow, it appears that they are giving members their money's worth. These organizations are serving the practice needs of their members who are serving the health care needs of the public.

A number of activities and programs that any profession should conduct or pursue are critical to and necessary for the continued functioning of the profession. The activities include (1) Assuring a continuing supply of qualified individuals who are interested in pursuing careers within the profession; (2) Creating an educational system to supply the profession with qualified practitioners; (3) Evaluating and assuring the quality of professional educational programs; (4) Defining what professionals do in their practice; (5) Assuring the public that professionals are competent; (6) Performing work force studies and analyses; and (7) Conducting media and public relations programs.

A major disadvantage of pharmacy's multi-organizational structure is that, in the past, no one pharmaceutical organization has gained sufficient size and wealth to implement these strategies. They were simply too costly and/or complicated. As a result, for many years, most of these initiatives were left undone. That has begun to change. While many have, with justification, decried the fractured nature of organized pharmacy, multiple initiatives of collaboration, synthesis, and synergy have grown up within organized pharmacy over time.

Assuring that the profession has enough qualified individuals who enter the profession is a major responsibility of all professions. Again, here is a responsibility that all professional organizations recognize, but none has the resources or drive to carry out on its own. All major national organizations in the profession came together in the late 1980s to pool their time, talents, and treasure to form the Career Information Clearinghouse (CIC). The CIC has maintained the profession's ability to recruit widely on a national level and provide resources for state and local associations and societies and colleges and schools of pharmacy to mount student recruitment activities. During the recent downturn in pharmacy's application pool, CIC produced videotapes about careers in pharmacy and coordinated a nationwide effort to place pharmacy before young people as a viable and rewarding career opportunity. The subsequent upturn in applications to pharmacy colleges and schools is a direct result of CIC initiatives.

In 1935, when it became clear that professionally based standards were needed in pharmaceutical education, AACP, NABP, and APhA pooled their resources and talents to create and fund the American Council on Pharmaceutical Education (ACPE) to evaluate and accredit professional education programs in pharmacy. That collaborative effort resulted in the establishment of an accrediting body that was then and continues today unique in the health professions. All other accrediting bodies are intimately connected with the relevant profession's practice organization. ACPE stands today as an independent agency of the pharmacy profession. As such, it has served us well through the years.

In 1977 and again in 1982, a coalition of pharmaceutical associations including AACP, APhA, NABP, and, in 1982, ASHP, pooled their resources to conduct task analyses of the profession in order to develop a psychometric definition of what pharmacists do in daily practice. These efforts served as the bases for curricular change in pharmacy schools, developing the Standards of Practice in 1977, practice competencies for the NABP licensing examination (NABPLEX) in 1977 and 1982, and the creation of the pharmacy technician certification process. Such studies are expensive, and any one pharmaceutical association may hesitate to embark on such a venture on its own. Approached in a consortial way, however, such endeavors not only become affordable, but also make it possible to conduct vitally needed projects within the profession more frequently.

In 1987, when it became obvious that the profession was woefully lacking in information about its own practitioner work force, a confederation of practitioner organizations, including the Pharmaceutical Research and Manufacturers of America and under the leadership of AACP and NABP, formed the Pharmacy Manpower Project (PMP) that conducted a census of the profession. In 2000, the project updated its census with a study to determine the demographic characteristics of the profession. Recently, the Pharmacy Manpower Project established and funded the Aggregate Demand Index so that we would have accurate assessments of the changes in demand for pharmacists over time. Their most recent contribution was to convene a conference to assess and characterize the need for pharmacists in 2020.

The most well-known example of transprofessional collaboration is the Joint Commission of Pharmacy Practitioners (JCPP) which was created in 1977. Composed of eight national practitioner associations: AMCP, ACA, ACCP, APhA, the American Society of Consultant Pharmacists (ASCP), ASHP, the National Community Pharmacists Association, and National Council of State Pharmacy Association Executives, and three liaison member associations (AACP, ACPE, and NABP), JCPP has served as a forum on matters of common interest and concern to its member organizations. It has been the place where important issues before the profession are discussed and debated in an open, frank, and respectful atmosphere. The member organizations may not always agree, but they always engage in comprehensive discussions of the issues before them. JCPP sponsored three out of the last four Pharmacy in the 21st Century strategic planning conferences held every five years since 1984.

To make the point of intra-professional collaboration even more emphatically, the following initiatives are being pursued cooperatively by two or more pharmaceutical organizations:

- The Alliance for Pharmaceutical Care designs, staffs, and conducts the pharmacy exhibit at the annual meeting of the National Council of State Legislators. All major national pharmaceutical associations and trade groups participate in this activity.

- The National Institute for Standards in Pharmacist Credentialing, composed of APhA, NABP, and the National Association of Chain Drug Stores, develops and administers certification examinations for pharmacists engaged in specific disease management practices.

- The Council on Credentialing composed of most JCPP member organizations develops standards for those groups in pharmacy that credential practitioners and programs.

- The Pharmacy Technician Certifying Board, created in 1995 by APhA, ASHP, the Michigan Pharmacists Association, and the Illinois Council of Health-System Pharmacists (now including NABP) develops and administers the certification examination for pharmacy technicians.

- AACP, ACCP, AMCP, APhA, ASCP, ASHP, the National Pharmaceutical Association, and the National Consumers League, in response to President Clinton's national health care reform proposal, created the Coalition for Consumer Access to Pharmaceutical Care. This consortium funded research by Johnson and Bootman that identified the enormous cost of drug-related illness.

These examples provide a convincing argument that pharmaceutical associations are achieving significant accomplishments through collaborative efforts to achieve common goals. In each of these examples, pharmacy has adopted a federated approach to solve common problems. It appears that organized pharmacy has become comfortable in working through federated mechanisms. They offer significant advantages. Organizations may or may not participate according to their desires, missions, or financial means. Costly projects could be undertaken at reduced individual cost to individual federation members. The more organizations that participate, the less is the incremental cost per organization. Collaborative approaches stimulate inter-organizational discussions, idea sharing, and the merging of concepts. It is not unusual that the resulting goal of a federated effort is more complete, comprehensive, and targeted than any of the individual participants.

There are disadvantages as well. Collaborative initiatives require each participant to provide sufficient staff or member input to ensure representation of the association's viewpoint. With so many federated systems within the profession, inevitably there will be duplication and dilution of effort. Most importantly, however, federations succeed best when one organization assumes the role of secretariat to staff the initiative, assure continuity, and achievement of outcomes. Unless such an association steps forward, or unless the coalition agrees to hire staff, the effort tends to muddle along and decline slowly over time.

A review of the topics covered by the large assembly of collaborative activities that I have listed reveals: (1) No collaborative activities currently occur in some areas such as media relations. (2) Federated approaches are falling short of covering the entire range of need in some areas such as government relations and credentialing. (3) Some activities that each organization funds and performs could be performed by one federated organization for all such as meeting planning and publications). (4) Enormous efficiencies in staff use and application could be realized by collapsing many individual coalitions into one.

As organized pharmacy has become comfortable with conducting its activities by means of federated structures, is the time here and appropriate that pharmacy examine whether it should adopt a profession-wide federated structure? This is not a novel idea, and it is not originally my idea. It has been discussed through the years, most recently in 1999 at a JCPP retreat. More specifically, the question is whether APhA should expand or reconstitute its structure to become pharmacy's federation governed and funded by a board of directors consisting of the associations participating in and contributing to the federation.

The Federation of American Societies for Experimental Biology may serve as a model for pharmacy. This federation is composed of a number of societies representing various facets of the biological sciences. It lobbies, arranges meetings and workshops, publishes journals, and provides a comfortable headquarters in Rockville, Maryland.

It is not the purpose of this address to design this federation. Our professional and trade organizations should do that. While it would not appear necessary for APhA to disband as a membership society, it would have to take on new responsibilities and the costs associated with fulfilling them. A formal federated structure in pharmacy would enable it to accomplish those heretofore unapproachable initiatives such as media and public relations. Yes, each organization performs a public relations function and maintains a public relations staff. The conclusion remains unassailable, however, that the profession's media coverage is virtually nonexistent and each organization's public relations activities are associated with preparing and issuing press releases about the most recent election results or testimony submitted to congress. Clearly, we need to do much more and we will not have the resources without a collaborative initiative.

The most important responsibility of professions is continual self-examination in order to inform themselves and society about who they are and what they do. This responsibility is critical to four key functions that professions perform: (1) Educating future professionals. (2) Providing information to states that license professionals to practice. (3) Providing the means for practitioners to maintain their own competence. (4) Educating the public about what pharmacists do in general and specialized roles.

Throughout its history, U.S. pharmacy conducted four national studies of pharmacists' functions: the W.W. Charters study in 1927, the Elliott Survey in 1948, the Standards of Practice Project in 1977, and the Scope of Practice Project in 1992. Each study identified the major functions that pharmacists perform in general practice. Each demonstrated that the responsibilities and functions of pharmacists had changed over time to keep pace with advances within the profession and public health needs. Each resulted in changes in the licensing examination, pharmaceutical curriculum, and the profession's definition of itself. Each demonstrated that the profession's responsibilities and functions have changed substantially from one study to the other. These studies were lengthy and expensive. External support was required for three of the four. Each required energy and persuasive power to organize and conduct. More than 20 years separated the Charters study from the Elliott survey; almost 30 years separated Elliott from the Standards of Practice Project; and almost 15 years elapsed between the Standards and the Scope of Practice Project.

We can ill afford to wait this length of time before we study ourselves again. In today's rapidly changing health care system, how can we assure that our current definition of pharmacy practice, including descriptions of knowledge, skills, and abilities required of practitioners, remains valid in terms of actual practice? Health care and the roles and responsibilities of those who practice within it are changing too rapidly for any profession to enjoy the luxury of studying itself every 20 or 30 years. Certainly, pharmacy cannot. We need a system that frequently studies and defines the profession as a whole and in its integral, discreet entities. Our licensing agencies need these data; our colleges and schools need them; and our professional societies need them. A national federation of pharmaceutical associations remains the best option for the profession to fulfill its responsibility to society and itself to understand how it is changing. A federation can amass and provide the financial backing, impetus, and staff to launch and maintain such an initiative.

And this brings us to a discussion of contemporary competence. At the dawn of the 20th century, pharmacists were educated and/or trained to practice a profession that was defined at the time by public need, public demand, and the dictates of organized pharmacy. As licensure laws became prevalent, state boards of pharmacy assumed the responsibility of examining pharmacy graduates to determine their competence to enter the profession. Board members created the examinations based on their own definitions of what pharmacists entering the profession should know and be able to do. The modern science of psychometrics, which dictates that examinations be based on sound analyses of what practitioners do, provided a valuable tool to state pharmacy boards in developing and administering their licensing examinations.

The evolution of the national examination by the NABP leaned heavily on psychometrics. In 1977, NABP, APhA, and AACP collaborated in a project to outline pharmacists' tasks at the generalist level. The resulting Standards for the Practice of Pharmacy served NABP as the psychometric benchmark for the NABPLEX, with APhA as the basis for professional continuing education programs, and colleges and schools of pharmacy as the basis for designing and revising their curricula. A subsequent scope of practice study in 1992 provided additional information to AACP, APhA, ASHP, and NABP and, with the addition of a technician survey, data on which to base the Pharmacy Technician Certification Board's technician certification examination.

Earlier, I discussed the four major studies that the profession carried out to define the practice of pharmacy in 1927, 1948, 1977, and 1992. These studies demonstrated that the definition of practice, in terms of the functions that pharmacists perform, changed during the intervals between studies. This prompts the question: How are practitioners, who were graduated and licensed under one definition, to assure the public, their employers, their peers, and themselves that they are competent to practice according to a more current definition or standard of practice?

Up until now, we have viewed the matter as a regulatory one and deferred to state pharmacy boards. The state boards responded by requiring practitioners to show evidence of continuing education in order to renew their licenses. However, as recently as 1998, the Pew Charitible Trusts Health Professions Commission issued a report, *Strengthening Consumer Protection: Priorities for Health Care Workforce Regulation*. The report recommended that: "States should require each board to develop, implement, and evaluate continuing competency requirements to assure the continuing competence of regulated health care professionals."

The PEW report was wrong. NABP attempted to implement this recommendation through individual state boards of pharmacy, but most pharmaceutical associations opposed its proposed strategy, and NABP abandoned the effort. Unfortunately, in opposing NABP's continuing competency initiative, pharmacy's organizations offered no alternative strategy to resolve the problem of assuring the public that practitioners were competent to perform according to the most recent definition of practice. These organizations owe it to practitioners, our state regulators, and the public to develop feasible alternative methods to assure contemporary competence.

One element in the profession's response must be its commitment to create a mechanism to redefine the practice of pharmacy at frequent, periodic intervals. Currently, practitioners assure their patients, their employers, and themselves that they perform according to the contemporary definition of practice by participating in continuing education activities, certificate programs, and/or certification in a disease management area or a specialized area of practice. The vast majority of practitioners have used continuing education as the means of maintaining their contemporary competence. Unfortunately, continuing education, as valuable as it is, is not designed to ensure competence across the broad array of contemporary practice. Only a psychometrically designed assessment could achieve that outcome.

There are several scenarios that describe how such an assessment instrument could determine competence:

- Practitioners could assess themselves periodically to demonstrate to themselves, employers, patients, peers, and the public that their knowledge, skills, and abilities comply with the national definition of practice.

- Employers could require their pharmacist employees to provide evidence that their knowledge, skills, and abilities comply with the national definition of practice. Periodic assessments can provide such evidence.

- State pharmacy boards could require practitioners, as a condition for relicensure, to provide evidence that their knowledge, skills, and abilities comply with the national definition or with definitions developed by specialty practices. Periodic assessments, including certification, can provide such evidence.

The matter of pharmacists' contemporary competence is too important for the profession not to give it prompt and close attention. The profession, including its regulators, must engage in a comprehensive dialogue about the issue before it identifies and pursues specific strategies. Some questions that are relevant and may prompt reasoned discussion include:

- Is it important that pharmacy maintain a contemporary definition/standard of practice that is consistent with what pharmacists do and patient care needs?
- Who should be responsible for updating this definition/standard?
- What assessment strategies could be employed to ensure that practitioners are practicing in accord with the contemporary definition/standard?
- Who should be responsible for creating and distributing these assessments?
- Should contemporary competence assessments be voluntary or a requirement for relicensure?
- Would the profession be well served or not by becoming the first major health profession to embrace publicly the need for regular reexamination based on contemporary standards for licensure?
- What roles should the Commission on Credentialing in Pharmacy and/or JCPP play in moving this dialogue forward?

This is not just a regulatory matter. Our difficulty is that we have treated the issue as a regulatory/legal matter, when we should treat it as a public policy and professional issue. It is a leadership opportunity for the entire profession. No other health profession is discussing contemporary competence on a professionwide basis. Simply restated, the profession must periodically redefine itself; recast that definition in psychometric terminology; and create mechanisms through which practitioners may demonstrate to themselves, their patients, their colleagues, and their employers that their performance is compatible with that definition.

Out of the vast number of people who, through the years, have influenced me, I cite a very few by name. Two Redwood City, California, pharmacists, John and Peter Ryan, hired me as a sweep-up boy, delivery agent, and stock clerk in 1949. They taught me the importance of treating people in a caring, professional manner and encouraged me to select a career in pharmacy. William S.

Apple, executive director of APhA when I joined the staff in 1966, was an enormous influence. He was a mentor and taught me the critical nature of verbal and written communications and the value of standing by principles. As important as these people have been, it is my wife, Laura, and children Terri, Anna, and Richard, who have exerted the most profound influence in my life and career. These blessed people have been and continue to be the reason why everything in my life makes sense. They may not have played a direct prominent role in pharmacy, but to the extent that I have been influential in the profession, they share a major portion of the credit. One of the sublime benefits of working in organized pharmacy is the opportunity to meet, know, and work with such an incredible group of members. Through the years, these interactions have inspired, sustained, and invigorated me. These interactions are today as engaging as an excellent novel that you can't put down once you begin reading. And in the process of these interactions, we've accomplished much on behalf of the profession. I look back on these opportunities and these people with pride, humility, and profound affection. Spending a career in pharmaceutical association, working in pharmacy's vineyard, has provided me the opportunity of associating with a large number of talented and dedicated staff colleagues from throughout organized pharmacy. The interaction with these individuals has sharpened my focus, expanded my thinking, and clarified my understanding. Compared with the number of practitioners in the profession, the number of association staff is minuscule. However small, the impact that this group has on the profession is profound. As in a vineyard, the effort of the workers is considerable, but the production of results, the fruit, is bountiful. For me, working in pharmacy's vineyard has been a stimulating, educational, fulfilling, and (sometimes) emotional experience. Few interactions with fellow staff occurred that did not change, in some respect, my understanding of the issue under discussion. It is the nature of pharmaceutical association staff to feel passionately about and interact passionately on issues. Such interactions are always respectful of other opinions; for other opinions and views are what stretch our thinking; and stretching our thinking is what education is all about. I am especially grateful to the 14 individuals who serve on the AACP staff. Their dedication, support, and hard work made it possible for AACP to achieve so much. I am eternally thankful to be able to call these superb people my colleagues and friends. It is to this incredibly talented and dedicated group of staff from across the pharmaceutical association spectrum that I dedicate this Remington Award. ■

2003 Remington Medalist

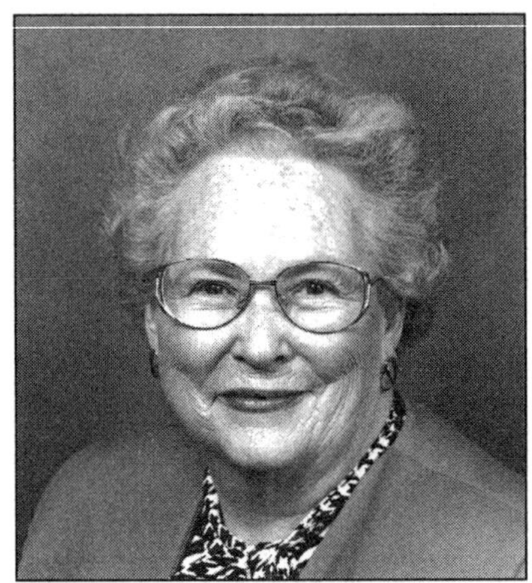

Mary Louise Tigue Andersen

Mary Louise Tigue Andersen was born in Wilmington, Delaware, July 28, 1930, and received her B.Sc. in Pharmacy in 1952 from the Philadelphia College of Pharmacy and Science. She joined her father in community pharmacy practice in Wilmington, Delaware, 1952-1970; developed with David Krigstein the first legislation to create a community pharmacy formulary in 1964; served as Delaware Pharmaceutical Society president in 1965; and as health planner for the Model Cities Wilmington 1970-1972. She joined government service as U.S. Public Health Service public health advisor 1974-1977; Office of the Assistant Secretary for Health executive intern 1978; Bureau of Medical Services Division of Hospitals and Clinics director of operations 1978-1980; Office of Assistant Secretary of Health special assistant to the director 1981-1994; Center for Substance Abuse and Treatment special assistant to the director 1995-1996; and Health Resources and Services Administration Bureau of Primary Health Care deputy director from 1996 until her retirement in 1999.

Andersen joined the American Pharmaceutical Association in 1949 and has served as APhA vice president 1967-1968, APhA House of Delegates speaker 1969-1971, member of the Pharmacists Insurance Trust board of trustees, and APhA honorary president 1997-1998. After her retirement from government service, Andersen helped found the Community Health Leadership Network of which she serves as a board member, as well as vice president of the Delaware Health Foundation, and a board member of the Westside Health Program, a community health center in Wilmington.

Between the 'No Longer' and the 'Not Yet'

Mary Louise Tigue Andersen

The 2003 Remington Medal was presented March 30, 2003, during the American Pharmaceutical (now Pharmacists) Association annual meeting in New Orleans, Louisiana, March 28 - April 1, 2003. Andersen's address was published in the *Journal of the American Pharmaceutical Association*, Supplement 1, pp. S6-S9, September-October 2003.

I look at tonight as an opportunity to have a conversation with the most important and influential persons in pharmacy and America's health scene in our society today. But first let me introduce you to the most important people in my life. Roger and I will have been married 50 years this summer. May you all be as lucky as I have been to have a spouse who is loving, loyal, and always there for you, as Roger has been for me. We also have some outputs from this union: Karen, Kenneth, Keith, Eric, Joan, Jane, and Kathleen. I am incredibly proud of each of them and want to say publicly that they are good people and good parents to our 13 grandchildren, with big hearts, who are wonderful to their mother and dad.

Leaders are called to stand in that lonely place between the "no longer" and the "not yet." We are not called to be popular; we are not called to be safe; and we are not called to follow. We are the ones called to change attitudes to risk displeasures. We are the ones called to gamble our lives for a better world.

I wrote those words in April 1970 when I was speaker of the APhA House of Delegates. The Policy Committee had made the recommendation that "the Association work for the repeal of the Anti-substitution laws in America." This was going to be one hell of a House meeting. The interests were many and passionate. The pharmaceutical industry had built its marketing strategy on the branding of drug products. Pharmacy associations, both national and state, depended on the financial support of industry. Community pharmacy's prescription reimbursement was based on a percentage of the cost of the drug product dispensed. Everyone felt threatened. The reference committee hearings were packed. The lobbying was continuous and pressing.

I knew how to count votes and went into that House meeting with some trepidation. The vote on this issue, which had never before been considered by the House, would determine the independence of pharmacy as a profession for decades to come. You all know the outcome. Pharmacy began that stay in the lonely place between the "no longer" and the "not yet."

Do I believe that the results have been worth it? You bet I do. Bill Apple's driving goal was the "emancipation of the profession of pharmacy," and Donald Brodie defined the profession as a "knowledge system" in a critical study completed about the same time. It was the courage to take these visions and turn them into policy decisions that led to the stature of the profession today.

I have seen the "not yets" become the everyday reality of today. Some of that reality is in my own family. Our daughter Karen and her husband John are decision-making pharmacists at Walter Reed Army Hospital and the federal Food and Drug Administration. They are partners with dispensing pharmacists, pharmacists in industry, prescribers, and researchers across the broad spans of the profession. They work in a knowledge system and are emancipated. So are all the new professionals who fill this meeting. Their future is no accident. It happened because there were people with a vision who put a stake in the ground and made their future happen.

We are all products of genes and environment. I am one lucky lady. I had a handsome, charming pharmacist father who saw himself and the profession as exemplified in the painting, *The Pharmacist*, and I still have it. Framed prints were distributed by Owens Bottling Company a long time ago. It shows the family of a very sick child at home at night, while another child waits at the pharmacy as the pharmacist prepares the medicine that the sick child needs. What do I think Daddy saw in that picture? He saw a professional whose first commitment was to his patient and responsibility was to assist whenever needed. My dad also was emancipated. He did business as Paul C. Tigue, Pharmacist.

My mother was smart and wise. She knew that education was the personal and societal basis for all excellence. She hosted seven foreign exchange students because she believed that long-term peace in the world would come from knowing one another. She recognized that the Social Security System, enacted during her lifetime, would free my generation and make it the first one in history that would not have to care for its parents financially. She taught me that there is an important ethic in how a nation spends its money. She taught me that voting is a privilege and one that I should never miss.

That's the genes, but the environment is also special. My personal life and professional life have been intertwined from birth. Roger and I met in college; Linwood Tice was my dean; David Krigstein was first my teacher and then my lifelong friend; Bill Apple was a special mentor and teacher; and then there are my friends from service to APhA.

Mother always said, "Show me your friends, and I will tell you what you are." Well, they are Grover Bowles, Lloyd Parks, Gloria Francke, Larry Weaver, Joseph Oddis, George Griffenhagen, Jere Goyan, Bob Johnson, Max Eggleston, and Dick Penna. These are winners and keepers. They had visions and passion, and I thank each for the gifts that they have shared with me. Does this recall have a purpose other than an old lady's memories? My purpose is to challenge all of us to the next "no longer" and "not yet" that we are facing.

For the last 30 years, I have worked with developing health services programs that were targeted because of vulnerable and underserved populations, whether the result of geography or social standing. These programs focused on the basic needs of primary care in communities that lacked them.

I spent a good amount of time in Appalachia, on Indian reservations, and in some inner-city neighborhoods, settings that are all different, yet all the same. The people living in these places share one tragic common thread: they are sicker and die younger than do the rest of us. Their primary diseases are diabetes, hypertension, heart disease, cancer, and asthma.

Every one of these chronic diseases are treatable with drug therapy. We can provide all the physicians in the world to these communities, but without comprehensive pharmacy services, there is no comprehensive primary care. Jimmy Mitchell in Health Resources and Services Administration's Office of Pharmacy Affairs has made this truth a mantra in the Agency. The demand for prescription drug coverage for Medicare beneficiaries proves that our nation understands that fact.

Access to pharmacy services was mostly a problem of the poor and geographically isolated. Many of the rest of the country had some form of third-party reimbursement with small co-payments for their prescription drugs. This is no longer true. Our health system in the United States is built on employer-provided health benefits. It is collapsing rapidly. You and your families may soon be uninsured or underinsured based on the corporate decisions of the next few years. Very high co-payments and deductibles may leave many of us effectively uninsured or underinsured. And this country does "not yet" have any system to take its place.

For the past five years, I have worked with community coalitions across America that have decided to tackle the issues of access and health status disparities. As many as 600 communities have convened to address these issues. They can no longer wait for a national solution. They know they can have better health care for more people for less cost. They have the measurable goals of 100 percent access to care and no health status disparity.

These coalitions include medical societies and group practices, hospitals, county commissioners, United Way chapters, health departments, academic medical centers, community health centers and, sometimes, the pharmacists. They examine a lot of the local issues that have an impact on the uncompensated care and the poor health statistics in their community. It is in this manner that the players find the critical role that each entity uniquely can play, and they recognize that not one of them can do it alone. Not the hospital, not the health department, not the community health center, nor the practitioners. If they are to improve health care in their community, they have to recognize their interdependence. Only then does the patient become the center of all that they do.

The coalitions look at how people are enrolled in public insurance programs, how many times the same data are collected and entered into myriad databases, and how many financial surveys result in how many sliding fee scales. Then they look at what happens to providers. Almost all providers take on some uncompensated care; it is one of the unknown costs of doing business. They work together to identify the population in real need and equitably share the load. They set up support systems to relieve individual providers of the administrative burdens of taking care of this population, and they make it easy for providers to participate. They establish specialty banks so that primary care physicians are able to get specialty services for needy patients. They move patients from costly emergency rooms to primary care offices and save significant systems dollars. They cooperate on case management for those high users of the system to see if they can get better compliance and better health outcomes. And they know that without comprehensive pharmacy services, there is no comprehensive health care.

Is this lady on the road to Oz? No, but I have been to Buncombe County, North Carolina; Middlesex, Connecticut; and Pittsburgh, Pennsylvania. I have seen pharmacists who provide comprehensive pharmacy services and make a difference as full partners with the physicians and hospitals in their towns where each contributes in his or her own way.

With very few exceptions these community plans call for organized, integrated, affordable, comprehensive pharmacy services. The pharmacists who are graduating from our colleges and universities are practicing in exciting environments. They are being recruited and challenged to help these communities design such systems. They are required to understand the health care disparities, the language implications of drug therapy, formulary development with quality standards, and procurement systems that take advantage of the various favorable pricing structures. It is most exciting to see pharmacists come together as a group in a community to work with all providers and community leaders to address their local needs.

Communities know that drug products are not free, and they have learned to seek resources for medications as part of their development process.

In these systems, I have seen newly emancipated pharmacists serving as independent, essential, valued, and equal partners in the care of the patient community. When working with Middlesex, Connecticut, the community brought to my attention how Peter Tczykowski of Pelton's Pharmacy had contributed to the development of their health system that serves the underserved.

When the community first organized to form a community health center, his pharmacy joined into the planning and found how he could help. It has remained a core linkage in this town as the programs have grown from health centers to health systems. Peter studied the drug pricing laws, became a contract pharmacy to help the health center with the complexity of pharmacy practice, found ways to use this benefit to serve as many people as possible, and learned how to leverage his work in the community to benefit all his patients in Middlesex. This community knows that there is no primary care without comprehensive pharmacy care because Peter has shown them.

When APhA leadership under executive vice president John Gans put a stake in the ground about the clinical role potential for the profession, it was one of those "not yets." The Association was not being safe or popular. APhA was making a statement that would affect every pharmacist yet to be educated. They were establishing a minimal level of care that every patient has a right to receive. That vision has been realized, and pharmaceutical care is gradually becoming the standard.

The national debate continues about the financing of health care for all Americans. We see the issue in every newspaper and hear it on the commentators' tongues. So how soon can we expect to have this issue settled for us again to be secure in our coverage?

I personally believe that we may never have a national system of health care in this country. The policy issues at the national level are very divisive and fraught with vested interests and require very large amounts of money. I do believe that we can have a national system that assures access for all persons through community organized and managed health systems. Community-driven reforms mandate cooperation in ways that recognize their own local cultures and values. Some depend on volunteer support; others are led by the local government efforts. Some institute small sales taxes; some develop small employer packages; and some reapportion the savings. All such emerging systems need support for the required infrastructure and financing of care for the truly needy.

The integration of these systems today comes as a result of the information systems that are being implemented in the community. All providers have access to common information, scheduling availability, and feedback to referral sources. When the pharmacist participates, this knowledge system of pharmacy is integrated no matter where the drug product is obtained.

Our challenge is to make our knowledge system accessible to the community at large and to make its value understood and appreciated. We can demonstrate in cold, hard terms the economic value that pharmacists contribute to the system in terms of improved health outcomes and the impact on costs. As more and more of the responsibility for health care is transferred to the patient and more medications become available without a prescription, self-medication will increase exponentially. Insurers will demand that only those drugs that really require physician oversight in their use will carry the *Rx Legend* because they will generally pay only for prescription drugs. It is happening now. The site of decision making about drug product selection has moved from the doctor's office, to the prescription counter, to the shelves of retailers. We have all discussed the pharmacist's role in assuring safety in this self-medication world.

I have seen the real life challenges of many patients: those who are illiterate or do not speak or read English; those whose dietary customs are not familiar to the rest of us and cause problems with some products; those with diabetes who continue to use corn pads until they have the amputation; or those with hypertension or glaucoma who continue to take the ephedrine-type drugs, and I have wondered why they are still having more troubles. They deserve better from us. And we can give them better.

I began these remarks by discussing the combination of genes and environment. During the next 25 years, while we will still have our genes, we will be required to create a response to change that will test our ethics and our value structures. I grew up in the last century in a United States that was predominantly white, Judeo-Christian, and English speaking, with a two-party political democracy and opportunity open to all.

As we enter this new millennium, dramatic change is the norm, especially in health care. Our society will be vastly different from that which we have known. It will be as multilingual as that of Europe, with mosques and Buddhist temples in the community, as well as churches and synagogues. The role of democratic government will be debated in every system, including health, education, communication, and transportation. Threats of terrorism challenge the civil rights we once took for granted. The people we now refer to as minorities, African Americans, Latinos, and Asian Americans, will outnumber whites.

The real numbers, as well as the percentage of those vulnerable populations, will grow. Doing nothing is inviting a disaster of social unrest that none of us can contemplate.

I mentioned Oz. I think there is a road map here for us as individuals and for APhA as an association. You remember the cowardly Lion who wanted Courage, the Scarecrow who wanted a Brain, and the Tin Man who wanted a Heart. We have a need for some new answers, and sometimes I feel like the Scarecrow who sang, "If I only had a Brain." The most critical part of the brain allows us to see the opportunities and to understand the power of the different choices. It gives us the ability to think of the consequences. But it will take more than a brain to answer these questions. It takes the Tin Man, who knows that knowledge is not enough. We need the right understanding with a commitment to care.

The cowardly Lion should have thought a bit about what he wished for, because he just might get it. Courage is tough to live with because it is the personal and organizational quality that makes a difference. It is what lets you stand in that lonely place between the "no longer" and the "not yet." Once courage is present, you have no choice but to act. You know the options and the consequences, and you care about those at risk. You begin traveling down the road of small, directed choices to do what is right. You work with others, value the differences, and take risks.

There are plenty of brains and very good hearts in this room. I am asking you to go home, each to your own community, and see who is organizing for change. Then, I ask you to have the courage to join and to bring your community into the movement for 100 percent access to care and no health status disparity. Know that we can have better health for more people at less cost. Make it happen, and remember that there is no comprehensive primary care without comprehensive pharmacy services.

Lead the way because leaders are called to stand in that lonely place between the "no longers" and the "not yets." We are not called to be popular; we are not called to be safe; and we are not called to follow. We are the ones called to change attitudes and to risk displeasure. We are the ones called to gamble our lives for a better world. ■

Index of Personalities

This Index is limited to personalities mentioned in the Introduction, the Remington lectures, and the medalists' biographies. It includes noted non-pharmacist personalities, but does not include family members with the same last name as the Remington recipient. Remington medalists and the pages for their lectures are printed in bold face.

Subject Index

This Index includes agencies, associations, businesses, colleges and universities mentioned in the Remington lectures. Organizations are listed under their most current name. Subjects that are mentioned in the biographies of the Remington medalists are printed in bold face.